Human
spatial
orientation

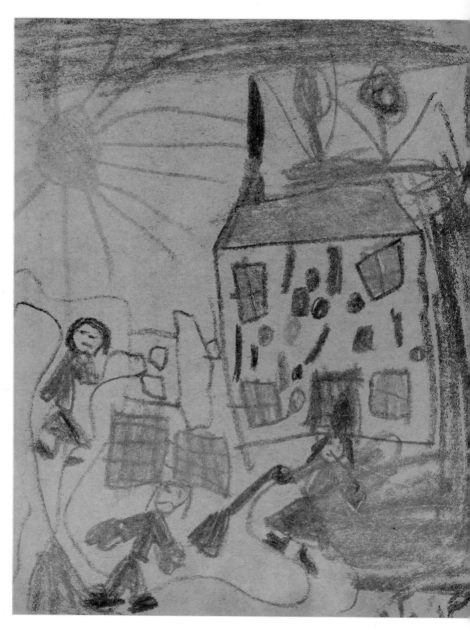

Hansel and Gretel drawing by a four year old child demonstrating the use of two horizontal frames of reference in the same picture

Human spatial orientation

I. P. Howard and W. B. Templeton

University of Durham, England

1966   John Wiley & Sons

London   New York   Sydney

Library of Congress catalogue card number 66-18106

Set in 11 on 12 point Monotype Bembo. Made and printed in
Great Britain by Hazell Watson & Viney Ltd., Aylesbury

Acknowledgments

The authors wish to record their appreciation of the help of the following people who read and criticized parts of the book: Brian Craske, Robert Davidon, Lila Ghent, James J. Gibson, Douglas Graham, Rae Harcum, David McFarland, Irvin Rock, Herman A. Witkin, Joachim Wohlwill; and of the U.S.Government in supplying research reports; and of the University of Durham in providing financial support; and of Mrs. Joyce Wood in preparing the typescript; and of Jill McFarland in reading the proofs.

The authors would also like to thank the following publishers for permission to reproduce the figures and other material mentioned: Edward Arnold (10.1, 10.2); Brain Books (5.7, 5.8); Cambridge University Press (5.9); Grune and Stratton (9.3); Hong Kong University Press (4.1); The C.V. Mosby Company (3.2); Sir Isaac Pitman and Sons (9.1, 9.2); Plenum Press (15.3); W. B. Saunders (15.1 15.2, quotation on p. 381); Charles C. Thomas (3.1, 3.3); University of Louvain (12.7). They would also like to thank the editors of the following journals: *Acta oto-laryng., Stockh.* (5.4, 5.5, 5.10, 5.11, 5.12, 5.13); *Amer. J. Psychol.* (7.5, 8.5, 8.6, 8.7, 8.8, 11.5, 12.2, 12.9, 12.12, quotation on p. 197); *Anat. Rec.* (5.2); *Ann. Acad. Sci. Fenn.* (12.4); *Arch. Ophthal., N.Y.* (3.9, 3.10, 3.11); *Brit. J. Psychol.* (table 5.3); *Confin. Neurol., Basel* (5.3, 5.6); *Int. Rec. Med.* (5.14); *Jap. J. Psychol.* (13.1); *J. comp. physiol. Psychol.* (15.6); *J. exp. Psychol.* (7.4, 9.4, 9.5, 9.6, 9.7, 9.8, 12.5, 15.5, table 7.3); *J. Psychol.* (14.1); *Percept. mot. Skills* (11.4, 12.6, 15.4); *Physiol. Rev.* (4.2); *Z. vergl. Physiol.* (3.8). And they would like to thank the following authors: E. E. David (6.13); F. A. Firestone (6.2, 6.3); L. A. Jeffress (6.4); A. W. Mills (6.5, 6.6, 6.7, 6.8, 6.9); E. P. Reese (7.2, 11.2); R. G. Rudel (6.11); C. I. Sandström (14.2); W. A. Van Bergeijk (6.14, 6.15, 6.16, 6.17); J. Zwislocki (6.10).

The senior author collected the material for the book and wrote most of the first draft. The final version emerged after the junior author had made extensive contributions and revisions both of content and style

Contents

1

Introduction

1.1 The scope of the book

This book is about those aspects of human behaviour which are determined by the angular position of the body (or head) in relation to any stable external reference system. Strictly speaking, this definition of the book's scope excludes judgments of the inclination of lines to gravity, for there only external reference axes are directly involved. However, this topic is important for an understanding of body orientation behaviour and is included for that reason. Other topics, such as the discrimination and recognition of shapes, are discussed only in so far as the relevant behaviour is affected by orientation variables. Geometrical illusions, figural after-effects, and judgments of visual angle, length, distance, and movement are omitted.

Chapters 2 to 6 introduce the four modalities most concerned in human spatial orientation. The tactile modality has been omitted, as its role in orientation is of minor importance. These chapters, while providing an up-to-date and fairly detailed review of present-day knowledge, are by no means comprehensive. Chapters 7 to 15 bear on the central topic of the book. They are intended to cover the literature comprehensively, either directly or by reference to existing reviews. The final chapter is a review of material on orientation in zero-g conditions. This material, while not classified as secret, is not generally available. We cannot claim that the chapter is comprehensive, for much material has not been available.

1.2 Orientation defined

The fundamental geometrical concepts required are *two lines* in a plane, the *sign of rotation* of a point moving about a fixed point in the plane and the *polarity of a line* i.e. the sign of a movement along the line. It is usual to specify the sign of rotation of a point about a fixed point in a plane as 'clockwise' or 'anticlockwise' depending on whether the movement is congruent with the movement of the hands of a clock or not. The polarity of a line will usually be given by whichever aspect of the physical world the line represents e.g. if it represents gravity one movement along the line will be up, the other down; if it represents a man one movement will be towards the head, the other towards the feet. These basic concepts are illustrated in figure 1.1.

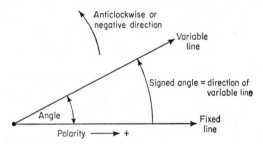

Figure 1.1 The basic geometrical concepts of lines, angle, sign of rotation, polarity, and direction

If one line is specified as fixed (e.g. gravity) and the variable line (e.g. a man) is coincident with it, and the polarities of the two lines are in a specified relationship, and this position is designated the zero position of the variable line with respect to the fixed line (e.g. the man standing upright on a bar), then if a point on the two lines is specified as the intersection of the two lines (e.g. the man's feet), and any other point in the variable line (e.g. the man's head) rotates about the intersection until it again lies in the fixed line, the lines will again be coincident but with the relationship between polarities reversed (e.g. the man hanging head down from the bar) and the variable line will be said to have moved through 180 degrees of angular rotation. It is then possible, by dividing this angular distance into 180 equal segments, to construct a protractor which when applied to the intersection between any two lines will produce a signal corresponding to the angular separation of the lines. If the rotation of the variable line from the zero position has a clockwise (or anticlockwise) sign, then the direction of the variable line is given by the signed (clockwise or anticlockwise) value of its angular separation from the zero position (e.g. a man is tilted θ degrees clockwise from the upright).

A *direction* is thus the signed angle which a variable line makes with a reference line, as measured by a protractor. A directional system is any system to which the operations of directional measurement may be applied.

A directional system may have one or more equilibrial states to which it will return when a disturbing force is withdrawn. This self-restoring process is called 'orientation' and one line is said to be oriented with respect to the other. In most systems the parallel congruence of the lines constitutes an equilibrial state.

1.3 Primitive orientation mechanisms

Wind-vane and plumbline–gravity systems are examples of orientation devices. Such devices have no means of recruiting energy to overcome an external disturbance and maintain equilibrium.

A device which is able to maintain an angular position against disturbances can do so either because it is so rigid that the disturbing force is too weak to affect it, or because it is a *servo-orientation system*, and therefore capable of recruiting energy (e.g. a man). Servos are superficially similar to rigid angular systems, but are quite distinct when considered part by part. The power which provides the restoring torque is isolated from the power providing the disturbance. A control link is introduced between them in such a way that a slight deviation from the equilibrium position caused by the disturbing force controls a valve (amplifier) which allows the restoring torque to operate and restore the balance. This is the negative feedback loop of the system. Ideally, the system maintains absolute stability; in practice, there are time lags which cause the system to oscillate, and power limits which determine the range of effective stability. For a fuller treatment of servo theory, with special reference to biological systems, see Grodins (1963).

In the living system any disturbance of the normal equilibrium between the body axis and an external reference system may affect the sensory system. The neuromuscular system acts as amplifier and driving force in the restoring responses. But behaviour consequent upon a disturbance of the normal orientation of the animal is not necessarily concerned with restoring the body's position. A disturbance of equilibrium affects behaviour in many ways: for instance, it may affect judgments of the position of stimulus objects in relation to other external systems and in relation to the observer's body. However, the simplest behavioural response to disturbed orientation is the reflex, righting response. In their most primitive forms such reflexes occur in response to stimuli arising in one sensory modality. They are typified in the orientation behaviour of invertebrates.

Fraenkel and Gunn (1940) have classified the mechanisms by which invertebrates aggregate and orient themselves. The simplest mechanism is the orthokinetic response. An example is the aggregation of wood lice (*Porellio scaber*) in damp places. Their rate of movement is inversely proportional to humidity, and it is solely on account of this simple relationship that they aggregate in humid places. Fraenkel and Gunn next describe the klinokinetic response. The planarian, *Dendrocoelum lacteum*, aggregates in dark places simply because the rate at which it changes its direction of movement is a function of light intensity, and because it adapts to light. Both these response mechanisms are aggregations rather than orientations.

The simplest orientations are the taxes, by means of which the animal aligns itself with the direction of a given stimulus gradient. In klinotaxis the animal, for instance the fly larva, possesses a single anterior light-sensitive region by means of which it successively compares the light intensity on either side of its body as it swings its head from side to side. Any asymmetry between successive light strengths on the eye spot induces an asymmetry in the body swinging in such a way that the body comes to point away from the light source. In tropotaxis the animal has a bilateral pair of sense organs which are capable of simultaneously comparing the light intensity on the two sides of the body. These two taxes are similar in that they both result in the animal aligning itself with the direction of the stimulus. Neither demand an image-forming eye. If two lights of equal intensity are put on at the same time these mechanisms will cause the animal to align itself with the line bisecting the angle between the two lights. By means of Fraenkel and Gunn's final mechanism, telotaxis, an animal with an image-forming eye can select one of several light sources as the effective stimulus towards which it orients its body.

Our point of departure is a human being, with an image-forming eye, and vestibular, kinaesthetic, auditory, and touch senses. (The senses other than vision and audition will sometimes be referred to collectively as the postural senses.) The human postural mechanisms are basically tropotaxic and the human visual system basically telotaxic, but the great variety and complexity of human orientation behaviour cannot profitably be described in terms of these simple mechanisms.

1.4 The classification of human orientation behaviour

Orientation behaviour may be classified according to the scheme shown in figure 1.2 (a)–(h). According to the basic definition in section 1.2 two lines or axes are required for the specification of an orientation. For convenience, one axis will be referred to as the standard, and one as the variable, depending

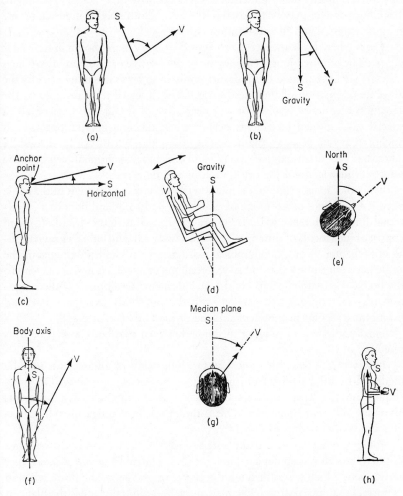

Figure 1.2 A classification of human orientation behaviour. (a) Judging angles; (b) Judging direction (e.g. inclination, compass direction); (c) Setting a point to eye level (horizontal); (d) Gravitational orientation of the body; (e) Geographical orientation of the body; (f) Egocentric orientation—setting a line parallel with the body axis; (g) Egocentric orientation—setting a point to the median plane; (h) Relative orientation of body parts

on which is more usually under the subject's control in an actual experiment. Both lines or axes may be external to the body, both may be internal, or one may be external and the other internal.

Cases where both axes are external to the observer are shown in figure 1.2 (a)–(c). The required judgment may be of the relative orientation of two lines (case a); we have treated this judgment only in so far as it is influenced by the absolute orientation of the lines (section 2.72). One of the axes may be the direction of gravity (case b) or any derivative of it (e.g. the horizontal); a special case of such judgments occurs when the non-gravitational axis is anchored at one point to the body (e.g. the judgment of eye level, case c). These tasks are discussed in chapters 7 and 8. All these judgments can be made without knowledge of the orientation of any body axis.

The other main group of orientation tasks involves judgment of the angle between two lines or axes, one of which is a body axis and the other an external line or reference axis. These are illustrated in figure 1.2 (d)–(g), and consist of judgments of the angle between a body axis and either a gravitational axis (chapter 9) or a geographical axis (chapter 10) and judgments of the angle between a body axis and an external line or axis anchored at one end to the body. This latter group consist of judgments traditionally called 'egocentric', viz. setting a line parallel with the mid-body axis (page 194) and positioning a point in the median plane of the body (chapter 11).

Finally, the task of judging the angle between two body axes (case h) is discussed in chapter 4.

In any of the tasks mentioned so far, judgments or adjustments may be mediated by information from more than one sensory modality. One may enquire into the degree of correspondence between judgments or adjustments involving different modalities. This is the problem of intersensory localization and is discussed in section 14.2.

For specifying the principal planes and axes of the human body we have adopted the axis system depicted in figure 1.3. The mid-body or Z axis is that vertical axis which passes through the centre of gravity of the body when in its normal standing posture. The median or mid-sagittal plane is the plane of bilateral body symmetry containing the mid-body axis (an approximation when the plane of symmetry does not contain the centre of gravity). A para-median or para-sagittal plane is any plane parallel to the median plane. The mid-frontal or coronal plane is a vertical plane at right angles to the median plane, and containing the mid-body axis. A frontal plane is any other plane parallel to the mid-frontal plane. The mid-transverse plane is the plane at right angles to the frontal and median planes, and passing through the centre of gravity. A transverse plane is any other plane parallel to the mid-transverse plane.

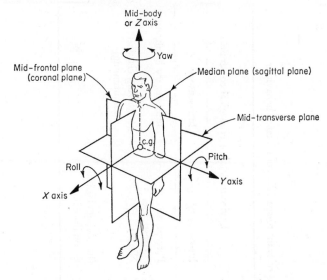

Figure 1.3 Body coordinate system and axes of rotation

1.5 Spatial orientation and a theory of constraints

Spatially coordinated behaviour is construed as the development and maintenance of a repertoire of response patterns which are moulded and conditioned by the spatial characteristics of the body and of the physical world in such a way that objectives may be rapidly and accurately achieved. Spatially coordinated behaviour is only possible because there are many predictable features of the body's structure and of the structure of the world. These predictable features or redundancies set a limit to chaos, and in that sense they are constraints; they are also constraints in the sense that, unless behaviour is conditioned by them, it will be non-adaptive. These constraints may be classified according to table 1.1.

Spatial behaviour, then, is conditioned by (1) the *internal constraints* of the body, that is, by the way in which the human body is constructed and normally develops and by (2) the nature of the physical world, that is, by *environmental* or *ecological* constraints.

The analysis of spatial behaviour is fundamentally a description of the way in which behaviour is moulded and conditioned by internal and ecological constraints. These two constraint systems provide the basis upon which spatial behaviour must develop if it is to be adaptive. These constraints are defined in physical, anatomical, or physiological terms. The different types of constraint are set out in table 1.1. The most fundamental body constraints are

Table 1.1 A classification of body and environmental constraints relevant to spatially coordinated behaviour

	Body constraints	Body–environment constraints	Environmental or ecological constraints	
	Sensory–motor	Motor–sensory	Intrasensory	Intersensory
Motor	Reflexes, particularly postural reflexes	Normal reafference due to: (a) self-observation and (b) locomotion (Involving operant conditioning)	Perceptual constancies Norms (Involving classical conditioning)	Intersensory localization (Involving classical conditioning)
Mechanical constraints in joints Tendo–muscular insertions				
Myogenic reflexes Response stereotypes				

provided by the mechanical structure of the neuromuscular system. Each joint has a limited direction and range of movement and every movement is controlled by contraction in particular muscles. This is the basic structural matrix of all operant behaviour. Furthermore, responses are patterned and controlled by neural mechanisms such as the myogenic reflexes and reciprocal inhibition. These constraints may be called functional in that, although they depend on the structure of the system, they are not purely mechanically determined. These mechanisms are discussed in chapter 4.

The second category of body constraints is what we have called sensory–motor constraints. These are the reflexes (excluding the myogenic reflexes which are an integral part of the motor system). The most important reflexes for spatial behaviour are the postural reflexes which are discussed in chapter 9.

The other main category of constraints in spatially oriented behaviour is composed of the motor–sensory constraints. The basic concept here is that of reafference—a term coined by von Holst to denote the consequences of self-produced movement on stimulation of the exteroceptors. One type of re-afference is what may be called *locomotor reafference*, that is, the reafferent stimulation produced by the movement of a sense organ relative to the out-side world. For instance, when a person walks about inside a room the retinal image of a given part of the room moves over the retina in a fashion fully determined by the movement of the person. This relationship between the self-produced movement and the movement of the retinal image is deter-minate and in that sense is an invariant or motor–stimulus constraint.

The second type of reafference is that involved when a person moves a part of his body relative to a sense organ, for instance, when a person observes his own moving hand. It is now not the sense organ which is moving, but rather a part of the body with respect to the sense organ. This may be called *self-observation reafference*.

As we shall see in chapter 15, both von Holst and Held have given a central place to reafference in explaining the development and control of spatially oriented behaviour and we must certainly agree that it is a very powerful source of information to the developing animal regarding the relation between its own body movements and the stimulation of the extero-ceptors. However, its importance should not blind us to the possible impor-tance of other sources of spatial information directly contingent on the structure of the environment itself. The learning paradigm for the behavioural mapping of self-produced movements in terms of their sensory consequences is that of operant conditioning.

The typical environment of man consists of solid objects in more or less consistent spatial relationship to one another together with some objects which change their positions. The visible world contains many redundancies or constant features, for example, most lines are either vertical or horizontal and most objects have a 'top'; these aspects of the visible world are discussed in chapters 7 and 12 respectively. Furthermore, the very static nature of this background provides a stable geographical environment within which man may orient himself or navigate. This set of environmental constraints and its behavioural significance is discussed in chapter 10.

The so-called 'perceptual constancies' are a further example of environmental constraints or ecological invariances. They arise as the result of relative movement between objects and an observer. For instance, the invariant relationship between retinal-image size and object distance, or the invariant relationship between body tilt and retinal-image tilt.

When these environmental constancies or constraints are considered within a single modality—what we have called 'intrasensory constraints'—a further set of constraints becomes apparent, viz., the so-called 'norms'. A norm is a uniquely specifiable value of a physical stimulus dimension which has special behavioural significance. Examples are the vertical orientation of a line, the straight-ahead position of a point, eye level. A norm is the physically neutral value or fulcrum point in a physical stimulus dimension; most intensity dimensions, such as light intensity, do not have a norm. The judged value of a norm may not correspond to its physical value; for instance, exposure to an asymmetrical stimulus value usually shifts the judged norm towards the side of asymmetry. This is the well-known process of *normalization*. Norms are thus behavioural constraints in two ways—they provide a natural anchor for relative judgments and form the basis for the normalization process. These matters are discussed further in chapters 8 and 11.

Finally, there are the intersensory constraints. An intersensory stimulus constraint is any recurrent combination of a stimulus in one modality with a stimulus in another modality. For example, the sight of a bell ringing is usually paired with the sound of the bell, the sight of a ball coming straight towards one is usually paired with the subsequent tactile impact. When a spatial dimension such as the azimuth dimension is considered it is apparent that the stimulus values in one modality normally correspond with those in another. On the basis of this physical correspondence an observer is able to judgmentally or behaviourally map one modality on to another. This intermodal spatial mapping is known as intersensory localization, and is discussed in chapter 14. The learning paradigm of this type of mapping is classical conditioning, in contrast to the operant conditioning paradigm for motor–sensory or re-afferent constraints already discussed.

This piecemeal motor and modality classification of constraints is convenient but there is a further class of constraints that may be called 'superordinate'. For instance, a movement of a limb is constrained by the joints and muscle, it disturbs balance, and invokes postural and other reflexes; it also produces unique proprioceptive, visual, and perhaps auditory inputs. In other words, body and stimulus constraints occur in clusters or patterns. We can ask questions about the behavioural additivity or combinability of information derived from related constraints or stimulus combinations, and we can ask whether behaviour based upon one type of stimulus constraint transfers to other stimulus conditions. These types of question are discussed in chapters 14 and 15.

In all this discussion we have assumed that the constraints are capable of influencing or generating behaviour. An important question refers to the manner in which information regarding stimulus constraints is presented. There is one important distinction here: between 'continuous' display and 'terminal' or 'anticipatory' display. In continuous display the conjunction of stimuli is continuously and simultaneously presented, whereas in terminal display one member of a stimulus pair or movement–stimulus pair is presented before the other. For instance, one may continuously observe one's hand while moving it, or one may see it only at the termination of a reaching movement. An important practical question arises here as to which is the most advantageous type of display for rapid learning of coordinated behaviour with respect to a given constraint. This matter is discussed in chapter 15.

In the normal environment of man, therefore, body movements, their sensory consequences, and external stimuli are patterned because of the way in which the body and the world are constructed. Adequate spatial behaviour implies a matching of the behaviour repertoire to the given constraints of the body and world. However, normal constraints may be disturbed experimentally, for instance by transplanting tendons, or wearing prisms before the eyes. Such disturbances may be random perturbations or systematic shifts of normal relationships. In either case they provide a powerful tool for the analysis of normal spatial behaviour. Chapter 15 is devoted to the discussion of such disturbances.

The above theoretical discussion indicates that our point of departure in analysing spatial behaviour is in the physical nature of the body and impinging stimuli and from there to the analysis of the way in which behaviour is moulded or conditioned by these physiological and physical constraints. We do not start from mentalistic concepts or questions, such as, 'why does the world appear as it does?' In this sense our approach is behavioural—but it is not behaviourist in the narrow sense, in that our analysis of response mechanisms includes reference to judgments.

2

The retina and visual direction

2.1 Basic concepts

The *visible world* consists of light sources and reflecting surfaces which emit or reflect light into the eye. The total panorama of visible sources and surfaces available to an observer at a particular location will be referred to as that observer's *visible surroundings*.

For any particular position of the eye, head, and body, only part of the visible surroundings is in view; this part will be called the *field of view*. The field of view thus consists of those sources and surfaces in the visible surroundings from which light enters the entrance pupil of the eye. The orbital ridges and nose set a limit to the practical field of view and it is this practical field of view which will be generally implied by the term 'field of view', and it may be further restricted and determined by optical devices such as prisms or artificial pupils. The complete specification of the field of view would include the wavelength and emission–absorption characteristics of the sources and surfaces, their distances from the observer, and the optical properties of the atmosphere or other intervening media. However, none of these features of the field of view is pertinent to the subject of this book, so that for our purposes, the field of view may be regarded as a two-dimensional array of areas of light and shade.

The monocular field of view is the sum total of distal visual stimuli that contribute to the bundle of light rays which enter the entrance pupil of the eye. All the 'information' regarding the distal visible stimuli is contained in this bundle of light rays, which will be referred to as the *optical array*. In other words, the field of view is that array of sources and surfaces which would be imaged by a lens at the position of the observer's eye and with the same entrance pupil. The optical array is completely specified by the field of view with one exception: a lens or prism may distort the relationship between the field of view and the optical array. Lenses and prisms do not of course affect the distal stimuli but they may shift the boundaries of the field of vision, and they may cause the observer to erroneously conclude that the distal stimuli have been changed.

The image produced by the observer's eye is defined as the retinal image. It may also be referred to as the proximal stimulus. The specification of the retinal image is ideally the task of the objective techniques of ophthalmic optics, although, in practice, it may be specified by psychophysical methods, that is, methods involving reports from the observer. However, it is not a psychophysical concept—but is physical—like the field of view.

Ideally the retinal image is completely specified by the optical array and the dioptric system of the eye. The optical system of the eye may locally distort the retinal image, so that it is no longer a simple projective transformation of the field of view. Behaviour is normally polarized towards the distal stimulus; it is this which ultimately shapes the observer's behaviour. Our basic concepts are thus anchored in physics and the other sciences which contribute to the objective specification of light sources, reflecting surfaces, and image formation.

Terms like 'visual world' and 'visual field' will be avoided. As used by

Gibson (1950a) they are psychophysical constructs, which contrast informationally degraded visual judgments which ignore depth, visual stability, constancies, etc. with judgments based on all the usable information in the optical array together with past experience. This simple dichotomy of psychophysical categories does little justice to the infinite variety of psychophysical judgments which may be made on the basis of the optical array. There are an infinite number of ways in which the information may be degraded; every experiment involves a particular set of instructions which require the subject to pay attention to one or other aspect of the field of view and to ignore other aspects. There is no heuristic value in selecting one type of judgment from this variety and reifying it by naming it the 'visual field'. The psychophysical counterpart of the physical concept 'field of view' in any particular experiment will be specified in terms of the responses which the subject makes to the field of view in accordance with the instructions he is given and the relevant past experience which he has had. The description of these responses, resulting from particular instructions and experiences related to the directional aspects of the field of view constitutes the subject matter of the greater part of this volume. When we talk of the field of view or the optical array we refer to physically defined variables; on the psychophysical side we shall talk of the judged or apparent field of view. The relation between the physical, independent variables and the dependent, psychophysical judgments is determined by the experimental instructions, the subject's past experience, and the state of his end-organs and nervous system.

2.2 Visual direction

So far as direction is concerned, the human visual system has three main tasks. The first is to provide information which will enable an observer to know where a seen object is in relation to the body and to stimuli in other modalities, and to know whether or not it is moving. The second task is to maintain the accurate functioning of the above mechanisms in spite of changes in the position of the eyes, the head, and the body of the observer. These two aspects of the problem of visual direction will be dealt with in this chapter and chapter 3 respectively.

The third task for the visual system is to provide a metric of judged relative directions and distances more or less isomorphic with physical space over the whole field of view. This is the problem of pattern vision which is dealt with only in so far as it is affected by the orientation of the distal stimulus or the observer (chapters 12 and 13).

The retina is a two-dimensional array of receptors upon which the lens focuses an image of those light-reflecting surfaces which constitute the field of view. Each point in the receptor mosaic is normally associated with a unique subjective visual direction relative to the eye's position at the time (oculocentric direction). The oculocentric directional value of each receptor is not coded in the neural discharge but rather in the spatial position of the receptors and their isomorphic projection on the visual cortex. This precise affine (point for point) neural projection through the visual chiasma, geniculate body, and optic tracts (Clark, 1932) is sufficient to account for how visual spatial information is conveyed to the CNS. It does not, however, tell us anything about how the CNS integrates this information, as the eyes move, to give egocentric directions, nor how this information is related to spatial information from other modalities, nor how motor behaviour is spatially organized in relation to visible objects. Walls (1951b) has argued that the precise, anatomical, spatial organization of the visual system proves the innateness of oculocentric visual direction; this may be so but all it proves is that the way in which visual spatial information is conveyed to the CNS is innately determined; it tells us nothing regarding the innateness of behaviour associated with this information, and this is the significant problem.

Although the oculocentric directional value of a point stimulus is not conveyed as a specific modulation of the neural discharge, it is now known that the direction in which a small light moves over the retina is coded in this way. Barlow and Levick (1963) found that the discharge of a retinal ganglion cell varied according to the direction in which a light spot was moved over the receptive field of that ganglion cell. The receptive field of a ganglion cell, that is, the receptor area feeding one ganglion cell, may be several degrees in diameter, although the movement necessary to fire the ganglion cell had to be over only a small fraction of this distance. This suggested to Barlow and Levick that there are smaller directionally sensitive subunits between the receptors and the ganglion cell—perhaps the bipolar cells. Such a mechanism resembles one suggested in 1911 by Wohlgemuth to account for the after-effect of seen movement.

Hubel and Wiesel (1959) have recently detected cells in the cat's visual cortex, some of which are selectively sensitive to the orientation of the visual stimulus, and some to its direction of movement.

The history of attempts to account for the oculocentric directionality of visible objects is fascinating. Various laws of 'projection' have been proposed, such as, that a person estimates objects to be in the direction of the rays of light striking the retina, or of the line at right angles to the retinal image. Clearly the visual system cannot possibly detect the direction of rays of light; projection theories are at best a geometrical description of the optics of vision, they are not theories of how information is coded physiologically. These 'projection' theories are described in Carr (1935), Helmholtz (1962, vol. III,

p. 268), and Walls (1951a). They are of historical interest only and will not be discussed here.

Hering (1861) was the first to set out in detail what has come to be accepted as the correct general psychophysical account of visual direction, although he acknowledged earlier, less detailed accounts by Johannes Müller (1840) and Prevost (1843) (see Hering, 1942). The following analysis is our own but embodies Hering's ideas and at the same time attempts to extend them.

The basic concept in the analysis is what Hering called 'visual lines'; *a visual line is the locus of all points fixed relative to the eye which stimulate a given point on the retina*. It defines the basic oculocentric direction. The visual line of the fovea is the principal visual line or 'visual axis'. For any given position of the eyes, all points on a particular visual line are normally judged to be in alignment, that is, to be geometrically superimposed even if at different distances. We shall call this the law of oculocentric visual direction; it states simply that *objects producing superimposed retinal images for a given position of the eye are judged to be in alignment*. This law says nothing about the plane or point of the observer's body with which the objects are judged to be in alignment, it states merely that they are reported to be superimposed, ignoring distance. The next stage in the analysis is to assume that for every retinal point in the binocular field of one eye there is a corresponding point in the retina of the other eye, such that when both are simultaneously stimulated there is judged to be a superimposed pair of objects, or if the stimulus objects are identical, a single 'fused' object. These *corresponding retinal points* are said to have identical oculocentric and egocentric space values, and all objects on the visual lines of a pair of corresponding points will be reported to be in spatial alignment. For any angle of convergence of the eyes there is a surface in space which an object must occupy if it is to stimulate corresponding retinal points. This surface is known as the *horopter*.

Hering stated these facts as *the law of identical visual directions* in the following words, 'For any given two corresponding lines of direction, or visual lines, there is in visual space a single visual direction line upon which *appears* everything which *actually lies* in the pair of visual lines' (Hering, 1942, p. 41). The truth of this statement was demonstrated by Hering in the following way. 'Let the observer stand about ½ meter from a window which affords view of out doors, hold his head very steady, close the right eye, and direct the left to an object located somewhat to the right. Let us suppose it is a tree which is well set off from its surroundings. While fixing the tree with the left eye a black mark is made on the window pane at a spot in line with the tree. Now the left eye is closed and the right opened and directed at the spot on the window, and beyond that to some object in line with it, e.g. a chimney. Then with both eyes open and directed at the spot, this latter will appear to cover parts of the tree and the chimney. Both will be seen simultaneously, now the tree more distinctly, now chimney, and sometimes both equally well, according to which eye's image is victor in the conflict. One sees therefore, the spot on the pane, the tree and the chimney in the same direction' (see figure 2.1).

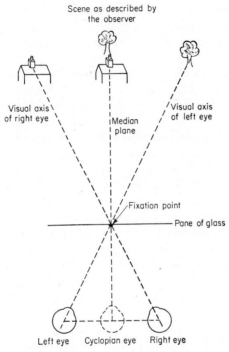

Figure 2.1 Diagrammatic representation of Hering's law of identical binocular directions, assuming symmetry of function of the visual system

The next step in the analysis is to assume that all objects on a visual line are judged to be, not merely in alignment, but also in line with a point of reference or projection centre in the head of the observer, and that this centre is common to all visual lines. In other words, *all visual lines of both eyes are judged to point to one and the same projection centre.* This projection centre is commonly assumed to lie at the centre of the axis joining the centres of the two eyes, that is, the interocular axis. It is often referred to as the cylopian eye (Duane, 1931). It is as if the directions of objects on the visual lines of each eye were judged as though they were seen by an eye midway between the actual eyes. A corollary of this is that a line which actually lies on the median plane of the head lies across non-corresponding visual lines of the two eyes except at the fixation point and will therefore be seen as a cross, intersecting at the fixation point. This 'cross' is easily observed simply by holding a card with a line on it horizontally so that one end of the line touches the bridge of the nose. It is as if the subjective space of each eye had slipped scissor-fashion about the fixation point over the subjective space of the other eye, apparently transferring the objects on the visual axes to the median plane and, for each eye, objects in the objective median plane to the visual axis of the opposite eye.

Thus, according to Hering, for symmetrical convergence all visible objects which are imaged on the fovea are judged not only to have the same oculocentric direction but also the same egocentric direction—namely the median plane of the head. This does not follow logically; if the point of fixation p is in the median plane and if this point is correctly localized by the observer, it follows from the laws of monocular direction and identical directions that all objects on the same visual lines as the point p must also be reported to be *aligned* with p. This does not necessarily imply that all the aligned objects would be reported to be in the *median plane*, they could be apparently in any plane passing through p. However, the only plane which is symmetrical with respect to the two eyes is the median plane of the head and therefore this is the plane one would expect them to apparently occupy in a balanced visual system. Even if they do apparently occupy the median plane, the apparent median plane and objective median plane may not coincide.

With symmetrical convergence, objects on the visual axis of an eye are usually judged to be in the median plane even when only one eye is open or when, because of an obstruction, the object can be seen by only one eye. This was demonstrated by Hering in the following manner. Several inches in front of the right eye a card was held with a pin hole at its centre (see figure 2.2). A black dot p, on a pane of glass was fixated by the left eye and by the right eye through the pin hole. A small object a was placed beyond the glass on the visual axis of the left eye. Although the object was seen by only the left eye and was situated to the right of the subject's median plane, it was reported to be in the median plane behind the point p. If the right eye was closed the subject's report remained the same; only if the eyes changed their position did the apparent position of a change. Hering claimed that persons such as microscopists who are used to using one eye are not subject to this illusion. Such people always report that objects on a given visual line have the same alignment (i.e. obey the law of visual direction) but do not necessarily report them to be in the median plane. All Hering's demonstrations reveal that visual lines are judged not according to their oculocentric directions but rather to a common egocentre.

Here then are three laws or principles of visual direction.

1. The law of visual oculocentric direction states that coincident retinal images give rise to a judgment of alignment or superimposition. A corollary of this law is that non-coincident retinal images give rise to a judgment of spatial separateness. There are occasions when this law does not hold; a single

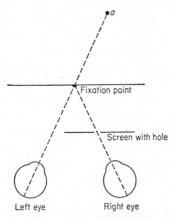

Figure 2.2 Arrangement described by Hering to demonstrate the law of cyclopian projection for an object on the visual axis of only one eye

object seen monocularly sometimes evokes a judgment that there are two objects in view. This condition is known as monocular diplopia and is discussed in section 2.3. There is another condition in which objects on different visual lines may be reported to be spatially superimposed. Such cases are discussed in sections 2.7 and 11.33.

2. The law of identical visual directions states that every retinal point in the binocular field of one eye has a partner in the retina of the other eye with identical directional value. Monocular diplopia provides an exception to this law also, for in this condition a point in one retina has a direction value identical with two retinal points of the other eye. In the condition known as binocular diplopia, which is a normal consequence of squint, the corresponding visual lines cannot be converged on to a visual object, and therefore the images of that object fall on non-corresponding retinal points and the object is reported as double.

3. The law of cyclopian projection states that objects on the visual axes of the two eyes in symmetrical convergence are judged to be in the median plane of the head. A more general form of this law for symmetrical conver-

gence is that objects on any corresponding pair of visual lines are judged to be in a plane passing through a point midway between the eyes and the point in the horopter contained in both visual lines. For asymmetrical convergence the simplest interpretation of Hering's law of cyclopian projection is that objects on corresponding visual lines are judged to be in a plane passing through the objective fixation point and a point midway between the eyes. The point midway between the eyes is the *cyclopean projection centre*. It is generally assumed that objects on corresponding visual lines are not only judged as being in line with the cyclopian projection centre but also as being in the objective plane passing through this centre and the objective position of the point of fixation. The extent to which objects on visual lines are in fact judged to be on planes passing through the cyclopian centre has been the subject of empirical investigations. We shall see later that these studies have revealed that the actual projection centre often departs from the position of the ideal cyclopean projection centre.

Hering's analysis of visual direction was meant to account for the way in which directional judgments are made about objects at different distances. The fact that the directions of objects at different distances along visual lines are judged in relation to a common egocentre means that the directions of all objects other than the one being fixated are misjudged. This would seem to be intolerable from the behavioural point of view; however, one's attention and behaviour are not usually directed to objects far outside the point of fixation, so that the illusory directions of such objects are of little consequence. Objects within a short distance of the fixation point are not seen as double and their direction is usually correctly judged. Consider, for instance, a short rod, such as a pencil, pointing towards the face and inspected binocularly. Its direction from the face is usually not judged incorrectly even though its far end is perceptibly double. We combine the binocularly disparate information to estimate the true direction of the pencil.

A further discussion of the projection centre or egocentre is given in chapter 11.

2.3 Monocular diplopia

If a person with one eye open reports that he sees two points of light where there is only one, he is said to have monocular diplopia. It occurs in three types of abnormal condition. (a) Physical conditions in the eye, such as irregular cornea, defective pupil, dislocation or refractive irregularities of the lens, entoptic bodies, and detached retina. We shall not discuss these causes further. (b) The development of anomalous correspondence in strabismus. (c) Lesions of the occipital lobes, cerebellum and oculomotor centres.

The most common circumstance in which monocular diplopia develops is when a strabismus or squint has been surgically corrected. It also occurs in bitemporal hemianopia, possibly due to the shift of normal fixation which this condition induces (Kubie and Beckman, 1929). Javal (1865) was the first to report a case, but it was not until 1898 that the significance of the condition was pointed out by Bielschowsky who worked with Hering. The condition is rare, even among squinters. Worth (1903) found only four cases among 2,000 squinters. Tschermak (1899), himself a squinter, suffered from monocular diplopia when he converged his eyes with only one of them open.

The usual explanation is that normal binocular correspondence becomes inhibited and is replaced by a new 'anomalous' correspondence. The new correspondence enables the image of an object on the fovea of one retina to have the same space value as the image of the object on an extrafoveal point in the deviating eye. The normal functional linkages which associate the cortical projections of corresponding retinal points are inhibited and gradually replaced by new linkages between the new corresponding projections. Anomalous correspondence takes years to develop; the apparent separation of the binocular disparate images gradually decreases until the angle of the new correspondence or 'angle of anomaly' equals the angle of deviation. The binocular disparity will then be absent. If the deviating eye is straightened after anomalous correspondence has developed, the new correspondence is no longer appropriate. The patient will rapidly reestablish, or disinhibit, the normal correspondence linkages; normal correspondence will be reestablished before the anomalous correspondence has been inhibited. Each point in the corrected eye will now have two space values, one determined by the anomalous correspondence, and the other by the normal correspondence.

Some squinters can straighten their eyes voluntarily. Morgan (1955) described a patient who could squint at will and who had monocular diplopia whenever she did so. Cases have been reported in which there was monocular diplopia in both eyes (Purdy, 1934; Cass, 1941; Lewis, 1944) but normally it is restricted to the corrected eye.

Evidently anomalous correspondence does not function in the same way as normal correspondence. In anomalous correspondence involuntary fusion movements of the eyes do not occur, although the accommodation–convergence reflex is intact. This lack of the fusion reflex is probably not a consequence of anomalous correspondence but of a general lack of such reflexes in squinters. In fact Worth (1903) and Bielschowsky (1931) suggested that deficient fusion reflexes are a major causative factor in the development of squint. Whether or not this deficiency of fusional reflexes is a consequence of anomalous correspondence, there are other deficiencies which apparently are caused by it, for instance, no depth effect is reported by a person with anomalous correspondence when he inspects stereograms in a stereoscope. If the stereograms are not identical, double images are reported by such a person, whereas the person with normal correspondence can tolerate some disparity before reporting two images (Panum's areas). According to Purdy (1934) binocular colour mixture does not occur with anomalous correspondence; instead, the subject reports the two colours as separately occupying the same place, presumably in alternation. It has been generally concluded from these differences that normal binocular correspondence is innately determined and that anomalous correspondence is an adaptation which overcomes binocular diplopia, but can never operate like normal correspondence in any other way. The extrafoveal image in monocular diplopia is dim compared with the one related to the normal position on the retina, and this may be a consequence of the innate preference for the normal space values.

The classical theory of monocular diplopia in squinters is a reasonable one. However, it is possible that monocular diplopia is not really monocular. We propose the following possibility. We shall assume that when an optical image is present in the visual system of one eye, a similar pattern of neural activity is induced in the corresponding cortical visual area of the other eye. This 'transferred' activity is not normally reported because it has the same space value as the image in the other eye. When a squint is present, new linkages form between the central areas of the two eyes. Some induction occurs across these new links while the old linkage is inhibited. When the squint has been corrected, induction occurs across two linkages. One of these, the normal one, corresponds spatially to the stimulus, but the other does not and is seen as a weak 'ghost' image. We can think of no test which would distinguish this theory from the classical one, though interocular transfer or induction is known to occur in certain circumstances (Howard, 1959).

Whichever theory is adopted, one has to assume that new functional linkages develop which are different to the preferred, original ones. Werner (1942) has suggested that the sufficient condition for the development of anomalous correspondence is 'that the binocular unity of disparate points is so strong that the tendency towards unification of anatomical corresponding points is of little or no effect.' He demonstrated that some degree of anomalous correspondence may be induced in normal people if the above principle is applied. If, for instance, the vertical parallel lines of figure 2.3 are employed, the tendency towards unification is strong because the disparity is relatively small and is the same at all points, and because no other lines of different or normal correspondence are in view. The lines of figure 2.3 are reported as occupying the same frontal plane, in other words the new correspondence serves as a new 'zero' of relative depth. This same 'equidistance tendency' has been reported by Harker (1962) and by Howard and Templeton (1964a), although not interpreted in the same way.

If anomalous correspondence may be induced in normal people, then monocular diplopia should also arise. Werner claimed to have shown that this is so. The stereogram of figure 2.3 was presented strobostereoscopically so that the two half-images appeared one after the other in rapid succession. When f_1 and f_2 were focused, a and b were usually seen displaced towards each other. Often, however, line a, seen only by the left eye, appeared double. It needs to be demonstrated that eye movements were not occuring before Werner's evidence can be accepted without reservation.

Monocular diplopia may also arise as a consequence of damage to the cerebellum, occipital lobes or oculomotor centres (Gerstmann and Kestenbaum, 1930; Klein and Stein, 1934). The reasons are complex and not well

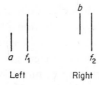

Figure 2.3 Stereogram used by Werner (1942) to demonstrate monocular diplopia in normal vision

understood. One possibility is that nystagmic eye movements resulting from damage to oculomotor centres, together with abnormal tonic balance in the extraocular muscles due to cerebellar or vestibular damage, cause monocular diplopia (Bender, 1945; Bender and Teuber, 1946). Other references to this subject are given in Purdy (1934).

Ronchi (1961) claims that normal subjects report double images of circular spots of light seen briefly 7° nasally against an adapting field in the mesopic range of luminances. The cause of this phenomenon is obscure, unless it is due to poor accommodation coupled with the peripheral position of the stimulus.

2.4 Spatial disorientation with homonymous visual defects

Damage to the visual system further back than the optic chiasma often results in loss of vision in the corresponding half of each eye. The patient is said to be suffering from homonymous hemianopia, and is blind in either the left or right half of visual space. In some hemianopic patients, a new centre of vision—a pseudo-fovea—develops. Clarity of vision decreases in all directions from this centre, even towards the true fovea. Fuchs (1922) investigated the nature of a pseudo-fovea. One of his patients could fixate with his true fovea, and when he did so nothing on the right could be seen. When a horizontal row of letters was shown to him at a distance of one metre, the clearest letter was about 6 cm to the left of the fixation point. Visual acuity was higher at the pseudo-fovea than at the true fovea. As the viewing distance increased to 3 metres the point of clearest vision shifted 6·8 cm to the left whereas according to the visual angle it should have been 18 cm left of fixation. Fuchs concluded that the pseudo-fovea is not anatomically fixed.

When the observation distance was held constant, the pseudo-fovea was found to be nearer the fixation point for small letters than for large letters. It was not even in the same place for small near letters and large far letters which projected retinal images of the same size. It was concluded that the apparent size was the important factor determining the position of the pseudo-fovea. When one small and one large letter were presented and moved together, the distance at which each was most clearly seen was the same as it would have been had each been presented singly. Voluntary shifts of attention had no effect on these relationships. When a sectional letter 'E' was presented piece-meal at the position of greatest clarity of the whole, the parts were not clearly seen until the whole figure was complete and recognized as an 'E'. These observations demonstrate the complex functional nature of a pseudo-fovea.

Fuchs* (1920) described another case of hemianopia, in which the right half of each retina was normal, the upper left was blind, and the lower left was amblyopic. Objects seen on the sound side were correctly localized, but objects in the amblyopic quadrant were displaced to the right and downward. A strip or row of dots half in the amblyopic quadrant and half in the opposite normal quadrant were displaced as if they had been entirely in the amblyopic region. In other words, things lying in the competent area were displaced provided they formed a composite pattern with things seen in the amblyopic area. With a weakly organized pattern, the parts were reported as sometimes displaced and sometimes not.

Fuchs explained these displacements by assuming that the new centre of attention, or pseudo-fovea, serves as the new centre of reference for direction in hemianopics. Kanzer and Bender (1939) described a hemianopic patient and confirmed that the area of clearest vision is shifted towards the competent side, and that visible objects are mislocated towards the opposite side.

Bruell (1958) applied the Bruell and Albee motor theory of visual direction (see section 11.31) to explain the visual mislocations in hemianopia. The mislocations, they argued, are the same as those reported by normal people when presented with an asymmetrical visual field. They develop immediately, both in normal and in amblyopic subjects, and are different in this respect from the corrective shifts in space values which occur in

* An English translation of Fuchs' papers is given in Ellis (1938)

strabismus, which take years to develop. This theory is similar to an earlier formulation by Metzger (1927).

2.5 The stability of judgments of visual direction (autokinesis)

2.51 Introduction

There are many reasons why a steadily fixated stationary point of light may be reported as moving. If a moving visual display has been exposed for some time, the well-known movement after-effect may be reported. For a review of this topic see Wohlgemuth (1911). If there has been no previous motion in the field of view, any apparent movement of stationary visible objects is known as autokinetic movement.

In 1799 the astronomer von Humbolt noticed that stars seen through a telescope appeared to drift about. He was convinced that the stars were actually moving, and it was not until 1858 that Schweizer demonstrated the subjective nature of the phenomenon by noting that different people reported different movements of the same star at the same time. In 1886 Charpentier rediscovered this phenomenon independently. Aubert also rediscovered it in 1887 and called it 'autokinesis', by which name it is now generally known. The early literature on the subject is reviewed in Adams (1912), Guilford (1928), and Grosvenor (1959), and will not be dealt with in detail here.

It is difficult to measure autokinesis, for any introduction of other visible objects disturbs the effect. The subject may be asked to give a verbal estimate of the apparent movement but, as the distance of the target from the subject is ambiguous, so will be the estimates of distance moved. It is not easy to make judgments in terms of visual angle. Guilford and Dallenbach (1928) asked the subject to trace the course of the apparent movements on paper, but such a procedure assumes that people can draw accurately in the dark. Bridges and Bitterman (1954) provided the subject with a lever which permitted him to move the autokinetic stimulus in the frontal–parallel plane. The subject was told that the light would be moved and he was to return it to its starting point. A permanent record of the direction and extent of the subject's tracking of his own autokinetic movement was thus obtained. To what extent this procedure contaminates the results is not known: it is certainly dependent on the subjects remembering a consistent starting point.

Not everyone reports autokinetic movement. Carr (1910) found that one person out of four did not report it. Voth (1941) tested 270 subjects, and obtained a J-shaped curve relating the amplitude of the reported movement (as drawn) to the number of cases. However, as the measure was in centimetres it cannot be known by how much the results reflect differences in the distance away which the subjects assumed the light to be.

Several theories of autokinetic movement have been proposed, but it is misleading to regard them as alternatives: they are best regarded as possible contributory mechanisms.

2.52 Autokinesis and eye movements

Any involuntary eye movement, such as nystagmus or passive movement of the eye by the finger, certainly produces an illusion of visual movement. The crucial question is whether appropriate eye movements of sufficient magnitude occur during autokinetic movement.

Exner (1896) and Schilder (1912) found that a small light and a surrounding frame may be reported as moving in different directions at the same time. If this were true it would demonstrate that at least one of the apparent movements was not due to eye movements. Bourdon (1902) and Simon (1904) could not find evidence of simultaneous opposed autokinetic movement, and although Skolnick (1940) confirmed Exner's effect he explained it by saying that the disc momentarily fades from view because of adaptation, and reappears when the eyes have changed position, giving the illusion of an apparent shift of the central location of the spot in the frame. This type of explanation would appear to be meaningful only if based on the differential latency of the centre and periphery of the visual system.

A more direct approach to the role of eye movements in autokinesis is to record the eye movements directly while the subject fixates a light. Carr (1910) found that eye movements did occur when the subject felt that the eye fixation was not following the movement of the light, but that when the subject reported autokinetic movement in which his eye seemed to remain fixated on the light, eye movements did not occur.

Guilford and Dallenbach (1928) also photographed the eye during autokinetic movement, and found no trace of related eye movements. However, Skolnik (1940) pointed out that only horizontal eye movements were recorded, whereas autokinesis is largely vertical, and that in any case autokinesis could be induced by eye movements too small to be detected by Guilford and Dallenbach's camera. Spontaneous eye movements are said by Brandt (1940) to occur mainly in a horizontal direction, so that Skolnick's claim (backed by Matin and MacKinnon, 1964) that vertical autokinesis is more marked than horizontal autokinesis does not accord with an eye-movement theory.

Skolnick himself claimed that small nystagmic eye movements do accompany autokinetic movement, although he could not predict the direction of the autokinetic movement by looking at what the eyes were doing.

A new approach to the problem of the role of eye movements in autokinetic movement has recently been reported by Matin and MacKinnon

(1964). They compared the amount of autokinetic movement of a point of light in each of the eight principal directions with normal viewing and when horizontal retinal-image movements consequent upon eye movements were compensated for by the 'stopped-image' technique. The horizontal movement was markedly reduced in the stopped-image condition compared with the normal viewing condition. Presumably the small drifts and saccades which are known to occur even during steady fixation contribute to autokinesis.

There is still some doubt whether or not eye movements always accompany autokinesis; there can be no doubt that involuntary eye movements can induce apparent visual movement when they do occur.

2.53 Autokinesis and motor strain

Whether or not actual eye movements occur during autokinesis, it may be that changes in muscle tonus occur. This would be hard to prove, but it is possible to demonstrate that induced tonus asymmetry can cause autokinesis. Carr (1910) found that his own autokinetic movement was in the same direction as a previous fixation of the eyes up to an asymmetrical position of 30° in the head; for larger angles of fixation asymmetry the apparent movement was in the opposite direction. Furthermore, the instruction, 'imagine you are looking to the left', produced a corresponding autokinetic movement; jaw contraction induced a downward movement; and sound to one side induced an apparent movement in that direction (see also Corso and Soloyanis, 1962). Carr concluded that the 'autokinetic illusion is mainly determined by the changing neuromuscular conditions involved in a continuous fixation.' Absence of a visual frame and elimination of head movements are important in weakening the eye–body link essential for visual localization. Gregory (1959) has recently produced evidence which confirms Carr's findings (Gregory and Zangwill, 1963).

Adams (1912) had his subjects fixate lights at various positions with the head held in a central position. The autokinetic movement increasingly tended to go in the direction of gaze as the eccentricity increased. Luchins (1954b) reported a similar effect. Battersby, Kahn, Pollack, and Bender (1956) reported that turning the head and trunk 40° to the side induced an opposed autokinetic movement.

Carr (1910) found that when only one eye is open the autokinetic movement of a light in the median plane is towards that eye. Crovitz (1962) confirmed this effect and suggested that the eyes tend to fixate a point directly in front of the open eye, and that it is this tendency of the eye to move from the objective median plane which causes the autokinesis to drift in that direction. This suggestion accords with Carr's finding that merely thinking of looking sideways causes autokinesis to the same side. It also accords with the fact that people with eye paralysis who 'intend' an eye movement experience an apparent visual movement in the same direction.

This theory would imply that when the open eye fixates eccentrically away from the median plane the eye-movement tendency, and therefore the autokinetic movement, is back towards the median plane, a prediction contradicted by the findings of Adams and Luchins (see above) that the more eccentric fixation is, the greater the apparent movement in the same direction.

Section 3.5 contains a discussion of the implications of these facts, and Bruell and Albee's theory of egocentric localization, which is discussed in section 11.31, is also relevant.

Goldman (1953) working within the framework of the sensory–tonic theory (see section 7.1), found that the more the subject was prevented from moving the more marked was his reported autokinetic effect. He concluded that this reciprocity supports 'the postulate of vicarious channelization, according to which an inverse relation is expected between the amount of perceptual movement and motor activity.' But Carr's simpler statement, that lack of movement weakens the eye–body link through sensory adaptation, accounts for Goldman's finding more directly and parsimoniously.

Intact labyrinths are evidently not essential for autokinesis; indeed Miller and Graybiel (1962) found that patients with bilateral labyrinthine defects reported more autokinesis than a comparable group of normal subjects.

2.54 Autokinesis and the visual frame

Clearly the most important factor determining the autokinetic movement is the absence of a visual frame of reference, including the absence from sight of the orbital ridges and nose. Royce, Stayton, and Kinkade (1962) studied the role of the visual frame quantitatively. As the number of lights in a multiple-light configuration was increased, the frequency of reported autokinesis declined. A $\frac{1}{4}$ inch concentric circular band of light also reduced the apparent movement of a central point, irrespective of the radius of the circle. The brighter the circle the more the reduction of the movement. Luchins (1954c) controlled the amount of visual field by gradually illuminating the inside of a box in the centre of which the autokinetic light was situated. As the illumination was increased the apparent movement became less until the light became stable at a value of 20 foot-candles.

Luchins and Luchins (1963) found that when one eye was focused on the autokinetic light on a dark background, while the other eye looked at an illuminated room, the light appeared to move even at a value of 150 foot-candles. Under these conditions there are no corresponding stimuli upon which binocular convergence could anchor itself. The apparent movement of point against background most probably reflected the 'hunting' vergence movements of the eyes, and Luchins and Luchins are probably wrong in identifying this effect with the autokinetic phenomenon.

Autokinesis may still be reported when a large number of points of light are in view. Edwards (1954b) suggested that this may be because a pattern of dots is highly redundant. In a later experiment (Edwards, 1959) he tested this idea by comparing the movement in a regular array of dots with that in an irregular array. Both patterns produced the same autokinesis, and therefore Edwards rejected his stimulus–redundancy hypothesis. He suggested that autokinesis is not apparent in a full visual field, which his patterns were not, because of the anchoring effect of the orbital ridges and nose seen against the objects at the edge of the visual field. It seems that nobody has tested this idea.

Larger single patches of light are reported as moving less than smaller patches (Honeyman, Cowper, and Rose, 1946; Edwards, 1954a; Luchins, 1954a). The effect of size may be due to the increase in the amount of light flux rather than the area of the stimulus: increasing the brightness of a light of constant area has been found to decrease the autokinetic movement (Karwoski, Redner, and Wood, 1948; Spigel, 1963).

Black points in a homogeneous light field also show autokinetic movement but of smaller magnitude than light points on a dark field (Schweizer, 1858; Luchins, 1954c). This reduced effect could be due to the fact that when the whole field is bright, the edges of the field come into view and provide an anchor or standard of reference.

In spite of all the evidence that autokinesis increases as the visual frame is weakened, apparent movements may be observed even in a full and varied field of view if steady fixation is maintained for some time (Marks, 1949; Honisett and Oldfield, 1961). The whole field may appear to move or parts may move relative to other parts. These effects are particularly marked if one steadily fixates a large pattern of regular black lines. The lines bend and contort, and at the same time appear to drift as a whole across the visual field. Stable visual directional values would seem to require constant eye movements as well as a full field of view.

Inspection of a simple outline figure prior to the exposure of a single light point has been found to reduce autokinesis equally in both directions (Crutchfield and Edwards, 1949) particularly if the prior pattern is presented to the side opposed to the prevailing direction of reported movement (Edwards and Crutchfield, 1951). No differential directional reduction of autokinesis has been found to result from the prior inspection of asymmetrical figures (Edwards and Crutchfield, 1951; Conklin, 1957). There is thus no obvious relationship between autokinesis and figural after-effects.

2.55 Autokinesis and entoptic streaming

Guilford (1928) and Guilford and Dallenbach (1928) reported that their subjects when in the dark saw a veil of streaming entoptic cloud-like material against which background the stationary point of light appeared to move like the moon through moving clouds. Ferree (1908) and Eldridge-Green (1920) had proposed a similar explanation of autokinesis. This entoptic streaming is elusive, for other investigators have never reported that their subjects saw it. Streaming is very obvious if one has just fixated a regular line pattern (Erb and Dallenbach, 1939) or if one looks into a flickering field of light (Smythies, 1959a, 1959b). It is especially evident in the field of a closed eye when the other eye is inspecting a flickering field (Howard, 1959). However, nobody has ever reported whether or not the direction of autokinesis is affected by the direction of these streaming effects. A casual observation by the senior author suggests that it is not.

Autokinetic movement is not limited to vision; Bernadin and Gruber (1957) and Anderson and Moss (1964) have reported an autokinetic effect in audition.

The direction and extent of autokinetic movement has been found to be affected by the shape of the stimulus (Adams, 1912; Honeyman, Cowper, and Rose, 1946), and by reinforcement (Haggard and Rose, 1944; Haggard and Babin, 1948; Hoffman, Swander, Baron, and Rohrer, 1953; Farrow and Santos, 1962). It is well known that suggestion and social influences also affect autokinesis but a discussion of these matters is beyond the scope of this book.

2.6 Visual acuity and the orientation of stimulus and observer

2.61 Introduction

The claim has repeatedly been made that even in the absence of clinical astigmatism, visual acuity is highest for vertical and horizontal lines, lower for lines at 45°, and lowest of all for lines at intermediate angles. Shlaer (1937) named this effect 'retinal astigmatism'. This name begs the question of whether the effect is retinal in origin; 'meridional astigmatism' is a better name. Hartridge (1950) was of the opinion that Shlaer had been the first to report this effect; in fact it was reported in 1925 by Emsley, who noticed it incidentally while studying clinical astigmatism. He wrote, 'This marked preference for lines in a certain direction, after the optical defect of the eye has been fully corrected, constitutes a kind of residual astigmatism . . . . . the reason for it is to be sought in the lens substance or humours or at the retina or even farther back along the optic nerve.'

Meridional astigmatism could have practical consequences; for instance, Hartridge (1950) pointed out that it could account for the fact that certain letters are more easily confused than others: there would be confusion between P and R, because the distinguishing line is at an oblique angle, whereas T and L would be easily distinguished, because the distinguishing lines are horizontal. A further practical consequence of meridional astigmatism was suggested by Higgins and Stultz (1948). They claimed that printers take account of this fact when they arrange the rows and columns of dots in half-tone prints along oblique axes in the picture and thus ensure that the dots are less easily seen that if they were aligned vertically or horizontally. We doubt whether printers are in fact aware of meridional variations in acuity; it is more likely that they arrange the dots obliquely so that the rows and columns do not form interference patterns with the predominantly vertical–horizontal orientation of most of the lines in pictures. Non-parallelity has been shown to be more easily detected when the lines are horizontal or vertical rather than oblique (Mach, 1897; Rochlin, 1955). Rochlin also found that the constant error in setting two lines to be parallel when they sloped from top left to bottom right was different from the constant error when the lines sloped the other way. He suggested that these differences are a function of laterality, but did not put this idea to experimental test. Finally, meridional astigmatism may account for the fact that a steadily fixated line is least likely to disappear when it is either vertical or horizontal (Craig and Lichtenstein, 1953).

There are several possible classes of explanation of meridional variations in acuity.

1. Perceptual theories, based on any factors which operate at a higher level than the eye.

2. Eye-movement theories, based on differences in the amplitude or frequency of physiological nystagmus between the various planes in which the eyes move.

3. Retinal theories, based on variations in either the density of the retinal receptors or in the functional properties of the retina.

4. Dioptric theories, based on meridional variations in the dioptric apparatus of the eye which remain after clinical astigmatism has been corrected.

We shall consider the evidence relative to each of these theories.

2.62 Perceptual theories

One possibility is that acuity is always better for lines which are vertical or horizontal irrespective of the orientation of the eye. If this were true it would involve a high-level mechanism. Ogilvie and Taylor (1958) tested this hypothesis by measuring meridional variations in acuity when the observer's head was at 45° to gravity. The orientations of the line stimulus which gave the best acuity measures were now at 45° to gravity. The effect was 'attributed to the structure of the visual system.' Luria (1963) recently confirmed this finding, but noted that the meridional differences were not as marked when the head was tilted.

2.63 Eye-movement theories

With regard to eye-movement theories, Brown (1949) suggested that meridional variations in acuity could be explained by assuming that the eye is suspended by two pairs of elastic muscles; an involuntary 'jump' of the eye would be followed by damped vibrations, predominantly in the horizontal and vertical planes. Higgins and Stultz (1950) put Brown's eye-movement theory to experimental test. A grating test-disc was exposed in various orientations for less than 1 msec so that no eye movements were possible. The superiority of the horizontal and vertical meridians was clearly demonstrated. There was a mean difference of about 1 min of arc between these two meridians and the oblique meridians. The fact that the astigmatism is still present with such short exposures shows that eye-movement theories such as Brown's cannot account for the effect.

Nevertheless, since the visibility of contours is affected by motion of the retinal image (Riggs, Ratliff, Cornsweet, and Cornsweet, 1953) and since the eye does not move uniformly in all directions (Nachmias, 1959) the visibility of contours should be related to orientation. Although Higgins and Stultz had shown that meridional astigmatism persists when there are no eye movements, eye movements may yet contribute to the effect when they are present. In a recent study by Nachmias (1960) the background luminance against which a fine wire could just be detected was determined as a function of the orientation of the wire and the duration of exposure. At the same time the eye movements were photographed. The data did not reveal any relationship between meridional variations in acuity and eye movements. Nachmias pointed out that he recorded only eye movements of small amplitude and may therefore have missed an effect due to differential eye movements of large amplitude.

2.64 Retinal theories

Shlaer (1937) first proposed a detailed retinal theory to account for meridional astigmatism. He argued that if, as Hecht (1928) suggested, the retina is composed of elements with different thresholds, then those with the lowest thresholds may be more numerous along the horizontal and vertical meridians. He supported this argument by two observations. First, the effect is greater at lower intensities where only low threshold receptors are stimulated, and practically disappears at higher values where all the receptors are active. Secondly, he found that the positions of the stimulus for which acuity was best were not constant for different levels of illumination. In terms of Shlaer's theory, this last fact would be explained by supposing that the distribution of low threshold receptors is not symmetrical about the meridian of highest concentration. Shlaer's arguments are very tenuous, there are other explanations of his findings, as we shall see later.

Using Landolt's C test in green light, Hartridge (1950) found that the gap was more easily resolved when in the vertical or horizontal position. He suggested that this effect is due to the way in which green receptors are clustered round the point in the retina which functions as the fixation point in green light. Hartridge acknowledged the similarity between his own theory and Shlaer's. He argued that the astigmatic effect would alter as the fixation point modifies its situation. Shlaer's results with various illumination levels were quoted to support this argument, although it is not clear from Hartridge's account how a change in illumination could modify the situation of the fixation point.

Foley (1962) proposed that retinal spatial summation is indicated by the ratio of the slope of the CFF–log area function to the slope of the CFF–log luminance function. If retinal summation is less along oblique meridians, the above ratio for these meridians should be less than for horizontal and vertical meridians. This ratio was found not to vary with the orientation of the targets. Foley concluded that this is evidence against a retinal theory of meridional astigmatism. In fact, it is evidence only against a retinal theory which depends on the assumption that there is differential retinal summation.

2.65 Dioptric theories

It is usually assumed that the lens aberrations of the eye increase as the pupil size is increased. This may not be a valid assumption: most artificial optical systems are designed to function optimally at intermediate apertures. However, if the assumption is valid, and if dioptric factors are important, then the extent of the meridional variations should increase with an increase in pupil size. Hamblin and Winser (1927) and Leibowitz (1952, 1953) found an increase in meridional variations as they increased pupil size, although Higgins and Stultz (1950) reported the opposite effect.

Shlaer found that intense illumination eliminated the meridional variations, and cited this evidence in support of his retinal theory (see section 2.64).

Leibowitz (1952, 1953, 1955), on the other hand, found that the meridional differences persisted at high levels of illumination, and argued that this fact supports a retinal theory on the grounds that, at high luminance, dioptric factors would be ineffective in changing acuity. It is odd that two apparently contradictory findings were both used as evidence for the retinal theory.

There seemed to be no way of resolving these contradictions, nor of deciding between the retinal and dioptric theories, until, in 1959, Weymouth published a paper which may have solved the problem. He reminded his readers that, according to Gullstrand (1901) and Boeder (1944), light from each point of an object is not reassembled in points in the image of the eye, but in caustic surfaces of complex form. The refracted pencil of light from a single luminous point is typically a star with long vertical and horizontal rays and short oblique rays. The lens is responsible for this effect, which is absent in aphakic subjects. Figure 2.4 demonstrates how, in the case of an image of an

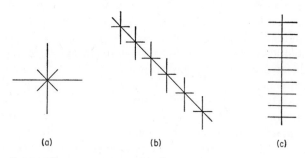

(a)   (b)   (c)

Figure 2.4 To illustrate Weymouth's theory of how the caustic-ray images from point sources cause differential contrast in the images of lines in different orientations. (a) Single point: typical caustic-ray pattern in the image from a point source; (b) Oblique line: all the major rays are outside the line and reduce contrast; (c) Vertical line: half the major rays outside the line and contrast not reduced so much as in (b)

oblique line on the retina, all the caustic rays lie outside the central part of the image of the line and thus reduce contrast more than is the case with a vertical or horizontal line, where only half the major rays lie outside the centre of the image. Weymouth's theory will thus account for meridional variations in acuity for lines, grids, and gratings. However, no figures have ever been presented to show what proportion of people see four-rayed patterns when looking at a point of light, nor what proportion of people seeing such patterns see them in a vertical–horizontal orientation. If most people do see such patterns in such an orientation, this in itself would require an explanation. The theory does not account for the finding that points of light are better resolved when on vertical or horizontal retinal meridians (Leibowitz, 1953; Leibowitz, Myers, and Grant, 1955a).

All these theoretical issues are somewhat premature, for no one has yet laid down an effective practical procedure for distinguishing between meridional and clinical astigmatism. Five procedures have been suggested and these will now be considered.

1. Weymouth pointed out that meridional effects do not show unless the test lines are very fine, whereas the effects of clinical astigmatism show on wide lines as well as fine. Weymouth implied that this is a basic difference, but all it necessarily means is that the meridional effect, if it exists, is small, whereas clinical astigmatism may be a small or a large effect; we still have the difficulty of distinguishing between meridional effects and small clinical effects.

2. The second suggested difference between the two effects is that clinical astigmatism can be diagnosed by both subjective and objective tests, whereas meridional astigmatism can only be diagnosed by subjective tests. But this may be only because objective tests are not as sensitive as subjective tests.

3. The third procedure is to define meridional astigmatism as the residual effect after clinical astigmatism has been fully corrected. But this assumes that clinical astigmatism can be fully corrected. Eastman (1958) questioned this assumption, and suggested that meridional astigmatism may be nothing other than residual, uncorrected clinical astigmatism. It also assumes that lenses do not correct for, nor modify, meridional astigmatism, and this assumption also may be incorrect.

4. If there are two types of astigmatism, the directions of their axes may not correspond. If this lack of correspondence could be detected, we would have a method for distinguishing between the two types of astigmatism. But such a method would depend on a perfect compensation for clinical astigmatism; for example, a lens which over-compensated for clinical astigmatism would cause an apparent shift in the direction of the astigmatic axis. However, if we could be sure of exactly correcting for clinical astigmatism, this test would be redundant.

5. The four tests which have been mentioned so far seem to be incapable of proving the existence of two basic types of astigmatism. It seems that the only reason for believing that there are two types is that clinical astigmatism usually has only one axis, whereas meridional astigmatism has two main axes. Weymouth's caustic-ray theory provides the most plausible explanation of this difference.

6. Finally we propose a new possible explanation of meridional astigmatism. It is well known that the optic axis and the visual axis are at an angle to each other, the so-called angle a. It is also a fact that, in any optical system,

points of light which come to a focus outside the optic axis of the system suffer an astigmatic distortion (see Hertzberger, 1963). This astigmatic effect has two main axes, one in the plane containing the ray path and the optic axis and the other at right angles to the first. This means that the angle α could account for meridional astigmatism if this angle is in a vertical or horizontal plane. A way of testing for astigmatism due to this effect would be to see whether it disappears when the visual target falls on the optic axis of the eye.

In section 7.2 evidence will be presented that the inclination of a line is most accurately judged when it is in either a vertical or horizontal orientation. Perhaps this phenomenon is related to meridional differences in acuity, and Taylor (1963) has argued in favour of this view.

2.66 The orientation of the observer

That visual thresholds are affected by body position as well as by stimulus position on the retina was first noted by McFarland, Holway, and Hurvich (1942). Charnwood (1950) claimed that visual acuity was higher in the seated position than in the supine position, although White and Jorve (1956) failed to confirm this finding. Pigg and Kama (1962) found that the four positions, standing upright, lying prone, lying supine, and standing inverted, gave a progressive loss of visual acuity. The loss of far acuity was greater than that of near acuity.

2.7 Visual anisotropy

Judgments of physical magnitudes vary from one part of the field of view to another. In other words psychophysical or subjective magnitudes are not homogeneously related to physical magnitudes for all positions and orientations of the distal stimulus relative to the observer. This lack of visual spatial homogeneity is known as visual anisotropy. A detailed account of anisotropy is beyond the scope of this book. The following is a brief account of the more important types.

2.71 Radial asymmetries of apparent length

It has been known since the last century that the apparent length of a line is affected by its radial position on the retina. Valentine (1912) and Ritter (1917) have reviewed the early literature. Ritter (1917), Shipley, Nann, and Penfield (1949) and Pollock and Chapanis (1952) found that the position of maximum apparent length of a line varied for different subjects but was commonly in the neighbourhood of the vertical position, on average at the 5 o'clock position, with the position of minimum apparent length at about the horizontal position. This overestimation of vertical relative to horizontal distances is the well-known vertical–horizontal illusion.

It is important in demonstrating this effect to avoid contamination from other illusions. For instance, the figure often used to illustrate the illusion is ⊥, but part of the effect here is due to the fact the horizontal line is bisected whereas the vertical line is not; bisected lines appear longer than unbisected lines (Finger and Spelt, 1947; Künnapas, 1955; Suto, 1960). An ⌊ or + shape should be used in which the vertical line is alternately standard and variable.

Four factors have been advanced to account for this illusion.

1. Gravity acts in a vertical direction and so a greater sense of effort is associated with this direction.

2. The field of view is oval-shaped especially when both eyes are open. A vertical line thus occupies a larger proportion of the total width of the field than does a horizontal line of equal length, and may accordingly be judged to be longer.

3. Eye movements occur less often in a vertical direction than in a horizontal direction.

4. Differential concentration of receptors over the retina.

The first, rather vague theory has not really been tested but it has been shown that the illusion is largely a function of the orientation of the test lines relative to the retina rather than to gravity, so that the name 'vertical–horizontal illusion' is a misnomer (Künnapas, 1958; Morinaga, Noguchi, and Ohishi, 1962). But the differential concentration of receptors which could explain the retinal association has yet to be demonstrated.

With regard to the influence of the oval shape of the field of view, Ritter (1917) found that varying this shape artificially had no effect on the illusion, although more recently Künnapas (1957) has shown that the vertical line is overestimated less when the limits of the field of view are eliminated by having the lines in dark surrounds. He also showed (1959) that the illusion may be reduced by introducing an artificial oval field with its long axis vertical, although the illusion never reversed in sign as it would have done if the shape of the field of view were the only factor operating.

The effects of eye movements on this illusion do not seem to have been systematically investigated. An illusion analogous to the visual vertical–horizontal illusion has been demonstrated in the tactile modality (Hatwell, 1960; Liddle and Foss, 1963) and in motor kinaesthesis (Reid, 1954).

Another radial asymmetry of judged length is the apparent difference of length between right and left of the fixation point. The usual procedure is for the subject to place a point mid-way between two other points in the frontal plane. This 'partition' experiment was first performed by Kundt (1863) using himself as the only subject. His two outer points were 100 mm apart in a plane 226 mm from the subject. Kundt found that he set the partitioning point on average to a position 50·33 mm from the left-hand point with left-eye viewing, and to 49·85 mm from the left-hand point with right-eye viewing. In other words the left side was underestimated with the left-eye and overestimated by the right eye. Münsterberg (1889) repeated the partition experiment, taking greater care to ensure that the head was fixed. His findings were the reverse of Kundt's, the right eye overestimated the right side and the left eye overestimated the left side. Fischer (1924) reported that his left eye had a symmetry discrepancy in the Kundt sense, and his right eye a discrepancy in the Münsterberg sense, i.e. overestimation of the right side throughout. Considering that each of these investigators used only himself as subject, the differences between their results only demonstrate that the symmetry discrepancy differs for different people and Brown (1955) found that it was not stable even for the same person. There seems to be no general agreement about which side tends to be overestimated with binocular viewing. Other early partition experiments are reviewed in Stevens and Ducasse (1912) and Wolfe (1923).

Brown (1953) conducted a partition experiment on six subjects who were asked to bisect a luminous white line 255 mm long at a viewing distance of 200 cm. Although he did not find any consistent difference between the left and right sides of each eye, his results showed that with the left eye a length on the left was relatively underestimated compared with the right eye, and with the right eye a length on the right was relatively underestimated compared with the left eye. In other words, apparent size was less to the right for the right eye than for the left eye. Brown explained his results in terms of the shape of the horopter, which is convex towards the subject at the viewing distance used. The reason for this convexity could be in the dioptrics of the eye or in the spatial distribution of receptors over the retina. For further details the reader is referred to Brown's paper.

2.72 Radial asymmetries of the apparent size of angles

Helmholtz (1962, vol. 3, p. 173) presented subjects with a pair of straight lines intersecting at right angles, one being vertical and the other horizontal. Most of the subjects judged the upper right and lower left angles as obtuse when using the right eye, but judged these angles as acute when using the left eye. Helmholtz went on to say that the amount of error made in estimating a right angle depends on the inclination of the sides of the angle to the retinal horizon. One leg of the right angle had to be 18° counterclockwise from the vertical for the right eye or 18° clockwise for the left eye in order for the angle to be judged a right angle. The apparent distortion of the right angle was greatest when the legs were at 45° to the vertical and horizontal. He also cited a study by Volkmann (1864) in which a line was repeatedly adjusted first to the vertical, then to the horizontal. The means for the two sets of adjustments made an angle of 91·1° for the left eye and 90·6° for the right eye.

Biehler (1896) also adjusted a line to appear normal to a second line which was set at various inclinations to the vertical. Both constant and variable errors tended to be lowest near the vertical and horizontal.

In recent times Onley and Volkman (1958) working at Holyoke studied the effect of angular position on the judgment of right angles. They used the three visual patterns of figure 2.5.

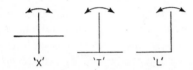

Figure 2.5 Patterns used by Onley and Volkman to study the effect of angular position on judgments of right angles

One arm in each pattern was variable; the subject had to set it so that it was at right angles to the other line in the pattern. Four subjects were used for each stimulus pattern. Each pattern was presented in 80 positions (except for the '+' pattern which has only 40 distinguishable positions).

The mean constant errors were of the order of 1° which, the authors pointed out, is better than for adjustments of single lines to a given inclination (Reese, 1953). It is, however, not less than the mean error obtained by other workers for adjustments of lines to the horizontal and vertical (see section 7.2). Individuals were consistent in the direction of their constant errors at all angles. The variability of the judgments increased rapidly as a function of angular deviation from the vertical and horizontal axes of space, but was somewhat less again at the 45° positions. Variability was least for the '+' pattern, next best for the 'T' pattern and worst for the 'L' pattern, except at the horizontal and vertical positions where they all gave similar, low variability.

Helmholtz reported (1962, vol. 3, p. 175) that when he observed a 30° angle with one of its sides horizontal and drew a third line through the same vertex in an attempt to make an adjacent angle of equal size, the new angle was more than 34°, regardless of which eye was used. For Helmholtz horizontally oriented angles thus appeared to be larger than others, a conclusion supported by his judgment that the vertical angle of the equilateral triangle was smaller than the base angles.

Weene (1962), using a technique adapted from Békésy, had his subjects bisect a right angle as it was rotated through 360°. For one 'typical' subject zero deviations of the adjusted from the true bisector occurred close to the vertical and horizontal, at 105°, 128–187°, 255°, and 349°, whereas peak deviations of up to 10° occurred at 57°, 115°, 225° and 295°. The direction of the deviations indicated that angles closer to the horizontal were judged larger than those closer to the vertical. Weene suggested that this results from a sort of permanent satiation gradient produced by a predominance of horizontal contour in the everyday environment.

Patients with damage to the visual areas in the occipital lobes often complain that shapes appear distorted when in that part of the field of view corresponding to the damaged visual area. These distortions are known as metamorphopsia and take a variety of forms. Visual space may be severely asymmetrical as revealed by the partition experiment (Holmes, 1919); objects may appear to be enlarged (macropsia) or reduced in size (micropsia); solid objects may appear flat; shapes may appear elongated, compressed, or skewed. Similar symptoms may also arise through damage to the parietal or temporal lobes (Brain, 1941b; Bender and Teuber, 1947, 1948, 1949).

3

Eye movements and visual direction

3.1 The extraocular muscles

The extraocular or extrinsic eye muscles control the position of each eye in its socket. They may be grouped into three pairs, the medial and lateral recti, the superior and inferior recti, and the superior and inferior obliques. Each pair of muscles forms an antagonistic pair. Their positions in relation to the orbit are shown in figure 3.1. All the muscles except the inferior oblique are inserted into the circular tendon of Zinn at the apex of the orbit. The superior oblique passes over a pulley-like structure, the trochlea, which deflects its direction of action on the eye. The inferior oblique is inserted in the medial wall of the orbit.

At first glance it would appear that the vertical recti elevate and depress the eye, the horizontal recti adduct and abduct it, and the obliques rotate it about the visual axis. But these statements are approximately true only for small movements from the eye's straight-ahead or primary position (see figure 3.2). Figure 3.3 demonstrates that when the eye moves far from the

H.S.O.—4

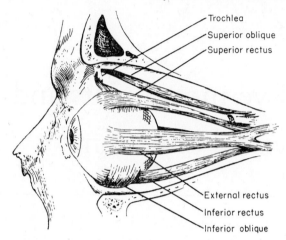

Figure 3.1 Origins and insertions of the extraocular muscles. [From Cogan, D. G., 1956. *Neurology of the Ocular Muscles.* Courtesy of Charles C. Thomas, Publisher, Springfield, Ill.]

primary position there is a change in the planes in which the pairs of muscles move the eye relative to the head.

Pairs of muscles, one in each eye, which act together in carrying out conjugate movements, are known as yoke muscles or synergists. It is obvious

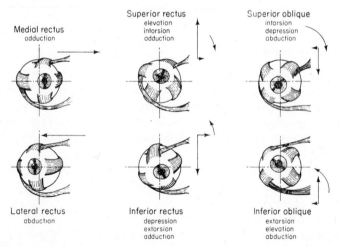

Figure 3.2 Diagrams illustrating the action of the three pairs of antagonistic eye muscles. [From Adler, F. E., 1965. *Physiology of the Eye*, 4th ed. The C. V. Mosby Company]

that synergists are not geometrically corresponding or homologous in the two eyes. Thus, the lateral rectus of the left eye and the medial rectus of the right eye are involved in looking to the left.

The extraocular muscles are innervated by the third, fourth, and sixth cranial nerves. The nuclei from which these nerves arise are in the upper brain stem, although their detailed disposition is not known. There are important pathways between these nuclei and the cerebellum, vestibular apparatus, and superior colliculi; the functional significance of these connections will become apparent in what follows.

There are two main cortical areas concerned with eye movements: the occipital and preoccipital areas on the one hand, and the *frontal eye fields* in

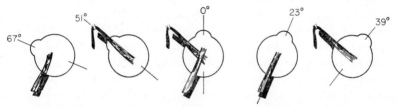

Figure 3.3 Diagrams illustrating the positions and actions of the vertical recti and oblique muscles in different positions of gaze of the right eye. [From Cogan, D. C., 1956. *Neurology of the Ocular Muscles.* Courtesy of Charles C. Thomas, Publisher, Springfield, Ill.]

the frontal lobes on the other. These two areas are linked by intracortical tracts. Consistent patterns of eye movements have been observed when loci within these cortical areas have been electrically stimulated (Bender, 1964).

The extraocular muscles are finer than any other voluntary muscles, and they contain an unusually high ratio of motor nerve fibres to muscle fibres. Certainly the movements which these muscles control are the fastest, most accurate, and most complex in the body.

3.2 The geometry of eye movements

Movements of the eyes considered separately are known as *ductions*. The various ductions are named and illustrated in figure 3.2. Normally the eyes work as a pair: a movement of one is accompanied by a movement of the other. This fact is known as *Hering's law of equal innervations*; its significance will be discussed later. Movements of the eyes in the same direction are known as *versions or conjugate movements*. Movements in opposite directions are known as *vergences or disjunctive movements*.

The centre of rotation of the eye is not fixed, either with reference to the eye itself, or with reference to the orbit (Park and Park, 1933). In other words, the eye translates a little as it rotates in its orbit. However, for most purposes the eye is assumed to rotate about a fixed centre 13·5 mm behind the cornea.

An eye has no fixed axes of rotation. Therefore, in order to specify the movements of an eye geometrically, any one of several axis systems may be adopted. The choice is arbitrary; it is not a question of which is, or is not, correct. However, for any particular purpose one axis system may have practical advantages. In the *Helmholtz axis system* the horizontal axis is assumed to be fixed to the skull, and the vertical axis is assumed to rotate gimbal-fashion with the horizontal axis. The position of a short reference line on the eye is expressed in terms of elevation (λ) and azimuth (μ). In the *Fick system* it is the vertical axis which is fixed, and the position of a short reference line is expressed in terms of latitude (θ) and longitude (φ). The Fick system is simply the Helmholtz system turned to the side through 90°. The *polar-coordinate or perimeter system* expresses movements of the eye in terms of the angles of eccentricity (π) and meridional direction (K) of a point at the centre of the pupil, in relation to a spherical scale fixed with reference to the head and having its zero point on the visual axis of the eye when the latter is pointing straight ahead. This system is formed by simply turning the fixed axis of either of the other two systems through 90° to the front and for simplicity will be ignored in what follows. The relationship between the Fick and Helmholtz systems is shown in figures 3.4, 3.5. and 3.6. In each system rotation

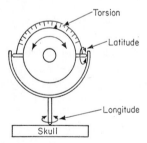 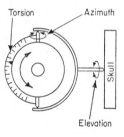

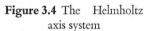

Figure 3.4 The Helmholtz axis system

Figure 3.5 The Fick axis system

of the eye about the visual axis is known as *torsion*, although the baseline from which the torsion angle is measured varies according to the system used.

When the eye is gazing straight forward it is said to be in the *primary position*, when it is straight up or down, or to left or right, it is said to be in a *secondary position*, and when it moves in an oblique direction, it is said to be in a *tertiary position*.

Listing proposed that any movement of the eye could be regarded as having occurred about a single axis in the mid-vertical or equatorial plane (Listing's plane) of the eye (plane $HD'D$ in figure 3.7). For elevations and depressions of the eye this axis is the horizontal axis, for lateral movements it is the vertical axis, and for oblique movements the axis is between the horizontal and vertical axes. In other words, the axis of rotation in Listing's

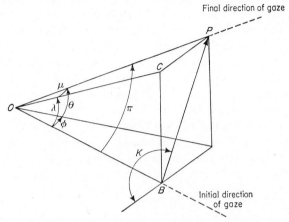

Figure 3.6 The relationships between elevation (λ) and azimuth (μ), latitude (θ) and longitude (φ), and eccentricity (π) and meridional direction (K)

plane is at right angles to the plane containing the initial position and the final position of the visual axis (plane OPB in figure 3.7). Only one axis is assumed to exist in this system; it always lies in Listing's plane, but has no fixed position within that plane. The extent of such a movement is given by the angular separation of the initial and final positions of the centre of the pupil (i.e. the angle of eccentricity π in the case of movements from the primary position); its direction is given by the angle which the meridian joining these two positions makes with an objectively vertical or horizontal meridian ($\delta 1$ or K in figure 3.7).

It follows that if Listing's system is to provide a comprehensive description of an eye movement, then torsional rotations of the eye about the visual axis, with reference to the meridian along which the visual axis travels, must be assumed not to occur. Helmholtz called this 'Listing's law'. If an initially horizontal, short reference line is substituted for the point marker then this assumption may be tested: $\delta 2$ should always equal $\delta 1$. The assumption appears to be correct for the case of versions including oblique versions (Quereau, 1954). But it is only for such conjugate eye movements that Listing's law holds; when the angle of convergence between the eyes changes, torsion in Listing's sense, does occur (Allen, 1954.)

If, on the other hand, movements of an eye are referred to either the Helmholtz or the Fick axis systems, the positions which a line marker assumes during oblique version movements can only be accounted for by assuming that torsion has occurred. But this merely means that torsion has been redefined. Torsion on the Listing system is defined in terms of the angle $\delta 2$ of figure 3.7, that is, the angle which a horizontal marker makes with the meridian (BH) along which the line of sight moves. This remains constant according to Listing's law. Torsion on Helmholtz's system is the angle which the marker makes with the plane of regard $(D'PD)$, that is, angle ρ. In Fick's system torsion is the complement of angle ρ. These angles (ρ in figure 3.7, or its complement) are a function of the angle $\delta 1$ and the angle of eccentricity (π) and are not constant according to Listing's law. Clearly, also, these systems can encompass torsion which occurs without any change in the position of the visual axis, whereas Listing's system cannot.

In general, then, a one-axis system, such as Listing's, can encompass only two types of eye movement; whether torsion is obtained in a given situation depends on the meridian with respect to which torsion is defined, and on the particular axes used in the system (see table 3.1).

Table 3.1 Types of eye torsion and their inducing conditions

Name	Inducing conditions	Listing's law
Oblique gaze torsion	Function of meridian of movement and eccentricity	Holds
Countertorsion	Head tilt	Does not hold
Optokinetic torsion	Visual patterns rotating in frontal plane	Does not hold
Cyclofusional torsion	Torsional disparity	Does not hold
Cyclophoric torsion	Release from cyclofusion	Does not hold
Convergence torsion	Convergence of lines of sight	Does not hold
Spontaneous fluctuations of torsion	Unknown	Does not hold

Donder's law originally stated that the torsional position of the eye depends only on the direction of gaze. Donders revised his law when he became persuaded by his assistants that torsional eye movements occur when the head tilts (see section 3.42). Donder's law is now taken to mean that the torsional position of the eye in whichever system it is defined is independent of the manner in which the eye is brought to a particular position.

Torsion, as defined in any of the systems mentioned, does occur in many

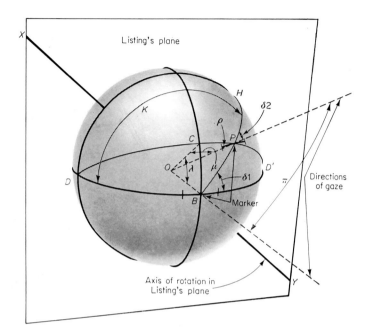

Figure 3.7 Diagrammatic representation of the geometry of eye movements. The direction of gaze is assumed to have moved from the primary position OB to an oblique position OP through an angle of eccentricity, π. The movement has occurred along the meridian BH which is at an angle K to the original horizontal meridian DBD'; which is equivalent to it having occurred about axis XY in the equatorial frontal plane (Listing's plane). The horizontal marker (between the small vertical bars) initially makes an angle $\delta 1$ with the meridian along which the visual axis moves and, according to Listing's law, this angle remains constant ($\delta 1 = \delta 2$). The eye can also be regarded as having moved on Helmholtz's axes, through an angle of elevation, λ, and an angle of azimith, μ. For angle $\delta 2$ to remain equal to $\delta 1$, the eye (and marker) must tort through angle ρ relative to the final plane of regard DCD'

circumstances. These circumstances are listed in table 3.1. Some of these types of torsion will be discussed at various places in this section.

For further details of the geometry of eye movements see Helmholtz (1962, vol. 3, p. 37), Lancaster (1943), and Fry (1945, 1947a, 1947b).

3.3 The positional stability of the eye

When a person fixates a small visual target, his eyes show low amplitude involuntary movements, sometimes referred to as physiological nystagmus. They are measured by photographing a beam of light reflected off a mirror attached to a contact lens (Ratliff and Riggs, 1950). Tremor movements of the eye with an amplitude less than one minute of arc, and frequencies of between 30 and 80 c/s occur all the time. Superimposed on this tremor are slow drifts of up to 5 minutes of arc, and rapid flicks or saccades which tend to restore the visual axis to the fixation point. These corrective saccades are in part visually determined, for the amplitude of the slow drift is increased when no fixation point is in view (Nachmias, 1959, 1961).

Special devices have been made which eliminate the motions of the retinal image induced by these eye movements (Ditchburn and Fender, 1955; Riggs, Ratliff, Cornsweet, and Cornsweet, 1953; Ditchburn, 1963). Light from the visual target is reflected off a mirror mounted in the frontal plane on a contact lens. The light is then reflected into the pupil so that as the eye moves one way, the beam reflected back into the pupil moves in the opposite direction through the same angle. The effects of the movements of the eye are thus cancelled. Torsional movements are not cancelled, but if circular, radially featureless targets, concentric with the fixation point, are used, the retinal image is not affected by torsional movements. Visual acuity is improved when retinal-image movements greater than 20 seconds of arc are not allowed (Riggs, Ratliff, Cornsweet, and Cornsweet, 1953; Ditchburn, 1955). Thus, as far as acuity is concerned physiological nystagmus is a hindrance. However, a stabilized retinal image soon fades from view due to the rapid adaptation of the receptors to the constant conditions of stimulation (Ditchburn and Ginsberg, 1952). In the earlier reports the image was noticed to return to view at intervals, especially after a rapid flick movement of the eye. Recently Barlow (1963) has suggested that this return of vision is due to incomplete stabilization resulting from slippage of the contact lens. When this is sucked on to the eye in the way suggested by Yarbus (1957) the fading may be permanent. The blood vessels overlaying the retina are a perfectly stabilized image, and these never become visible unless special methods of viewing are adopted.

The physiological tremor has been thought of as an evolved mechanism serving to compensate for loss of vision by adaptation. However, it seems unlikely that a living eye could have evolved to be more stable than it actually is. Evolution has probably been concerned to reduce eye tremor as far as possible rather than to generate it. It is more likely that other features of the visual system, such as the mean diameter of the receptors, the rate of adaptation, and the optical resolving power, have evolved to suit a degree of tremor which could not be reduced beyond a certain minimum.

3.4 Types of eye movement

3.41 Introduction

The conditions under which the eyes move may be classified as shown in table 3.2.

Table 3.2 A functional classification of eye movements

General type	Specific type
Maintaining constant position of retinal image	Utricular and proprioceptive reflexes Vestibular nystagmus—slow phase Optokinetic nystagmus—slow phase Foveal pursuit movements (in foveate eye only)
Restoring central position of eyes	Centring movement (nystagmic quick phase)
Changes of fixation (foveate eyes only)	Reflex and voluntary changes of fixation
Movements serving stereopsis	Versions and vergences (only in eyes with corresponding projections)

Most eye-movement reflexes are designed to maintain the retinal image in the same position on the retina. This is the basic task of the eye muscles, and in lower animals, they probably serve no other function (Walls, 1962). Utricular eye-movement reflexes and nystagmus are the principal image-stabilizing eye movements.

Nystagmus is any rhythmic movement of the eyes. Such movements can occur in a vertical, horizontal, or oblique direction, or in the frontal plane (torsional nystagmus). Normal nystagmus is induced by a variety of conditions the most common of which are stimulation of the vestibular apparatus and movements of the visual field. These are known as vestibular and opto-kinetic nystagmus respectively. Vestibular nystagmus is discussed in section 5.3.

Clinical nystagmus shows itself as an involuntary and persistent to-and-fro movement of the eyes. Many neurological conditions may give rise to this symptom; for further details see Cogan (1956).

If the animal is to decode the information received by the retina, the image must be kept still for some time in spite of movements of the animal's head and movements of the visual target. Utricular and neck-muscle reflex eye movements and the slow phase of vestibular nystagmus serve to compensate for head movements. The slow phase of optokinetic nystagmus compensates for movements of the retinal image. All these compensatory reflex eye movements are involuntary and very primitive. They occur even in animals whose eyes have no fovea. *Foveal pursuit movements* may occur in response to movements of a small part of the field of view. They occur only in foveate eyes and serve to maintain the object which is fixated on the area of clearest vision. If only one object in the field of view moves, that object tends to be fixated and pursued. If more than one object moves, factors of vividness, size, speed, etc., determine which is pursued.

The second type of eye movements (see table 3.2) is the *eye-centring reflex* which serves to return the eyes to central gaze after they have deviated to a certain extent as a consequence of vestibular or visual pursuit reflexes.

The third type of eye movements occurs only in animals with foveate eyes. It includes the reflex and voluntary changes of fixation. The term *saccade* refers to any quick movement of the eyes, whatever the stimulus conditions.

The final class of eye movements includes those which involve the simultaneous movement of both eyes. These are the conjugate versions and disjunctive vergences. It was the last type to evolve, and occurs only in those animals with stereoscopic vision, and serves to keep similar images on corresponding parts of each retina, i.e. parts which project to equivalent points in the visual cortex. Hemidecussation of the optic nerve fibres is a prerequisite for the development of projection correspondence, although not all animals which have incomplete decussation have stereoscopic vision (Walls, 1962). Versions and vergences will not be discussed further, as they are not relevant to the subject of this book. The other types of eye movements will now be discussed in more detail.

3.42 Utricular eye-movement reflexes

When the head is inclined backwards or forwards the eyes tend to remain horizontal; similarly when the head is tilted to one side the normally vertical meridian of the eye tends to remain vertical. The former reflex is known as the *doll eye movement* and is present in man only in the first few days after birth (Peiper, 1963, p. 155). The latter reflex is known as *countertorsion* and is the only clearly defined, entirely involuntary, utricular reflex in man. Stimuli for both the reflexes probably arise from the canals as well as from the utricles and neck muscles, although the residual effect present when the head is held in the inclined or tilted position can be due only to stimuli arising in the utricles and neck muscles.

Countertorsion is defined as a reflex eye torsion that accompanies a sideways tilt of the head. It has sometimes been called compensatory eye torsion, or 'counterrolling'. This latter term is a translation of the German *Augenrollung* but in English the word 'rolling' refers to the rotation of a circle or sphere over a surface, which is not the idea being conveyed here. The term should be dropped in favour of 'countertorsion'. John Hunter (1786) was the first to describe countertorsion. He reported that when he tilted his head in front of a mirror he could see his eye rotate about its optic axis in a direction opposite to the direction of the head tilt. This occurred more strongly as the head was tilted up to a certain angle, at which point the eye rotated back again.

Several investigators could not confirm the existence of countertorsion (Ritterich, 1843; Ruetes, 1846; Donders, 1846; Aub and Knapp, 1870; Contejean and Delmas, 1894) while several others (Tourtual, 1840; Burow, 1841; Krause, 1843; Javal, 1865; Skrebitzky, 1871; Woinow, 1871; Breuer, 1874) were able to observe it. Hueck (1838) and Graefe (1854) observed countertorsion in animals but denied that it was present in humans.

Donders, who had previously (1870) denied the existence of countertorsion, became convinced that it was a fact (1875) when Mulder (1874) and other researchers working in Donders's laboratory in Holland developed more refined methods of observation. Wide individual differences in the extent of the effect, combined with inadequate observations, probably accounted for the earlier conflict of opinion.

Nagel (1896) reviewed the earlier literature and the methods available at that time for recording eye torsion. He presented positive evidence for countertorsion from observation on both human and animal subjects.

In the present century, landmarks have been the quantitative studies of Kompanejetz (1928), Fischer (1930 a and b), and Walton (1948). All authorities now seem to be agreed that countertorsion does take place (Duke-Elder, 1939; Lancaster, 1943; Emsley, 1946).

Several of the standard methods of recording eye movements, such as the corneal reflex method and electro-oculography, cannot be applied to eye torsion. Special methods have been devised (see Howard and Evans, 1963 for a review). One method is to impose an after-image of a line of light on the retina and ask the subject to align an external thread with the after-image before and after a change in the torsional position of the eye has occurred (McCord, 1953). The blind spot boundary and the axis of astigmatism have been used in lieu of an after-image by some investigators (Walton, 1948; Quereau, 1955). These are all subjective procedures, that is, they depend upon the subject's ability to align an external thread with some feature attached to his eye. These methods cannot be used to record rapid fluctuations of torsion and it is not possible to get an accurate estimate of their validity.

Several objective procedures have been proposed which overcome the disadvantages of the subjective methods. Fender (1955) and Davies and Merton (1958) recorded torsion by the movements of a beam of light reflected from a small mirror mounted in the sagittal plane of the eye, on a contact lens. Various photographic procedures have been proposed. The problem is to find suitable features on the eyeball and head to serve as reference markers. Brecher (1934) and Free and Jones (1960) used iris marks but these are very indistinct and, because of their proximity to the axis of rotation, provide an inconveniently short reference line. Graybiel and Woellner (1958) sewed a black silk suture on to the conjunctiva, apparently not realizing that the conjunctiva is not attached rigidly to the eyeball. Howard and Evans (1963) used for eyeball marker, the fine episcleral blood vessels well out in the corner of the eye and, as head marker, lines on a plate mounted on a bite.

The results of the principal investigators are set out in table 3.3. Walton (1948) is the only one to have used a considerable number of subjects, but he obtained figures only for head tilts of 15° and 30°. He employed an objective as well as a subjective method for recording torsion but, as the results from the two agreed closely, the combined means are entered in the table. His figures are much higher than those of the other investigators.

Woellner and Graybiel (1958) relied on conjunctival markers in their method and, as the conjunctiva is known not to be attached to the eyeball, it is not surprising that they recorded less countertorsion than the others.

It is clear that all the investigators observed countertorsion in the direction opposite to the head tilt for all angles of head tilt. All the results show that the ratio of eye torsion to head tilt decreases as the angle of head tilt increases. Mulder and Nagel who both used an after-image method show very good agreement; they both recorded maximum torsion at about 70° of head tilt, and a subsequent levelling-off. Fischer got his maximum effect at 60° (he did not test at 70°) but recorded a falling-off in the effect at larger angles. Schöne's data are the most complete and are shown graphically in figure 3.8.

Thus there is agreement on the main point; the differences between the

Table 3.3 The extent of countertorsion, in degrees, obtained by various investigators for increasing amounts of head tilt

Investigator	Degrees of head tilt												
	0 to 10	11 to 20	21 to 30	31 to 40	41 to 50	51 to 60	61 to 70	71 to 80	81 to 90	91 to 100	101 to 120	121 to 160	161 to 180
Skrebitzky (1871) self	—	2·0	2·6	4·2	5·5	6·8	7·7	—	—	—	—	—	—
Mulder (1874) self	—	2·4	4·0	5·1	5·8	6·2	6·1	6·6	6·5	6·6	—	—	—
Nagel (1896) self	1·3	3·8	5·2	5·4	6·3	6·7	6·8	8·0	8·1	8·6	—	—	—
Fischer (1930a) self clockwise	—	—	2·9	—	—	3·9	—	—	2·9	—	0·4	0·75	2·5
Fischer (1930a) self anticlockwise	—	—	6·2	—	—	6·3	—	—	5·9	—	4·7	3·5	2·0
Walton (1948) 31Ss	—	5·0	9·8	—	—	—	—	—	—	—	—	—	—
Woellner and Graybiel (1958) 5Ss	—	—	2·8	—	3·2	—	4·2	—	—	—	—	—	—
Schöne (1962)	2·3	3·8	4·8	—	—	6·0	—	—	5·9	—	5·7	2·9	0·75

various investigators probably represent mainly individual differences in the effect since most of them studied only their own eyes. Several investigators noted a considerable variation in the readings from the same observer under similar conditions. Fischer reported an average deviation of about one degree for himself. Whether this is variation due to the uncertainty of the method or whether it represents spontaneous torsion is difficult to say. However, Howard and Templeton (1964b) have also demonstrated a variation in torsion of about one degree, and in this case errors of measurement were known to be only of the order of 0·1° (Howard and Evans, 1963). Such a large 'spontaneous' eye torsion must surely be of great significance in vision but no one has suggested what this significance can be. Howard and Templeton have

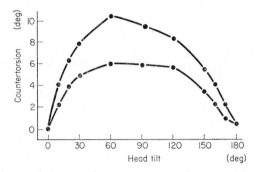

Figure 3.8 Countertorsion as a function of head tilt under 1·0-*g* (lower curve) and under 2·0-*g* (upper curve). [From Schöne, 1962]

suggested that the spontaneous torsion arises when the eye is in the dark or semi-dark, as it usually is when torsion is being measured. When a full field of visual objects was introduced the amount of 'spontaneous' torsional variation was found to be about half what it had been when only a vertical line of light was visible.

Fischer (1930a) found that the countertorsion was different for his two eyes, and that it depended on the direction from which the tilt of the body was achieved (see table 3.3). Nagel (1896) and Miller (1962) were not able to detect any 'hysteresis' effect of this kind.

Sideways turnings about the vertical axis of the head and tilting in the sagittal plane have been shown not to produce countertorsion (Mulder, 1874).

Using the after-image method Mulder (1874) observed a temporary countertorsion of the eyes in excess of the normal amount, when the head was tilted rapidly. This temporary torsion soon subsided to the normal amount associated with the particular angle in which the head had come to rest.

Mulder also reported that when he bent his head forward until his face was horizontal, a turning of the head in the horizontal plane produced a large temporary countertorsion which left no permanent residue when the head was stopped, thus showing that the stimulus for temporary torsion may be present when the stimulus for permanent torsion is not. This large temporary countertorsion was also noticed by Merton (1956, 1958), and Davies and Merton (1958) when they looked at the subject's eye through a microscope. Like Mulder (1897) they noticed only the temporary torsion if the subject was rotated about a gravitationally vertical axis when lying on his back. They concluded that the semicircular canals are responsible for the temporary torsion and the otoliths for the residual torsion.

The decay of initial rapid countertorsion took place in jerks. Nystagmic-type jerks were also noticed by Mulder while the head was turned slowly. Two, six, or eight such jerks occurred while the head was tilted through 45°. These intermittent nystagmic movements whereby the eyes tended to catch up with the head were not present when the subject fixated something which rotated with the head. This tendency to intermittent eye movements is typical of slow voluntary sweeps of the eye in a lateral direction, and here too the effect disappears when the subject's gaze follows a moving stimulus. Davies and Merton (1958) also noticed the nystagmic nature of countertorsion.

It is probable that the temporary countertorsion and nystagmic movements help to maintain good visual acuity as the head moves. The nystagmic movements are probably partly of vestibular origin, just as they are in the case of ordinary rotational nystagmus. However, purely optically driven torsional nystagmus also occurs (see sections 3.43 and 8.5).

Mulder (1874) adapted the after-image method of measuring torsion so that he could find out whether countertorsion persists when the head is maintained for some time in the tilted position. The head was put at an angle of 86° to the right, and an after-image of a horizontal line formed, either immediately or at some later time. The head was then returned to the vertical. If the eye had had no torsion when the after-image was formed, then the latter would have been inclined 4° to the right (90°–86°) after the head was straightened. The extent to which it deviated from this position was a measure of the countertorsion which had persisted for the given duration of head tilt. Mulder found that his countertorsion had decreased from 6° to 5° after forty-five minutes, and a second subject had his torsion reduced by 2° during this time. Fischer (1930a) used a similar method and found that countertorsion was not substantially altered after five minutes of maintained head tilt.

Kompanejetz (1924) suggested that mechanical intertia resulting from the fact that the eye's centre of gravity is below its centre of rotation is a contributory cause of countertorsion. But clearly the chief mechanisms involved must be neuromuscular. Nagel (1896) observed considerable countertorsion in fish, frogs, and rabbits. When both labyrinths were removed from each of these animals the countertorsion ceased to occur, a result confirmed by Kompanejetz (1925) on deaf mutes. Nagel did not know which part of the labyrinth was responsible for initiating torsion, but he concluded that an inertial rather than a gravity mechanism must be responsible for the countertorsion produced by tilting the head when lying on the back.

Kompanejetz (1928) found more torsion when the head was tilted to the right than to the left and from this fact, together with his assumption, based on some evidence by Bárány that the right otolith dominates the left, he concluded that the countertorsion of the eyes to the left when the head is tilted to the right depends on the right otolith.

The results of studies by Woellner and Graybiel (1958, 1959), also stress the importance of the otolith organs for countertorsion. They compared the amount of countertorsion produced by tilting a subject with the amount produced by displacing the direction of force acting on the body to an equivalent angle by spinning the subject in a centrifuge. The torsion was found to be a function of the sine of the angle of body tilt or, in the centrifuge, of the magnitude of the centrifugal force i.e. in both cases a function of the force acting at right angles to the body axis. Thus the torsion was greater in the centrifuge, for there the laterally acting component of force is greater than for the equivalent degree of body tilt. Schöne (1962) also found that increased g enhances countertorsion and concluded from the shape of the curves relating countertorsion to body tilt at different g strengths, that countertorsion is dependent on the shearing force in the utricle. These views accord with modern physiological evidence about the functioning of the utricles (see section 5.14).

Further indirect support for the view that the utricles are mainly responsible for countertorsion comes from an observation by King and Wade (1961). They noted that in zero-g conditions pigeons do not show the usual reflex head countertorsion when turned about the longitudinal body axis. Now that zero-g conditions for human subjects are easy to obtain, human countertorsion and the Aubert and Müller phenomena ought to be measured under these conditions.

3.43 Optokinetic nystagmus

When a series of objects are moved in one direction across the field of view there results an involuntary, conjugate, rhythmical movement of the eyes. Slow movements in pursuit of the moving stimuli alternate with quick return jerks. These alternating movements are known respectively as the slow and quick phase of optic or optokinetic nystagmus (OKN). It may easily be observed in a person who is looking at the passing scene out of the window of a moving train. Helmholtz (1962, vol. III, p. 247), who was apparently the first to describe it, noticed it under these circumstances, and Bárány (1908) called it *Eisenbahn* (railway) nystagmus. It is one of the most basic and phylogenetically primitive orienting responses. It occurs in mammalian and many submammalian species. Functionally it can be understood as an attempt to keep a stable image on the retina for as long as possible during movements of the whole field of view (Bárány, 1921, 1922).

OKN is most obviously elicited in a horizontal direction. It has been claimed that it is more readily elicited by left to right motion than vice versa (Roelofs and van der Bend, 1930), although the frequency varies only slightly with varying direction of rotation (Mackensen, 1954). A frequency difference of more than one oscillation per second is considered pathological and is known as directional preponderance (Cords and Nolzen, 1928). Vertically moving stimuli also elicit OKN (Walsh, 1957, pp. 266–268; Smith, 1962). Vertical responses are, if anything, more readily elicited by targets moving downwards (Stiefel and Smith, 1962). According to Walsh vertical OKN is not so well sustained as horizontal OKN. It is less well known that OKN can occur as a torsional movement of the eyes in response to stimuli rotating in the frontal plane (Noji, 1929; Brecher, 1934; Howard and Templeton, 1964b).

Three main procedures have been used to record the nystagmic eye movements: mechanical, photographic, and electrical. Ohm (1925, 1927b, 1928) used the mechanical system first proposed by Rählmann (1878), in which a lever is attached to the eyelid or rests directly on the cornea. Cords (1926a) criticized this method on the grounds that it introduces artefacts due to the intertia of the moving parts (but see Ohm, 1927a).

There are various photographic procedures. Direct ciné photography has been used on newborn infants by McGinnis (1930). The standard corneal reflection method has often been used, and also the more recent photoelectric method which makes use of the differential reflection of cornea and sclera (Pfaltz and Richter, 1956; Rashbass, 1960). It is not easy in using photographic methods to avoid introducing extraneous visual stimuli. Dodge (1921) used a system in which a concave mirror is rested lightly against the closed lid of one eye, over the apex of the cornea. The mirror is displaced as the cornea moves beneath it. A beam of light is reflected from the mirror towards a moving film. The other open eye is stimulated by the moving pattern. The method is thus limited to monocular viewing, and relies on the conjugate nature of OKN. The method was used by Dodge and Fox (1928) and Fox and Dodge (1929) to study variations in OKN due to blinks, pulse, head movements, and fatigue, as well as clinical conditions.

Contemporary studies of nystagmus usually involve a method which has come to be called electronystagmography. The eyeball carries a corneoretinal potential of a fraction of a millivolt (Mowrer, Ruch, and Miller, 1935). Because the eyeball is an electric dipole, movements of the eye are reflected in changes in potential recorded from the orbit, although it is still not clear whether these action potentials evoked by eye movements are solely corneo-retinal in origin (Pasik, Pasik, and Bender, 1959). This method introduces no extraneous visual stimuli, allows free movements of the head, and gives a record of the amplitude, speed, and frequency of nystagmus in the vertical and horizontal directions simultaneously. There is a linear relationship between eye movements up to 15° and periorbitally recorded potential changes (Jung, 1953, Henriksson, 1955b; Law and DeValois, 1958).

The usual stimulus used in the clinic or laboratory is a pattern of complex shapes or simple black and white stripes moving across the subject's visual field. The subject may be placed at the centre of a hollow vertical cylinder which rotates around him, and the inside of which is covered with vertical stripes. It is important that the moving pattern fills the visual field or, if it does not, that no inhomogeneities are present in the stationary parts of the field, upon which the subject can anchor his gaze. Ohm (1927b) has shown that the area of moving pattern need subtend an angle of only 2·1°, although according to Roelofs and van der Bend (1930) larger fields are more effective in proportion to their size. Fine lines near the limit of acuity (Smith, 1937), or a single moving object (Ter Braak, 1936), may elicit OKN.

It has been claimed that OKN may be induced by stimulation of the periphery of the retina (Fox and Holmes, 1926; Dodge and Fox, 1928; Ohm, 1931a). However, Kestenbaum (1947) claimed that peripheral stimulation does not elicit OKN if there is a scotoma involving the entire macula.

Cogan and Loeb (1949) have claimed that it is impossible to inhibit OKN, although Blomberg (1960) found that some of his subjects could inhibit it. Mackensen (1953) reported that accommodating out of the plane of the stimulus reduced the amplitude of OKN. It is not difficult to inhibit OKN by fixating and focusing the attention on a stationary object in the field of view.

OKN is apparently influenced by hypnotic suggestion. Erickson (1962) has reported that when subjects in a trance were instructed to develop hypnotic blindness, there was a slow diminution and eventual total disappearance of OKN. Two normal subjects under hypnosis were told they were on a train and were asked to 'direct their attention' to the fence posts, trees, etc., along the track. Both subjects showed OKN, but after a while one of them showed a cessation of the nystagmus; when asked about this he explained that the train had stopped at a station.

Torsional nystagmus is almost certainly beyond voluntary control, for no torsional eye movements have been found to be under voluntary control. It would be interesting to discover whether hypnosis could be used to induce torsional nystagmus in the absence of a moving stimulus or to inhibit it when a stimulus is present.

Not only is it difficult or impossible to inhibit OKN, but it is also impossible to move the eyes in this fashion in the absence of a steadily moving stimulus (Khomskoya, 1962). The quick phase may be imitated *in vacuo* but if a person attempts to move his eyes slowly and smoothly in one direction without the aid of a moving target, the result is a series of saccadic jerks.

The latency of the slow phase of OKN is about 0·2 sec (Lebensohn, 1931; Dodge, Travis, and Fox, 1930; Westheimer, 1954b).

The amplitude and speed of the slow phase have been found to increase when the speed of the moving stimulus is increased up to a certain value, above which the amplitude and speed fall off (Grüttner, 1939; Rademaker and Ter Braak, 1948; Mackensen, 1954). The frequency of OKN has also been found to be a function of the speed of the stimulus. At higher speeds the graph connecting these quantities levels off (Ehlers, 1926).

Dodge, Travis, and Fox (1930) studied the 'adequacy' of the slow phase of OKN. By adequacy was meant the extent to which the speed of the slow phase is related to the speed of the moving stimulus. The slow phase was found to be more or less adequate up to a speed of about 90°/sec. When the stripes moved faster than this, the eye failed to keep up with the stimulus and moved through a smaller amplitude and became irregular. Westheimer (1954b) found that the eyes followed adequately up to only 30°/sec, but he was probably using a more stringent criterion than that used by Dodge *et al.*

Dodge *et al.* found that when the stripes moved at speeds over 100°/sec, the OKN sometimes ceased altogether (fusion limit). The stripes in this study were spaced at 40° intervals and passed one at a time across a 30° aperture. Therefore there were between two and three transits per second at the speed where the responses became inadequate. This is well below flicker fusion frequency, and therefore the inadequacy must have represented the limit of the eye's capacity to follow the stimulus, rather than of its capacity to detect it. More recent studies by Smith, Kappauf, and Bojar (1940) and Blomberg (1960) have confirmed that the optokinetic fusion limit occurs below the flicker fusion frequency. Neither is the capacity of the eye to follow moving stripes limited by the speed at which the eye can move, which for saccadic movements is over 800°/sec.

Blomberg found that at the higher speeds before the fusion limit slight distractions stopped the OKN which would not then start again unless the speed of the stimulus was reduced. An increase in the width of the moving stripes has been found to increase the fusion limit slightly (Roelofs and van der Bend, 1930).

Westheimer (1954b) found that if the stimulus stripes were moved sinusoidally through 30° to and fro across the field of view, the eye movements were at first an irregular sequence of slow pursuit movements and saccadic jerks. After some practice, the eye movements began to follow the stimulus smoothly in both directions as long as the stripes did not oscillate at more than 3c/s. This demonstrates how adaptable human pursuit movements can be: the quick phases were inhibited leaving only slow pursuit movements. A cybernetic approach to the whole problem of visual pursuit is outlined in Young and Stark (1963).

OKN has been found to persist for some time after the lights are put out. This is known as optokinetic after-nystagmus or OKAN (Ohm, 1927b; McLay, Madigan, and Ormerod, 1957; Mackensen and Wiegman, 1959). Shanzer, Teng, Krieger, and Bender (1958) have found that oculomotor dysfunction in monkeys may cause a loss of OKAN while not affecting OKN. Attempts have been made to ascribe the movement after-effect to OKAN (Helmholtz, 1962; Leiri, 1927). However, movement after-effects may be induced in several directions at the same time, and this fact excludes OKAN as the cause.

Several earlier investigators reported that OKN does not occur during the first few days of life in the human infant (Bartels, 1920; Ohm, 1931b) or even during the first few weeks (Kestenbaum, 1930a). On the other hand, Bárány (1921) and Lebensohn (1931) observed it in infants only a few hours old. McGinnis (1930) in a careful study found that OKN occurs the first time the eyes are opened, both in its quick phase and its slow phase. The number of eye movements was found to be influenced by the number and speed of movement of the stimulus stripes and only to a slight degree by the experience of the child. In spite of this, fully successful ocular pursuit was not exhibited by any subject during the first two weeks of life. The evidence from animal species is apparently contradictory. Warkentin and Smith (1937) found that OKN took 14 days from birth to develop in the cat irrespective of the time at which the eyes first opened. They concluded that its development was independent of learning or experience. On the other hand, Mowrer (1936) found that OKN did not develop immediately in pigeons after they had spent the first 5 weeks in the dark after hatching; they concluded that OKN is learned. This latter experiment involves such an acute procedure that the conclusion is probably not warranted. On balance, the best evidence suggests that OKN does not depend on learning or experience and that, in human beings at least, it functions in the new-born infant.

The nervous pathways involved in OKN are not fully known, but it is clear that the slow phase involves a mechanism distinct from that responsible for the quick phase. With lesions in various parts of the oculomotor pathways, the slow phase or quick phase may be absent. When the slow phase is absent, there is no movement of the eyes. When the quick phase is absent, the eyes are conjugately deviated to the side towards which the visual display is moving.

In seeking an explanation of OKN we shall first consider the contribution of retinal factors. In submammalian species and low mammals (e.g. the guinea pig), covering one eye abolishes OKN towards the seeing eye. In other words, in these animals the slow phase towards the right is controlled by the left eye and vice versa (Smith and Bridgman, 1943; Fukuda and Tokita, 1957; Fukuda, 1959c.)

If this were true of man then, since the human optic paths hemidecussate at the chiasma, one might expect that OKN would be abolished towards the side of a hemianopia (Bárány, 1921). However, it is now generally agreed that hemianopia is not a determining factor in abnormal OKN in man, unless it is accompanied by damage to the occipital lobes or efferent pathways (Ohm, 1932). OKN may show no abnormal directional preponderance even in the presence of complete hemianopia (Brunner, 1922; Ohm, 1922, 1932; Stenvers, 1924; Fox and Holmes, 1926). OKN persists in man when only a small portion of the perimetric field remains intact (Fox and Holmes, 1926).

At the level of the central nervous system, knowledge is fragmentary and confused. There has been some dispute as to whether OKN depends on the cerebral cortex. Smith and Bridgman (1943) found that decortication in the cat leaves OKN intact as long as the stimulus is a repetitive pattern and not merely a single moving stripe. This finding has given rise to the distinction between a subcortical OKN, dependent on movement in large parts of the visual field, and a cerebral OKN which may occur in response to single moving stimuli (Rademaker and Ter Braak, 1948). Only the higher mammals are said to be capable of the latter type of OKN. However, it seems that neither type of nystagmus occurs in monkeys unless the preoccipital and occipital eye fields are intact. Furthermore, neither type of nystagmus occurs in man when the occipital lobes are not functioning as the result of occlusion of the cerebral artery (Velzeboer, 1952). Therefore no purely subcortical OKN would appear to be present in primates.

The generally accepted view is that in man the slow phase depends primarily on the occipital cortex which acts via the basal ganglia and oculomotor centres in the brain stem (Cords, 1926b). Fox (1932) and Fox and

Holmes (1926) claimed that the oculomotor centres of the frontal lobes are also involved. However, Henderson and Crosby (1952) and Cords (1926b) deny that they play any important role. Many human cases have been described in which there was a directional preponderance of OKN away from the side of a unilateral cerebral lesion in occipital, temporal, or parietal lobes (Stenvers, 1924; Strauss, 1925; Cords, 1926b; Kestenbaum, 1930b; Fox, 1932; Smith and Cogan, 1960). Enoksson (1956), in a survey of 58 clinical cases, concluded that if directional preponderance of OKN occurs in cases of cerebral lesions, it is in the direction away from the side of the lesion. Lesions in the region of the cerebellum and acoustic nerve were reported to produce preponderance to the side of the lesion.

The neurology of the quick phase is particularly enigmatic. Whether it involves cortical or purely subcortical centres is not known. Duke-Elder (1949) favours the view that it depends on cortical centres acting via the brain stem. This phase is abolished in anaesthesia and deep sleep. However, against this evidence and in favour of a subcortical centre is the evidence of Wycis and Spiegel (1953) that it persists when the hemispheres are removed. The mechanism of the quick phase has been located in the pons (Bárány, 1907b), near the vestibular nucleus (Ohm, 1939), and in the reticular substance and basal ganglia (Bartels, 1941). Lorente de Nó (1931) located it in the reticular formation on the evidence that the quick phase was abolished by a lesion there, although Spiegel and Price (1939) observed that this loss was temporary. Whatever the centres involved, Bender (1955) pointed out that the quick phase is not simply a fixation reflex in response to stimuli entering the field on the opposite side, for it occurs when only one stripe has moved over the field and no other stripe appears (Ter Braak, 1936).

Kestenbaum (1947) and Bender (1955) equated the quick phase with what Bender called 'the eye-centring system'. This is the reflex tendency of the eyes to return to the position of central gaze. This response has been called the 'orientation of the optical axes reflex' by Brown (1922) and the 'mid-positioning of eyes' by Weinstein and Bender (1948). Bender suggested that it may take part in righting reflexes, supplementing vestibular and neck-muscle reflexes. He described a clinical state known as 'fixation nystagmus' in which pathological spontaneous nystagmus occurs only, or is most marked, when the eyes are in the position of forward gaze. This condition was contrasted with nystagmus due to vestibular defects, which usually occurs only when the eyes are deviated in the direction of the quick component. This latter type was attributed to an interaction between abnormal vestibular impulses and the normal eye-centring system. The first type was ascribed to a defective eye-centring system, consequent upon damage to the oculomotor centres of the cortex or the brain stem.

The neural mechanisms involved in the eye-centring response have been placed in the frontal, parietal, occipital, and temporal lobes as well as in subcortical centres in the upper medulla, pons, pretectal region, and vermis (Weinstein and Bender, 1948; Bender, Teng, and Weinstein, 1954; Hyde and Eliasson, 1955). Particular attention has been paid to the brain-stem reticular formation. Arousal of this system has produced awakening coupled with eye centring. This finding squares with the observations, already noted, that the quick phase is abolished in sleep and barbiturate anaesthesia (Bender and O'Brien, 1946). It also squares with the fact that habitutation to vestibular nystagmus can be prevented by keeping the subject awake (see section 5.52) although Carmichael, Dix, and Hallpike (1954) advanced reasons for supposing that OKN and vestibular nystagmus depend on distinct and separate centres; Ohm (1936) had claimed that the vestibular nuclei form the nervous mechanism common to both types of nystagmus.

The study of OKN has practical uses. For instance, it has been used in the objective determination of acuity (Smith and Bojar, 1938); as a test for malingering blindness (Snell, 1939); and as a test of eye dominance (Enoksson, 1961, 1963). Its use as a tool for the diagnosis of lesions of the central nervous system is a subject of some debate (Cogan, 1956; Smith and Cogan, 1960; Jung and Kornmuller, 1964).

No attempt has been made to give a comprehensive review of OKN in this section. A complete bibliography would run to many hundreds of titles. For a bibliography of work from 1954 to 1960 see Reinecke (1961), and from 1946 to 1954 see Kestenbaum (1957), and for more recent literature see Jung and Kornmuller (1964). For earlier work see the review by Smith and Bojar (1938) and the standard reference books (Cogan, 1956; Walsh, 1957; Bender, 1964). Nystagmus and head movements, may also be elicited by a rotating sound field (Hennebert, 1960).

3.44 Eye fixations

Changes in fixation occur in response to peripheral visual objects which attract attention. The movements always involve both eyes, even if one of them is covered. Once the visual axis has centred on the new object it is maintained there, against movements of either subject or object, by the pursuit phase of vestibular or optokinetic nystagmus. When an eye changes its fixation it does so with a single, rapid, and remarkably accurate, saccadic movement. This movement is initiated after a latent period of between 0·12 and 0·18 sec, following the first appearance of the new fixation light.

The velocity increases to a maximum and then declines as the target is reached. The maximum velocity and the total duration of the movement both increase as a function of the amplitude of movement (Westheimer, 1954a; Hyde, 1959). A 15° movement is completed in about 0·05 sec. Velocities as high as 830°/sec may occur. A typical velocity–time curve for a 20° saccade is shown in figure 3.9. When the subject is uncertain about where the target

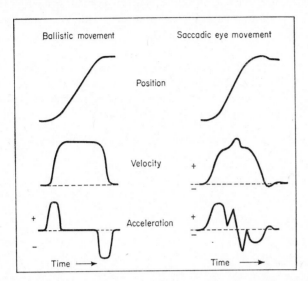

Figure 3.9 Schematic diagram of position, velocity, and acceleration changes during a hypothetical ballistic movement (left) and a typical saccadic eye movement (right). [From Westheimer, 1954a]

will appear his total duration of movement will be greater than when he knows where it will appear (Hackman, 1940; White, Eason, and Bartlett, 1962).

Westheimer concluded that saccadic movements 'are brought about merely by a change in torque which the extraocular muscles are applying to the eyeball, the latter coming to rest in a position representing an equilibrium of the forces applied.' The movements are probably triggered-off as a unit by the central nervous system; proprioceptive and visual feedback are not involved. It is a 'dead-reckoning' system stabilized by the pattern of reciprocal innervation in the muscles, viscous fluid damping, and friction. A differential linear equation was derived and applied with some success by Westheimer, although the system is not altogether linear. Because the load which the eye muscles have to move is constant, unlike the typical load on skeletal muscles, the eye can develop a dead-reckoning system to a high order of accuracy. The physical conditions of the muscles may change with fatigue, age, etc., and the muscle spindles in extraocular muscles are more likely to be concerned with compensating for such long-term changes rather than with feedback control during eye movements. The former type of control is based on 'parametric' feedback, for it involves a change in the constants or parameters of the system rather than a change in its moment-to-moment behaviour (Ludvigh, 1952b). How such parametric adjustment occurs is not known, but it may involve adjustment of the γ-fibre outflow to the extraocular muscles (see section 4.23).

When the point of fixation changes to a target which is at a different distance as well as in a different direction, a complex sequence of movements is necessary. A schematic representation of these movements is shown in figure 3.10. This figure describes data from actual eye-movement records

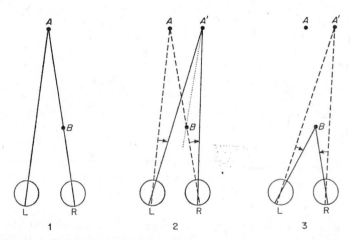

Figure 3.10 Schematic diagrams illustrating sequence of movement in changing fixation from A to B.
(1) Binocular fixation of A; (2) Conjugate lateral movement without change of convergence to A', so that bisector of angle of convergence passes through B; (3) Convergence movement from A' to B
Steps (2) and (3) are to some extent superimposed; but in view of their time characteristics, they are easily distinguished. [From Weistheimer and Mitchell, 1956]

(Westheimer and Mitchell, 1956; Alpern, 1957). The conjugate and convergence movements which are necessarily involved are entirely separate responses, and occur in sequence, not simultaneously. The two eyes first move to a new direction of conjugate lateral gaze so that the bisector of the angle of convergence passes through the new fixation point. A convergence movement then occurs, bringing the two lines of sight to intersect in the new fixation point. The two eyes always move together, as Hering's law of equal innervation demands, even if only one eye is open. In the example given, if the left eye had merely changed its direction of gaze until its visual axis intersected the new fixation point, the right eye would not have had to move. The whole movement would have been much simpler, but Hering's law would have been violated. One might ask why the movements are apparently more complex than they need to be. The answer is probably that the repertoire of 'programmes' for saccadic eye movements in the central nervous system need not be so extensive if the movements obey Hering's rule of equal innervations. Economizing on the number of movements in particular cases would involve an uneconomical extension of the central repertoire. It should prove possible to demonstrate this principle geometrically or by set theory.

Hering's law does not hold for slow pursuit movements (Breinin, 1955; Blodi and Van Allen, 1957). Such movements do not depend upon set programmes but are guided by visual feedback. Therefore the need to economize on a central repertoire does not apply.

In reading, the eyes move in a series of saccadic jerks interspersed with fixation pauses. Over 90% of the total time is taken up by the fixation pauses; the duration of any particular pause is governed by the nature of the material at that point (Tinker, 1946). A skilled reader makes few backward or regressive movements, and takes shorter pauses.

While no thorough review of the subject of eye movements exists, reference may be made to the following sources for further details: Helmholtz (1962), Hering (1942), Duke-Elder (1949), Davson (1962), Scott (1962, 1963), Bender (1964). The methods by which eye movements are recorded are reviewed in Lord and Wright (1950).

3.5 The stability of visual direction during eye movements

If an observer moves his eyes when viewing a stationary object he will normally report that the object remains stationary, in spite of the movement of the retinal image. If the object is moving, the observer is able to judge its speed even when his eyes move so as to cancel out the movement of the retinal image. These achievements imply that the observer takes account of movements of his eyes as well as of the image on his retina in making judgments about movements in the visible surroundings. He must combine these two sources of information in a way which enables him to achieve correct judgments. We shall assume that this type of judgment depends on activity in a neural centre which we shall call the *visual-stability centre*. We shall review what is known, first about how signals regarding eye movements reach this centre, and then about how signals regarding movements of the retinal image reach it.

Signals regarding eye position and movements could be derived from kinaesthetic and tactile receptors in the extraocular muscles and membranes, and/or from the central outflow to the eye muscles. The following evidence suggests that the motor outflow is the main source of eye-movement signals available to the stability centre.

1. When the eyeball is moved passively by the finger, a stationary visible object is reported to move. This fact was known to Helmholtz, Mach, and Hering in the 1860's (see Helmholtz 1962, vol. 3, pp. 243–245; Hering, 1942, p. 165). A series of related observations were made by Karrer and Stevens (1930), who seemed to be blind to the fact that their observations disproved the role of kinaesthesis in visual stability, for they concluded that graded kinaesthetic impulses are an essential component. Passive movement of the eyeball must stimulate muscle spindles in the extraocular muscles, and if the afferent inflow from these spindles were the crucial information that the vis-ual-stability centre required, the world would be reported as stationary when the eye is moved passively. What of course is lacking with passive movements is the motor outflow from the eye-movement centres. It must be concluded that the visual-stability centre is informed of the motor outflow. Certain eye movements occur, apparently without sending information to the visual-stability centre. Among these are vestibular nystagmus and pathological nystagmus of recent onset. When the eyes move in any of these ways, the surroundings are reported to move (see sections 5.4 and 7.45). In these cases the kinaesthetic feedback is no different to that in voluntary eye movements and if kinaesthesis were sufficient to indicate eye movements to the stability centre, the surroundings would be reported to be stable for involuntary as well as voluntary eye movements.

2. If the eye muscles are paralysed, any attempt to move the eyes results in an apparent movement of the stationary surroundings in the same direc-tion as the attempted movement (Helmholtz, 1962; Mach, 1886; Hering, 1942; Kornmuller, 1930). In this case, the motor-outflow information reaches the visual-stability centre, but is not accompanied by any movement of the retinal image. The situation is one which would normally arise if the visible surroundings were to move with the eyes, and this is what the observer reports. Similar disturbances of visual stability may arise as a result of partial loss of function of eye muscles in paresis (Ludvigh, 1952b). William James (1890, p. 507) suggested that a voluntary attempt to move a paralysed eye would result in movement of the other eye and for this reason the role of kinaesthesis is not disproved by observations on paralysed eyes such as Helmholtz reported. Hughlings Jackson, and Paton (1909) showed by care-

ful clinical observation that movements of the other eye could not account for the reported visual movements produced in a paralysed eye. William James's objection is therefore groundless, and his theory that kinaesthesis is the basis of the eye's sense of position is not supported.

3. If an after-image is formed, and the eye closed and moved voluntarily, the after-image is reported to move with the eye. Motor-outflow information is again not accompanied by the usual movement of the retinal image. If the eye is moved passively, the after-image is reported to be stationary. In this case there is neither outflow information nor retinal-image motion.

All this evidence supports the theory that the visual-stability centre receives information regarding the motor outflow to the eye muscles rather than kinaesthetic feedback from those muscles. One might have concluded that there are no muscle spindles in the eye muscles, if it were not known on histological evidence that there are (Sherrington, 1898; Buzzard, 1908; Daniel, 1946; Cooper and Daniel, 1949; Cooper, Daniel, and Whitteridge, 1955; Christman and Kupfer, 1963).

William James was not the only worker to believe in the sensory role of kinaesthesis in the eye muscles, in spite of all the evidence to the contrary. Sherrington (1918) and Hoffmann (1934) also continued to believe that the position sense of the eye depends on proprioception. Sherrington claimed that his experimental results supported such a view. His procedure was to anaesthetize the conjunctiva, to ensure that tactile inputs were removed. The subject was asked to direct his gaze to points on a screen to which his hand had been passively moved. The light was then switched on, and the point to which the gaze was directed was noted. He gave no quantitative results but claimed that, 'The power to direct the gaze under these circumstances has been found to be good.'

Merton (1961) has criticized Sherrington's procedure. He pointed out that the accuracy with which Sherrington's subjects could do the test would depend as much on the position sense of the arm as of the eye. In any case, the task could be performed on the basis of motor-outflow information as well as that from kinaesthesis.

Merton repeated Sherrington's experiment, with improvements. Under the conditions of Sherrington's experiment, errors of the order of 5° are made, which Sherrington could not have called 'good'. Under the best conditions, the gaze could be redirected in the dark towards an object previously fixated with lights on, with a standard deviation of successive attempts around their mean position of roughly 1° in both horizontal and vertical directions. Even this performance would have to be improved by a factor of 12 to equal the ability of the eye to maintain fixation with lights on. Ludvigh (1952a) had reported a similar experiment. The subject, with head clamped, saw a disc of light in an otherwise dark room. The light was presented in one of several fixed positions to the side or up or down by amounts equivalent to the introduction of 2, 5, and 8 dioptres. On each presentation, the subject had to fixate the light and report whether his gaze was directed to the left or to the right of the median plane. The results indicated that ocular movements in excess of 6° either way must occur for the observer to state with high reliability whether the eye was directed to the right or to the left. It is not necessary to conclude that even this coarse position sense depends on kinaesthesis; motor-outflow information could serve.

A direct test of the kinaesthetic sense of the eyes must be performed under conditions where the motor outflow is either absent, or known not to serve as a position sense. Such experiments have been done.

Irvine and Ludvigh (1936) have demonstrated that, (1) persons with paralysed eye muscles cannot judge the position of their closed eyes, (2) persons with clinical nystagmus or nystagmus induced by vestibular stimulation may believe that their eyes are stationary and that the environment is moving, and (3) normal persons in the dark whose eyes are moved passively by pulling on the anaesthetized conjunctiva with forceps do not report the movement. Rivers reported a similar finding in 1900, and it has been confirmed in recent years by Brindley and Merton (1960) who found that simultaneous passive movements of both eyes through as much as 30° were not reported. Passive movement of one eye did not induce reflex movements in the other eye, which suggests that conjugate eye movements are not controlled by proprioceptive feedback. When a subject was asked to deviate his occluded eyes to left or right he was unable to report whether his eyes had been allowed to move or whether the experimenter had applied mechanical restraint. In both cases he reported having the impression that he had succeeded. This evidence does not prove that position sense in active movement is not served by the muscle spindles.

Ludvigh (1952a, 1952b) concluded that, although kinaesthetic receptors in the eye muscles do not send impulses to the visual-stability centre, they may induce 'parametric adjustment' of the eye muscles. In other words, they may signal to the oculomotor centres the length and state of tension of the various eye muscles so that the motor outflow may be adjusted to move the eye accurately to a new fixation. The scheme which Ludvigh proposed is shown in figure 3.11. This scheme equates the visual-stability centre ('space representation') with the centres for ductions; we have talked as if they are not the same.

Whether or not the kinaesthetic receptors induce parametric adjustments, there is little doubt that they do not serve to indicate the position or movements of the eyes directly to the visual-stability centre.

Information regarding movements of the image on the retina could arise from one of two features of the proximal stimulus. It may be the change of location of identifiable objects, or it may be movement across neighbouring receptors which is coded. Small quick discontinuous movements are indistinguishable from smooth movements. However, discontinuous movements of low rates of intermittence may be expected to reveal the demands of the stability mechanism. MacKay (1958) has shown that if the eye is pressed

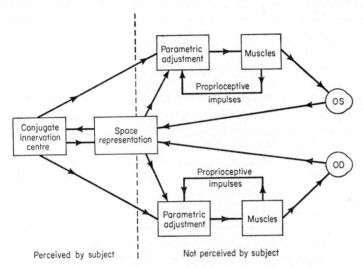

Figure 3.11 Ludvigh's proposed scheme for the role of proprioceptive feedback in the control of eye movements and the appreciation of visual movement. [From *Arch. Ophthal.*, N.Y., 1952, **44**, 446]

with the finger when a room is illuminated stroboscopically at rates of about 15 per sec, i.e. close to flicker fusion frequency, the surroundings are judged to move, just as they would be in steady illumination. However at rates of about 5 per sec the room is reported as stable, while continuously self-luminous objects continue to be unstable. Gregory (1959) has reported a similar finding. The visual-stability centre seems therefore to require signals from a relatively smooth, continuous movement.

We may finally conclude that the ability to judge seen movements depends on the interplay of information from the centres which are responsible for the voluntary control of eye movements, and information from the visual centres indicating image movements on the retina. Apparently the outflow from the subcortical centres which control involuntary eye movements does not reach the visual-stability centre. When the movement of the retinal image which results from a voluntary eye movement has such speed and direction as normally accompany that motor outflow, the visible surroundings are judged to be stationary. If the retinal movement is more than this, the surroundings are judged to be moving in the opposite direction to the eye, and if it is less, they are judged to be moving in the same direction.

MacKay (1958) proposed what he claimed to be an alternative theory. He wrote, 'Briefly, the argument is that if perception is the adaptive "keeping up to date" of an organism's state of organization for activity in its world, then what requires informational justification is not the maintenance of stability but the perception of change. The internal state of organization, which implicitly represents the perceived world, should remain unaltered unless sufficient information (in the technical sense) arrives to justify a change, by indicating that the current state of organization is significantly mismatched to the state of affairs sampled by the receptor system.

'Thus the retinal changes resulting from voluntary movement evoke no perception of world-motion, because they are not an awkward consequence to be compensated, but part of the goal to be achieved.'

The 'cancellation theory', and what we shall call the 'evaluation theory' of MacKay, both account for the facts which have been outlined, and on the face of it, the two theories seem to be operationally equivalent. However, MacKay insists that, 'The operational difference comes in the details of the computing operations carried out when the incoming signals are integrated with the motor outflow' (private communication). More research into the neural computing mechanisms involved is clearly called for.

4

Kinaesthesis

4.1 Kinaesthesis defined

Sherrington (1906) introduced the terms 'proprioception' and 'intero-
ception' to include all those sensory systems which respond to stimuli arising
in the 'deep field' of the body as opposed to the 'surface field'. They include
the visceral, muscular, arthrodial (joint), and vestibular afferent systems. In
this chapter we are concerned with only the muscular and arthrodial afferent
systems of this complex i.e. those parts generally thought to be involved in
kinaesthesis. Kinaesthesis is best understood as a behavioural term. It includes
the discrimination of the position of body parts, the discrimination of movement and amplitude of movement of body parts, both passively and

actively produced. Visual and auditory information is assumed to be absent. As well as afferents from muscles and joints, touch, stretch, and pressure signals from the skin serve these discriminations. The pattern of motor innervation is almost certainly also available as a source of information for kinaesthetic judgments. We define kinaesthesis, therefore, as the discrimination of the positions and movements of body parts based on information other than visual, auditory, or verbal. The immediate stimuli arise from changes in length and from tension, compression, and shear forces arising from the effects of gravity, from the relative movement of body parts, and from muscular contraction.

4.2 Structure and physiology of kinaesthetic receptors

4.21 Muscle spindles and Golgi tendon organs

Charles Bell postulated a 'muscular sense' as early as 1826. Muscle spindles, which are now known to be the source of the afferent discharge from muscles, were recognized histologically by Hassell in 1851 (Hellebrandt, 1953) but more convincingly by Kolliker in 1862, and Kühne in 1863. The detailed histology of the spindles was not known until 1898, when Ruffini published what has become the classic description of their structure.

Tendon receptors were first described by Golgi in 1880, and have come to be called Golgi tendon organs.

Sherrington (1894) established by experimental means the function of muscle spindles as sensory end-organs. Many papers appeared on this topic at the turn of the century, but a detailed knowledge of the function of muscle spindles and tendon organs had to wait until electronic amplifiers were available, and adapted by Adrian for recording from single sensory nerve endings. With this technique Matthews (1931a, 1931b) was able to investigate the activity of single muscle spindles in the frog. In 1933 Matthews used the same procedure to study mammalian muscle spindles. It is the elaboration and further use of electrophysiological techniques that has led to present-day knowledge.

Modern knowledge of the structure and innervation of muscle spindles and tendon organs is depicted in figure 4.1; their detailed histology is reviewed in Hinsey (1934), Barker (1948, 1962a), Lissman (1950), Tiegs (1953), Boyd (1962), and Matthews (1964).

The spindles are interspersed among, and parallel with, ordinary (extrafusal) muscle fibres, which they resemble in many respects. In fact, a muscle spindle is a specialized form of muscle fibre, containing contractile elements (intrafusal fibres) as well as sensory endings. Spindles occur in most if not all of the muscles of the human body and not, as previously thought (Fulton,

1946), merely in the anti-gravity muscles. Each spindle consists of a central equatorial region, an elongated proximal pole and an elongated distal pole. Sometimes there are two or more equatorial regions in tandem, spaced out along the length of the spindle (Barker and Ip, 1961). The outer sheath of the spindle in the central section of each equatorial region swells out to form a

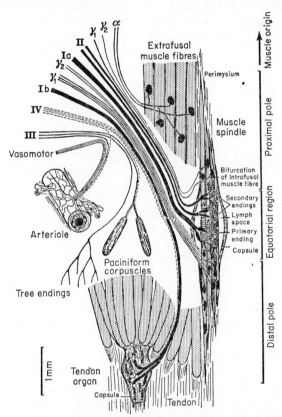

Figure 4.1 Schema of the innervation of mammalian skeletal muscle, based on a study of the cat. [From Barker, 1962a]

lymph-filled capsule surrounding the sensory end-organs, which are confined to this region. This capsule presumably serves to protect the end organs from the effects of mechanical shocks and pressures, and ensures that their adequate stimulus will be a change of tension along their length.

The sensory endings are of two kinds, primary and secondary. Usually the primary endings have an *annulo-spiral* structure, and the secondary endings a *flower-spray* structure. In man the two types of endings are not always

H.S.O.—6

distinguishable by their shape, but the primary endings are always confined to the equatorial region and the secondary endings to bands, known as myotube sections, close to the proximal and distal ends of each equatorial region. Primary endings are always present; secondary endings may be absent. The primary endings are innervated by large diameter (8–12 μ in the cat), fast conducting, low-threshold, group I afferents (Sherrington, 1894; Eccles and Sherrington, 1930; Lloyd, 1943). The secondary endings are innervated by smaller (6–9 μ in the cat), higher-threshold fibres. The primary

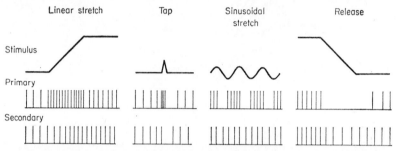

Figure 4.2 Diagrammatic comparison of the responses of the 'typical' primary and secondary endings to various stimuli according to Matthews (1964). The responses are drawn as if the muscle were under moderate initial stretch and as if there were no gamma-fibre activity

endings have a low-frequency resting discharge. Muscle-spindle receptors respond to changes in the length and tension of the spindle; chemical or other incidental changes in muscle during contraction do not affect them (Barker, 1948).

Cooper (1959, 1961) found that discharge from secondary endings during the application of stretch hardly exceeds that during maintained stretch, whereas the primary endings discharge particularly heavily during the 'dynamic phase of stretch'. Harvey and Matthews (1961) confirmed these findings and also found that the secondary endings, but not the primary endings, show after-discharge when tension is released. Bessou and Laporte (1962) and Bianconi and van der Meulen (1963) have presented the response profiles of the different endings under impulsive and vibratory stimulation. The primary endings were found to be particularly sensitive to high-frequency low-amplitude vibration. These differences between the two types of endings are summarized diagrammatically in figure 4.2. Thus when a muscle is stretched the primary endings signal both the instantaneous length of the muscle and the rate of stretching, while the secondary endings signal mainly instantaneous length. Matthews (1964) has pointed out that the velocity-dependent response of the primary endings implies that somewhere in the causal chain from mechanical deformation to nerve response there is a 'differentiation' of the signal. He presents very good arguments for concluding that this differentiation depends on the mechanical-damping properties of the nuclear-bag region in which the primary endings are situated.

During isotonic (i.e. constant load) contractions and during submaximal isometric (i.e. constant length) contractions the resting discharge i.e. the discharge due to applied steady tension, may cease in both types of ending. This is the so-called 'pause' which covers the period during and just after contraction. A similar interruption occurs in the electromyographic record from a muscle during active contraction, and this is known as the 'silent period' (Hoffman, 1922). The silent period is due in part to the pause in spindle firing but also to autogenetic inhibition (see below) and central factors (Granit, 1955, p. 210). The pause demonstrates that the muscle spindles are in parallel with the muscle fibres, as first pointed out by Fulton and Pi-Sũner in 1928. When the muscle contracts, the tension on the spindles is released and its sensory end-organs cease firing until the slack in the spindle is taken up by contraction of muscle fibres inside the muscle spindle.

The fact that the pause occurs during isometric as well as isotonic contraction is thought to be due to the elasticity in the tendons and muscles which allows some release of tension in the spindles to occur. If the tension in the muscle has already taken up the elastic slack, then the pause will not occur in isometric contraction when additional muscular tension is induced (Matthews, 1933). The spindle discharge is a very sensitive indicator of changes of tension in a muscle. Tension changes in a contracting muscle become evident in the afferent spindle discharge before they are evident by recording at the tendon. The pause after a stretched muscle has been released could be due either to the slow viscous return of the spindle to its normal length (Matthews, 1933) or to post-excitatory depression (a phenomenon common to all sense organs), or both.

The discharge in primary spindle endings is approximately proportional to the logarithm of the load (i.e. the amount of stretch) applied to the passive muscle, but adaptation is rapid and therefore the maximum discharge reached will depend as much on the rate at which the muscle is stretched as on the absolute tension. Furthermore, the viscous and elastic properties of the spindles probably differ from those of the surrounding muscle tissue, and these differences will affect the silent period and the relation between discharge frequency, tension, and the rate at which the muscle is passively stretched.

The balance of evidence now suggests that spindle afferents feed into the spinal cord by way of the sensory or dorsal roots. Once inside the cord, they initiate monosynaptic reflexes (e.g. the stretch reflex). The spindle afferents also project up to the cerebellum in the spino–cerebellar tracts but do not reach the cortex (Granit, 1955; Rose and Mountcastle, 1959).

The tendon organs are innervated in the main by lower-range group I fibres. The pattern of discharge of the tendon organs differs in several respects from that of the spindles. They have a higher threshold to external stretch, and do not show any resting discharge. Therefore at low tensions there will be a proportionately greater discharge from spindles; as the tension is increased, more and more tendon organs will contribute to the total discharge. Tendon organs discharge during the spindles' silent period. They thus behave as if they are in series with the contracting muscle fibres, and anatomical evidence supports this conclusion. They respond to the total tension in the muscle, whether this be produced by active contraction or passive stretch.

The tendon-organ afferents feed into the spinal cord by way of the dorsal roots and provoke monosynaptic, inhibitory reflexes (McGough, Deering, and Stewart, 1950; Granit, 1955; Rose and Mountcastle, 1959). The well-known 'clasp-knife' reflex or lengthening reaction is due largely to inhibition from the Golgi organs overriding the facilitatory stretch reflex initiated by the spindles as muscle tension mounts. Reflexes originating thus in muscle or tendon receptors are called 'myogenic' (for details of myogenic reflexes see Granit, 1955 and Hunt and Perl, 1960).

It is generally agreed that the large, group I afferents from spindles, apart from entering into spinal motor pools, ascend in the dorsal tracts to the cerebellum. They do not reach the cortex by any direct route (Lloyd and McIntyre, 1950; Lundberg and Oscarsson, 1956; Holmqvist, Lundberg, and Oscarsson, 1956; Laporte and Lundberg, 1956; Laporte, Lundberg, and Oscarsson, 1956a, 1956b). The group I fibres from the tendon organs follow the same path (Oscarsson, 1956). Direct stimulation of muscle spindles by stretching produces no detectable response in the post-central somaesthetic areas of the cortex (Mountcastle, Covian, and Harrison, 1950; Mountcastle, 1957). Small, group III sensory fibres from muscles project to the cortex, but these are thought to arise from pain and vascular receptors. Rose and Mountcastle (1959) consider that the cortical responses which Gardner and Morin (1953) produced by stimulation of group I and group II muscle afferents, were due to afferents from joint receptors intruding into the muscle nerves.

4.22 The gamma-fibre system

The literature on this topic was thoroughly reviewed by Granit (1955). The following is an account of the main facts and of work since 1955.

Each muscle spindle contains several contractile muscle fibres (intrafusal fibres). The nuclei of these fibres are arranged in *nuclear chains* in the polar regions, and in *nuclear bags* in the equatorial region. The fibres are striated in the polar regions but not in the equatorial region, and it is thought that they are contractile only in the polar regions (Barker and Gudumal, 1960; Cooper and Daniel, 1956). The efferent fibres which supply the intrafusal fibres are known as gamma (γ) fibres. They are 2–8 μ in diameter in the cat, being smaller than the main motor efferents or alpha (a) fibres which are 8–20 μ in diameter. About one third of all the motor fibres in the lumbo-sacral ventral roots are γ fibres (Kuffler and Hunt, 1952). Boyd and Davey (1962) have claimed that there are two groups of γ-fibres, a larger-diameter group innervating the nuclear bag, and a small-diameter group innervating the nuclear chains. Barker (1962b) doubts the validity of this claim. It is now well established that all small-diameter (2–8 μ) motor neurons innervate exclusively intrafusal muscle fibres. It is generally agreed that large diameter motor neurons innervate exclusively extrafusal muscle fibres (Eccles and Sherrington, 1930; Kuffler and Hunt, 1952); the evidence that the spindles receive collaterals from a neurons is reviewed in Matthews (1964). A single γ fibre innervates several spindles (Kuffler, Hunt, and Quilliam, 1951; Hagbarth and Wohlfart, 1952). On the other hand, a single spindle receives branches from several γ efferents (Hunt and Kuffler, 1951a, 1951b). Each efferent fibre branches extensively within the spindle, each intrafusal fibre receiving several terminal boutons (Barker, 1948).

The threshold for the γ efferents is on average 3·9 times the threshold of the a efferents, but full γ activation requires 12 to 23 times the a threshold. Efferent discharges in the γ neurons cause the intrafusal muscle fibres to contract. This stimulates the spindle sensory endings which in turn affect the contraction of the extrafusal muscles. A complete feedback loop is thus established.

It was shown in 1934 by O'Leary, Heinbecker, and Bishop that stimulation of the muscle-spindle efferents does not add significantly to the muscle tension caused by activity in the main a system. However, it was not until 1945 that Leksell demonstrated conclusively that stimulation of the γ system causes an enhancement of afferent spindle discharge in frog's muscle, but no noticeable contraction of the muscle as a whole. Kuffler and Hunt (1952) and Kobayashi, Oshima, and Tasaki (1952) demonstrated the same relationship in a mammal (the cat).

Jansen and Matthews (1961, 1962) and Matthews (1962) have produced evidence that there are two types of intrafusal muscle fibres which they have called 'static' and 'dynamic'. Stimulation of both types of intrafusal fibre increased the afferent discharge from the primary spindle end-organs. When the spindle was stretched during stimulation of the 'static' fibres the normal 'dynamic response' of the primary endings was absent. When the spindle was stretched during stimulation of the 'dynamic' fibres the 'dynamic response' of the primary spindle receptors was increased. Whether these two types of intrafusal fibre are innervated by distinct fibres is not known, and the functional significance of these findings is still obscure.

4.23 Gamma-leading and the effects of deafferentation

It is thought that in normal muscular contractions, activity in the γ system precedes or leads activity in the α system. The spindle muscle fibres contract before the main extrafusal fibres. This spindle contraction sets up afferent discharges from the spindle end-organs which reflexly facilitate, or perhaps initiate, contraction of the main muscles (Whitteridge, 1959). When the extrafusal muscles have 'caught up' with the contracted spindles, the tension in the spindle is relieved, and facilitation of muscular contraction ceases. The spindles are, in effect, 'misalignment detectors', signalling the difference in length between muscle and spindle. Eldred, Granit, and Merton (1953) were able to demonstrate the 'γ-leading' (our term) process by recording from the spindle discharge in a cat's gastrocnemius–soleus muscle. An acceleration of spindle discharge was found to precede the contraction of the main muscle. After deafferentation of the muscle, acceleration of the spindle discharge occurred as before, but the muscular-contraction response to the particular stimulus used (ear twitch) was abolished. Not that deafferentation always abolishes muscular responses. Hyde and Gellhorn (1949) were still able to elicit muscular contractions from the gastrocnemius muscle of a cat after section of the appropriate dorsal roots, although the response was weaker than with intact afferents. Furthermore, the responses were still graded in strength in accordance with the strength of the electrical stimulus applied to the motor cortex, showing that gradations in muscle responses are not entirely dependent upon proprioceptive recruitment. Conditioned motor responses, in particular conditioned forelimb flexions, have been found to survive limb deafferentation (Knapp, Taub, and Berman, 1958, 1959; Taub, Bacon, and Berman, 1965) although not without some change in the pattern of the response (Górska and Jankowska, 1959, 1960, 1963).

However, Hyde and Gellhorn found that deafferentation did abolish the recruitment which the electromyographic response of the muscle normally shows when the muscle's initial length is increased by passive stretching (Gellhorn, 1948, 1949). Deafferentation also abolished the reflex co-contraction which is normally found in an antagonist when activity is high in an agonist. Breinin (1957) found also that the fine regulation of reciprocal innervation in the agonists and antagonists in the eye is lost if the afferent activity is disturbed by separating the muscles from the globe.

4.24 Cerebellar and brain-stem control of muscle spindles

Granit and Kaada (1952) in an extensive series of experiments found that the γ system could be activated or inhibited both by stimulating the anterior cerebellum and by stimulating the diencephalic reticular formation. It is also known that in the absence of the anterior lobe of the cerebellum γ firing no longer facilitates α contraction (Eldred, Granit, Holmgren, and Merton, 1953; Granit, Holmgren, and Merton, 1955). Muscular contraction may still occur, but when it does, the spindle discharge shows the silent period as it does when the limb is moved passively. A drop in the level of the γ control of tension is also revealed in the slower spindle discharge from the resting muscle. Reflex activity is still intact, however, and the conclusion is that in this case the direct α route is used to initiate muscle contraction without facilitation by γ outflow. In the intact animal either route is available; one could speculate that the fast, direct, α route is for ballistic or well-practised movements, and the indirect γ-leading route for exploratory movements. The cerebellum apparently controls whether the γ control system or the direct route is used.

The spindle control system, like any control system which depends upon negative feedback, is potentially unstable. This is because the error signal takes time to generate a corrective response, which means that in the absence of any compensation, the corrective signal guiding a limb to its target would arrive at a time when the limb had moved on to a new position. Thus, overshooting of the limb would result from conduction and synaptic delay, and from the delay involved in overcoming the inertia of the limb. A second correction would have to be applied which would also result in overshooting, and the limb would oscillate about the target position. In order to correct this state of affairs, the movement of the limb must be damped. Purely mechanical damping is provided by the 'in series' elastic elements in muscles (the fibres themselves and the tendons) and the viscosity of the muscle tissues and joints (T. D. M. Roberts, 1963). Sensory adaptation in spindle receptors, coupled with the inhibitory control from the tendon organs also helps to provide damping (Partridge and Glaser, 1960). Another way of stating the role of damping is to say that the reflex control system must have an output determined by both position error (length misalignment) and the rate of change of muscle length. With rate-of-change information available, the system is able to anticipate the future position of the limb, and the corrective signal can be adjusted to suit the state of affairs at the instant when the corrective adjustment can be made. Adaptation in spindles may provide the rate-of-movement information, as long as the movement is not impulsive (Partridge and Glaser, 1960). The cerebellum probably controls this rate-dependent adjustment by timing γ outflow in relation to the α outflow, for Higgins, Partridge, and Glaser (1962) found that after cerebellar ablation cats were ataxic and, although they recovered to some extent, they were never again normal (Higgins and Glaser, 1964). Tremor due to cerebellar disease in man may represent a disturbance of the same system.

Single-pulse or low-frequency stimulation of thalamic nuclei has been shown to depress muscle-spindle activity in the cat. High-frequency stimulation had the opposite effect. A stronger depressing effect was obtained when the low-frequency stimulus coincided with the EEG wave (Hongo, Kubota, and Shimazu, 1963). These relationships are probably part of an arousal or alerting mechanism.

To summarize, the prime function of the γ system (γ fibres and intrafusal spindle fibres) is to maintain the tension of the spindle in a constant relationship with that of the muscle. If this were not done the spindle would become flaccid during muscular contraction, and would cease to function; the gamma system also keeps the spindle in trim and maintains its threshold at a usable level. As a consequence of achieving this prime function the γ system can carry out at least two other functions. In the first place, it helps to initiate and control reflex activity, especially the stretch reflex, which serves to maintain the animal's posture and grade the strength of muscular contraction in relation to variations in external load. In the second place, the γ system serves to initiate, or at least facilitate, voluntary contraction by the process of γ-leading, and contributes to the stability of muscular control.

We have already discussed how muscular contraction is inhibited by the release of tension in the spindles, and by increased discharge from Golgi tendon organs. But muscular contraction is also reflexly inhibited by activity generated in recurrent collateral, or antidromic fibres which run back from motor axons via the ventral horns into the motoneuron pools of the spinal cord. This system was described by Renshaw (1941), and is known as the Renshaw loop. Its precise physiological function was established by Eccles, Fatt, and Koketsu (1954) and Holmgren and Merton (1953). Not only are the active motoneurons inhibited by these antidromic discharges, but inactive motoneurons are also inhibited. The reflex involves one synapse, but its latency is shorter than that of the spindle stretch reflex, and the two reflexes are distinguishable on this basis (Holmgren and Merton, 1953). These mechanisms of γ leading and antidromic inhibition have an important bearing on the problems of the normal and pathological reflex control of movement, and in particular the knee jerk and stretch reflex. These matters are beyond the scope of this book; for details see particularly Granit (1955) but also Granit and Suursoet (1949), Granit (1950), Hunt (1952), and Hammond, Merton, and Sutton (1956).

4.25 Receptors in the joint capsule and skin

The articular surfaces of free-moving, or diarthrodial joints are lined with cartilaginous material and a limiting synovial membrane. A fluid, the synovial fluid, is secreted into the joint and lubricates it. Ligaments bind the joint to form the joint capsule (for further details of joint physiology, see Gardner, 1950).

The ligaments of mammalian joints are well provided with sensory endings (Leriche, 1930; Gardner, 1944; Andrew and Dodt, 1953; Skoglund, 1956). There are two main types of sensory end-organ. The commonest are the 'spray-type' endings which resemble the Ruffini endings in the skin. They are located in the connective tissue of joints, and are innervated by myelinated, low-order, group I sensory fibres (6–9 μ in the cat). The second type of endings are the Golgi-type endings, similar to those found in tendons. They have a similar innervation to the Ruffini type and similar discharge properties. Smaller, unmyelinated fibres also innervate joints, usually in conjunction with fine blood vessels, and are presumed to be of sympathetic origin and unconnected with the movement of the joint.

It has been demonstrated that the discharge from joint receptors in the cat is related to the movement and position of the joint (Andrew and Dodt, 1953; Boyd and Roberts, 1953; Cohen, 1955; Gardner, 1948; Skoglund, 1956). Andrew (1954) isolated the medial ligament in the knee joint of a cat and recorded from individual afferent fibres while tension was applied. No resting discharge was found at zero tension. *In vivo* the ligaments are always under tension, so this lack of resting discharge in isolated tissue does not reflect normal functioning. When tension was applied to the isolated ligament slowly adapting discharges were found in one or two large fibres. After an initial decline in response frequency during the first few seconds, these fibres discharged steadily for the whole period of three minutes during which a steady tension was applied. The application of rapidly developing tensions of up to 200 g revealed the presence of endings which discharged very briefly at only the onset and the release of tension.

Receptors in the joint capsule are probably not affected by tensions in the muscle, and are thus isolated from the effects of variations in tonus and external load.

Cutaneous receptors have been shown to fire in response to deformations of the skin, so that they could serve to indicate changing skin tensions resulting from changes in the position of a limb (Adrian, Cattell, and Hoagland, 1931).

The afferents from joint receptors (and skin receptors) are known to project via the dorsal root into the lemniscal system, the thalamus, and up to the sensory cortex. This has been demonstrated both by mechanical stimulation of the receptors (Mountcastle, 1957; Mountcastle, Covian, and Harrison, 1950) and by electrical stimulation of joint afferents (Gardner and Haddad, 1953). The discharge patterns of various neurons, both in the nerve and at the cortex, show a range of types. Most show an initial high transient discharge followed by a slowly adapting discharge when the joint is held at a particular angle. Some units are active at any joint position, others are maximally active for small joint angles, and yet others are maximally active at large joint angles (Berry, Karl, and Hinsey, 1950). Mountcastle, Covian, and Harrison (1950) report that some pairs of spatially related cortical cells are reciprocally related, one cell being active as the joint moves in one direction and the other being active when the joint moves in the other direction.

4.3 Kinaesthetic judgments

The various types of kinaesthetic judgments are set out in table 4.1. Those that are relevant to the subject of this book will now be discussed.

Table 4.1 A classification of types of kinaesthetic judgment

Passive movement	Threshold of movement Judgment of position (indication of when previous position is regained) Threshold of direction of movement Accuracy of direction judgments Judgment of amplitude of movement Judgment of speed of movement
Active movement	Steadiness and fineness of movement Judgment of position Accuracy of direction of movement Accuracy of amplitude of movement Accuracy of pressure production Accuracy of speed of movement

4.31 Kinaesthetic sensitivity to passive movement

Various determinations of sensitivity to passive movement have been made, perhaps most thoroughly by Goldscheider (1889) some of whose data are given in table 4.2. He found that the sensitivity of a joint is directly related to its proximity to the trunk and that it is not much affected by the position of the joint, suggesting that the stretch of muscle is not important. More recent determinations have been made by Laidlaw and Hamilton (1937a, 1937b) and Cleghorn and Darcus (1952). These latter authors found that passive movements of 0·8° in the elbow joint could be detected 80% of the time, for speeds of approximately 0·2°/sec but that a movement had to be 1·8° before the subject could identify its direction 80% of the time.

Table 4.2 To show thresholds of passive movement obtained by Goldscheider for several joints, together with the speed of movement during the determinations

Joint	Threshold (deg)	Speed of movement (°/sec)
2nd Interphalangeal	1·03–1·26	—
1st Interphalangeal	0·72–1·05	12·4–12·8
Metacarpo–phalangeal	0·34–0·43	3·6
Wrist	0·26–0·42	3·1–8·7
Elbow	0·40–0·61	0·7–1·4
Shoulder	0·22–0·42	0·5–1·0
Hip	0·50–0·79	1·6–3·2
Knee	0·50–0·70	1·0–2·5
Ankle	1·15–1·30	1·9–3·5

Extension movements were detected by the subjects more easily than flexion movements in most of the studies (Pillsbury, 1901; Winter, 1912; Cleghorn and Darcus, 1952), although Goldscheider found the reverse to be true of the elbow joint. The subjects often reported an arm movement when none had occurred. These 'false positives' were most often described as occurring in the same direction as the preceding movement.

Very few studies have been devoted to the ability to judge the extent of passive movement. Von Skramlik (1933) moved the subject's arm a given distance passively at 60 cm/sec, and asked the subject to indicate the same distance when his arm was moved passively at between 1 and 5 cm/sec. The distance of the faster movement was underestimated relative to that of the slower movement.

4.32 Kinaesthetic position sensitivity with active movement

Two procedures have been suggested for measuring the active position sensitivity of a limb. The first procedure is to ask the subject to place his unseen finger on a reference point by initially groping and then to lower the arm and regain the same position either with the same hand or the opposite hand. Klingelhage (1933) used this procedure, and found that errors were greater in a vertical direction than in a horizontal direction. The dominant hand was superior to the non-dominant hand. Cohen (1958a) used a similar procedure and reported a mean average error of 3·3 cm (about 2°) at the finger tip of the fully extended arm for the standing subject.

Accuracy was less away from the straight-ahead position of the arm, although he found no consistent pattern of accuracy for the different directions of pointing. The errors reported by Cohen would reflect not only arm sensitivity but any unsteadiness in the posture of the subject as well as his sensitivity to any sway which occurred. The errors would in any case be the sum of the sensitivity of initial registration of position and the accuracy of subsequent re-aiming. The procedure also involves a time error, as it is necessarily a sequential task. Merton (1961) used a similar procedure but allowed the subject to leave his arm extended near the target. A pin the subject was holding was replaced after one second with a mean horizontal constant error of 0·1° and a mean vertical constant error of 0·2°. After five seconds the variability had doubled. Clearly these errors are much less than those of Cohen; any absolute measures of active position sensitivity are meaningless unless the precise conditions of measurement are specified. Merton for instance does not tell us whether his subject was sitting or standing.

The second procedure for studying active position sensitivity overcomes some of these disadvantages. In it the subject is asked to point the unseen fingers of the two hands to the same place. Horsley (1905) and Slinger and Horsley (1906) used a test of this kind in which the blindfolded subject was asked to point to the same location on two scales on opposite sides of a plate of glass. They found that accuracy diminished with increased distance out from the surface of the body and with increased angular displacements from the mid-sagittal plane of the body.

A related procedure to the one just discussed is to ask the subject to point the two hands to symmetrically opposite points about the median plane of the body. Hall and Hartwell (1884) asked their subjects to move their hands to symmetrical points. The dominant hand was found to be moved out further than the non-dominant hand, especially when the movement was ballistic. Stock (1933) used a similar procedure both with the hands moving to their own side and with them crossed over the body line. The latter condition gave the greatest error.

The kinaesthetic position sense may be influenced by a previous movement or posture, Hoff and Schilder (1925), Selling (1930), and more recently Nachmias (1953) have shown that if a subject holds two arms horizontally in front of him and is then asked to raise one 45° above the horizontal for about 30 sec, the arm remains above the other when the subject is asked to restore the horizontal position. Such 'postural persistence' was demonstrated with a greater variety of 'exposure' positions by Jackson (1954) who showed that exposures as short as 5 sec were sufficient to influence subsequent posture. Whether this effect is due to the persistence of muscular tension and innervation, to physical after-effects in the muscle tissue, to sensory adaptations, or to central processes, is not known. Related to the phenomenon of postural persistence are kinaesthetic figural after-effects (Köhler and Dinnerstein, 1947; McEwen, 1958) and post-contraction (see Hick, 1953).

4.33 Accuracy of distance production

Woodworth (1899) reported a now classic study of factors related to the accuracy of voluntary movement. Initially, pencil strokes of a particular length were made to the beat of a metronome varying between 20 and 200 beats per minute. Up to 40 beats per minute accuracy was constant; above that point accuracy gradually decreased as movements became more ballistic i.e. fine terminal adjustments became less possible. With eyes shut this trend was to some extent reversed showing that whereas visual control declines with rate, muscle control is, if anything, improved. An exception was that the non-dominant hand was adversely affected by rate whether or not the eyes were open; the difference in accuracy between dominant and non-dominant hands increased with rate.

The rate variable was then broken down into its two components, the speed of movement and the interval between movements. The results when only speed of movement was varied, closely paralleled the effect of the rate variable as a whole; in addition, with eyes shut, faster movements were drawn too long and slower ones too short. When only the interval was varied, accuracy tended to increase with decreasing intervals, due to 'a certain momentum of uniformity' and 'ease of rhythm'. The duration of the interval was said to affect the 'initial impulse' while movement speed affects 'current control'. Thus the combined variable of rate has two simultaneous and opposed effects on accuracy, and the fact that the net effect is similar to the effect of movement speed alone suggests that, 'in the situations which permit great accuracy, that accuracy is due mostly, not to the initial adjustment of the movement as a whole, but to the current control, consisting of finer adjustments' (p. 62).

Woodworth also investigated accuracy as a function of distance moved, with movement time held constant. Error increased with distance at a rate lying between the functions given by Weber's proportionality law and

Fullerton and Cattell's square-root law. With eyes closed, the rate of increase was less and approximated the square-root prediction.

Woodworth tried to separate the two elements of 'perception error' and 'movement error'. He reported an experiment by Fullerton and Cattell in which visual lengths were estimated and then produced; the results indicated that the perceptual error was greater than the movement error. Woodworth found that the combined error in copying a line at some distance from the drum on which it was displayed was greater than the sum of the errors in a task in which perceptual errors were virtually excluded by having model and copy close together and a task in which movement error was reduced by allowing the subject time to lay off the distance deliberately. This residual error was attributed to 'inaccuracy of intention', a failure in translation from the perceptual to the motor side.

In another experiment Woodworth compared the accuracy with which standard movements could be reproduced with various limbs, at different positions and speeds. He found that although accuracy decreased with increasing difference between the character of the standard and the reproduced movement, performance was always reasonably accurate, indicating that length judgments are not based on any single factor e.g. time taken or position sense.

Woodworth concluded that the accuracy of voluntary movement depends on the acuity of the sense modality used, the level of sensory–motor coordination, the steadiness of muscular control, and the degree of deliberateness allowed. When the use of more than one sense is possible, the most accurate predominates e.g. with eyes open the muscle sense is not attended to. But if the muscles can provide the required degree of accuracy, as in typing or piano playing, then vision is ignored.

Hollingworth (1909) studied various factors related to the accuracy of reproduction of linear movements of the finger. He found that when the standard movement was delimited by a physical stop, the subject greatly overestimated the distance when attempting to reproduce it. This 'illusion of impact' depends on the force of impact, and on the related factor of the proportion of the intended movement actually completed when the stop is reached—the closer the stop is to the intended terminus of the movement the smaller the overestimation. The constant error was several times greater than that made when a standard distance of comparable length was freely produced by the subject. He also demonstrated the central tendency or series effect—the longest standards in a series are underestimated and the shortest overestimated, with a correctly reproduced indifference point near the mean of the series. He showed how the central tendency would break down if sufficient time were allowed between successive judgments.

He found that the extent and duration of a movement could be reproduced with similar accuracy and that the errors in the two tasks were correlated. He concluded that neither factor was more fundamental than the other
in the reproduction of movement.

4.34 Accuracy of movements in different directions

Siddall, Holding, and Draper (1957) studied the speed and accuracy of
horizontal movements from a starting position to a target on the left or the
right, or closer to or farther away from the subject. They found that errors
of extent were greater than errors of direction. The former were mainly
over-shoots, the latter mainly to the right. The four directions were equally
accurate but left–right movements were the fastest. (Almost all subjects were
right handed and used their right hands.) This last result contradicted an
earlier finding (Brown and Slater-Hammel, 1949) of a slight tendency for
left–right movements to be slower than right–left. But Searle and Taylor
(1948), using simple corrective tracking movement in the same four directions as Siddall, Holding, and Draper, also found that left–right movements
were the most rapid, followed by movements away from the body, right–
left movements and, slowest of all, movements towards the body.

Corrigan and Brogden (1948, 1949) found that the precision of horizontal
linear pursuit movements of constant velocity was trigonometrically related
to the direction of movement. The precision was best in the right–forward
(away from the subject) and left–backward (towards the subject) directions,
and worst in the left–forward and right–backward directions. Since the right
arm was used, this means that the least precise movements are made when the
forearm translates along the line of its long axis, the most precise when it
translates in a direction normal to its long axis. Brogden (1953) using the
same apparatus, found that there was no consistent directional bias in the
errors of linear pursuit movements in the various directions. Begbie (1959)
suggested that this may have been due to the nature of the task, in which the
subject received immediate kinaesthetic feedback of errors and had time to
correct for any tendency to wander in a particular direction. Begbie's own
work confirmed the approximately trigonometrical relationship between
direction and errors. He had his subjects link up pairs of dots by means of
ballistically produced straight lines. The lines were of various lengths and in
various orientations. In the case of short lines, there was agreement with
Corrigan and Brogden that the relationship was biphasic (in 360°) with the
line of least error running from right–forward to left–backward; in the case
of the longest lines the relationship was quadriphasic. No really consistent
relationship emerged between direction and constant error or bias. Increasing

length had the effect of increasing total error—a direct proportional relationship with the eyes open, and a square-root relationship with eyes shut—though not by the same amount for all directions. Closing the eyes decreased the difference between subjects, between lengths, and between directions, but increased the total error, the bias, and the distinction between the error patterns of the short and long lines.

Brown, Knauft, and Rosenbaum (1948) used visually presented distances between 0·6 cm and 40 cm which had to be produced by movements of a slider in various directions relative to the body. In general the short distances were overestimated, the longer distances underestimated—a result confirmed by B. Weiss (1954, 1955)—irrespective of whether the movement was towards or away from the centre of the body. The exception was the consistent overshooting in all movements downwards in the vertical plane, a result which was ascribed to gravity, although it was not matched by a corresponding under-shooting in upward movements. There was also a tendency for outward movements to be more accurate than inward movements. Also the 0·6 cm distance was overestimated to a lesser extent than a 2·5 cm distance; it was suggested that this might be due to momentum, on the somewhat implausible assumption that only the fingers and hand were involved in the shorter movement whereas the arm also was involved in the longer movement.

B. Weiss (1954, 1955) studied a task in which the subject had to use a lever to return a spot to the centre of an oscilloscope screen with delayed visual feedback. Relative accuracy was increased by increasing the range of distances to be moved but was not affected by changing the range of lever pressures required. (For any given range, pressure and displacement were linearly related.) This suggests that distance is a more informative cue or is better remembered than pressure.

4.35 Accuracy of movement under different loads

Hollingworth also attacked a problem which had caused considerable controversy around the turn of the century—the question of whether a movement is judged differently depending on the part of the range of rotation of the joint at which it occurs. Loeb (1890) had claimed that movements were relatively underestimated when they occurred under conditions of slight contraction and overestimated when under conditions of greater contraction. He suggested that the same innervation produced larger and smaller movements under the two sets of conditions due to the greater difficulty of further contraction when the muscle was already in a state of contraction. Angier (1905) denied the existence of the effect but Delabarre (1891) found it to occur, though only with large differences of contraction, and he agreed that it was due to varying difficulty though this did not involve 'innervation feelings'. Kramer and Moskiewicz (1901) confirmed the widespread occurrence of the illusion but ascribed it to the fact that the extent of movements under different degrees of contraction cannot be directly compared because the difference in the sensation complex is so great. The comparison is therefore made on the basis of apparent duration, the only quality shared in common by the two movements. But movements in the less familiar condition of greater contraction will be slower, and hence will be shorter in extent, than movements of the same duration made in a position of less contraction. This elaborate theory was unsupported by the necessary time measurements.

Woodworth (1899) found that of the subjectively equal segments of a line, the objectively longest occurred not at the beginning but in the middle, while the shortest (those overestimated) occurred at the two extremes, which were therefore said to be the most difficult segments of the line. Hollingworth had his subjects divide the total linear excursion into several apparently equal segments and found, in agreement with Woodworth, that the longest segments occurred in the middle of the range. He also measured the duration of the segments and found that although the intermediate segments were the longest, the durations were more homogeneous than the extents, in agreement with the conjecture of Kramer and Moskiewicz, presumably because the judgment of duration, unlike extent, is based on factors elsewhere in the organism which are uninfluenced by the movement of an arm. However, Hollingworth argued that this reliance on duration could not be the whole explanation since there was in addition a tendency to reproduce the movement as a whole, in both its temporal and spatial aspects, and performance was a compromise between these two tendencies, extents in the extreme position being too short and durations too long. He concluded that all the factors mentioned by earlier workers were probably involved—the slowness of movement at the beginning and end being due to inertia (at the beginning), and degree of contraction (at the end), and relative unfamiliarity with the cues to extent. In addition the increase in the intensity of associated sensations would cause the movement to be judged greater than it really was.

Hollingworth firmly rejected any theory which would attribute the accuracy of voluntary movement solely to joint sensation or to another single type of sensory information and, together with Woodworth, leaves us with a picture of a distinct sense, based on a multiplicity of cues, and not reducible to a sense of force or duration or of initial and terminal position.

Recently, several workers have studied the effect of loading the moving limb on the production of distances. Weber and Dallenbach (1929) found that the application of various loads to a stylus had no consistent effect on the production by free arm movements of visually presented areas. The authors concluded that this resulted from the great variability caused by the cross-modal nature of the task. In later experiments they had subjects compare the sizes of pairs of figures, using the constant stimulus method. Both members of each pair were perceived by movements of the stylus along contour guides, the load being different for the two members. The chief effects of increasing load were the enlargement of a sensed area, decrease in size of a traversed angle and increase in curvature of an arc. These effects are presumably due to the greater apparent length of lines under load, and the greater effort required to negotiate an acute angle or a tight curve.

Hick (1945) reported the pattern of errors made by subjects who, pushing or pulling against a force of one to five pounds, are required to change their pressure by an increment or decrement indicated on a visual display. Errors were of the order of 5 to 15% chiefly in the direction of over-shooting. This was most marked in the case of relaxations, especially relaxations from a steady pull.

Bahrick, Fitts, and Schneider (1955) failed to find any consistent improvement in spatial accuracy of rotary or triangular movements as a result of spring loading the control, but with extended practice and knowledge such an improvement was found for the case of rotary arm movements (Bahrick, Bennett, and Fitts, 1955). Accuracy increased with increasing percentage force change and increasing basic force.

Gibbs (1954) used two types of joystick to control the position of a spot on a screen; the subject had to either continuously correct the spot's position to keep it in the centre of the screen or else move it in a discrete step from one position to another, at the same time correcting for a tendency to wander. The free-moving stick, giving isotonic muscle contraction, yielded a significantly poorer performance than a heavily spring-loaded stick giving virtually isometric contraction. Clearly a spring-loaded stick provides a position-dependent signal to the subject whereas the free-moving joystick does not.

4.4 The afferent and efferent conditions for kinaesthetic judgments

4.41 Techniques

For the sake of analysis the receptors which may serve kinaesthesis will be classified into: (1) the muscle spindle receptors along with their γ efferents, (2) Golgi tendon organs, (3) receptors in the joint capsule, (4) skin receptors. Kinaesthesis may also be served by (5) the motor outflow, or what Helmholtz called 'sensations of innervation'. The main questions are which of these five potential sources of information are used in kinaesthetic judgments and what types of judgment does each serve.

There are various techniques for isolating certain of these sources of information. These are summarized in table 4.3. In addition to these tech-

Table 4.3 Procedures for isolating sensory and motor components of kinaesthesis and the known judgments possible in each case

Receptors left active	Procedures	Known types of judgment possible
Spindle–tendon receptors	Passive movement of tongue, eye or joint with anaesthetized capsule	No passive kinaesthesis
	Direct stimulation of motor neurons	No information available
Joint receptors	Passive movement with severed tendons	No information available
Motor outflow	Active movements with anaesthesia of all afferents	No passive kinaesthesis
		Active appreciation of amplitude of movement as long as the limb is not loaded

niques, there are electro-physiological procedures for recording the discharges in each of these systems as the limb is moved. Knowledge derived from these latter procedures has already been summarized in section 4.2; in this section, the behavioural significance of this work will be discussed, but in the main the discussion will be about psychophysical measurements.

4.42 Joint receptors versus muscle spindles and Golgi tendon organs as kinaesthetic receptors

No adequate means exists of inactivating all factors other than muscle spindles and Golgi organs. Neither is there an easy way of inactivating only spindle and tendon receptors. It has not been possible, therefore, to study directly the role of these receptors in kinaesthesis. The eye has no joint receptors and, once the conjunctiva has been anaesthetized, it makes an ideal organ for studying the role of muscle spindles and tendon organs. This work has been reviewed in section 3.5, and the conclusion is that there is no position sense for an eye on the basis of spindle and tendon receptor activity alone. But although these receptors cannot signal position unaided, it may be that they form an essential component of the direction-sensitivity mechanism, in partnership with the voluntary motor outflow. To test this hypothesis one would have to deafferent the eye muscles, and test position sense with voluntary movements. Such an experiment has not been done. We predict that the spindle–γ system and tendon organs are an essential component of the total position sense system even if not sufficient in themselves. Even if it were shown that spindle–tendon receptors were not necessary for position sense in the eye, one could not conclude that they are not necessary for position sense in skeletal muscle. There is a good reason for supposing that eye movements and skeletal movements differ. The eye does not have to work against a variable load: for any position, the required innervation is constant. The eye can therefore afford to work on a 'dead-reckoning' basis. Parametric adjustment would be needed to compensate for long-term changes due to such factors as fatigue and ageing, but the moment-to-moment control could be independent of spindle–tendon feedback; indeed, saccadic movements must be independent of moment-to-moment feedback, and pursuit movements can rely on visual feedback. Skeletal muscles, on the other hand, are constantly required to operate against unpredictable load changes, and length–tension feedback is essential if desired amplitudes of movement are to be accomplished.

The tongue may provide a more suitable organ than the eye, for it too has no joint receptors, and is probably not a purely dead-reckoning device. Merton has claimed that it is impossible to tell where the surface-anaesthetized tongue is, but his observation was qualitative, and only on one subject. We have tried to repeat the experiment, but found it impossible to completely anaesthetize all the skin of the tongue, particularly the skin at the root of the tongue, which is affected most by tongue movements But even if the surface-anaesthetized tongue were shown not to have any position sense when moved passively, this would not be conclusive evidence against the necessary or sufficient role of spindles and tendon receptors. The experiment would prove that the patterns of spindle–tendon receptor discharge produced by passive movement are not sufficient to indicate position, but it would not prove that the pattern of such discharge in active movement is not sufficient or necessary. Even if the pattern of discharge from spindle–tendon receptors in passive and active movements were the same (and this is very unlikely), one could only conclude from the experiment that spindle–tendon receptors are not sufficient for position sense; one could not conclude that they are not necessary, as we showed in the case of the eye. We are assuming that the surface-anaesthetized tongue, like the surface-anaesthetized eye has both active position sense and amplitude of movement sense (although no one has done the experiment to prove it).

When we come to movements of skeletal members, the evidence for the role of spindle–tendon receptors is even more unsatisfactory. It is essential to anaesthetize the receptors in the joint capsule. The skin over the joint should also be paralysed, although this has usually not been done.

Goldscheider (1889) was the first to study the effects of anaesthetizing the joint capsule on the threshold of passive movement. He found that anaesthetizing the joints of the index finger reduced the sensitivity to passive movement, and concluded that movement is sensed on the basis of impulses arising in ligaments, tendons, and muscles, but mainly from those arising from the articular surfaces of joints. Angier (1905) agreed with this conclusion, for he found that sensitivity to movement was not much affected by the position of the limb and hence by the condition of stretch of the muscle. Strümpell (1903) found that large muscular lesions did not affect position sensitivity and this too supports Goldscheider's thesis that the joint afferents are most important, although Strümpell himself did not come to this conclusion.

Pillsbury (1901) criticized Goldscheider's conclusion that the articular surfaces are involved in the sense of movement. He could find no histological evidence that receptors exist in these surfaces, and even today such evidence does not exist. Pillsbury and later Winter (1912) reported that passive movement sensitivity at the elbow and knee joints was reduced by passing electric currents through the joints but also, and by about the same amount, when the current was passed through the ankle and wrist respectively i.e. distal to the joint moved. The effect of the current therefore could not have been due to its effect on the articular surfaces, but must have been due to its effect on stretch receptors in tendons and ligaments at either end of the insertion of the muscles.

In spite of this criticism, Goldscheider's results demonstrate that receptors in, or close to the joint capsule play an important role in position sensitivity. More recent evidence by Browne, Lee, and Ring (1954) also supports Goldscheider's general thesis. The metatarso-phalangeal joint of the great toe of human subjects was moved passively at two speeds (1 and 2°/sec). The subjects had to indicate when they felt the movement, which was found on average to be when the toe had moved through about 4°, although some subjects required movements of up to 15°. One of those requiring a large angle had laxity of the capsule, and some of those with high sensitivity had mild thickening of the joint. Appreciation of downward movement was found to be grossly disturbed by anaesthesia on the upper aspect of the capsule, which suggests that the end-organs concerned are stretch receptors. All sense of position and passive movement was lost when the whole capsule was anaesthetized with procaine. When the subjects tensed the muscles of the leg, the sense of movement in the passively moved toe was restored, and

Browne *et al.* concluded that passive movement in the relaxed limb is appreciated on the basis of tensions in the joint capsule, whereas passive movements of the tensed limb are appreciated both by capsule receptors and impulses from muscles and tendons.

Provins (1958) repeated the experiment by Browne *et al.* using the index finger. He could find no evidence that tensing the anaesthetized finger restored the sense of position or passive movement, and therefore rejected the suggestion that relaxed passive movement and tensed passive movement are served by different receptors.

Cohen (1958b) asked blindfolded subjects to place a finger on a reference point, then to lower the arm and bring the finger back to the same point. In order to interfere with any contribution which tactile receptors might have made, adhesive tape was stretched over the skin at the shoulder joint, and in order to interfere with musculo–tendon receptors, some trials were run with a 1 kg weight in the subject's hand in the test pointing. The weight was found to cause a small but significant increase in mean error of pointing, and Cohen concluded that, as the weight affected only the musculo–tendon receptors and not the joint receptors, the musculo–tendon receptors must have been making a small contribution to position sense in active movement. Cohen may not be justified in assuming that the weight would have no effect on joint receptors; Skoglund (1956) found that a change of tension in the leg muscles of the cat modified the afferent impulses recorded from the knee joint. But in any case, his conclusion is completely unwarranted. The fact that a load affected the accuracy of active pointing was probably due, not to the effect it had on the muscle receptors, but to the effect it had on the motor outflow. Indeed, the muscle receptors probably prevented the disturbance from being worse than it was. Evidence discussed in the next section supports this interpretation.

The only other evidence which bears on the relative contribution of joint receptors and muscle–tendon receptors is the observation made by Sarnoff and Arrowhead (1947). They applied procaine to the lumbar region of the spinal cord of human subjects. Vasomotor, pain, and stretch reflexes were blocked, while motor power, touch, and position sense were unimpaired. This suggests that position sense and stretch reflexes depend on different afferents and, although Sarnoff and Arrowhead's experiment did not identify the afferents in either case, it does suggest that position sense does not depend on muscle–tendon receptors, for these presumably serve the stretch reflex.

In conclusion, it may be stated that receptors in the joint capsule contribute to the sense of position and of passive movement, but whether they are the only receptors involved is not known. It seems, on balance, doubtful whether muscle–tendon receptors serve the passive movement sense; it is more likely that they are involved in judgments of the amplitude of active movement, but the evidence is by no means clear.

Further work is necessary to clarify these questions. Experiments on animals are needed in which sensitivity to passive movement is recorded by a conditioning procedure, before and after the tendons are severed. Only by severing the tendons is it possible to isolate the joint receptors. On the other hand, we need a technique for inducing activity in muscle–tendon receptors in the absence of joint receptors and motor outflow. Passive movement with anaesthetized joint receptors is one way of doing this. But passive movement probably does not induce the same discharge pattern as active movement, and although such experiments demonstrate that spindle–tendon receptors are not sufficient to signal passive movement, they do not indicate the role of these receptors in active movement. For this purpose it would be necessary to induce spindle–tendon activity typical of active movement but without motor outflow. Perhaps it would be possible to stimulate the distal end of severed motor neurons or motoneuron pools in the cord, which have been isolated from tracts descending from higher centres. The muscle afferents would be left intact, the joint receptors anaesthetized, and the sensitivity to movements investigated by use of a conditioning procedure.

4.43 Kinaesthesis and the motor outflow

The best 'preparation' for studying the role of motor outflow in kin-aesthesis is one in which all afferent pathways are anaesthetized or severed. The only recorded experiments on such a preparation are those of Lashley (1917) on a patient with anaesthesia of most of the leg afferents due to a bullet wound to the spinal cord. The patient had no appreciation of passive move-ment at the knee; he could not maintain his lower leg in one position for long, and yet was unaware that he had failed to do so; and he could not actively return his leg to a position into which it had been passively placed. Lashley realized, as few have realized since, that the above tests do not exclude the possibility that muscle receptors may still be active and serve to indicate amplitude of movement, if not position. He tested for this possibility by asking the patient to move his leg through a given angle against various spring loads. The patient was not able to compensate for the different loads, although he had the impression that he had done so. In concluding that this result showed the absence of spindle–tendon afference, Lashley was assuming that load compensation is the only kinaesthetic function of these receptors; he was probably right but not necessarily so.

When the leg was not loaded the patient could make movements in the right direction and through consistent amplitudes on command, even though the specified distances in inches were not accurately achieved. In fact his ability to reduplicate a given amplitude of movement was as good as that of a normal person. Lashley concluded that motor innervation provides an accurate source of information of the amplitude of active movement, as long as the limb is not loaded. The accuracy did not depend on the speed of movement in the way it would have done had the patient been basing his estimates of movement amplitude on the time duration of the movement.

Motor outflow is obviously of prime importance in ballistic movements, especially in well-practised ballistic movements such as are involved in piano playing. Such movements are so rapid that kinaesthetic feedback has no time to act during the actual movement (Chernikoff and Taylor, 1952), although it may be involved in the preparatory adjustments.

5

The vestibular apparatus

5.1 The structure and physiology of the labyrinths

5.11 The receptors and their stimuli

The vestibular apparatus, or labyrinths, consists of sense organs in the cavities of the inner ear. These evolved along with the auditory cochlea from ancestral organs in primitive vertebrates. These primitive organs consisted of cells covered with sensory hairs or cilia situated in pits in the skin of aquatic animals. They were mechano-receptors, sensitive to vibrations or movements of the fluid filling the depressions. At a later time these depressions became specialized and linked by canals under the skin to form the lateral-line and vestibular organs of fish and, by further specialization, the vestibular-cochlear organs in the bony cavities of the inner ears of mammals. Four subdivisions evolved, which in mammals are represented by the *spiral cochlea*, sensitive to high-frequency vibrations; the sac-shaped *utricle*, sensitive to linear acceleration; the three circular *canals*, sensitive to angular acceleration about any head axis; and the saccule. The function of mammalian saccules is not known; they are probably vestigial and will not be discussed further. Under artificial conditions each of the three remaining receptors may be stimulated by any type of mechanical disturbance. They are 'tuned in' to their normal, or adequate, stimuli as a consequence of the inertia and damping of their associated structures, which filter off or attenuate the effects of other, or inadequate, stimuli.

This division between organs sensitive to rotary acceleration and organs sensitive to linear acceleration is very primitive. But the significance of the division has often been misunderstood. Many writers have distinguished between static or head-position receptors (the utricles) and dynamic or head-movement receptors (the canals). This is a false distinction, as Jongkees and Groen (1946) pointed out. Einstein's theory of gravitation tells us that gravity, accelerative movement, and centrifugal force are indistinguishable as stimuli. The utricle is sensitive to linear acceleration, however it is produced. It is therefore as much a dynamic receptor as the canals, which are sensitive to rotary acceleration. Both receptors also have a static aspect: the utricles are responsive to the direction of linear acceleration, as well as to its amount, and similarly the canals, as a triplet, are sensitive to the direction of rotary acceleration about any head axis as well as to its amount. Both organs are therefore both dynamic and static receptors.

It is to be expected that rotary acceleration will have some effect on the utricles, and that linear acceleration will have some effect on the canals. De Kleyn and Magnus (1921) found some response to linear acceleration when only the canals were intact; destruction of the canals eliminated this response. Gernandt (1950) recorded regular responses from the horizontal canal as a function of centrifugal (linear) acceleration. Corresponding to this finding are observations by Gray and Crosbie (1958) and Gray (1960) that the oculogyral illusion, which is thought to be induced by canal activity, is affected by varying the radius of rotation while maintaining constant angular velocity, that is, by changes in linear acceleration when there is no change in angular acceleration. However, Graybiel, Niven, and MacCorquodale (1956) found the oculogyral illusion unaffected by the radius of turn, and we shall assume for the sake of convenience that the canals and utricle do have separate, though overlapping functions.

5.12 The vestibular canals

The canals are usually called the semicircular canals, but the prefix 'semi' is misleading; although the canals share a common cavity in the utricle, each one is functionally a complete and independent fluid circuit (see figure 5.1).

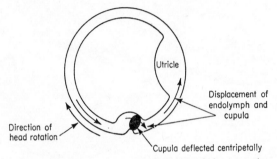

Figure 5.1 Schematic diagram of a vestibular canal showing the complete fluid circuit. The arrows depict the consequences of a clockwise rotation of the head in the plane of the canal

The anatomical arrangement of the structures is shown in figure 5.2. The canals, sacs, and cochlea are suspended in a fluid, the perilymph, which fills the cavity between them and the bone. Inside, the organs share a common cavity which is filled with endolymph fluid. Ducts join the utricle–canal system with the saccule, and the saccule with the cochlea. Another duct runs from the utricle to a lymphatic reservoir, the endolymphatic sac. In man, the canals lie in planes approximately at right angles to each other. There is a laterally placed canal making 30° to the horizontal, a vertical superior canal making 55° to the frontal plane open in front, and a vertical posterior canal making 45° to the frontal plane, as in figure 5.3. Each canal has a contra-lateral parallel partner. A canal and its contralateral partner form a synergic pair, for instance, the right superior and left posterior.

At one point of each canal, near its junction with the utricle, is a swelling or *ampulla*, which contains the sensory epithelium or *crista ampullaris*. The structure of a crista is shown in figures 5.4 and 5.5. It is a ridge of epithelium protruding into the cavity or *lumen* of the ampulla, and carrying many multi-ciliated sensory cells interspersed with structural cells. The cilia of all the cells project into a common gelatinous mass or *cupula* reaching to the far side of

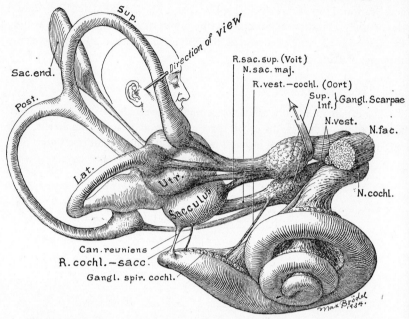

Figure 5.2 Diagram of the inner ear, showing the semicircular canals, utricle, saccule, and cochlea, together with the nerves innervating them. [From Hardy, *Anat. Rec.*, 1934, **59**, 412]

the ampulla which is arched at this point so that the cupula may swing from side to side like a swing door. At the same time, the cupula forms an effective seal preventing any leakage of endolymph past that point. In effect, the cupula is a damped, spring-loaded pendulum.

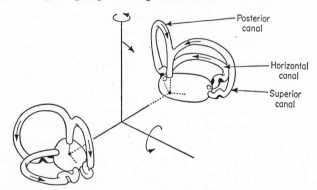

Figure 5.3 The arrangement of the vestibular canals on each side of the head. [Adapted from Groen, 1961]

The general *hydrodynamic theory* of the canals, the theory that stresses the importance of movements of the endolymph, was outlined independently by Mach (1875), Breuer (1874), and Crum Brown (1875) (see Dusser de Barenne, 1934, and Wendt, 1951, for the early history of the subject). The cupula is a difficult structure to see because it has the same refractive index as

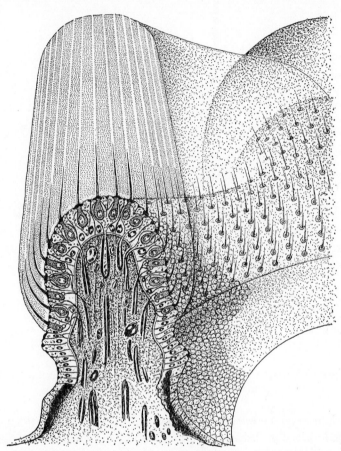

Figure 5.4 Schematic drawing of one half of a crista ampullaris, showing innervation of its epithelium. Thick nerve fibres forming nerve calyces round type I hair cells at the summit of the crista; medium calibre fibres innervating type I hair cells on the slope of the crista; medium calibre and fine nerve fibres forming a nerve plexus innervating hair cells of type II. The sensory hairs pass from the hair cells into fine canals in the cupula, which is separated from the epithelium by a narrow subcupular space. [From Wersäll, 1956]

the endolymph. For this reason, the early theorists did not realize that the cupula seals the lumen of the ampulla; they thought that the endolymph flowed over the cristae. It was not until 1931 that Steinhausen observed the functioning of the cupula *in vivo* by injecting Indian ink into the endolymph

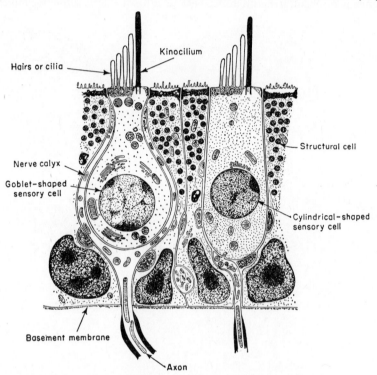

Figure 5.5 Diagrammatic representation of the detailed structure of the crista ampullaris. [From Engström, 1961]

of a fish (the ray). Developing some earlier work by Schmaltz (1932), Steinhausen described the behaviour of the cupula by the well-known differential equation for the torsion pendulum:

$$H\ddot{\xi} + \pi\dot{\xi} + \Delta\xi = 0,$$

where $H =$ moment of inertia of the cupula
$\pi =$ moment of friction at unit angular velocity
$\Delta =$ directional momentum at unit angle
$\xi =$ angular deviation of the endolymph
$\dot{\xi} =$ angular velocity of the endolymph
$\ddot{\xi} =$ angular acceleration of the endolymph

Little direct study of the behaviour of the cupula has been made, but by the use of behavioural indices it has been confirmed that within limits this equation adequately describes the behaviour of the end-organ (Mayne, 1950; Van Egmond, Groen, and Jongkees, 1949a). The limits of the equation's applicability have recently been investigated by the use of transfer functions by Niven and Hixson (1961), and Hixson and Niven (1961, 1962). The lag of the nystagmic eye-velocity response behind a sinusoidal angular-acceleration stimulus was used to quantify the transfer function of the skull-acceleration-to-cupula-displacement transducer system. The system was found to become non-linear as the frequency of stimulation approached the low value of 0·02 c/s, that is, when the cupula deflection was greatest. At higher frequencies the rapid alternation of acceleration and deceleration prevents the cupula from being deflected through a large angle. The cupula's range of linearity has also been studied, using as a measure the duration of the apparent visual movement produced by rotation (Mann, 1952b).

Apart from the limits to linearity (applicability of the torsion pendulum formula) set by the mechanical properties of the end-organ, the non-linearities in the end-organ-response-to-behaviour transformation must be considered. This transformation may be severely non-linear, and therefore the torsion pendulum formula only partially accounts for the behavioural consequences of rotations of the body; inputs from other modalities, and central inhibitory processes complicate the behaviour in natural circumstances, as we shall see later. Both the methods discussed above rely on the assumption that the non-linearity is in the stimulus-to-cupular-response part rather than the cupular-response part of the function. Thus it may be that the torsion pendulum formula is actually a better fit for the first leg of the system than is realized.

It is clear from what has been said that the cristae discharge when the canals move relative to the endolymph. Because of friction between the endolymph and the canal wall, the fluid catches up with the movement of the wall during a period of rotation at constant angular velocity. When this has happened the cupula will return to its resting position and the discharge will cease. If the body is now decelerated and brought to rest, the cupula will be displaced in the opposite direction. Because it is heavily damped it will take up to about 30 sec to regain its central position. During this recovery period the subject will behave as if he is decelerating. He will fall to one side, his eyes will move nystagmically (see later), and he will report turning sensations and nausea.

If an acceleration is followed immediately by a deceleration, as is usually the case when a person voluntarily turns his body, the two opposed deflections of the cupula cancel out, leaving no residual deflection and no after-effects. Provided that the movement does not last more than about 3 sec, a person is able to judge accurately the angle of turning (Mulder's law).

All this assumes that the subject does not move his head while he is rotating. If he does, he will modify the effects which the rotation has on his vestibular canals. If he rotates his head about the same axis as the applied rotation, he will momentarily increase or decrease his total angular acceleration. If he turns his head about any other axis, his own angular velocity will interact with the applied velocity in a complex way. Anyone who has tried to turn the axis of a spinning wheel at right angles to itself will have noticed that the axis tends to rotate at right angles to both itself and to the manually applied torque. This is known as *precession*, but we shall refer to the effect as *cross-coupling*. Groen (1961) has analysed the effects of cross-coupling on the vestibular system. In figure 5.6 the two horizontal canals are in the plane of

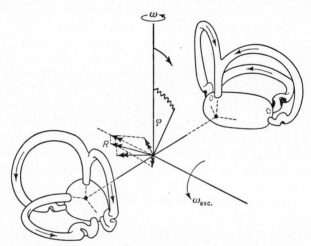

Figure 5.6 Demonstrating cross-coupling between head tilt and body rotation. The head is rotating round a vertical axis, angular velocity ω. The lateral canals are in a horizontal plane. The head is suddenly inclined forwards over the angle φ. A momentum excess $\omega_{exc.}$ results, driving the endolymph clockwise; hence a counterclockwise sensation, equivalent to a stimulus intensity

$$\omega_{exc.} = \omega \sqrt{(1 - \cos \varphi)^2 + 2 \sin^2 \varphi}.$$

[From Groen, 1961]

rotation (ω); the vertical canals are perpendicular to the plane of rotation and so are not affected by it. When the head is quickly tilted forwards through an angle φ the vertical canals project themselves as narrow ellipses in the plane of rotation and become subject to a momentum component of that rotation of $\omega \sin \varphi$. The horizontal canals each lose a fraction of their original angular momentum equal to $\omega \cos \varphi$, and therefore have a final momentum of $\omega (1 - \cos \varphi)$. The three momenta in the three canals add like vectors; the resultant momentum over the three canals just after the head has reached its new position is therefore given by

$$\omega \sqrt{(1 - \cos \varphi)^2 + \sin^2 \varphi + \sin^2 \varphi}.$$

This effect can be very powerful and its behavioural and subjective effects are very distressing. It has often been confused with the Coriolis effect which properly refers to the acceleration effects in a rotating system when a mass is submitted to *linear translation* (see section 16.51). Guedry and Montague (1961) gave a misleading analysis of the effects of head rotations in a rotating vehicle. This analysis was entirely in terms of the Coriolis effects produced by the relative radial movements of different parts of each canal. These effects must be small compared to cross-coupling effects, and on Guedry and Montague's admission do not account for the differential effects produced by different directions of head movement. Cross-coupling does account for what these authors regard as anomalous results.

5.13 The vestibular end-organ potential

The microstructure of the sensory epithelium of the cristae is shown diagrammatically in figure 5.5. There are two types of sensory hair cell. One is flask shaped and almost totally enclosed in a goblet-shaped nerve chalice. These endings are innervated by the largest diameter fibres in the cristal nerve. Any one nerve fibre may branch to supply several sensory cells. The second type of sensory cell is cylindrical, and innervated by several knob-shaped nerve endings (Wersäll, 1956; Engström, 1961).

Each sensory cell projects about 70 fine cilia into the cupula mass; these *stereocilia* are distinguishable from a single, larger *kinocilium* in each cell. The cilia membranes and cell membrane are continuous. A resting potential of about 160 mv exists across the membrane; the cell interior is negative with respect to the contents of the cupula. Whether this potential is maintained by an active 'ion pump' or because the cilia membrane is an insulator is not known; but in any case the whole structure is a 'charged condenser'.

Microelectrode studies have revealed that a centripetal cupular deflection is accompanied by a decrease or depolarization of the resting 'condenser' potential across the cilia membrane, and that a centrifugal deflection is accompanied by an increase in the resting potential (Trincker, 1961, 1962; Gernandt, 1959). It is thought to be the shearing movement of the cilia produced by the bending of the cupula which alters the charge on the 'condenser'. Lowenstein (1961) suggested that these changes in the membrane potential are due to a piezoelectric effect, that is, the effect by which potentials are induced in crystals that are subjected to shearing forces. However, such a mechanism could not generate the large changes in potential which occur across the membrane, and Lowenstein had to postulate an amplifier mechanism at the membrane. Dohlman (1959) suggested that the slight movement of the cilia in the cupula substance induces a differential migration of small positive potassium ions and large negative polysaccharide ions.

A mechanism something like that suggested by Dohlman has recently been shown to exist in the vestibular end-organ by Vilstrup and Jensen (1961). It had been known for some time that the cupula contains a muco-polysaccharide, potassium hyaluronate, which has interesting mechanical and electrical properties. The molecules are thread-like and extremely long (several thousand Å). They form a stroma-like network, the meshes of which contain a solvent. The molecules are poly-electrolytes; each one carries a thousand or so electronegatively charged side-chains along its length. Positive potassium ions in the solvent maintain the electroneutrality of the system. Solutions of this substance possess a peculiar structural viscosity known as 'flow viscosity'. If they are displaced they show a tendency to return to their original position. Jensen, Koefoed, and Vilstrup (1954) found that if a solution of potassium hyaluronate in a glass column is displaced into an elastically strained position, the advanced front of the column becomes positive with respect to the back, with a potential difference of over 100 mv. This potential persists as long as the column is deflected, at least for several days. This potential was called the 'displacement potential'. What seems to be happening is that during bending, the electronegative ions bonded to the hyaluronate molecules become concentrated on the concave side of the column and chase out the mobile positive potassium ions. Christiansen (1964) has suggested a way in which an electromechanical transducer based on displacement potentials in muco-polysaccharides could be bidirectional in the way that the vestibular end-organs are known to be. Each muco-saccharide molecule could be anchored at one end to a cilium of a hair cell, so that the molecules are all kept in orderly arrangement. Their geometrical disposition is not known but it could be that deflections of the cupula induce a migration of positive ions at right angles to the cilia in one direction or the other. The resulting effect on the hair cell would then be bidirectional provided there was some transverse asymmetrical feature of each hair cell.

Lowenstein and Wersäll (1959) found that the kinocilium is always situated on that side of the stereocilia that points in the direction of depolarizing (excitatory) cupula deflection. Here then is the required asymmetry: the kinocilium could 'register' the increase or decrease in the positive ion concentration as the cupula is deflected one way or the other, resulting in depolarization or hyperpolarization of the hair cell.

Consider now the sequence of events in the right horizontal canal when the head is rotated to the right in the plane of the canal. The inertia of the endolymph causes it to lag behind the canal walls, and flow to the left, relative to the walls of the canal. The cupula is deflected centripetally (ampullopetally) relative to the utricle (see figure 5.1). This results in a depolarization of the hair-cell membrane and a consequent increase in the frequency of firing in the sensory neurons. There occurs simultaneously a centrifugal (ampullofugal) deflection of the left-hand cupula which induces an increase in the resting potential (hyperpolarization), and a decrease in the frequency of the afferent discharge. The effect on each side is of course reversed for a head rotation to the left. The end-organs are thus bidirectional, although the sensory membrane as a whole is known to be more sensitive to depolarization than to hyperpolarization at least in some animals. This means that in the horizontal canals, centripetal deflection is a more effective stimulus than centrifugal deflection. In other words, body rotation stimulates the ipsilateral horizontal canal more intensely than the contralateral canal (see table 5.1).

Table 5.1 Summarizing the consequences in the horizontal canal of rotating a person to the left

Right ear	Left ear
Ampullofugal deflection	Ampullopetal deflection
Increased resting potential (hyperpolarization)	Decreased resting potential (depolarization)
Decreased frequency of afferent firing	Increased frequency of afferent firing
Less sensitive response according to Ewald's second law	More sensitive response according to Ewald's second law

In the vertical canals, depolarization is produced by centrifugal deflection, which is therefore the more effective stimulus. This pattern of directional preponderance in the three canals is known as Ewald's second law of vestibular function (his first law states that cupula deflection is the proximal stimulus for rotary acceleration). He inferred his second law by observing nystagmus in a pigeon as he deflected a cupula either way by means of a 'pneumatic hammer' inserted into the lumen of one of the pigeon's vestibular canals (Ewald, 1892).

This law cannot describe the behaviour of individual sensory cells of the cristae. Most of these are bidirectional, but some give an excitatory response and some an inhibitory response to deflection in a given direction (Gernandt, 1949). Possibly these different types, and intermediate types, form a continuum, and differ because of the value of a bias mechanism, analogous to the bias on a thermionic valve (Lowenstein, 1956b). Ewald's law, in so far as it depends on peripheral mechanisms, could be an expression of the average bias over the whole population of cells in each crista.

Another possibility is that it could be a reflection of the fact that there is a lower limit of nerve discharge but no obvious 'ceiling'. If this last mechanism were the cause of peripheral directional preponderance, preponderance should become more evident with more intense stimuli. Groen (1960a) has claimed that this is so. The behavioural implications of Ewald's second law are discussed in section 5.23.

5.14 The utricles

The utricle or statolith organ is a sac at the junction of the three vestibuarl canals. It contains a sensory mechanism, the macula, which responds to the extent and direction of linear acceleration, including the direction and extent of gravity. Organs sensitive to position with respect to gravity are very old in the evolutionary scale. They are represented in every animal phylum. Their general mode of functioning is remarkably constant. In invertebrates they are known as statocysts. One of the neatest ways of studying their function is provided by the crayfish's habit of moulting the linings of its statocysts every so often. The crayfish uses its chelae to replace grains of sand in the new cavity. These grains serve to stimulate the sensory cells as the crayfish moves about. If iron filings are the only small particles available, the crayfish will place these in its statocyst cavity. If a magnet is now moved about, the crayfish will alter the orientation of its body accordingly. For further details of the comparative study of otolith organs see Lowenstein (1950, 1956a).

The utricle of mammals is filled with endolymph which has a specific gravity of about 1·02. The *macula* or receptor organ is situated on the anterior and medial walls of the utricular cavity. When the head is erect, the macula is in an approximately horizontal position (see figure 5.7). The macula consists of an epithelium of ciliated sensory cells. The cilia protrude upwards from the macula surface and are embedded in a gelatinous substance containing calcium carbonate particles—the otoliths or otoconia (see figure 5.8). The specific gravity of the otoconia is about 2·95 and is thus greater than that of the surrounding endolymph. Such an organ is clearly suited to respond to displacements of the heavy otoconia induced by changes in the extent and direction of linear acceleration.

There has been much dispute about the precise way in which the otoconia stimulate the hair cells. Magnus (1924) claimed that tension acting vertically on the macula by the weight of the otoconia is the effective stimulus. Recently Trincker (1962) has recorded the potential changes inside the sensory cells of the macula of the guinea pig. Only shearing forces produced

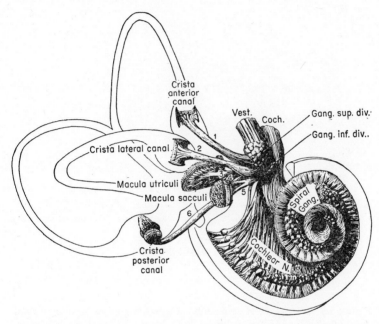

Figure 5.7 Lateral view of vestibular and cochlear nerves and their branches in relation to their receptor organs. Of the membranous labyrinth, only the sensory epithelia are shaded. [Adapted from Krieg, J. S., *Functional Neuroanatomy*, 1953. Brain Books, Box Nine, Evanston, Ill.]

by tangential displacements were effective in producing sensory responses. Pressure or tension applied at right angles to the macular epithelium had no effect. Békésy (1953) had found a similar state of affairs in the organ of Corti in the cochlea. Shearing forces at first rise steeply as the head and the utricle are tilted away from the upright. Pressure forces, on the other hand, change only slowly at first. In other words, the shearing force theory predicts that the utricular response is a sine function of the angle of tilt, whereas the pressure theory predicts that it is a cosine function of tilt. Trincker was able to demonstrate the sine function in actual recordings from the tilting macula of the guinea pig (see figure 5.9).

The operation of the utricle is presumably multidirectional but no attention seems to have been paid to this aspect in the literature.

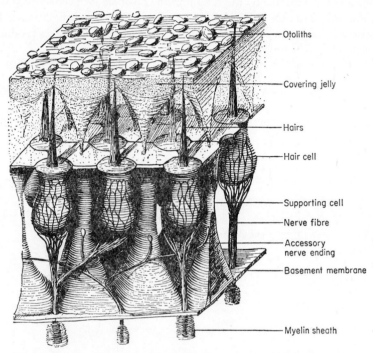

Otoliths

Covering jelly

Hairs

Hair cell

Supporting cell

Nerve fibre

Accessory nerve ending

Basement membrane

Myelin sheath

Figure 5.8 Stereogram of epithelium of macula and associated endings of vestibular nerve. [Adapted from Krieg, J. S., *Functional Neuroanatomy*, 1953. Brain Books, Box Nine, Evanston, Ill.]

Wing (1963) was not able to record any consistent potential changes in the mammalian vestibular ganglion in response to head tilt. He suggested that the utricle is largely vestigial in higher mammals, where vision and kinaesthesis are dominant in maintaining balance.

5.15 Labyrinthine pathways

The vestibular part of the eighth nerve on each side passes to the four vestibular nuclei, which sit astride the cerebellar peduncle on one side of the medulla. The vestibular nuclei on the right are connected to those on the left directly as well as by fibres running through the reticular formation.

Other fibres from two of the vestibular nuclei form the medial longitudinal fasciculus which ascends to the oculomotor centres of the brain stem to mediate the vestibular-nystagmus reflex. Yet other fibres descend into the spinal cord as the vestibulo-spinal tract, which terminates in motoneuron pools in the cord and mediates vestibulo-spinal reflexes. Some fibres pass

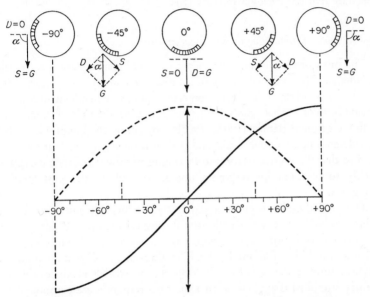

Figure 5.9 Stimulation of the macular sensory epithelium by shearing force, and the characteristic curve representing information input. *Above:* schematic drawings of the utricle, with its macula and statolithic membrane, undergoing tilting in both directions around the horizontal rostro-occipital axis of the head. Forces on the sensory epithelium represented as vector parallelograms. G, gravity; S, shearing force (the component of gravity, acting tangentially on the epithelium); D, pressure (or tension), the component, acting vertically on the macula. In a normal position, $S = 0$; at 90°, $D = 0$. *Below:* the relationship of shearing force (continuous line) and pressure (broken line) to degree of inclination (abscissa): shearing gives a sine relationship, while pressure gives the cosine. [From Trincker, 1962]

directly to the cerebellum and reticular system. Although doubted for a long time, it is now established that the vestibular apparatus projects to the cerebral cortex, principally contralaterally to the superior ectosylvian fissure. As always with afferent cortical projection, this pathway runs via the thalamus (Gernandt, 1964).

The foregoing account of the complex ramifications of the vestibular afferents throughout the central nervous system suggests that the behavioural consequences of vestibular stimulation may be equally complex. However, the paucity of cortical projections suggests that these behavioural consequences are largely at the unconscious reflex level. What follows will demonstrate that these suggestions are true.

5.16 Methods of stimulating the vestibular apparatus

The most obvious way to stimulate the vestibular apparatus is to utilize the 'adequate' (i.e. normal) mode of stimulation, namely rotary acceleration. In order to avoid the difficulty of observing a subject when he is rotating, use is made of the fact that vestibular responses outlive a period of deceleration.

In the original Bárány (1907a, 1907b) procedure, the blindfolded subject is accelerated in a rotating chair, and is then rotated for 20 sec at a constant speed so that the cupula restores to its resting position, and then decelerated quickly to rest and his responses noted, particularly the post-rotational nystagmus.

This procedure has been criticized on two counts. The initial acceleration which produces the cupular deflection during rotation (per-rotatory stimulus) is of the order of $45°/\text{sec}^2$, which is a massive stimulus in comparison with the threshold of about $1°/\text{sec}^2$. The after-effects of such a stimulus do not have time to decay before the deceleration (which produces the post-rotatory stimulus) is applied, so that the final responses are compounded of the opposed after-effects of the per-rotatory and post-rotatory stimuli. The second criticism is that the deceleratory stimulus is excessively massive; the end-organs are being 'sledge-hammered' in a very atypical way.

Buys (1937) modified Bárány's method to overcome these objections. The acceleration is kept below threshold value, so that the per-rotatory after-effects are eliminated. The deceleration may be controlled so that any value of deceleration over any desired period of time may be applied. Even this method is not without its critics. Fukuda, Hinoki, and Tokita (1957) have suggested that the accelerations used are not really sub-threshold. Other refinements of Bárány's method have been suggested (e.g. Fukuda, 1959a, 1959b), and a vast clinical literature has grown up.

A modern development of the above method is known as cupulometry. In this technique, the duration of nystagmus, or of other vestibular responses following rapid deceleration, is plotted as a function of the velocity reached before deceleration (Van Egmond and Groen, 1955; Groen, 1957; Ek, Jongkees, and Klijn, 1960). The resulting graph is known as a cupulogram, and is ideally a linear function.

In so far as the duration of post-rotational nystagmus represents the time which the cupula takes to return to equilibrium, the slope of the cupulogram is equal to π/Δ (see page 102). Ideally, this is a method of determining some of the constants of the differential equation of cupular function. However,

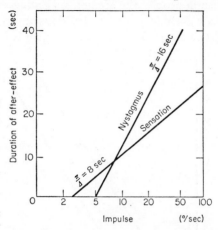

Figure 5.10 Cupulograms for normal subject showing different slopes for sensation and nystagmus. [From Groen, 1960b]

the cupulogram slope changes with practice, and it is unlikely that this is due to a change in cupular deviation. Figure 5.10 shows the averaged cupulogram from ordinary people, and figure 5.11 the averaged cupulogram from practised aviators. Clearly, nystagmus is not a simple function of cupular restoration. A cupulogram may be obtained by plotting the duration of

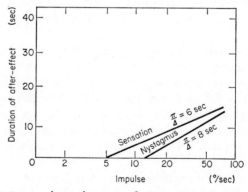

Figure 5.11 Averaged cupulograms of 18 experienced aviators showing unusually low value of $\dfrac{\pi}{\Delta}$. [From Groen, 1960b]

post-rotational after-sensations (vertigo) instead of nystagmus. Any difference between the slopes of the two kinds of cupulogram in the same person must be due to effects in the central nervous system. The interesting point is that the slopes for the different effects are more alike in people susceptible to motion sickness than in people who are not, suggesting that people subject to motion sickness are not able to modify the effects of vestibular stimulation by central control (see figure 5.12). The cupulogram from the experienced

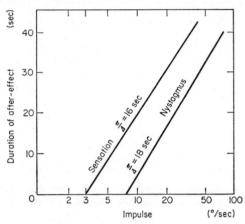

Figure 5.12 Cupulograms for an individual sensitive to motion sickness showing similar slopes for sensation and nystagmus. [From Groen, 1960b]

aviators is lower than normal, reflecting a high degree of cortical suppression of vestibular after-effects. This could be because aviators learn to suppress these after-effects, or because only those with low cupulograms become aviators.

Several investigators have suggested that the speed of the slow phase of vestibular nystagmus is a better indicator of cupular deflection than is the nystagmus duration (Lorente de Nó, 1931; Dohlman, 1935; Hallpike and Hood, 1953; Van Egmond and Tolk, 1954; Dohlman, Henriksson, and Andrén, 1956; Henriksson, 1956; Benson, 1964). Such a measure does not have the indefinite 'end point' of the duration measure, although it requires more elaborate apparatus. There is dispute as to whether or not it changes during habituation.

For further details of cupulometry, see Van Egmond, Groen, and Jong-kees (1949a), and Cawthorne, Dix, Hallpike, and Hood (1956).

Electronystagmography (see section 3.43) is now the standard method of recording nystagmus, and this method may easily be applied to a rotating subject. Thus, per-rotatory methods are now in common use (Montandon, 1954; De Boer, Carels, and Philipszoon, 1963; Henriksson, 1955b).

The vestibular apparatus may also be stimulated by inadequate (i.e. unusual) stimuli. If the outer ear is irrigated with water above blood temperature, heat is conducted into the vestibular apparatus, reaching the most lateral part of the horizontal canal first, and then the lateral parts of the other canals. Temperature gradients, and hence specific gravity gradients, will come to exist across the ampullae; if a particular canal is not in a horizontal plane, convection currents will be induced in the endolymph which will displace the cupula. If cold water is used, a temperature and specific gravity gradient will be induced in the opposite direction and will deflect the cupula the other way. This theory of caloric vestibular stimulation goes back to Bárány (1906c), and has received support recently from the results of an experiment by Bergstedt (1961a) which showed that the intensity of vestibular nystagmus induced by caloric stimulation is increased by centrifugally increasing the gravitational field and hence the convection currents. If the heat acted directly on the end-organs, centrifugal force would make no difference, because in itself it does not stimulate the canals.

With this method it is possible to stimulate the vestibular system on either side of the head, and any one canal in either direction. The procedure of caloric stimulation has been standardized for both clinical and research use by Fitzgerald and Hallpike (1942).

An electric current, either a.c. or d.c., may be passed through the skull or to inserted electrodes. Faradic (a.c.) stimulation produces a single-phase nystagmic response. Galvanic (d.c.) stimulation produces nystagmus with the slow phase directed towards the anode. Reversing the polarity of the current reverses the direction of the nystagmus (Spiegel and Scala, 1943). In animals, the cristae may be stimulated directly by inserting a small piston or pneumatic hammer into the lumen of the canals (Ewald, 1892). All these inadequate modes of stimulation have the advantage over rotation that the various cristae and maculae may be stimulated separately. For a full review of methods of stimulating the labyrinths see Arslan (1955) and Aschan (1956).

5.2 Vestibular thresholds

5.21 Thresholds for rotary acceleration

There are three manifestations of vestibular canal activity which have been used to determine threshold values. These are: (1) reports of feelings of rotation, (2) nystagmus, and (3) the oculogyral effect (the apparent movement of a point of light in the dark). It is misleading to regard each of these thresholds as measures of a single underlying end-organ threshold; they each reflect threshold functions at various levels of partially distinct control systems. Some of the many determinations of these three thresholds are shown in table 5.2. On the whole, the threshold for the first report of rotation is higher than that for the first appearance of nystagmus, which in turn is higher than the threshold for the first appearance of the oculogyral illusion (see later).

Table 5.2 Thresholds for various vestibular functions

Method	Investigator	Threshold value (deg/sec^2)
First reports of rotation	Mach (1875)	2·0
	Dodge (1923c)	2·0
	Tumarkin (1937)	0·2
	Hilding (1953)	Less than 1·0
	Clark and Stewart (1962)	0·12
Nystagmus	Dohlman (1935)	1·0
	Buys (1937) Buys and Rijlant (1939) }	0·8
	Montandon and Russbach (1955)	0·8
	Ek, Jongkees, and Klijn (1959)	0·04 (in pigeon)
Oculogyral illusion	Christian (1939, 1940)	0·13
	Groen and Jongkees (1948) (using after-sensations)	0·5
	Graybiel, Kerr, and Bartley (1948)	0·12

It is not surprising that there is so much variation between the different determinations, even of the same threshold. It is not easy to accelerate a human subject smoothly, and avoid all extraneous sources of stimulation, and experimenters have differed in the extent to which they were successful. In any case, there are many factors which modify the results, such as the psychophysical method used and the duration of the stimulus. In addition, it is to be expected that the utricles would be stimulated by the centrifugal force induced by rotation about the body axis.

Ek, Jongkees, and Klijn (1959) reduced the level of background stimulation of the vestibular system in a pigeon by testing it in a quiet dark room, and were able to induce a detectable nystagmus with rotary accelerations as low as $0.04°/sec^2$. The threshold here, as in other modalities, is a function of the signal-to-noise ratio; reduce the 'noise' and one reduces the threshold.

The duration of the stimulus affects vestibular thresholds for two reasons. The first is that the product of the acceleration and the time required to reach threshold is constant. Thus for shorter times of application, greater accelerations are required to reach threshold. This relationship is analogous to Bloch's law in vision. The second reason is that vestibular reactions adapt like other sensory functions. Discussion of this topic is postponed until section 5.5.

5.22 Thresholds for linear acceleration

It is difficult, and perhaps impossible, to measure utricular thresholds by behavioural procedures. This is because, to a greater extent than rotary acceleration about the body axis any linear acceleration is appreciated also through the kinaesthetic and tactile stimulation which inevitably arises. Early attempts to establish utricular thresholds are reviewed in Bourdon (1914). A procedure often used to overcome this difficulty has been to immerse the subject in water, and ask him to point upwards or set a rod to the vertical when he is tilted at various angles. It is invariably found that the mean error in both tasks is increased compared with performance on land, although performance is found to be still above chance, especially when the head is up and forward rather than down and back (Stigler, 1912; Schock, 1959; Brown, 1961; Whiteside, 1960). Apart from these general findings there is little agreement on the mean error of localizing the vertical under these circumstances, but the precise nature of the task varied from study to study, and the extent to which extraneous cues to the vertical were present probably also varied.

Graybiel and Patterson (1955) measured the utricular threshold by noting the least change in centrifugal force, acting on a subject in a centrifuge, which gave rise to an apparent displacement of a visual target (oculogravic illusion). A value of $0.00034\ g$ was found to be effective for a subject in the sitting position, and a value of $0.002\ g$ for a subject in a supine position. Thresholds like these are of little significance as measures of the absolute thresholds of the end-organ, as they must also reflect the threshold of response of the visual system. Nevertheless, the relative values are of interest, and support Brown's findings with submerged subjects.

Gurnee (1934) claimed that he was the first to study thresholds of vertical movement. Three subjects were oscillated in a simple harmonic linear motion in a vertical direction. The amplitude was fixed at 8 cm, the period varied from 8 sec to 16 sec. Thresholds were expressed as the peak velocity correctly identified as a movement, and ranged from 1·7 cm/sec to 40 cm/sec. The threshold was lower for downward movement than for upward movement.

More recently Walsh (1962) has studied responses to linear motion in a horizontal plane. Mean threshold determinations were made for various amplitudes, frequencies, and body positions. The linear swing was started and allowed to slow down. The least motion that could be reliably detected (criterion not given) was taken as the threshold under each condition of swing and body position. The results are shown in table 5.3. Walsh also studied the phase relationships between the swing's oscillation and the subjects' reports of movement. At oscillations of $\frac{1}{8}$ c/s, the reports of movement came at the turning points of the swing; only at an oscillation of 1 c/s were the reports in phase with the stimulus. Walsh speculated that the nervous system is unused to handling slow oscillations, and applies an inappropriate phase correction to the input. He assumed that the natural resonance of the end-organ is well above any of the frequencies which he used. However, the resonant period of the human otolith is not known, and peripheral factors may account for Walsh's results.

5.23 Ewald's law of directional preponderance

According to Ewald's second law the horizontal canal in the direction of body rotation is more intensely stimulated than the contralateral canal. The physiological aspects of this law have already been discussed; the behavioural consequences will now be considered.

In persons with an intact vestibular system on each side of the body, one would not expect the behavioural consequences of rotation in one direction to be different from those of rotation in the other direction. Any directional preponderance in one labyrinth would be cancelled by a similar directional preponderance in the other. Only in persons with one defective labyrinth would one expect to detect the behavioural consequences of Ewald's second law.

Ewald's second law has not gone unquestioned; Van Egmond, Groen, and Jongkees (1949b) found little evidence of directional preponderance in persons with one labyrinth destroyed, although Groen (1960a) later reinstated Ewald's law for the case of intense stimuli. Cawthorne, Fitzgerald, and Hallpike (1942) found that patients, after unilateral labyrinthectomy, showed directional preponderance of nystagmus to ampullopetal endolymph

Table 5.3 Thresholds for the report of rhythmically repeated horizontal motion obtained by Walsh (1962)

Frequency (c/s)	Position				
	Supine	Prone	On right	On left	
1/3	3·7 ± 2·7	3·2 ± 3·1	3·0 ± 2·8	3·0 ± 2·7	⎫ Threshold expressed as amplitude of motion
1/9	50·2 ± 28·5	25·2 ± 15·4	42·5 ± 19·4	31·8 ± 22·9	⎬ (cm)
1/3	3·9 ± 2·8	3·4 ± 3·2	3·1 ± 2·9	3·1 ± 2·8	⎫ Threshold expressed as peak velocity
1/9	17·5 ± 9·9	8·8 ± 5·4	14·8 ± 6·8	11·1 ± 8·0	⎬ (cm/sec)
1/3	8·2 ± 5·9	7·0 ± 6·8	6·6 ± 6·1	6·6 ± 5·9	⎫ Threshold expressed as peak acceleration
1/9	12·2 ± 6·9	6·1 ± 3·7	10·3 ± 4·7	7·7 ± 5·6	⎬ (cm/sec²)
1/3	17·1 ± 12·4	14·7 ± 14·2	13·7 ± 12·8	13·7 ± 12·4	⎫ Threshold expressed as peak values for rate of
1/9	8·5 ± 4·8	4·3 ± 2·6	7·2 ± 3·3	5·4 ± 3·9	⎬ change of acceleration (cm/sec³)

Subjects—three young adults and two 10 year old children. With each subject the mean of four determinations was taken as 'threshold'. The values in this table have been averaged over the different subjects, the standard deviations refer to the 'between subjects' variance.

currents induced by caloric stimulation. However, they attributed this phenomenon to conversion of the normal bidirectional sensitivity of the ampullae into an abnormal unidirectional type, perhaps through disturbance of the symmetry of central interpretation of the input from the remaining labyrinth, rather than to a basic unidirectionality of the ampullae. Fluur (1961), on the other hand, attributed this effect to facilitation of efferent impulses reaching the vestibular nuclei from supravestibular centres in the cerebellum and reticular formation. He cited physiological and anatomical evidence in support of this idea. His view of the situation is that when both labyrinths are intact, inhibitory impulses act across from the vestibular nuclei on one side to those on the other, following routes through the cerebellum and reticular formation. When one labyrinth is removed the remaining vestibular nuclei are released from inhibition. Since he used only warm water irrigation, Fluur's own data showed only that the ampullopetal response was increased by unilateral labyrinthectomy. His theory would lead one to suppose that ampullofugal responses would also be facilitated; in other words, it does not account for directional preponderance after unilateral labyrinthectomy, but rather for heightened general vestibular reactivity resulting from unilateral labyrinthectomy.

Whatever its cause, directional preponderance is not a fixed pattern. As patients recover from unilateral labyrinthectomy, the directional responses to turning become again more or less symmetrical, as they are in the normal person.

We shall see later that in normal subjects, practice at turning in one direction may bring about a directional preponderance of vestibular responsiveness to the opposite direction of turning. In terms of Ewald's law this means that the normal preponderance in the ear to the side of the practice turning is decreased, or reversed, whereas the normal preponderance in the other ear is increased. One must distinguish between directional preponderance within a single canal (Ewald's law) and directional preponderance between directions of turning in an animal with two labyrinths (bilabyrinthine preponderance). Bilabyrinthine directional preponderance is usually taken as a sign of ipsilateral central-nervous pathology, although its diagnostic value is disputed (Anderson, Jepson, and Kristiansen, 1956).

Whatever the truth of Ewald's second law as applied to the behavioural aspects of labyrinthine stimulation in man, there seems little doubt that it is true of lower animals. Frogs, it seems, cannot respond at all to a decrease in the resting vestibular nerve potential; their directional preponderance is complete. Birds show some responsiveness to a decrease in the resting potential and man shows an equal or near equal responsiveness to increases and decreases in potential, at least for mild stimuli (Dohlman, 1960).

5.3 Vestibular nystagmus

5.31 Eye nystagmus

When a person rotates about his body axis the eyes execute rhythmic, conjugate, reflex movements. They move slowly in the opposite direction to the rotation (the slow phase) and quickly back (the quick phase). Vestibular nystagmus may be elicited in a horizontal direction, a vertical direction, or a rotary direction (torsional nystagmus), depending upon which of the three canals is in the plane of rotation. It may also be elicited, in pathological states, when the head is tilted; the so-called 'positional nystagmus' (Jongkees, 1960). That positional nystagmus is a response to utricular stimulation is suggested by the fact that its intensity is increased by centrifuging the subject (Bergstedt, 1961b). Positional nystagmus may be elicited in a normal subject, but only when he deviates his eyes to left or right (Jongkees and Philipszoon 1963). Thus, stimulation of any of the canals or of the utricle (and perhaps saccule) may initiate nystagmus, although in assessing the utricular contribution care must be taken to ensure that the responses are not due to neck-tonic reflexes, or to compression of the blood vessels serving the labyrinths (Keleman, 1926).

The whole nystagmic reflex occurs when the subject is in the dark, and it is therefore not dependent on vision. The slow phase has a latency of about 0·05 sec for passive head movements, but for active head movements the latency is zero. This means that in the latter case the head and eye movements are initiated together; these eye movements have on this account been called coordinate compensatory eye movements (Dodge, 1921).

The generally accepted view is that within normal limits the speed of the slow phase of vestibular nystagmus is a linear function of the cupular deviation as indicated by the rate and duration of acceleration of the subject's head (Buys, 1924; Henriksson, 1955a). The speed of the slow phase of vestibular nystagmus produced by a given stimulus is practically constant for a given individual, and is not correlated over individuals with the duration of post-rotational nystagmus (Henriksson, 1955a).

Vestibular nystagmus is clearly directed towards keeping a stationary image on the retina but the speed of the slow, compensatory phase is less than the speed at which the head turns, at least when the subject is in the dark (Wendt, 1936a). When the eyes are open, the nystagmus is more precisely geared to the speed at which the retinal image moves. It is thought that, although the vestibular response initiates the nystagmus, optokinetic or visually induced nystagmus takes command when the eyes are open (Dodge, 1923b). Optokinetic nystagmus is therefore dominant over vestibular nystagmus. Optokinetic nystagmus apparently evolved before vestibular nystagmus, the latter being present in only those animals with vestibular canals (Fukuda, Hinoki, and Tokita, 1957).

Another aspect of the dominance of vision over vestibular nystagmus is seen in the fact that the latter is almost entirely inhibited if the rotating subject fixates a visual target attached to the head (Travis, 1929; Mahoney, Harlan, and Bickford, 1957). In a similar way, post-rotational illumination of the room tends to inhibit nystagmus (Mowrer, 1935a; Fenn and Hursch, 1937; Guedry, Collins, and Sheffey, 1961). Vision during rotation also inhibits post-rotational nystagmus; Mowrer (1937) suggested that this may be a consequence of a conflict between post-rotational vestibular nystagmus and the persistence of optokinetic nystagmus, if the two types are out of phase in the post-rotational period. The subservience of vestibular nystagmus to influences from higher centres is further demonstrated by the results of an experiment by Spiegel and Aronson (1934) in which they showed that stimulation of cortical eye-movement fields inhibits vestibular nystagmus in the cat.

Perhaps vestibular and visual stimuli for nystagmus tend to summate algebraically but, if they do, it is not a complete summation during rotation, for, if it were, the speed of the slow phase of nystagmus would exceed the speed of rotation and become inefficient in stabilizing the retinal image (Mowrer, 1935a).

5.32 The neural centres for vestibular nystagmus

Vestibular nystagmus in both its phases is basically a subcortical mechanism; it is present in neonate infants (Peiper, 1963, p. 150) and De Kleyn and Schenk (1931) were able to elicit both phases in an anencephalic child. The fact that vestibular nystagmus disappears in anaesthesia is probably due to the effect of the drug on subcortical centres.

The vestibular end-organs are not essential for vestibular nystagmus, for it may be elicited by stimulation of the vestibular nuclei when both of the VIIIth nerves have been cut. It has also been shown that the rhythm of nystagmus does not originate in the oculomotor nuclei, although of course these nuclei are essential for vestibular nystagmus. Proprioceptive impulses from the eye muscles have been found not to be essential for vestibular nystagmus, just as they have been found not to be essential for optokinetic nystagmus (Spiegel and Price 1939; Spiegel and Sommer, 1944a). Spiegel concluded that the vestibular nuclei are the centres for both phases of vestibular nystagmus, discharging via the medial longitudinal fasciculus and some other bypath, to the oculomotor nuclei.

More recently Lachmann, Bergmann, and Monnier (1957) have demonstrated the existence of a nystagmogenic area in the diencephalon of the rabbit and, while they do not deny that the vestibular nuclei in the medulla are an essential part of the circuit, they conclude that the diencephalic centre also plays an important role (Lachmann and Bergmann, 1961). Stimulation of the right side of this centre gives a nystagmus with the rapid phase towards the left, and vice versa. The frequency of the beat depends upon the intensity of stimulation. The interactions between the effects of stimulating this centre and the effects of rotation, drugs, optokinetic nystagmus, etc. have been investigated by Jongkees, Oosterveld, and Zelig (1964).

Other electrophysiological evidence suggests that the main route from vestibular apparatus to eye muscles involves three neurons running via the medial longitudinal fasciculus, but that other, more complex pathways also exist (Szentágothai, 1950). By recording from particular eye muscles while particular ampullae were deflected in particular directions, Szentágothai found that each crista has a predominant connection with a pair of ocular muscles according to the following scheme:

$$\text{Horizontal canal} \begin{cases} \text{ipsilateral medial rectus} \\ \text{contralateral lateral rectus} \end{cases}$$

$$\text{Superior canal} \begin{cases} \text{ipsilateral superior rectus} \\ \text{contralateral inferior oblique} \end{cases}$$

$$\text{Posterior canal} \begin{cases} \text{ipsilateral superior oblique} \\ \text{contralateral inferior rectus} \end{cases}$$

In each case the response was only induced by deflection of the cupula in a single direction. The appropriate direction in each case was the one predicted from Ewald's second law (see section 5.13). This is a pattern of responses which had already been outlined by Högyes in 1880, and has since been confirmed in essentials by Cohen, Suzuki, Shanzer, and Bender (1964).

Behavioural confirmation of this supranuclear localization of nystagmic eye movements has been provided by Fluur (1962) who observed that patients with spontaneous vertical nystagmus could have a concurrently induced, horizontal nystagmus which caused no change in the vertical eye movements. The rapid phases in the two simultaneous nystagmic movements tended to coincide, although the slow phases behaved as if controlled by separate mechanisms. He concluded that the slow phases of nystagmus in different planes are controlled by different centres, but that the quick phase is elicited from a common centre. However, according to Koike (1959), the slow phase and the quick phase do not operate independently. He found that the speeds of the two phases are positively correlated, although these results contradict earlier findings by Dohlman (1935). The precise mechanism which is responsible for the transformation of the vestibular input into the rhythmic nystagmic response is still unknown.

Cortical influences may modify vestibular nystagmus, and Spiegel has produced evidence that this influence funnels through the vestibular nuclei (Spiegel, 1932, 1933).

5.33 Head nystagmus and body deviations

Vestibular stimulation not only induces nystagmus, but also motor deviations of the whole body or of the head or limbs. These reflex responses are known as cristospinal reflexes. Nystagmic head movements are common in subhuman species, and are especially evident in birds. In the post-rotational period in humans, walking will deviate in the same direction as the slow phase of nystagmus, that is, in the opposite direction to the previous rotation of the body. The presence of this deviation in the absence of previous rotation has been used as a clinical sign in the so-called 'stepping test' (see Fukuda, 1959a). Any marked deviation which occurs when a person attempts to hold his hands out straight in front with eyes closed has also been taken as a clinical sign; the procedure is known as Bárány's arm deviation test. The extent of sideways head deviation resulting from caloric vestibular stimulation has been analysed, and proposed as a clinical test (Henriksson, Dolowitz, and Forssman, 1962; Henriksson, Forssman, and Dolowitz, 1962; Dolowitz, Forssman, and Henriksson, 1962).

5.4 The oculogyral illusion

Everyone will have noticed that during or just after a period of spinning about the body's longitudinal axis, visual objects appear to move. There are several early reports of this phenomenon (Purkinje, 1820; Mach, 1875; Bárány, 1907b). Graybiel and Hupp called this visual phenomenon the 'oculogyral effect' (Graybiel and Hupp, 1946; Graybiel, 1952b). If a full field of objects is in view, more rotatory stimulation is necessary in order to produce the illusion than when only a single object or point of light can be seen (Guedry, 1950b). If the eyes are open during the rotation, the visual aftereffect is compounded of that due to vestibular stimulation and the after-effect of seen movement, that is, the effect which would be produced by rotating the visual field round the subject. The oculogyral after-effect as a vestibular phenomenon should therefore be studied with eyes closed or fixated on a target fixed relative to the subject during the period of rotation.

Graybiel and Hupp described two per-rotatory phases in the oculogyral illusion produced by fixation of a light stationary with respect to the subject: an initial apparent movement in the direction of turning and, when a constant angular velocity has been reached, a second phase in the opposite direction. They also described two phases in the post-rotational oculogyral illusion: a first phase lasting up to about 30 sec in which visible objects are reported as moving in a direction opposite to that of the original rotation of the body, followed by a second phase lasting about as long, in which objects are reported to be moving the other way. Sometimes a third phase occurs in which the direction of the visual movement is again reported to change.

When the illusory oculogyral movement is reinforced by a real movement of the visual object relative to the subject, the target is reported to be moving too fast to be compatible with the resulting displacement. When the illusory movement is in the opposite direction to a real movement, the subject reports the movement to be occurring in one direction and the displacement to be occurring in the other direction—a paradoxical report, but understandable if one assumes that the neural signal for movement is different from that for displacement (Graybiel, Clark, MacCorquodale, and Hupp, 1946).

The most obvious explanation of the oculogyral illusion is that it is caused by movement of the retinal image consequent on the slow phase of vestibular nystagmus. This was the explanation adopted by Graybiel, Clark, MacCorquodale, and Hupp (1946) and by Hallpike and Hood (1953). However, there are several features of the phenomenon which argue against this being the only, or even one of the contributory factors (Van Dishoeck, Spoor, and Nijhoff, 1954; Vogelsang, 1961). These features are listed below:

(a) Illusory visual movements are reported by subjects who are in the dark after rotation (Mann, Guedry, and Ray, 1951).

(b) The threshold for the oculogyral illusion is lower than that for nystagmus, which means that the illusion occurs before nystagmus becomes evident (Roggeveen and Nijhoff, 1956).

(c) The oculogyral illusion commonly outlasts post-rotational nystagmus (Guedry, Collins, and Scheffey, 1961).

(d) The illusion may be reported when nystagmus is inhibited by fixation or is otherwise absent, for instance, in patients suffering from paralysis of the eye muscles.

(e) The oculogyral illusion occurs with after-images (Göthlin, 1927, 1946), or with 'stopped' retinal images (Van Dishoeck, Spoor, and Nijhoff, 1954).

(f) The apparent speed of the oculogyral illusion is influenced by the direction in which the visual target (an arrow or aeroplane) appears to point (Morant, 1959a).

(g) The slope of the cupulogram (see section 5.16) for nystagmus is different from that for the oculogyral illusion (figure 5.13).

The cupulogram for the oculogyral illusion runs parallel to that for the reported sensation of rotation (figure 5.13), and most investigators now seem to agree that the illusory movement is a consequence of a misjudgment of the movement of the body during and after rotation, rather than to movements of the retinal image during nystagmus. In other words, these experiments provide a set of conditions conducive to unidirectional autokinesis.

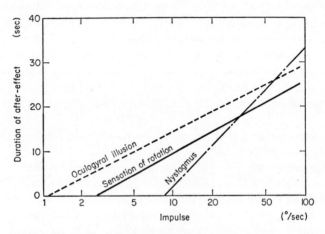

Figure 5.13 Averaged cupulograms showing how that derived from the oculogyral illusion runs parallel to that derived from the sensation of turning but not to that derived from post-rotational nystagmus. [From Van Dishoeck, Spoor, and Nijhoff, 1954]

A complementary illusion to the vestibular oculogyral effect is that in which people report that they are moving or rotating when the visible world is set in motion. A common experience of this kind is that of sitting in a stationary train and looking at a nearby moving train. Vision dominates: even when the body is actually moving in the opposite direction to that indicated by the visual movement, the subject interprets his movement in terms of the visual information (Warren, 1895). Very little experimental work has been done on this illusion (Gurnee, 1931), but a variant of it is the effect which a tilted line or visual frame has upon the judgment of the upright position of the body (see section 9.26).

5.5 Vestibular adaptation and habituation

5.51 The occurrence of vestibular habituation

If a steady rate of angular acceleration is continued for several minutes, the subject will report that the rotation is stopping or even reversing. This adaptation occurs even though the cupula remains deflected. It is not known whether it depends on a peripheral or a central process (Graybiel, Kerr, and Bartley, 1948; Hallpike and Hood, 1953; Guedry and Beberman, 1957; Ek, Jongkees, and Klijn, 1960). The most obvious explanation, in terms of neural adaptation, depends on the assumption that the vestibular nerves adapt; in any case it would be unlikely to provide a complete explanation. Guedry and Lauver (1961) found that adaptation of the subject's report of rotation is not necessarily accompanied by any adaptation of nystagmus, and this suggests that the former adaptation is due to the selective attenuation of a central mechanism which does not affect the oculomotor centres. If adaptation were peripheral, there would have to be one type of receptor which adapts and feeds to the centres which sustain the verbal report, and another type which does not adapt and supplies the eye-movement centres.

Adaptation effects are usually thought of as quickly induced and rapidly decaying. The effects of prolonged practice may last days or even months and are known as vestibular habituation. The distinction between the two processes is not clear however, and we shall assume that they are the same.

Abels (1906), a ship's physician, did the first experiments on vestibular habituation. He had noticed how sailors gradually cease to be sea-sick, and he found evidence in pigeons for the habituation of post-rotational nystagmus and dizziness. Bárány (1906a, 1906b, 1907a), Nobel prize winner and founder of clinical otology, claimed that the duration of post-rotational nystagmus is a reliable clinical index of the state of the vestibular system in man. In order to demonstrate its reliability he rotated one subject 50 times a day for 14 days, and got no habituation of nystagmus (Bárány, 1907b). He pointed out that Abels's results from pigeons should not be applied to man. He also found that professional dancers who habitually rotated one way, showed an average of 30 sec of post-rotational nystagmus for that direction as against the usual average of 41 sec. But they showed 49 sec the other way, so their mean value was normal. Dancers who rotated both ways showed a normal duration of post-rotational nystagmus, but Bárány admitted that they showed less dizziness than normal subjects.

On the authority of these findings, Babcock (1917) recommended that the United States government test every military aviator on the Bárány rotating chair, and reject those whose duration of post-rotational nystagmus was less than 16 sec (see Jones, 1918; Levy, 1919).

Mowrer (1934b) pointed out the double fallacy in this recommendation. In the first place, it had never been established that the vestibular organs are important in aviators' skill and safety; in fact, what evidence there was suggested that they were not important. In the second place, it cannot be claimed that because vestibular defects shorten the duration of nystagmus the converse is necessarily true, namely, that if the duration of nystagmus is short the vestibular system is defective. When several expert aviators were dismissed from service because of failure on the Bárány test given by army otologists, the psychologist Knight Dunlap began to suspect that a short duration of nystagmus may reflect the effects of practice. Consequently, he had tests done by an otologist on a group of professional acrobats and dancers in New York. In almost every case, contrary to Bárány's results, the nystagmus time was far below the minimum set for admission into the air service (Dunlap, 1919).

Dancers, and others practised at spinning round, normally forestall sustained cupula deflection by the habit of 'spotting'; as the body rotates they keep the head pointing towards the audience for as long as possible, and then flick the head round faster than the body until it again faces the same way. They thus overcome the need to execute eye nystagmus by substituting head nystagmus, and at the same time subject their cupulas to alternating clockwise and counterclockwise stimulation as the head successively accelerates and decelerates. The conditions necessary for post-rotational nystagmus are therefore not allowed to develop. Of course, dancers would not have been allowed to resort to this habit when they were tested by Dunlap's assistant. More recently, McCabe and Lawrence (1959) have also demonstrated that figure skaters are capable of suppressing dizziness and nausea even without spotting.

Dunlap then commissioned another psychologist, Madison Bentley, to do a controlled experiment on enlisted men (Bentley and Dunlap, 1918). Six men were rotated 50 times each way, each day, for 10 days. In each case, at the end of this period, the nystagmus time was reduced to about half what it had been at the start, and was finally below the otologists pass level of 16 sec. These results caused a storm of protest from the otologists (Fisher and Babcock, 1919), who nevertheless got similar results when they repeated the experiment. They argued that the effect was due to an increased control of the eyes by the eye-movement centres, rather than to any basic change in vestibular responsiveness. The psychologists had never denied the possibility of such an explanation, but were only anxious to show that the Bárány rotation test was invalid as a measure of aviators' fitness to fly. (See Mowrer,

1934b, and Griffith, 1929, for further details of this controversy, and of the early work in this area.) Subsequent experiments have confirmed that post-rotational nystagmus does habituate under the right circumstances, in both man and animals (Griffith, 1920, 1924; Dodge, 1923a; Holsopple, 1923a, 1923b; Mowrer, 1934b; Kraus, 1960). Other consequences of rotation, such as nausea, dizziness, and reports of visual movements have also been found to habituate; indeed, these effects often habituate fully, whereas post-rotational nystagmus rarely habituates by more than about 70%. Vertigo symptoms habituate more rapidly than nystagmus (Forssman, Henriksson, and Dolowitz, 1963). They also habituate fully; for instance, McCabe (1960) found that figure skaters could walk straight after being rotated in a chair; the tendency to veer had completely habituated out. Similarly, Graybiel, Guedry, Johnson, and Kennedy (1961) found that some subjects completely adapted out the oculogyral illusion during exposure to rotation. However, Collins (1965) found that such habituations occur only when the subjects are allowed to see after rotating.

The speed of the slow phase of nystagmus, as well as the nystagmus duration is said by some to be reduced during habituation. Indeed it is claimed that eye velocity is a more sensitive index of habituation than nystagmus duration (Henriksson, 1956; Henriksson, Kohut, and Fernández, 1961; Proctor and Fernández, 1963). On the other hand, Benson (1964) claims that the speed of the slow phase is unaffected by habituation.

There is habituation of the nystagmus induced by caloric stimulation as well as of that induced by rotation (Lidvall, 1961a; Fluur and Mendel, 1963). Caloric stimulation provides a means of stimulating and habituating one side at a time. It also provides a means of testing one side after habituation to rotation (Fluur and Mendel, 1964).

Brown and Guedry (1951) found that repeated rotations in darkness produced no habituation of the oculogyral effect, i.e. post-rotational apparent visual movement, whereas fixation of a faint object fixed relative to the body during and after rotation did produce habituation; this was further increased by the occasional, brief, post-rotational illumination of the environment, also fixed relative to the subject. They assumed that the oculogyral effect is a valid index of nystagmus; in this they were probably wrong (see section 5.4) and therefore their results probably do not apply to the habituation of nystagmus.

Forssman, Henriksson, and Dolowitz (1963) and Forssman (1964) compared the nystagmic habituation to repeated caloric stimulation in darkness and in light. They found that nystagmus had much shorter duration and lower maximum velocity and decayed more rapidly during habituation with vision. However, switching the light off or on suddenly during the course of habituation produced a corresponding increase or decrease in nystagmus, suggesting that light does not affect the rate of habituation but merely has a transitory and reversible effect on the degree of nystagmus shown in individual trials. This latter effect is presumably due to the stabilizing effect of the stationary field of view, or even the cancelling out of the vestibular nystagmus by an opposed optokinetic nystagmus induced by the apparent movement of the visible surroundings. This type of situation may be complicated even further by the fact that optokinetic nystagmus has its own after-effect which also habituates (Mowrer, 1934b). It is a wise precaution, when studying vestibular nystagmus, to keep the subject in the dark all the time. Forssman *et al.* found that vertigo showed a more rapid habituation than nystagmus and appeared to be totally independent of light or darkness.

5.52 *The mechanism of vestibular habituation*

There are several mechanisms which could contribute towards the habituation of post-rotational nystagmus. These have usually been discussed as 'theories' of habituation, which has resulted in a tendency to think that a particular 'theory' has been disproved when it has merely been shown that habituation occurs in the absence of the relevant factor. In order to avoid confusing 'the sufficient' with 'the necessary' conditions it is preferable to talk of possible contributory mechanisms. Five such mechanisms will be discussed.

a. Peripheral factors There are known to be efferent fibres to the cristae, and these may innervate contractile cilia or kinocilia (Carpenter, Bard, and Alling, 1959). Therefore, it is possible that central processes may control the activity of the peripheral sense organs directly (Groen, 1960b). This may contribute to habituation, although there is no direct evidence that it does.

Breuer (1875) accounted for vestibular habituation by assuming that the cupula undergoes non-elastic bending when repeatedly deflected one way, but there is no evidence that vestibular habituation involves any such structural change in the peripheral organ.

Hamberger and Hydén (1949) detected an increase of nucleoproteins within the vestibular ganglion of the rabbit following a moderate treatment of angular acceleration. These cytochemical changes persisted for two days, but there is no other evidence to suggest that they are causal agents in habituation, rather than merely incidental by-products.

b. Habituation and nystagmic disrhythmia Many experimenters have noticed that habituation of post-rotational nystagmus involves not only a reduction in the duration of nystagmus but also an increasing disrhythmia of nystagmus (McLay, Madigan, and Ormerod, 1957; Suzuki and Totsuka, 1960; Lidvall, 1961b; Fluur and Mendel, 1962a). Suzuki and Totsuka consider that this 'labyrinthine fibrillation' or fluttering accounts for the apparent reduction in duration after habituation; the nystagmus is not really reduced but rather transfigured by a central mechanism into a fibrillation.

   c. Habituation and arousal Vestibular habituation could be due to a general loss of 'arousal' activity in brain-stem nuclei consequent upon the declining arousal value of the repeated rotation. Certainly anything which keeps the subject in an alert state, such as mental arithmetic, delays or prevents habituation, while day-dreaming and lack of attention cause the rapid attenuation of nystagmus (Bach, 1894; Mowrer, 1934a; Wendt, 1951; Collins, Crampton, and Posner, 1961; Collins and Guedry, 1962; Collins, Guedry, and Posner, 1962; Collins 1962, 1963; Crampton, 1964). Pendleton and Paine (1961) and Collins (1962) have even suggested that vestibular nystagmus is a more sensitive index of a subject's state of alertness than the EEG.
   Another factor determining the rate of vestibular habituation is the repetitiveness of the stimulus. Lidvall (1962) found that repeated identical caloric vestibular stimulation produced more habituation of vertigo and nystagmus than stimuli varying in intensity and site of application. This would follow from the general arousal hypothesis if one assumes that repetitive stimulation is less arousing than varied stimulation. However, Lidvall claimed that the general activation level, as reflected in the EEG, was the same for both types of stimuli, and he concluded that specific stimulus parameters as well as general arousal contribute to habituation. However, if the EEG is a less sensitive index of general arousal than the sequelae of vestibular stimulation, his claim that the level of arousal for the two types of stimuli was the same, is invalid, and his conclusion suspect.
   A more serious objection to the general arousal hypothesis as the sole explanation of habituation comes from work by Crampton and Schwam (1961), who found that arousal restores post-rotational nystagmus in the cat, but not to its pre-habituation level; they concluded that habituation depends, to some extent, but not entirely, upon a reduction of arousal.

   d. Habituation and directional balance Bárány (1907a) claimed that repeated rotation both ways produced no habituation, and that repeated rotation in one direction diminished the nystagmus duration produced by this type of stimulation but lengthened that produced by rotation in the other, unpractised, direction. Habituation was seen as a shift in the point of balance between the effects of the two directions of turn, rather than an overall reduction in the response to vestibular stimulation. We shall refer to this idea as the 'directional balance mechanism'. If it could be shown that habituation to one direction of turn was not always offset by a corresponding increase in responsiveness for the other direction, Bárány's directional balance mechanism would cease to give a complete account of the facts, even though it might retain some explanatory value for some of them.

Before looking at the evidence, we must examine what is meant by 'rotation in one direction', for any rotation involves both an acceleration and a deceleration in the same direction. Holsopple (1924) demonstrated that the crucial factor is the difference in the duration of the successive rotation (acceleration-to-retardation) and rest (retardation-to-acceleration) intervals comprising the practice schedule. If the rotation interval is short, the practised-direction nystagmus will be reduced more than the unpractised-direction nystagmus: if, on the other hand, the rotation interval is long in relation to the rest interval, the practised-direction nystagmus will be less than the unpractised-direction nystagmus. In other words, the amount of habituation depends on the extent to which the post-rotational nystagmus has been allowed to run its course, uninterrupted by an opposing vestibular stimulus. That is not to say that habituation cannot occur for both directions of turn at once, but the training each way would have to fulfil the above condition i.e. both intervals would have to be long enough to allow the nystagmus in each direction to run its course.

Dodge (1923a) and Holsopple (1923a) confirmed that vestibular habituation is directionally specific, although Dodge found some reduction of nystagmic duration in the unpractised direction (cf. Bárány).

Individuals apparently differ in the extent of directional preponderance after one type of stimulation. Fluur and Mendel (1962a) found some subjects who exhibited directional preponderance after prolonged, unidirectional cupular stimulation induced by repeated monaural irrigation with hot water, or with cold water. In these subjects the direction of the preponderance could easily be changed by reversing the treatment (Fluur and Mendel, 1962b). Other subjects given the same treatment did not show directional preponderance, but rather a reduced nystagmus time to both types of stimulation in either ear. Lidvall (1962) also found that habituation was to some extent directionally specific, not only for the particular direction of turning, but also for the plane in which the turning occurred. However, there was some transfer of habituation to the unpractised direction and planes.

It thus seems that, like arousal, the mechanism of directional balance operates, but it cannot explain all the facts.

In so far as vestibular habituation involves a shift in the directional balance of nystagmus, one would expect that while the subject is unidirectionally habituated there would be spontaneous nystagmus when the subject is at rest. Several investigators have noted such spontaneous nystagmus (Guedry, Graybiel, and Collins, 1962; Guedry and Graybiel, 1962; Fluur and Mendel, 1962a). It is especially evident in darkness, and is a common accompaniment of directional preponderance due to brain damage (Koch, Henriksson, Lundgren, and Andrén, 1959).

Hood (1960) has pointed out that the possibility of directionally specific habituation has an important bearing upon our views of the nervous response of the cupula. According to an extreme view of Ewald's second law, ampullopetal movement is the effective stimulus for accelerations to the right. During these accelerations such movements can occur in the right vestibular apparatus only. Persons with only one labyrinth should not therefore habituate both ways. Hood found that three such patients could be selectively habituated to either ampullopetal or ampullofugal stimulation. The monaural caloric-habituation experiments of Fluur and Mendel demonstrate the same point. The single cupula must therefore be capable of signalling both types of deflection, a conclusion supported by physiological evidence (see section 5.13), and not denied by Ewald, whose second law was not stated in such an extreme form as Hood assumed. Hood believed that vestibular habituation or adaptation depends upon an attenuation of the peripheral signal. Ampullofugal displacement involves a decrease in the resting cupula potential, and therefore adaptation at this level would have to involve a relative increase in the discharge. Hood found this difficult to understand in terms of the usually accepted account of adaptation as a decrease in end-organ discharge. He postulated the existence of two independent sets of cells in the end-organ, one set inhibiting the resting discharge for ampullofugal displacement, and the other exciting the discharge for ampullopetal displacement. Adaptation and, by implication, habituation involve a reduction of the discharge of one or other of these sets of 'switch cells'. Such an elaborate peripheral mechanism is unnecessary if one abandons the idea that adaptation and habituation are peripheral in origin.

e. Habituation and learning The most commonly accepted view is that vestibular habituation is a form of learning. Animals do not often rotate one way for any length of time, and therefore the deceleratory stimulation of the cupulae usually cancels out the acceleratory stimulation. Post-rotational nystagmus gives rise to conflicting sensory inputs: the vestibular signals indicate rotation, while the proprioceptive and visual stimuli indicate no rotation. Learning probably involves a greater weighting of the visual information, or if the eyes are closed, of the proprioceptive information.

Nystagmus is thereby reduced, and nausea and dizziness prevented (Wendt, 1936b; Hood and Pfaltz, 1954; Collins, 1965).

A further feature of the central adaptive control of the effects of angular and linear accelerations is the well-known acclimatization to the movements of a ship. It is as if the body learns to anticipate each movement by producing a central 'copy' of the particular sequence and by partialling this out from the afferent signals as they come in. When one returns to dry land, the partialling-out process persists for hours or even days, for the firm ground seems to pitch and roll.

These then are five mechanisms which may contribute to vestibular habituation; but the main factor is probably the increased reliance on other modalities, particularly vision.

5.53 Vestibular habituation and age

People are subjected to rotations in the ordinary course of life, and it may be supposed that post-rotational phenomena are normally habituated to some extent. If this is so, newborn infants should manifest an unusually low threshold for, and an extra long duration of post-rotational nystagmus. This seems to be the case (Galebski, 1928; Groen, 1963) at least as far as the slow phase is concerned, which may be the only phase present in the first few weeks (McGraw, 1941). The infant, like the adult, must be kept alert in order that the nystagmus may be elicited (Pendleton and Paine, 1961).

There is some evidence that older people again develop a long duration of rotational after-effects (Guedry, 1950a), although this could be due to a loss of elasticity in the cupulae.

5.6 Effects of loss of labyrinthine function

Unilateral loss of vestibular function is followed by a period of acute discomfort. The patient is unable to move his head without feeling distressed, nauseated, and disoriented; the skin is pallid, pulse rate high, and vomiting frequent. He has nystagmus and falls to the healthy side (Cawthorne, 1946). After some days or weeks these symptoms subside and the patient recovers his normal behaviour (Cooksey, 1946). This recovery presumably depends on a change in the way in which the central nervous system makes use of an asymmetrical vestibular input (Fluur, 1960). An emotional disturbance causes the symptoms to recur (Boenninghaus, 1926). Ross and Olsen (1936) found that recovery in a unilaterally labyrinthectomized dog was not delayed by destruction of the cerebellar vermis or posterior spinal columns and concluded that the cerebral cortex is responsible for this recovery.

The threshold of appreciation of horizontal linear acceleration is adversely affected by unilateral labyrinthectomy, but evidently only when the patient is lying on his damaged side (Walsh, 1960).

Bilateral vestibular loss is not accompanied by nausea, distress, or nystagmus. For some time, the patient is unable to stand upright steadily when his eyes are closed but after a time stability is regained by the use of kinaesthesis and touch. A person with bilateral vestibular loss is just as likely to swim downwards as upwards when submerged in water, but here again some recovery of stability takes place. Invertebrates and lower vertebrates are more affected by labyrinthectomy than is man.

Men with bilateral loss of vestibular function are not susceptible to motion sickness (James, 1882; Graybiel, Clark, and Zarriello, 1960; Graybiel and Johnson, 1962). Because of the proximity of the cochlea to the vestibular apparatus, deafness is often accompanied by loss of vestibular sensitivity (Terawaza, 1927; Worchel and Dallenbach, 1948, 1950).

5.7 Motion sickness

Motion sickness is a state that develops in animals and humans when they are subjected to accelerations over which they have no control. It manifests itself in nausea, vomiting, and distress. It is of increasing practical importance to understand and be able to prevent motion sickness, as civilians and military personnel are increasingly subjected to accelerative forces at sea, on land, in the air, and in outer space.

The literature on this subject was reviewed by McNally and Stewart (1942) and Tyler and Bard (1949) and more recently by Chinn and Smith (1955) and Loftus (1963). There is abundant evidence that the vestibular apparatus is implicated in the etiology of motion sickness. Bilateral labyrinthectomy or sectioning of the vestibular-cerebellar tracts in animals renders them immune to motion sickness. We have already mentioned that bilateral loss of labyrinthine function in man gives him immunity. Caloric or electrical stimulation of the vestibular apparatus induces motion sickness.

McNally (1944) and others have concluded that changes in the direction of linear acceleration (utricular stimulation) rather than rotary acceleration (canal stimulation) are the crucial factor. However, the weight of modern evidence suggests that both organs may be involved. Low-frequency, high-amplitude oscillations seem to be more effective than high-frequency, low-amplitude oscillations (Alexander, Cotzin, Hill, Ricciuti, and Wendt, 1945).

However, the most potent stimulus seems to arise when there is a complex series of changes in the amplitude and direction of both linear and rotary acceleration (Noble, 1945). Even if a person is subjected to a simple rotation or swing, complex forces will act on his head every time he moves it (see section 5.12). These forces arise from the interaction between the angular velocity produced by the movements of the machine and that produced by the movement of the head. If the head is strapped in one position, symptoms are much reduced (Johnson, 1954, 1956; Johnson and Taylor, 1961). After a time most people adapt to sickness-inducing conditions, even to complex interactive stimuli. Graybiel, Clark, and Zarriello (1960) observed volunteers living in a slowly rotating room for many days. The initial distress and incapacity gradually diminished, provided the speed of rotation was not too great (Clark and Graybiel, 1961).

Thus complex stimulation of the vestibular apparatus is the main etiological factor in motion sickness. However, the fact that adaptation takes place suggests that central factors are also important. It is a common experience that motion sickness does not develop when one has control over the moving vehicle: the driver of a car is rarely sick, even though subject to sickness when he is a passenger. This suggests that the main factor in habituation to motion sickness is the learning of anticipatory schema. If this theory were correct one would not expect habituation to one form of motion to transfer to another form of motion. This experiment does not seem to have been done. An alternative theory is that habituation is due to a general suppressor effect produced by the central nervous system. The preventive effects of anti-motion-sickness drugs lend support to this theory. Both factors may play a role in habituation. Persons susceptible to motion sickness have been found to have a cupulogram with a steep slope (see figure 5.12). Van Egmond, Groen, and de Wit (1954) have suggested cupulometry (that is, the measure of the duration of post-rotational nystagmus as a function of the strength of the accelerative impulse) as a test for selecting individuals susceptible to sickness.

The utricular system probably has a natural periodicity, such that when it is rhythmically stimulated at this frequency its discharge keeps in step with the stimulus. At lower frequencies of stimulation it may be expected that the response would get out of step. Walsh (1961, 1962) has reported an effect of this kind. He oscillated the subject on a parallel swing, which he adapted from Jongkees and Groen (1946). At 1 c/s the blindfolded subject correctly reported the direction of travel at each part of the cycle, but at lower frequencies the subject's report was out of phase with the actual movement: he reported moving one way when he was in fact moving the other way. Walsh suggested that the slow movement of a ship may induce motion sickness because of this discrepancy between the felt movement and the actual, visually-detected movement.

In spite of the importance of vestibular stimulation it is not a necessary condition of motion sickness. There is a well-known fairground device known as the phantom swing. People enter what looks like a swing but instead of the carriage moving, the scenery outside the windows is moved to-and-fro. The occupants are convinced that it is the carriage that is moving, and exhibit all the symptoms of imbalance and nausea which a real movement would produce. The crucial factor is probably still discordance between visual and labyrinthine information; the effect may not appear in people with defective labyrinths, though this is not known. Other non-labyrinthine agencies which contribute to motion sickness are conditioned anticipatory responses associated with previous sickness-inducing situations, and clinical conditions such as migraine (Schwab, 1954).

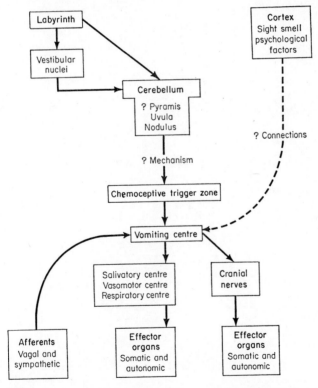

Fig. 5.14 Schematic representation of the central nervous pathways of motion sickness. [From Wang and Tyson, 1954]

There is evidence from work on animals that a vomiting centre exists in the dorsolateral reticular formation. Figure 5.14 shows the scheme which Wang and Tyson (1954) have proposed for the afferent and efferent connections of this vomiting centre.

This account of the vestibular system is by no means comprehensive, especially with regard to the earlier literature; a full account would involve reference to over ten thousand sources. The following reviews deal with the earlier literature: Maxwell (1923), Fischer (1928), Griffith (1922, 1929, 1932), Camis (1930), Dusser de Barenne (1934), McNally and Stewart (1942), Schilder (1942), Spiegel and Sommer (1944a, 1944b), Wendt (1951), Fischer (1956), Gernandt (1959), King and Wade (1961).

6

Auditory localization

6.1 The physics of auditory localization

6.11 Theoretical analysis

Under ideal conditions human beings are able to locate the source of a small sound to an accuracy of about one degree. When several sounds arrive at the same time from different directions, the listener is able to sort them out and locate the source of any one of them.

In trying to find out how these tasks are accomplished one naturally starts by asking whether both ears are necessary. It so happens that under certain circumstances sounds may still be localized with only one ear functioning, but much less accurately than when both ears are in use. The physics of these abilities will be considered before their behavioural aspects.

Clearly, if binaural hearing helps in auditory localization, this must be because the sound arriving at one ear differs from that arriving at the other according to the position of the sound source. A little thought reveals what these differences could be. Consider the case where a sound source is to the left of the listener. The left ear will be stimulated at a greater intensity than the right ear because the left ear is nearer the source and because, unlike the right ear, it is not in the 'shadow' of the head. If the source is a brief click, the sound from it will arrive at the left ear before it arrives at the right ear. The *intensity difference* and the *time difference* between the ears will depend upon the position of the source. When it is positioned anywhere in the median plane of the head (in front of, behind, above, or below the head), it will stimulate the two ears with the same intensity and at the same time, assuming the head and ears are symmetrical. As the sound source moves from the median plane to a lateral position, the intensity difference and the time difference will increase.

The intensity difference produced by the shadowing effect of the head will vary with the frequency of the sound. High-frequency tones have a shorter wavelength than low-frequency tones and will therefore cast a sharper 'shadow' when they pass an obstacle. The long waves of low-frequency tones 'get round' the obstacle to some extent; that is, they are diffracted more than short, high-frequency tones. From this physical fact it may be predicted that laterally placed high-frequency sounds will produce a larger intensity difference between the ears than low-frequency sounds. *The 'cue' of intensity should be more effective for high-frequency than for low-frequency tones.*

If the sound source is a continuous pure tone rather than a click, the crests of the component sound waves are likely to arrive at different times at the two ears. In other words, the sounds at the two ears will be out of phase. *This phase difference* between the sounds at the two ears will vary with the position of the source, just as the time difference does. A phase difference is

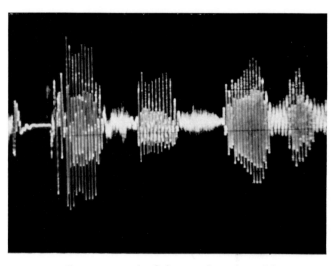

Figure 6.1 Oscilloscope record of the sound pattern of human speech, demonstrating transients and the concept of the sound envelope

[*To face p. 141*

expressed as an angle: when two sounds are in phase, the phase angle is 0°; when the crest of one coincides with the trough of the other, they are 180° out of phase.

If the difference in time of arrival at the two ears of a given crest of sound wave exceeds half the period between one crest and the next, the sounds at the two ears will begin to come into phase again as the sound is moved into a more lateral position. There will be a certain frequency of sound for which half the intercrest period is equal to the time difference introduced between the ears. This frequency has been calculated for the average head and is about 1,000 c/s. In theory, for frequencies above this the phase-difference cue will become ambiguous, since the interval between successive crests both between the left ear and the right ear and between the right ear and the left ear will be short enough to be compatible with a source on the left or with a source on the right. *Thus the phase-difference cue should become less effective for high-frequency pure tones.*

For pure tones, the intensity-difference cue should be most effective for high-frequency notes, and the phase-difference cue should be most effective for low-frequency notes. However, in real situations sounds do not consist of a single pure tone; real sounds have complex wave-forms which may be considered to be a synthesis of many sine waves of different amplitudes and frequencies. Figure 6.1 is a picture of the wave-form of a voice. Peaks occur in the wave-form at irregular intervals. These are known as *transients*, and the outline of the wave-form is known as the envelope. Even though the component sine waves of a sound may be above the frequency at which phase differences can be expected to serve localization, the frequency at which transients arise may be well below it. In real situations, therefore, time differences or phase differences between transients could be very important in localization.

Since sounds usually consist of different tones, some of low frequency, and some of high, the different component frequencies will be diffracted by different amounts; they will be phase-shifted by different amounts; and the transients will be delayed by different amounts between the two ears. Sound localization could thus depend upon the simultaneous comparison of the intensity, phase, and arrival time of two complex wave forms, and their envelopes, one received by the left ear, the other by the right ear. The nerve centres concerned could, as it were, carry out a complex *running cross-correlation* on the two sounds.

The situation is complicated further by the fact that there are usually many sounds occurring at the same time in different places. The listener would be hopelessly confused if some means were not available for keeping the different sound patterns separate, and for identifying, in each ear, those patterns which come from the same source. This is the well known 'cocktail party problem', which arises when a person selectively listens to one voice among many without becoming confused. Auditory localization under these circumstances must depend upon the mechanism of selective listening, that is, the mechanism of auditory pattern recognition.

So far it has been assumed that both ears are functioning. But people can distinguish the direction of sound sources, especially of complex ones, with only one ear. People can also discriminate the directions of two sounds which both lie in the median plane of the head; neither of these abilities should be possible on the basis of the mechanisms so far mentioned. One may predict how these things are done from physical principles. The simplest way to achieve localization of a source using only one ear would be to move one's head. One would then be able to compare successively the sound patterns for different positions of the head. Theoretically, one should be able to perform as well as a person with two ears. The other way is to learn how the complex wave form of a particular sound is affected by each position of the source relative to the head. In a sense this is the same mechanism that is used when one is allowed to move the head, except that one stores all the information for each head position over a long time, and does not have to move the head on each occasion. In practice, this ability is not so complex as it may appear. The learning does not have to be specific to each sound, for consistent types of change are produced in many complex sounds by changes of position. Once the general 'rules' are known the central nervous system should be able to decode any particular sound pattern accordingly.

Localizing of a complex sound which lies in the median plane of the head could be achieved on the basis of the 'shadowing' effect of the pinna or external ear, producing differential phase and intensity shifts for different component frequencies, and differential time shifts for different component frequencies and for any transients there might be.

6.12 Objective measurements

Theoretical calculations of phase and intensity ratios at the two ears for various azimuth angles have been made by Stewart (1920a, 1920b) and Hartley and Fry (1921). They assumed that the head is a rigid sphere with diametrically opposed ears, in a free field.

It is possible to check these calculations by taking oscilloscope recordings from microphones placed at the 'eardrums' of real or dummy human heads. Firestone (1930) checked them by measuring the interaural phase differences in a dummy head for the frequencies, 256, 1,024, and 1,944 c/s, at various distances and azimuth angles. His results are shown in figure 6.2. They agree well with the theoretical values computed by Hartley and Fry, and also with subsequent determinations made from microphones placed in the ears of living subjects by Feddersen, Sandel, Teas, and Jeffress (1957) and by Nordlund (1962).

The results of Firestone's additional investigations of interaural intensity

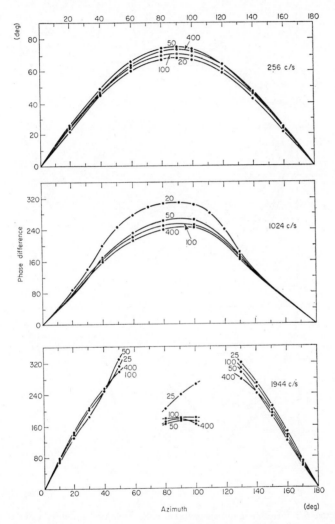

Figure 6.2 Firestone's measurements of phase difference as a function of azimuth at different distances between head and sound source, at three frequencies

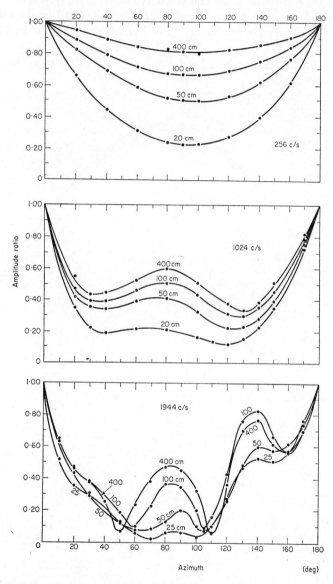

Figure 6.3 Firestone's measurements of the interaural intensity ratio as a function of azimuth at different distances between head and sound source, at three frequencies

ratios are shown in figure 6.3. It can be seen that the interaural intensity difference is greater the nearer the sound source is to the head, and the higher the frequency of the tone. The results fitted the computed values reasonably well for frequencies below 1,000 c/s, but became very irregular at the frequency of 1,944 c/s. However, Sivian and White (1933) found more regular functions at higher frequencies.

More recent measurements by Feddersen, Sandel, Teas, and Jeffress (1957), obtained from sound probes in human ears, deviated from calculated values at all frequencies. The intensity differences were found to be variable from one subject to another and showed many maxima and minima as the azimuth angle was varied. Feddersen *et al.* were at a loss to understand how intensity differences could serve to localize sounds, even high-frequency sounds.

The maxima in the intensity differences at various azimuth angles arise when there is a phase displacement of half a wavelength between the sound which reaches a given ear directly and the sound which reaches it after passing round the head. When this happens that ear is in a 'null region' where the two waves cancel. The other ear may not be in such a null region and will therefore be more intensely stimulated. These null regions cannot exist for sounds below about 1,000 c/s, for the diameter of the head is less than half a wavelength for those frequencies. The graphs of figure 6.4 show how the number of maximum points increases for frequencies of 1,000 c/s and above.

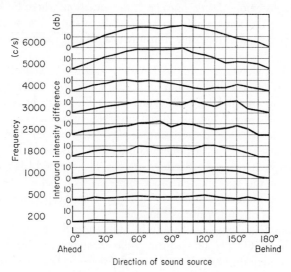

Figure 6.4 Interaural intensity differences as a function of frequency and direction (five subjects). [From Feddersen, Sandel, Teas, and Jeffress, 1957]

At very high frequencies the maxima do not show because their position becomes very variable due to slight head movements.

Thus, according to the results of Feddersen *et al.*, the same intensity difference can be registered at many azimuth positions, and this cue is therefore ambiguous. If the head is allowed to move the ambiguity should be eliminated for it should then be possible to detect which ear is approaching the sound and which is receding from it.

So much for the physics of auditory localization. These are the predictions which a physicist might make regarding the basis of auditory localization. The next question is whether these theoretical mechanisms operate in practice. But before that question can be discussed it is necessary to consider the experimental procedures which may be used.

6.2 Experimental procedures

6.21 Methods of stimulation

Experiments on auditory localization, like all experiments on sound, require the careful control of the acoustic properties of the immediate environment. There are three basic procedures; (1) diotic listening in a sound cage or anechoic chamber. (2) diotic listening in open-air or free-field conditions, and (3) dichotic listening. *Diotic listening* is the situation where both ears are stimulated by the same sound source. Small tuning forks or mechanical hammers were used at one time, but nowadays small loudspeakers are preferred.

The sound cage was a device used in early studies (e.g. Matsumoto, 1897); it consisted of a framework within which the sound source could be moved. The subject sat with his head at the centre and had to judge the position of the sound. The early sound cages produced disturbing echoes and they have been replaced by modern sound-proof and *anechoic* (echo-proof) chambers.

In the open-air or free-field method the subject sits on top of a tall building away from any sound reflecting surfaces. The method has many of the advantages of the anechoic chamber and was used before these became available (Stevens and Newman, 1934, 1936). It is cheaper to set up than a chamber, but is obviously not as convenient.

If the sounds at the two ears are to be independently manipulated, *dichotic methods* are used. Usually a close-fitting tube or ear-phone is placed over each ear. A sound may thus be delivered to each ear from separate sound sources. These may be mechanical sources feeding ear-tubes, or electronic sources feeding ear-phones. Dichotic listening is thus the situation where each ear is stimulated by a separate sound source. As long as the sounds do not differ too much the subject will report hearing one 'fused' sound, which may be called a *dichotic phantom*. If the sounds differ too much the phantom splits into two separate sounds in two different places. For example, when the frequencies differ widely (e.g. 800 c/s against 6,000 c/s) the sounds fail to fuse, suggesting that some input from a common region of the basilar membrane is required for fusion (David, Guttman, and Van Bergeijk, 1958; Deatherage, 1961).

Older mechanical devices for producing dichotic phase differences between the two ears consisted of tubes which could be telescoped to alter the length of the path along which the sound had to travel. It was difficult to vary phase independently of intensity in these devices. Electronic oscillators are now used which can generate alternating currents of known wave-form, frequency, amplitude, and phase angle and which, when fed into loud-speakers or ear-phones, produce corresponding sounds. The dichotic method is useful for studying the influence of time and intensity differences, but not so useful for studying more complex factors which operate under ordinary conditions of diotic listening.

When listening dichotically the subject will often report that the phantom is inside his head, and that it moves across from one ear to the other as the intensity difference, or some other difference, is varied. This type of judgment is known as *lateralization* as opposed to ordinary localization of diotic sounds outside the body. It is as if, in lateralization, the distance information were lacking in the sound. Perhaps this is due to the fact that the sound from ear-phones lacks the characteristics which sounds acquire by passing through the air. But there may be another reason: when dichotic sounds are delivered by ear-phones, movements of the head do not affect the position of the phantom. The subject may be interpreting this anomalous situation by assuming that the source is in the head, for real sounds in the head would behave in this way.

Two loudspeakers at a distance from the listener, one on his left and one on his right, also produce a phantom. This is the situation familiar as *stereophonic* listening. Each ear is stimulated more by its own speaker than by the speaker on the other side. There is only partial separation. The phantom is reported to be somewhere between the two loudspeakers and is localized at a distance rather than lateralized in the head. Hanson and Kock (1957) produced an 'in-the-head' phantom from two symmetrically placed speakers in antiphase. This effect was probably due to the presence of 'null regions' where the antiphase waves cancel. If one ear was in a null region and the other not, one ear only would be stimulated, which is the condition holding when a source is very close to one ear.

It should be obvious from the discussion so far that the nature of the sound source is of vital importance in an experiment. Clicks are useful for studying intensity and time differences. Pure tones are useful for studying intensity and phase differences, and head parallax. Complex sounds must be used for studying transients, differential sound defraction, and selective localization of multiple sources.

6.22 Methods of indication

In any experiment on auditory localization the experimenter must decide how the subject is to indicate where he judges the sound to be. The most obvious, and the earliest method used, is to ask the subject to point to where he thinks the sound is. The accuracy of the subject is limited by the accuracy with which he can position his hand, as well as by the accuracy with which he can localize the sound. A variant of this method is to ask the subject to indicate the direction of the sound on a chart (Ferree and Collins, 1911). Stevens and Newman (1936) asked their subjects to estimate the position of the sound in degrees out from the mid-line. Modern experimenters use one or other of the following three methods.

The first modern method uses a second diotic sound or a second dichotic phantom as a *sound pointer*. The position of the pointer is varied, until the subject reports that the pointer and the experimental source or phantom are in the same place. The tone of the pointer phantom should be very different from that of the experimental phantom so as to avoid interference between them. The 'pointer' is usually white noise, and some interference is inevitable in this method. A point of light may also be used as a 'pointer', but is unsatisfactory in practice, for people tend to equate the direction of a sound with that of a light, even when they are far apart (see section 14.3).

The second modern method is known as the *centring method*. It is used principally for studying the relationship of one variable to another. The phantom is first 'placed' in the subject's apparent median plane, which in a lateralization judgment will usually mean the middle of his head. The experimenter then 'moves' the sound by varying say the intensity difference, and asks the subject to restore it to the centre by varying another variable, say the phase difference. In this way one variable is measured in relation to another; one is said to be 'traded' against the other and the function obtained is known as a *trading function*.

A variation of the centring method is one in which the sound source is switched to an off-centre position and the subject has to report to which side it has been moved. This is the constant-stimulus method and is very useful for measuring the threshold of localization and the position of the subjective auditory median plane (Leakey, 1959). If it is used with dichotic stimulation, the thresholds of time and intensity differences may be obtained.

Kikuchi (1957) described what he called the 'nullity method' of locating the position of a dichotic sound image. The inputs to the two ears are rapidly reversed, the left input is switched to the right ear as the right input is switched to the left ear. If there is any detectable difference of time or intensity between the two sources the phantom will be reported as having changed its position at the time of the switch-over. Only when the two sounds are objectively identical, within the limits of discrimination, will the phantom be reported as stationary at the switch-over. What is being measured here is the objective physical equality of the two sound sources, *not* the subjective median position of the phantom as in the centring method. At the nullity point the phantom may be reported as not in the median plane; this reflects a difference between the two ears. Applied to unidimensional interaural differences, the procedure measures the subject's threshold of discrimination of the difference between the two sounds. The dispersion of readings is probably lower than for any other method. The results are not affected by any differences between the ears, hence constant errors in median plane settings are not directly reflected in the results. A similar procedure has been described by Jeffress and Blodgett (1962).

The nullity method has been used effectively to measure trading between interaural intensity and time differences (Harris, 1960).

6.3 Localization thresholds

Several stimulus factors have been shown to affect the threshold of localization, or JND of azimuth position, of an actual sound source. The azimuth angle relative to the centre of the head is 0° when the sound is straight in front of the subject, and is 90° when it is on the aural axis, that is, laterally in line with one ear (see figure 6.5). Factors affecting the threshold are:

(1) The azimuth position of the sound.
(2) The frequency and tonal purity of the sound.
(3) Interaural intensity differences.
(4) Interaural time differences.
(5) Interaural phase differences.
(6) Monaural localization.

6.31 Localization and azimuth

It is established that the resolving power of sound localization is highest or, in other words, the threshold for change is lowest, at the median plane or 0° and 180° positions (Pierce, 1901; Starch, 1905; Stevens and Newman, 1936; Wilcott, 1955; Mills, 1958; Jeffress and Taylor, 1961). Figure 6.6 shows the relations between azimuth angle and the minimum audible change of angle (derived from half the difference between the 25% and 75% points on the psychometric function expressing judgments 'to the right of the standard sound' as a function of change of azimuth angle). Changes in azimuth position of as little as 1° from the median plane can be discriminated. At the lateral position, on the other hand, a change of many degrees is necessary for discrimination.

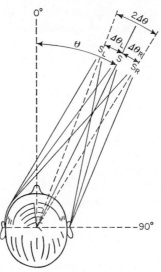

Figure 6.5 The minimum audible angle ($\Delta\theta$). The position of the sound source at the reference azimuth (θ) is indicated by S, and at each of the just noticeably different positions by S_L and S_R. The light lines indicate hypothetical sound paths to the ears from each source. [From Mills, 1958]

It is possible to distinguish whether complex sounds are in front of, behind, below or above the head, even though the ears are symmetrically stimulated in all these positions. Young (1931) demonstrated that if sounds are delivered to stethoscope ear-pieces this ability is lost. He concluded that the ear-pieces have this effect because of the elimination of differences between the diffraction patterns round the pinnae, of sounds in these different positions, and the elimination of the effects of head movements.

6.32 Localization thresholds and frequency

The localization threshold is also a function of the frequency of the sound. It remains fairly constant at about one degree at the median plane for fre-

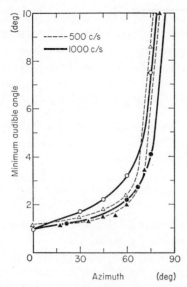

Figure 6.6 Average minimum audible angle as a function of azimuth at 500 and 1000 c/s. The outline symbols represent the results obtained with a horn source by Mills (1958), and the solid symbols those reported by Schmidt *et al.* (1953). [From Mills, 1958]

quencies up to about 1,000 c/s. Discrimination falls off and reaches a minimum at about 2,000 c/s but recovers again at higher frequencies (Stevens and New-man, 1936; Sandel, Teas, Feddersen, and Jeffress, 1955; Mills, 1958, 1960).

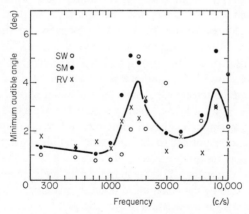

Figure 6.7 The minimum audible angle about the median plane as determined with a small source by Mills (1958)

These relationships are shown in figure 6.7. It will emerge in what follows that low-frequency tones are localized largely on the basis of interaural time differences, and high-frequency tones on the basis of interaural intensity differences. This may be called *the duplicity theory of auditory localization*.

6.33 Localization thresholds and interaural intensity differences

In an early study, Stewart and Hovda (1918) claimed that the reported azimuth position of a 256 c/s dichotic pure tone is related to the interaural intensity difference by the function:

$$\text{azimuth angle} = K \log \frac{I \text{ right}}{I \text{ left}}.$$

Stewart (1922) later reported that at some frequencies between 200 and 4,000 c/s interaural intensity differences were not effective in displacing a dichotic phantom. If such 'lapse regions' exist they could explain the contradictory results obtained by the different investigators who have studied the relationship between azimuth displacement and interaural intensity differences (Trimble, 1929; Halverson, 1922). However, Trimble (1935) failed to confirm their existence, and found that intensity differences were effective throughout the frequency range.

Mills (1960) investigated the role of interaural intensity differences in auditory localization in the following manner. He first measured the just noticeable interaural intensity difference of dichotic tone pulses as a function of their frequency. He then measured the objective interaural intensity differences produced by an actual single source, just noticeably displaced from the median plane, as a function of frequency. For those frequencies at which the two functions coincide it may be inferred that the actual source was localized by means of interaural intensity differences. The two functions are shown in figure 6.8. They correspond well between 1,500 and 5,000 c/s. At frequencies below 1,500 c/s diffraction around the head is so great that the resulting interaural intensity differences fall below threshold, which is in any case particularly high for low-frequency sounds. Above 6,000 c/s the subjects were able to discriminate dichotic intensity differences smaller than the differences that corresponded to the minimum audible angle. In other words, they were not making full use of the differences which were above threshold. This may have been because at these high frequencies large spurious intensity changes occur, due to the changing diffraction patterns of the small waves round the external ear as the head moves slightly.

Results published by Feddersen, Sandel, Teas, and Jeffress (1957), which were discussed in section 6.12, are at variance with those reported by Mills.

They measured the actual interaural intensity differences produced by sound sources at different frequencies, 50 cm away from the centre of the head. These were found to be below the intensity-difference threshold for *dichotic* localization in the case of tones below 5,000 c/s. In other words, they claimed that it is below 5,000 c/s, rather than 1,500 c/s, as Mills thought, that diffraction fails to produce intensity differences sufficient to serve as a basis for

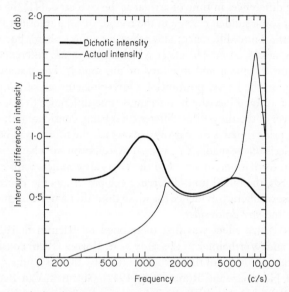

Figure 6.8 Idealized curves comparing thresholds for interaural differences in the intensity of dichotic tone pulses with the interaural differences in intensity produced by the minimum audible angle about the median plane. [From Mills, 1960]

localization. These results apply only to a sound 50 cm distant although sounds at a greater distance should produce even smaller intensity differences. Probe measurements of intensity differences vary with slight changes in the position of the probe microphone (Wiener and Ross, 1946). It is possible that actual sources produce greater intensity differences than those detected by the probes used by Feddersen *et al.*

The role of intensity differences in auditory localization is therefore very much a matter of dispute. Perhaps the contradictory findings are due to differences in the extent to which head movements were controlled.

It has recently been discovered that a pure tone in one ear can affect the lateralization of a pure tone in the other ear even when the first tone is a few decibels below the monaural intensity threshold (Guttman, 1962). This does not imply that the lateralization mechanism is more sensitive than the detection mechanism: there may be interaural facilitation.

6.34 Localization thresholds and interaural time differences

When one talks of interaural time differences in auditory localization, one refers to the differences in time of arrival at the two ears of (1) the start of the sound, or of some sudden change in the sound, or (2) a transient noise in the sound pattern. Time differences also affect interaural phase, but that is discussed in the next section. The effect which a given time difference will have depends upon the pitch and intensity of the sounds. For instance, there is more change in the lateral position of a low-pitched than of a high-pitched transient, for a given increase in interaural time difference (Teas, 1962).

Whichever of the above time differences is being considered, the ear which receives the prior signal is the ear towards which the source will be localized. Once the decision is made, the system is reluctant to change it, even if subsequent information conveyed to the two ears conflicts with its decision. In other words, the initial time-difference cue pre-empts the decision mechanism against conflicting evidence for some time after a noise is sounded. This is known as the *precedence effect*.

The precedence effect was first mentioned by Klemm in 1920, and by Hornbostel and Wertheimer in the same year. Boring (1926) considered that it is due to the inhibition of the second stimulus by the first; subsequent work by Wallach, Newman, and Rosenzweig (1949), Guttman, Van Bergeijk, and David (1960), and David (1959, 1962) has confirmed this view. Guttman *et al.* fed two pulses to one ear, and one pulse to the other. When the two pulses to the one ear were separated by, say, 10 msec, two phantoms could be heard successively as the single pulse was moved into appropriate time relations with each of the other two. For time intervals shorter than about 7 msec, only one fusion could be heard—that corresponding to the earlier pulse. This temporal masking effect was found to be decreased by background noise.

The argument that the precedence effect may be explained by temporal masking assumes that a masked noise is no longer available to the localization mechanism, and this may not be so: the fact that only the first of two closely spaced sounds is *reported* does not necessarily mean that the other one is lost to the localizing mechanism. The situation may be analogous to stereopsis, where, although only one 'fused' image of a pair of binocularly disparate images is discriminated, the observer is nevertheless able to estimate the position of the distal stimulus on the basis of disparity.

For complex noises, with complex 'envelopes', time differences may still serve localization, even when the component tones are well above the limit for phase-shift detection. It is now the transients in the frequency envelope which are 'timed' (Leakey, Sayers, and Cherry, 1958).

Intensity–time trading (see below) may still occur, although the functions probably differ from those obtained with pure tones (David, Guttman, and Van Bergeijk, 1959; Harris, 1960). Transients of low- and high-frequency context may be localized as a single phantom, as long as the frequency content to one ear is not too different from that to the other (Deatherage, 1961).

6.35 Localization thresholds and interaural phase differences

Time differences also affect the interaural phase difference. With dichotic pure tones of equal intensity which have been on for some time, only the phase difference can serve localization. Thompson (1877, 1878) and Rayleigh (1875, 1907) were the first to demonstrate that the lateral location of a sound was affected by the interaural phase difference. Identical in-phase dichotic sounds are localized in the region of the median plane; as the phase difference increases the phantom is reported to move laterally; for large phase differences the apparent source broadens and eventually splits into two sounds, one opposite each ear (Halverson, 1922; Hughes, 1939).

The same procedure which Mills used to study interaural intensity differences may be followed for studying the effectiveness of interaural phase differences in localization at different frequencies. The curve which shows the just noticeable interaural phase difference for dichotic tones as a function of frequency is plotted in figure 6.9, along with the curve showing the interaural time difference produced by an actual, single sound source. The two curves correspond well up to a frequency of about 1,500 c/s. Above this frequency the interaural phase difference becomes an ambiguous cue because the half wavelength of the sound approaches the dimensions of the head. In any case, this point probably represents the limit of resolving power for interaural time comparisons. Above this frequency interaural phase may be reversed without the subject noticing (Licklider and Webster, 1949). It is at about this frequency that interaural beats (successive phase summation and cancellation of a tone at one ear with a similar tone at the other) become inaudible, although the exact relationship between the two functions is a matter of some dispute (Licklider, Webster, and Hedlum, 1950; Zwislocki and Feldman, 1956).

There is now general agreement that the limiting frequency for phase-difference judgments with pure tones lies between 1,200 and 1,500 c/s (Stewart, 1920a, 1920b; Banister, 1925; Halverson, 1927; Klumpp, 1953;

Sandel, Teas, Feddersen, and Jeffress, 1955). Hughes (1940) obtained curves differing from those of other investigators, but Zwislocki and Feldman (1956) pointed out that Hughes' results were probably contaminated by re- action times.

If dichotic white noise is used, i.e. noise with all frequencies represented on an equal-energy basis, the phantom may still be localized by a phase difference as long as the two sources are correlated, that is, as long as their wave forms are identical from moment to moment when in phase. Pollack and Trittipoe (1959) found that subjects could identify above chance a change

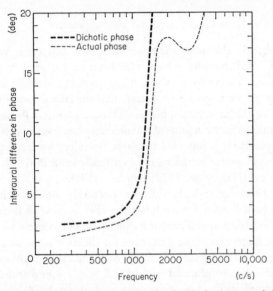

Figure 6.9 Idealized curves comparing thresholds for interaural differences in the phase of dichotic tone pulses with the interaural differences in phase produced by the minimum audible angle about the median plane. [From Mills, 1960]

in phase of 180° between diotic white noises correlated more than 0·66. Jeffress, Blodgett, and Deatherage (1962) obtained lateralization judgments even with a correlation of 0·1 between dichotic white noises. The highly correlated noises produced a tightly bunched phantom, and as the correlation was diminished the phantom spread out over a wider area. The discrepancy between the correlation thresholds in these two studies is probably due main- ly to the fact that diotic noises were used in one study and dichotic noises in the other.

The threshold for phase differences varies according to the intensity, frequency, and duration of the source. Figure 6.10 shows how the JND of dichotic phase for 1 sec pulses varies with sensation level at three different frequencies. It can be seen that the threshold is lowest at medium intensity levels and for low frequencies. Under optimal conditions it reaches a value of about 2°, which is equivalent to a time difference of 4 microseconds (μsec). Klumpp (1953) and Klumpp and Eady (1956) obtained time-difference thresholds for 65 db pure tones, wide-band (150–1,700 c/s) random

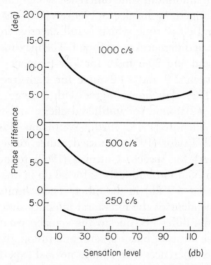

Figure 6.10 Just noticeable difference in dichotic phase as a function of sensation level at three frequencies. The curves represent the means of three subjects. [After Zwislocki and Feldman, 1956]

noise, and a 1 msec click. Of the pure tones, the 1,000 c/s tone gave the lowest threshold at 11 μsec. The random noise gave 9 μsec, and the click 28 μsec. The subjects were therefore more sensitive to phase differences in wide-band noise than in any pure tone. The threshold was much higher for the short click than for most of the tones and noises, which were sounded for 1·4 sec.

This last finding suggests that time-difference information is integrated over time. Tobias and Zerlin (1959) tested this idea by measuring the inter-aural time-difference threshold for white noises of varying duration. The function of time-difference threshold against duration became asymptotic at 0·7 sec, that is, time-difference information was being integrated over this period at the sound-pressure level used (65 db).

The fact that such small time differences serve for localization, does not mean that they are discriminated as time differences between successive noises. Kreidl and Gatscher (1923) rejected the time-difference hypothesis on the grounds that such small temporal intervals could not be discriminated. Their mistake was in confusing the role of time differences in localization with judgments of time intervals. For the early work on this problem see Mallock (1908), Aggazzotti (1911), Klemm (1918, 1920), Hornbostel and Wertheimer (1920), Pièron (1922), Hornbostel (1926).

So much for the minimum time difference which can be used as a basis for localization. Blodgett, Wilbanks, and Jeffress (1956) have determined the maximum interaural delay time which is still effective in dichotic localization. Wide individual differences were found. The maximum time difference was between 7·5 and and 20·6 msec for low-frequency-band noise (106–212 c/s), and between 2·5 and 14·2 msec for high-frequency-band noise (2,400–4,800 c/s). These last figures agree with a range of up to 15 msec, which Guttman (1962) found for unfiltered clicks, and with the results of earlier studies by Klemm (1918, 1920), Wittmann (1925), and Trimble (1928). Cherry and Taylor (1954) reported rather longer maximum time differences (25 msec) for speech. Guttman (1962) found the same time-difference limits for 36 db in both ears as for 36 db in one ear and the minimum effective level (− 2 db) in the other. These limits would therefore appear to be independent of the interaural intensity difference. The maximum interaural time difference due to the actual separation of the ears is about 1·5 msec. The limits of binaural temporal fusion, therefore, far exceed the maximum time differences met with in normal experience.

6.36 Monaural localization

Interaural differences in sensitivity, as revealed in audiogram measurements, must be considerable before having any detrimental effect on the ability to localize sounds (Sandel, Teas, Feddersen, and Jeffress, 1955; Nordlund, 1963). Evidently the auditory system is able to discount constant intensity differences and concentrate on the differential effects produced by changes of position. Jongkees and Van der Veer (1957, 1958) could find no consistent relationships between types of auditory defect and impairment of directional hearing. Even in patients with total unilateral deafness, directional hearing was found not to be completely lost and was normal in the case of one patient. For this reason it has been suggested that tests of auditory localization should be included in any comprehensive clinical examination of auditory functions (Sedee, 1957; Nordlund, 1963).

Monaural subjects cannot localize pure tones unless they move their heads (Angell and Fite, 1901; Wallach, 1940) but they can localize complex sounds, presumably by sensing the modifications of the partial tones produced by the head and pinnae (Mathes, 1955). The importance of the pinnae is demonstrated by an observation made by Holding and Dennis (1957). They found that auditory localization was improved when normal subjects wore a cap with earflaps. Evidently the flaps were enhancing the diffraction effects and hence interaural intensity differences.

The ability to localize sound monaurally is apparently improved if the inputs from a low-pass microphone at one ear and a high-pass microphone at the other are fed into the one ear (Mouzon, 1955).

6.4 Constant errors in auditory localization

Under many circumstances sounds are mislocalized or their reported position is unstable. The apparent position of a sound has been shown to be influenced by the following factors:

(1) Vestibular–kinaesthetic stimulation consequent upon rotation or tilt of the body.

(2) Eye movements and movements of the visual world.

(3) Random 'autokinetic' fluctuations.

(4) Auditory figural after-effects.

(5) Artificial displacement of the aural axis.

6.41 Vestibular–kinaesthetic influences on auditory localization

At one time it was suggested that auditory localization depends upon the semicircular canals. Diamant (1946) finally disproved this theory by showing that a patient with no functional labyrinths was still able to localize sounds adequately.

Even though the labyrinths are not the basic peripheral mechanism for auditory localization, stimulation of these structures does affect the apparent location of a sound. Münsterburg and Pierce (1894) first demonstrated that after a period of rotation about the body axis, subjects tend to misplace a sound in the direction of the previous rotation. A similar shift was reported by Clark and Graybiel (1949). They rotated their subjects at 20 rev/min for 6 turns. Before and after rotation, sounds were presented briefly at 10° intervals from 40° left to 40° right. The subject had to estimate the position of the sound in relation to the median plane. After rotation there was a 14° mean displacement of the sound in the direction of the previous rotation. This shift lasted from 20 to 35 sec and was accompanied by reports of apparent rotation of the body in the opposite direction i.e. there was an apparent shift of the median plane in the opposite direction to the apparent shift of the sounds. Very similar results were reported by Arnoult (1950) although a few of his subjects reported a displacement of the sound in the opposite direction to the previous rotation of the body. He relied on the subjects' pointing to the sound source, an unsatisfactory procedure, for pointing itself is affected by body rotation.

Goldstein (1925, 1926) found that patients with cerebellar or cortical lesions which resulted in tonus and postural disturbances on one side, mis-localized sounds towards the affected side.

Tilting the body sideways has also been found to affect the apparent position of a sound. Liebert and Rudel (1959) tested 70 blindfolded subjects between the ages of 5 and 17 years. They compared their subjects' settings of a sound to directly above their heads (i.e. on the main body axis) when they were upright, tilted 28° left, and tilted 28° right. The sound was reported to be displaced several degrees in the direction of the body tilt (see figure 6.11).

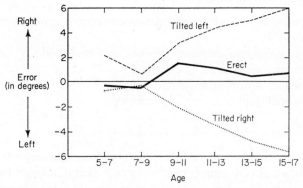

Figure 6.11 Effect of body tilt (left, erect, right) on localization of auditory mid-line as a function of age. [From Liebert and Rudel, 1959]

Graybiel and Niven (1951) found that subjects who were subjected to a displaced gravitational field in a centrifuge misjudged the position of a sound located in the same plane as that containing the initial and displaced direction of gravity. Graybiel and Niven related the judgments to the direction of the earth's gravitation. On this criterion, the direction of the sound was, on average, misjudged by 70% of the displacement of the direction of gravity. There appears to be some confusion over the direction of this effect. When the subject is facing the centre of rotation he has the same experience as if he were tilted backwards and one would therefore expect him to report stimuli as being above their true position relative to the apparent horizon. Graybiel and Niven actually report the effect as in the opposite direction to this expectation (p. 228) but we shall assume that this is a textual error. In any case, to use the earth's gravity as a reference is artificial; according to our analysis in section 7.46, this experiment is identical (side-effects apart) to one in which the subject is merely tilted. The error in terms of the resultant direction of gravity (the only one which meant anything to the subject) was 30% of the displacement angle, and it is this—the failure to behave 100% in accordance with the new direction of resultant force—which requires explanation. The centrifuge is entirely irrelevant, and to grace the effect with the name 'audiogravic illusion' is to give the misleading impression that a new phenomenon has been discovered.

6.42 *The effects of eye movements and visual movement on auditory localization*

Pierce (1901) and Goldstein and Rosenthal-Veit (1926) reported that fixation of the open eyes to one side produces an apparent displacement of a sound in the same direction, and that a sideways position of the closed eyes produces an apparent shift of a sound in the opposite direction. Neither quantitative data nor the precise instructions to the subjects were reported. Ryan and Schehr (1941) repeated the experiment, asking the subjects to report whether a sound was straight ahead, to the left, or to the right. The results were very variable. Some subjects showed the effects which Goldstein and Rosenthal-Veit reported, but others showed an opposite effect, and most subjects showed no consistent effects at all. Perhaps Ryan and Schehr's instructions were ambiguous: 'straight ahead' could refer to either the body median plane or the visual axis. In view of the different available criteria, and possible differences in the degree to which different people may adopt one or other of them, it is not surprising that large individual differences exist. An analogous situation holds in the case of judgments of the visual straight ahead in the presence of conflicting cues (see section 11.3).

Results of studies on the effects of visual movement on auditory localization are also contradictory. Gemelli (1951) found that most subjects, placed in the centre of a rotating striped cylinder, reported a sound as displaced in the opposite direction to the rotation of the stripes. However, this effect was only evident when the subject reported that the stripes appeared to move; when he interpreted the situation as one in which his own body was moving and the stripes standing still, the sound was not consistently reported as displaced in either direction. Arnoult (1952) did a similar experiment but found no significant effects in his subjects as a whole, but he apparently made no distinction between whether the subjects interpreted the movement as being of the visual stimulus or of themselves. Here again, therefore, the type of judgment a subject makes may depend upon the frame of reference he adopts.

The effects of the position of visual objects on sound localization are considered in section 14.3.

6.43 Auditory autokinesis and apparent movement

One would expect that the location of single small sounds in an otherwise noiseless and dark surround would seem to fluctuate in an analogous fashion to the well-known visual autokinetic effect. Bernadin and Gruber (1957) obtained unsolicited reports of spontaneous drifting of pure-tone sources of various frequencies sounded one at a time for 5 min each. The phenomenon does not seem to have been investigated by anyone else.

There have been reports of apparent auditory movement analogous to apparent movement in vision (Burtt, 1917; Bourdon, 1925). That is, two successive sounds some distance apart, are reported as a single moving sound. Burtt found an optimum time delay of between 10 and 50 msec—a similar range of values to that found for visual apparent movement.

Nobody, it seems, has attempted to discover whether there is a movement after-effect in auditory space, analogous to the movement after-effect or waterfall illusion in vision.

6.44 Auditory figural after-effects

There have been several reports dating back to the 20's to the effect that a sound is apparently displaced from the position of a previous nearby sound (Flugel, 1921; Bartlett and Mark, 1922; Jones and Bunting, 1949). More recently Krauskopf (1954) has considered this displacement after-effect in the context of Köhler and Wallach's (1944) theory of visual figural after-effects. Comparing Jones and Bunting's data with his own, he concluded that the auditory displacement effect, like the visual after-effect, exhibits a distance paradox, at first increasing as a function of the separation between the inspection and test sounds, and then decreasing as the angle of separation increases beyond a certain point. He also found that the after-effect decayed with time after the end of the inspection sound, in an analogous way to the decay of visual after-effects. Taylor (1962) reported experiments in which a more extended range of separations between inspection and test sounds was used. His results agree well with the corresponding results of Krauskopf, and direct evidence of a distance paradox was obtained. The effect increased as the separation between the sounds was increased to about 30°, thereafter it decreased to almost zero at a separation of 90°.

Pre-adapting one ear to white noise can disturb the balance of localization of dichotic white noise towards the unadapted ear. Carterette, Friedman, Lindner, and Pierce (1964) found that after pre-adapting one ear to a noise of over 60 db for 10 min, a 30 db brief noise in the adapted ear was not reported to be lateralized at that ear even though the noise level in the unadapted ear was zero. In so far as an inspection sound produces unequal intensities at the two ears, auditory figural after-effects could be due to a differential adaptation of the kind which Carterette *et al.* found. However, Krauskopf found that inspection of a sound in the median plane reduced the variability of subsequent determinations of the median plane. This effect could not be due to differential adaptation, nor even to equal binaural adaptation, which should increase variability rather than decrease it. More evidence is called for on this point.

6.45 *Artificial displacement of the aural axis*

As a child grows, the shape and size of its head changes. There will result a change in the relative effects which a sound source has on the two ears. Held (1955) argued that the growing child must constantly adjust its auditory-localization behaviour to compensate for these changes. If this is so, then similar systematic changes suffered by an adult may produce shifts of localization. Held fitted three adults with electric pseudophones which displaced the aural axis by 22° around the vertical axis of the head. At the end of seven hours spent in a normal environment, the subjects were tested without the pseudophones and reported that the test sound was simultaneously in two different directions from 8° to 21° apart. This doubling is analogous to binocular diplopia (see section 2.3). It demonstrates that a new frame of reference has been established, but that the old frame is still present. Perhaps the old frame remained because the pseudophones did not completely exclude direct sound to the ears, although Held reported that the direct sound was attenuated by 40 db. Freedman and Stampfer (1964) have recently confirmed that subjects adapt to a displacement of the aural axis.

6.5 Intensity–time trading

Consider the arrangement shown in figure 6.12. Two identical in-phase speakers are emitting the same pure tone at the same intensity. The listener reports hearing a single phantom in front of him. If the signal to one speaker is now delayed in time (phase) by, say, one millisecond, the phantom source is reported to move towards the other speaker. However, by increasing the intensity of the delayed signal it is possible to restore the position of the phantom to its original central location, although a 'spatial widening' of the sound will be reported. The intensity difference is said to have been 'traded' against the phase difference. As greater time delays are compensated for, the

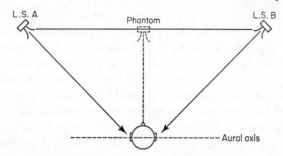

Figure 6.12 A simple arrangement for demonstrating intensity–time trading. [After Leakey and Cherry, 1957]

widening effect becomes more obvious, until the listener is unable to make a consistent judgment.

6.51 Methods of measuring trading

The method just outlined for studying trading has been used by Snow (1954), and Leakey and Cherry (1957).

In practice it is more common to measure intensity–time trading using dichotic stimulation, for it is possible to control the stimulation to each ear more precisely in this way. The technique described above of off-centring the phantom by introducing a time difference, and restoring with an intensity difference, is commonly used.

A second commonly used method is to match the position of an intensity-difference, pure-tone phantom with a simultaneous broad-frequency-band, time-difference pointer (Moushegian and Jeffress, 1959). These techniques will be referred to as the centring technique and pointer technique respectively.

A third method of measuring trading is to use the nullity method described by Kikuchi (1957) and applied to this problem by Harris (1960) (see section 6.22).

Precise methods of varying interaural phase have been available only since about 1940. Before that time phase was varied by altering the relative lengths of tubes, and it was difficult to exclude interaural intensity differences (Klemm, 1920; Halverson, 1922; Wittman, 1925; Trimble, 1929).

Whichever method is used the results are usually expressed as a ratio of the time difference which is equivalent to a unit intensity difference. Shaxby and Gage (1932) called this ratio a *trading relation*. It is expressed in microseconds per decibel.

An enormous range of trading ratios has been reported. Shaxby and

Gage reported 1·7 μsec/db. At the opposite extreme, Christman and Victor (1955) reported 100–150 μsec/db. It is now known that many factors affect the trading relation. Among these are the interaural intensity difference, the absolute intensity level, the frequency or frequency band, the duration of the sound, and the presence of masking noise. The effects that these factors have will be discussed in the following account of possible mechanisms underlying trading.

6.52 Cue summation

Several mechanisms may be responsible for the particular form of the trading functions. The most obvious assumption is that the two 'cues' of time and intensity cancel out when they are opposed and add when they are congruent. However, Trimble (1935) found that this simple model does not explain the data; when the two factors are varied congruently, the net change in localization is less than the change brought about by the more effective factor acting alone. It is a common experience of all investigators that when the factors are opposed, the sound is reported to be spread out, and judgments are consequently very variable.

The two factors obviously interact in a complex fashion. Some features of this interaction may be predicted on physiological grounds.

6.53 Physiological latency conversion

It is well established that the latency of a receptor's response is decreased when the stimulus intensity is increased. The latency of the cochlear response is affected in this way by the intensity of the sound stimulus. Pestalozza and Davis (1956), measuring at the cochlea, found a change of about 1 msec over an 80 db range. Similar changes have been recorded higher up the auditory pathways and in the auditory cortex (Thurlow, Gross, Kemp, and Lowy, 1951; Galambos, Rose, Bromiley, and Hughes, 1952; Rosenzweig, 1954). It follows that if one ear is stimulated more intensely than the other, it will respond more quickly. An intensity difference therefore becomes a time difference. Such a mechanism was first suggested by Hornbostel (1926) and could clearly explain why it is possible to restore an off-centre intensity-difference phantom by means of a time difference. We shall refer to this mechanism as *physiological latency conversion* to distinguish it from trading, which is a psychophysical concept that may or may not be explained in terms of physiological conversion.

Deatherage, Eldredge, and Davis (1959) studied in detail the factors which determine the latency of response in the cochlea of the guinea pig. They measured the latency of that part of the nerve action-potential recorded from the whole cochlear nerve which is well synchronized with the stimulus. The latency of this part was found to include two factors: (1) the time necessary for the travelling sound-wave to reach different parts of the basilar membrane of the cochlea, and (2) the neural delay (utilization time) required for the integration of sufficient energy to fire the neuron. Whitworth and Jeffress (1961) added a third delay factor: the time required for the displacement of the membrane to reach the stimulation level. Deatherage et al. (1959), and Deatherage and Hirsh (1959) were able to isolate the travelling-wave latency from the neural-delay latency by selective frequency masking of different parts of the cochlear membrane, by selective fatigue, and by the local injection of drugs. They concluded that nearly all the well-synchronized cochlear nerve action-potential is due to neurons which arise in the first turn or high-frequency end of the cochlea. The travelling-wave delay is a significant component only when the high-frequency response is suppressed.

This interpretation is supported by the observation made by Moushegian and Jeffress (1959) that people with high-frequency loss show higher intensity–time trading ratios than people with normal hearing. For those with high-frequency deafness, high-frequency tones are nearer the threshold and therefore give a longer latency and hence more potentiality for trade.

Whitworth and Jeffress also found that masking of the response from the first turn of the cochlea of one ear by high-frequency noise shifted the dichotic phantom click towards the opposite ear, in spite of the fact that the intensity of sound to the first ear had been increased by the masking noise. They concluded that the relative amplitudes of the whole-nerve action-potentials are less important than the relative modal time of their initiation, in determining the localization of a click phantom. This conclusion is perhaps not warranted, for the subject would probably discount that part of the intensity difference induced by the masking noise, in making the lateralization judgment of the click. In other words the subject may not have been unresponsive to the intensity difference, but may have merely treated it as irrelevant (which it was) to the task of localizing the click, in which case the latency difference would not be pitted against an effective amplitude difference.

Deatherage and Hirsh finally concluded that 'intensity, having made its contribution to neural "time", may drop out of consideration leaving the judgment of localization almost entirely dependent upon the results of a comparison of neural times.' Others had also come to this conclusion. (See Schubert, 1963, for a further discussion of unilateral masking and trading, and Leakey and Cherry, 1957, for a discussion of the effects of binaural masking.)

Whether or not this conclusion is justified, it is certainly true that peripheral physiological latency conversion accounts for many of the facts about trading, as the following discussion will show.

Figure 6.13 shows a set of functions obtained by plotting the trading ratio for high-frequency clicks as a function of the interaural intensity difference at different absolute intensity values. These results were obtained by David, Guttman, and Van Bergeijk (1959), and similar results were obtained by Deatherage and Hirsh (1959). It can be seen that the trading ratios are

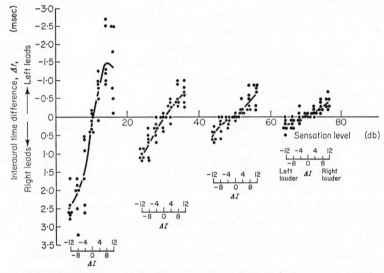

Figure 6.13 Set of trading functions obtained by David, Guttman, and Van Bergeijk (1959) by plotting the trading ratio for high-frequency clicks as a function of the interaural intensity difference at different absolute intensity values. The signs of Δt and ΔI with regard to sidedness are indicated. The long abscissa serves to locate the reference level only; datum points are to be referred to the subabscissae. The curves drawn through the plots were obtained from third-degree polynomial fits

higher for less intense sounds than they are for loud sounds. At lower sound levels the latency of the ear's response is long, and therefore there is a greater potentiality for change of latency with level. At high intensities the latency approaches its limit, so that there is no 'reserve' for physiological conversion. In so far as physiological conversion is the cause of trading, these facts explain the way the trading ratio varies with intensity level.

Moushegian and Jeffress (1959) found that trading functions for high-frequency tones tend to be less than for low-frequency tones. This may be due to the fact that a 1000 c/s signal produces a given displacement of the basilar membrane in half the time required for a 500 c/s signal of the same amplitude just because there are twice as many peaks. This should result in shorter latencies, and hence smaller reserves for latency changes, for the higher-frequency tone. Here again therefore, the latency hypothesis is able to explain the facts.

However, the following arguments have been put forward to show that intensity differences do function in their own right in spite of this physiological conversion.

(1) Intensity differences still operate at frequencies where phase differences can no longer be discriminated (Stewart, 1922).

(2) When an intensity-difference phantom is centred by a time difference the variability of judgments is greater than when sounds equal in intensity are centred. This would not be so if intensity differences and time differences were truly equivalent (Harris, 1960).

(3) When a constant intensity difference is traded against a variable phase difference the resulting trading function differs from that obtained by the reverse process, of trading a constant phase difference against a variable intensity difference (Moushegian and Jeffress, 1959). According to the latency-conversion hypothesis they should be the same.

(4) It is commonly reported that if there is a dichotic interaural intensity difference or phase difference, the subject will detect two phantoms (Trimble, 1935). One way to interpret this fact is to assume that one phantom is produced by the physiological latency-conversion mechanism, and the other by the intensity-difference information. This latency-conversion time difference will differ from the total (direct and conversion) time difference associated with the same intensity difference produced by a single sound source. Thus the dichotic sounds produce an atypical combination of time difference and intensity difference which the subject interprets as two phantoms. However, Whitworth and Jeffress (1961) have argued that both phantoms can be accounted for if one assumes that there are two peripheral latency-conversion mechanisms.

(5) Thurlow and Elfner (1959) found that when tones of slightly different frequency were presented to the two ears one of them was 'pulled-in' from the side position by increasing the intensity of the tone in the other ear. This effect, they argued, must be due to intensity differences as such.

(6) Blodgett, Wilbanks, and Jeffress (1956) have found that subjects can judge the sidedness of a dichotic phantom on the basis of a short time difference (1–4 msec) in spite of a large intensity difference of 15 db in the opposite direction.

Perhaps all these objections to the theory that only time differences are ultimately involved in localization will eventually be overcome.

Although both time–intensity and intensity–time trading can be accounted for by conversion of intensity differences into time differences, it is possible that there are peripheral mechanisms by which time differences are converted into interaural intensity differences. One possibility is that sound from one ear is conducted by bone conduction to the other, resulting in some summation of the direct with the indirect sound in each ear. The degree of this intensity summation will depend upon the interaural time or phase differences. In this way time differences could be converted into intensity differences (Wilson and Myers, 1908).

Boring (1926) suggested another way, viz. that the prior stimulus inhibits the second one at some point in the projection pathways where the impulses from the two ears meet. This possibility has already been discussed in section 6.34.

6.6 Localization of multiple sources

If several familiar complex noises are present at the same time, it is possible to judge the direction of each. This would not be possible if the different noises were not recognized as separate noise patterns: auditory pattern recognition must precede localization.

Cherry and Bowles (1960) measured the accuracy with which a dichotic speech source could be localized relative to a second dichotic speech source centred on the median plane. They then repeated the experiment using two complex independent white noises. The subjects could accurately discriminate when the two speech sounds were separated by means of a change in the interaural time difference of one of them. The two white noises could not be separated at all, but remained fused as one sound 'image'. Cherry and Bowles concluded that it is impossible for a subject to separate sound patterns with which he is not familiar: prior probabilities are essential.

This conclusion is not warranted, for no amount of prior knowledge would enable a person to separate two white noises; they do not have any pattern in them and Cherry and Bowles' experiment demonstrates this fact. It is not the lack of 'prior' probabilities which is important, but the lack of any sequential probabilities at all. They should have compared the ability to separate speech noises with the ability to separate unfamiliar modulated noises, that is, noises with a similar envelope pattern to that of speech but unfamiliar to the subjects. We predict that had they done this the 'prior knowledge' would have made little difference. In other words, people are very good at detecting sound patterns whether or not they have heard them before, just as they can detect unfamiliar visual patterns. The more complex and random the pattern gets, the less certain would be the separation, and experience with particular complexes may restore accuracy. But the experiments which would show this have yet to be done. Cherry is right, however, in insisting that a separation of sound patterns must precede, or at least accompany, the act of localization, and his experiments do demonstrate this fact.

Cherry and Taylor (1954) demonstrated that binaural fusion of a speech source breaks down if the interaural delay time is greater than about 15 msec, that is, about 20 times the maximum delay ever experienced by virtue of the separation of the ears. Within these limits the nervous system must possess the ability to relate the pattern arriving at one ear to that arriving at the other and integrate them as a single 'fused' image. This process is analogous to the process of binocular fusion and, as in that case, the word 'fusion' must not be taken as implying that the two messages lose their identity physiologically. This cannot be so, as time differences very much less than the fusion limit continue to serve as a basis for localization.

Even though the discrimination of auditory patterns must accompany localization, the fact that complex sounds occupy separate positions in space makes it easier to listen selectively to one of them (Koenig, 1950; Schubert and Schultz, 1962). Having selected one speech pattern for attention, it is as if the nervous system 'tunes in' to the particular time-delay features of that pattern arising from its particular spatial position, and 'filters off' patterns with different time-delay characteristics (Kock, 1950).

The threshold for binaural masking of speech by noise has been found to depend on the interaural phase difference of the speech relative to that of the noise. When these are the same, discrimination is most difficult (Hirsh, 1950). The threshold for masking of pure tones by white noise has been found to be affected by as much as 12 db by the relative interaural phase differences of the tone and noise (Jeffress, Blodgett, and Deatherage, 1952). Jeffress called a difference of threshold of this kind a 'masking level difference'.

In line with this evidence is the fact that patients with hearing losses are better able to discriminate speech from noise with a binaural hearing aid as compared with a monaural aid (Belzile and Markle, 1959; Lidén and Nordlund, 1960). For further details of the work by Cherry, see Cherry (1953, 1961), Cherry and Sayers (1956, 1959), Sayers and Cherry (1957).

6.7 The physiology of auditory localization

6.71 The neural centres involved in auditory localization

Both cochleae are represented in each auditory cortical projection area. Electrophysiological studies have revealed that stimulation of a cochlea evokes stronger responses in the contralateral cortex (Bremer and Dow, 1939; Tunturi, 1944, 1946; Rosenzweig, 1951). Earlier ablation studies by Luciani (1884) had shown the same thing. It seems that cats with bilateral ablation of the auditory cortex cannot localize clicks, even though they may be able to localize prolonged sounds. This latter ability probably does not depend upon binaural integration, but rather on changes consequent upon head movements. Earlier claims that localization is possible without the auditory cortex were based on the use of stimuli prolonged enough to allow head movements to occur (Ten Cate, 1934; Neff and Diamond, 1958).

In man it is unlikely that any form of auditory localization is possible with bilateral loss of auditory cortex. But with unilateral loss some localization is possible, even on the basis of interaural time difference (Walsh, 1957). Teuber and Diamond (1956) studied 20 patients with brain injuries, 14 of them unilateral. Compared with normal subjects these patients required larger dichotic time differences and intensity differences to shift a click from the median plane. Subjects with unilateral lesions in the right hemisphere required greater intensity in the left ear than in the right in order to judge a sound to be in the median plane, and conversely for subjects with left-sided lesions. Related to these findings are the observations made by Penfield and Rasmussen (1950): when stimuli were applied to the auditory cortex of one hemisphere, the human subjects reported a sound on the opposite side.

More precise information about the cortical correlates of binaural localization is supplied by Rosenzweig and Rosenblith (1950), Bremer (1952), and Rosenzweig (1954). Dichotic time intervals of one-tenth of a millisecond were found to affect cortical response amplitudes. The response in one hemisphere was found to be larger when the contralateral ear received the prior stimulus. These cortical events were found to parallel the corresponding psychophysical judgments in the following respects. When the dichotic phantom was in the median plane the activity in the two hemispheres was equal; when the phantom was heard at one side of the head the cortical activity was greater at the contralateral hemisphere, and the more lateral the apparent position of the sound, the greater was the difference between the activity at the two hemispheres.

Interactions of a similar kind were also recorded electrophysiologically at the inferior colliculus (Rosenzweig and Wyers, 1955; Erulkar, 1959), at the lateral lemniscus (Rosenzweig and Sutton, 1958), and at the superior olivary nuclei (Galambos, Schwartzkopf, and Rupert, 1959). However, no interactions have been recorded at the cochlea itself (Rosenzweig and Amon, 1955).

Thus, although the auditory cerebral cortex is necessary for auditory localization in man, the coding process seems to be initiated at the level of the olivary nuclei, and maintained from there up to the cortex. For a fuller discussion of this topic see Rosenzweig (1961).

It has been claimed that damage in areas of cerebral cortex other than the auditory cortex of the temporal lobes, results in impairment of directional hearing. For instance, Matzker and Welker (1959) reported that such impairment results from damage in the frontal, parietal, and occipital lobes as well as the temporal lobes. However, Greene (1929) and Sanchez-Longo and Forster (1958) found loss of directional hearing only in patients with temporal lobe lesions.

6.72 Models of auditory localization functions

Several models of the neural processes responsible for auditory localization have been proposed. Békésy (1930) proposed that there exists in the brain a nucleus consisting of neurons innervated by both ears. Nervous signals arriving from the left 'tune' these neurons 'left', signals arriving from the right 'tune' them 'right'. If the signal from one side is more intense it advances on a broader front; if it is prior, it reaches more cells in the nucleus than the signal from the other ear. The total number of cells 'tuned' each way constitutes the neural coding of localization. The model accounts for the way in which both time differences and intensity differences may affect localization; however, the mechanism of bidirectional 'tuning' does not accord with modern ideas of neural functioning.

Jeffress (1948) proposed a mechanism for the representation of a time difference as a locus of responses in neural tissue. Like Békésy he assumed that there is a centre where tracts from both ears make common synaptic connections. If the two ears are equally stimulated the impulses meet in the middle of the hypothetical centre; if one ear is stimulated before the other the impulses meet to one side or the other, depending on the relative times which the two impulses take to cross the common centre as they approach it from opposite sides. This model appears to take no account of intensity differences as such, and cannot, it seems, account for the localization of high-frequency tones, where time information is lacking. However, David, Guttman, and Van Bergeijk (1959) have suggested that such a model could account for localization on the basis of intensity, for there will be a higher probability of meetings on the side of the centre receiving the smaller number of impulses. This would produce the same sort of asymmetry which is produced when that side of the centre is receiving impulses later in time.

Van Bergeijk (1962) has proposed a similar but more sophisticated model. Relying on physiological and histological data by Stotler (1953) and Galambos, Schwartzkopf, and Rupert (1959), Van Bergeijk suggests that each cochlear nucleus sends inhibitory fibres to the ipsilateral accessory nucleus (medial superior olivary nucleus) and excitatory fibres to the contralateral accessory nucleus. The corresponding fibres from each cochlea converge on common cells in the accessory nucleus which then discharge to higher centres via the lateral lemniscus (see figure 6.14).

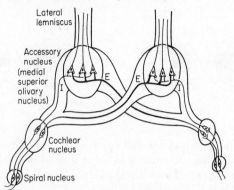

Figure 6.14 Outline of essential features of the model, proposed by Van Bergeijk (1962) to account for auditory localization. Cochlear-nucleus neurons send inhibitory fibres (I) to the ipsilateral, and excitatory fibres (E) to the contralateral accessory nucleus. Neurons of the accessory nuclei receive inhibitory fibres as well as excitatory fibres on their dendrites. See text for further details

The balance of excitation and inhibition of cells in the two accessory nuclei is assumed to be affected by interaural intensity and time differences. Simultaneous, equal-intensity clicks excite equal areas in the two nuclei as in figure 6.15(a). When one click leads, it causes a larger excited area on the

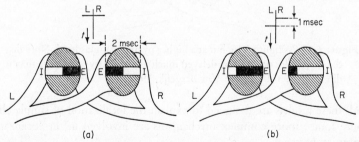

Figure 6.15 (a) Simultaneous, equal-intensity clicks excite equal areas (black) in the two nuclei, resulting in a centred image; (b) When one click leads, it causes a larger excited area on the contralateral side, resulting in an off-centre image. Inhibited area white, unaffected area hatched. [From Van Bergeijk, 1962]

contralateral side, resulting in an off-centre image (figure 6.15(b)). When the intensity at one ear is greater than at the other, the inhibitory and excitatory influences do not cancel over the whole width of the active areas in the two nuclei (figure 6.16(a)), resulting in binaural imbalance. This may be

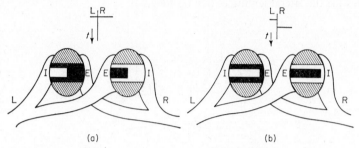

Figure 6.16 As figure 6.15, but with a stronger stimulus in R ear.(a) L and R stimulus simultaneous, resulting in binaural imbalance; (b) R stimulus delayed so that excited areas (black) are equal, resulting in binaural centre percept. [From Van Bergeijk, 1962]

restored by time trading as in figures 6.16(b) and 6.17. The model appears to account for most of the facts and is, unlike earlier theories, well grounded in physiology.

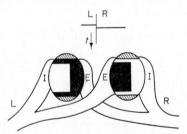

Figure 6.17 As figure 6.16, but at a higher overall stimulus level. Note that the R stimulus needs to be delayed much less to achieve a balance than it did in figure 6.16. [From Van Bergeijk, 1962]

All these models are designed to explain the localization of simple clicks or pure tones; more complex mechanisms are involved in the localization of complex noises.

This review is not fully comprehensive, especially with regard to the earlier literature. For further details see the following reviews: Pierce (1901), Ferree and Collins (1911), Stevens and Davis (1938), Boring (1942), Rayleigh (1945), and Békésy (1960).

7

Orientation to gravity I

7.1 Introduction

Gravity is the most constant, pervasive, and significant of all the features of man's environment to which he orients himself. Under normal conditions it is virtually constant, both in strength and direction, and affects practically every aspect of man's overt behaviour.

A man has a mid-body axis which is normally kept in line with the direction of gravity; any disturbance is corrected by many complex postural reflex mechanisms. Discussion will be limited for the most part to rotations of the body (head and trunk) and the eyes in the frontal plane. These are two of the basic variables as both stimuli and responses. Furthermore, man lives in an environment of visible objects and surfaces which usually maintain a constant relation to gravity and provide a visible frame of reference. However, the visible frame of reference may itself be tilted, which adds a third important variable.

The possible combinations between body tilt, eye tilt (torsion), and visible frame tilt are schematically depicted in figure 7.1(a)–(h). The squares in the 'eyes' depict the visible frame; its orientation is indicated by the position of the small pointer. The orientation of the two eyes are similarly indicated. The orientation of the head (and body) is indicated by the 'nose'. All directions are with reference to gravity which is considered to be in line with the sides of the page. There are thus four stimulus factors, (1) body tilt, (2) eye torsion, (3) visible-frame tilt, and (4) gravity, but only three degrees of freedom since gravity is always considered fixed. Ignoring differences of extent and direction of tilt, there are eight possible states of the system. This is the basic plan of stimulus conditions in terms of which judgments of, and motor responses to gravity will be discussed.

The responses to each of these stimulus conditions may be classified according to the plan set out in table 7.1. A man may set an external reference

Table 7.1 A classification of responses to gravity

Response or task	Influences
Eye torsion	Body tilt (countertorsion, section 3.42) Visible-frame rotation (optokinetic torsion, section 3.43)
Setting or judging the orientation of an external line with respect to gravity, by sight; by touch	⎧ Body tilt ⎫ (Aubert and Müller ⎨ Eye torsion ⎬ effects, section 7.4) ⎩ Visible-frame tilts (section 7.5) As above (section 8.6)
Setting or judging the orientation of the body with respect to gravity	Visible frame, and eye torsion in so far as it affects the apparent orientation of the visible frame (chapter 8)

line to alignment with gravity. But his performance is likely to be influenced by the tilt of his body axis, eye torsion, and the visible frame. Under normal

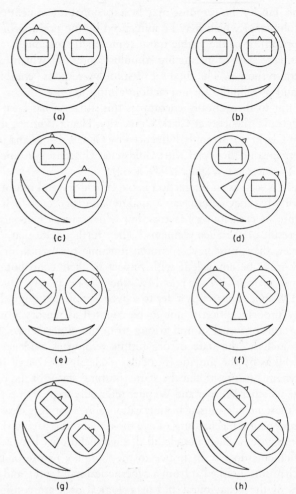

Figure 7.1 A classification of the relative positions of body, eyes, and visual frame. (a) Normal; (b) Eyes tilted (cyclophoria); (c) Body tilted, eyes erect (countertorsion); (d) Body and eyes tilted; (e) Frame and eyes tilted (optokinetic torsion); (f) Frame tilted; (g) Body and frame tilted, eyes erect (countertorsion); (h) Body, frame, and eyes tilted

circumstances the directions of these three factors coincide with gravity and any one of them may be successfully used as an index of the direction of gravity. When they do not coincide with gravity, the subject may use an inappropriate index or combination of indices. Secondly, his task may be to set his body to gravity, when he may be influenced by eye torsion, and the visible frame. Finally, his response may be a torsional movement of the eyes (always involuntary) which may be influenced by the position of the body (utricular torsion) or of the visible frame (optokinetic torsion).

We thus have a set of interacting stimulus conditions which may evoke one of several responses. The total set of stimulus–response combinations is very great and possibilities for interactions almost infinite.

An attempt to theoretically encompass this situation has been made by the 'sensory–tonic' theorists at Clark University. Heinz Werner, the former Chairman at Clark, was strongly influenced by Gestalt theory and in particular by the organismic theory of Kurt Goldstein. The sensory–tonic theory is outlined in Werner and Wapner (1949, 1952).

Perception is seen as an interaction between sensory and motor elements arising out of what they describe as 'a total dynamic process which might be analysable into its contributory factors, but which cannot be conceived as a summative result of the alien elements.' They further state that, 'If factors are to interact, they must have common dynamic properties; or, in other words, they must be equivalent with respect to their contribution to the total dynamic process' (Werner and Wapner, 1949, p. 91). By 'sensory' Werner and Wapner apparently refer to exteroception, although they never explain why proprioception is not to be counted as sensory nor do they explain the status of visual stimuli arising from the subject's own body. By 'tonic' they include 'the state of organismic tension as evidenced by the visceral as well as by the somatic (muscular–skeletal) reactivity.' It includes both 'the dynamic (motion) and the static (posture) status of the organism.' It is not clear whether Werner and Wapner refer only to proprioception here or whether they include muscular innervation also. Nor is it clear whether the stimuli and neural mechanisms of eye movements are part of the sensory or of the tonic system. Such a crude, ill-defined dichotomy between sensory and tonic elements does scant justice to the complex nature of behaviour control mechanisms. Looked at from a cybernetical standpoint, and when the complexities of the behavioural and neurological data are considered, the sensory–tonic theory is seen as a wordy, oversimplified, poorly-defined set of ideas.

Werner and Wapner attempted to give these ideas predictive value by suggesting that their validity may be tested by showing (1) that tonic factors interact with sensory factors in 'perceptual formation' and (2) that sensory and tonic factors are 'dynamically equivalent'. They wrote, 'Since any neuropsychological entity is neither sensory nor motor but a dynamic process prior to both, it may be affected in a similar way by stimulation through the receptors, as well as by direct stimulation of the muscles.' And 'if stimuli interfere, or are incommensurate with the organismic state, there emerges a tendency in the organism to change its state in the direction towards establishment of equilibrium between body and object' (Werner and Wapner, 1952, p. 325). These 'predictions' were claimed to have been borne out by a series of experiments conducted at Clark University. These experiments are described in various parts of this book (sections 2.53, 7.3, 7.4, 11.3). It will be shown that the theory has been used to predict contradictory results and even if these contradictions could be resolved, the theoretical formulations are so broad that almost anything would be predicted with suitable *ad hoc* assumptions. The theory is so general and untied to specific operationally definable variables that it is untestable.

Subjects certainly combine stimulus information from many modalities as well as from the state of innervation of muscles in making certain judgments, such as whether the visible world is stable, or whether a rod is upright. If this is what Werner and Wapner mean by 'dynamic equivalence', we agree—but why use esoteric language to describe a state of affairs which has been known for a long time and which can be simply described in ordinary language or, if necessary, in the technically precise language of control theory?

We shall attempt to describe the many complex interactions between stimuli and responses in the way people behave in relation to gravity, avoiding jargon where possible.

7.2 The judgment of inclination

Several investigators have reported on the accuracy with which a man is able to set a luminous line to the vertical. Reported average unsigned deviations from the true vertical are approximately: Jastrow (1892), $\frac{2}{3}°$; Neal (1926), 1°; Witkin and Asch (1948a), 1·5°; Mann, Berthelot-Berry, and Dauterive (1949), 1°; Kaufmann, Reese, Volkmann, and Rogers (1949), 1° or less. In all these investigations, only a luminous line was visible. Considering that the length of the line and other factors were not the same in the various studies, the results are in good agreement. Figures for the vertical and horizontal were found to be similar by Mann *et al.*

No large constant errors were found, except by Cohen and Tepas (1958) who found a constant error of 2·3° to the left of the true vertical (they gave no variance measures). Gibson and Radner (1937) found consistent constant errors varying from subject to subject. The errors ranged from a few tenths of a degree up to 2°, either clockwise or anticlockwise.

There is a good deal of evidence that the vertical and horizontal positions of a line are more accurately judged and produced than other positions. Table 7.2 shows the mean average deviations of the settings which five

Table 7.2 Mean average deviations of settings, produced by five
subjects, of lines to various inclinations (Gibson and Radner, 1937)

Position to be set (deg)	Vert.	30	45	60	Horiz.
Mean average deviation (deg)	0·28	1·99	1·44	1·74	0·52

subjects made of a line to various positions. It can be seen that the vertical and
horizontal positions were produced with least variability and the 30° and
60° positions with most variability. Results obtained by Jastrow are in substantial agreement with these results from Gibson and Radner (1937).

Takala (1951b, p. 31) asked subjects to set a variable line parallel to a
standard line. The two lines could be seen, one at a time, as often as the
subject wished. It was found that the positions of vertical and horizontal
standards were reproduced with greatest accuracy, and those of standards at
45° with least accuracy. In a second study, Takala (1951a) used a variety of
psychophysical procedures to study the judgment of inclination. In the first
series of experiments the subject had to set a line to be of equal inclination to
each of three standards of 30°, 45°, and 60°. The standards were presented
for 4 sec followed, after a further interval of 4 sec, by the variable. This was
done in an illuminated room with or without a reduction screen, or in the
dark. In the judgments made in the illuminated room, the variable was
placed too near the horizontal, particularly for the 30° standard. In judgments
made in the dark, there was a tendency for the variable to be placed too near
the vertical. Takala concluded that the horizontal is a stronger norm for
judgments made in the light, and the vertical is a stronger norm for judgments made in the dark. It is not clear how this method of reproduction
measures normalization, for no unaffected standard was provided by which
the effect could be measured.

In a second series of experiments, Takala asked his subjects to estimate
when a line was inclined at 30°, 45°, and 60°. These judgments were done
both in an illuminated and in a dark room. The inclinations were all set too
near the horizontal, in other words, the angle between the line and the
horizontal was overestimated compared with the angle between the line and
the vertical.

The most extensive studies of the judgment of inclination have been
carried out at Mount Holyoke College. Rogers, Volkmann, Reese, and
Kaufman (see Reese, 1953, pp. 9–16) asked each of 50 subjects to give 25
estimates of the inclination of each of 35 stimuli distributed between 10°
anticlockwise and 100° clockwise. The mean constant error was zero at the
vertical position, 1° at the horizontal position with maximum errors of 4°

at the 30°, 75°, and 100° positions. Intermediate errors were obtained at the 45° position (see figure 7.2). The within- and between-subject variances of judgments followed the same trends as the constant errors. Between-subject variance ranged from 5° to nearly 40°; within-subject variance from 2° to nearly 8°. The substitution of a 14 cm or a 4 cm line for the original 56 cm

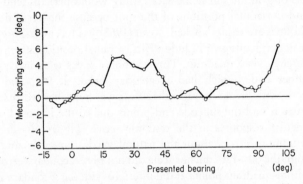

Figure 7.2 The results of Reese *et al.* (1953) showing the estimated bearing of a vertical line as a function of presented bearing; each point is based on 860 estimates from 33 subjects

line did not affect the results. But when the 4 cm line was placed at the edge of the circular screen, instead of having one end at the centre, both accuracy and consistency improved significantly. When the method of production was used, rather than the method of estimation, the constant and variable errors were less, but the pattern of errors for the various inclinations was similar for the two methods.

Muller, Sidorsky, Slivinske, Alluisi, and Fitts (1955) using an entire circular range of stimulus lines, found that identification of inclination was similar in each quadrant. Like Rogers *et al.* they found that accuracy was highest at the horizontal and vertical positions, but unlike Rogers *et al.* they did not find a secondary point of accuracy at mid-quadrant positions.

Leibowitz, Myers, and Grant (1955b) have also shown that bearings are most accurately judged at the primary positions. Their subjects had to inspect a spot of light which was 4·2° out from a spot at the fixation point, and at one of 36 positions round the clock. The spots were exposed for from 0·01 to 0·64 sec at various brightness levels. After the spots, a grid of concentric circles and radiating lines was exposed for 1 sec. The subjects had to judge the radial position of the critical spot on the grid. The average errors were found to be least for the vertical and horizontal positions, higher for the 45° positions, and highest for intermediate positions. These results are in agreement with those of previous workers. We wonder, however, to what extent the subjects could see the projection of the after-images of the spots of light on the grid. Leibowitz did not mention this possibility. The results were not affected by the changes in the exposure time or brightness of the spots, as long as the spots were visible.

The use of grid lines in Leibowitz's study would perhaps tend to favour vertical and horizontal positions of the spot because the vertical and horizontal grid lines are easily labelled. Keen (1963) has recently shown that the response categories allowed in judgments of radial position affect the differential accuracy over a quadrant. Three response scales were used; degrees, a letter–number code which had a category break at 90°, and a letter–number code with breaks at 60° and 120°. It was hypothesized that accuracy would centre round the subcode end-points due to the imposed salience of these particular responses in the response series. The results in each case showed minimum errors about the natural vertical and horizontal points, and although the 60°–120° anchor scale did not give secondary error-minima at these within-quadrant points, it did interfere with the secondary minimum which otherwise occurred at the 45° position. In other words, the normal vertical–horizontal categories exert their influence in spite of imposed category end-points, even though the imposed end-points may affect the within-quadrant distribution of error magnitudes.

Anchors have been found to affect subjective scales of inclination, just as anchors have been found to affect judgments of weight and other qualities. Rogers (1941) obtained a large number of judgments from four subjects of the inclination of a line varying in position between 10° and 40° from the vertical. Added to each series of stimuli was an anchor stimulus which was at one of several angles between 25° and 110°. A six-category scale was used. The width of the categories was found to increase as the inclination of the anchor was increased. Those categories closest to the anchor were affected most. Anchors inclined more than a certain amount ceased to affect the judgment categories. Presumably the point at which the anchor ceased to have any effect, was that point where the subject ceased to regard it as belonging to the main series of stimuli. This 'breakaway point' varied from subject to subject.

A continuously visible anchoring marker, known to the subject to be at 30° to the vertical, has been shown to reduce the constant and variable errors of estimation of the inclination of a line at that position and for a considerable distance to either side. Rogers, Volkmann, Reese, and Kaufman (1947) suggested that the vertical and horizontal norms, and to some extent the 45° norm, act like anchors in reducing errors of judgment.

Stevens and Galanter (1957) are of the opinion that the scale of inclination is a metathetic one i.e. that the subjective and objective scales are linearly related. Reese (1953, p. 19) found that when subjects were asked to repeatedly divide a quadrant to produce eight equal-appearing intervals, the resulting scale closely resembled the physical scale.

It seems that certain inclinations of a line are more rapidly identified than others. Katsui (1962) showed his subjects (300 children between the ages of three and eight years) a radius in a circle. The circle and radius were presented tachistoscopically with the radius in one of eight positions. The subjects were then shown eight circles, each with the radius in a different position, and had to select the one which was identical to the one which they had seen. It was found that there were least errors of identification for the vertical positions. Mirror-image reversals were the most common type of error, then 180° rotations; 45° rotations were the least common. The predominance of left–right reversals was explained by the assumption that left–right concepts are not well developed in children. It would surely be more reasonable to explain the late development of left–right concepts in terms of the difficulty of left–right discriminations. The difficulty of making left–right discriminations probably arises from the relative lack of left–right differences in most objects. This type of work should be repeated with adult subjects.

Sutherland (1957) showed that the octopus can readily discriminate vertical from horizontal rectangles, but confuses rectangles oriented obliquely in different directions. Rudel and Teuber (1963) found essentially the same differences of discriminability in children aged 3 to 4. In other words, when reinforced with the words 'right' and 'wrong' they soon learned to choose | from — but most of them could not learn to choose / and not \ . Furthermore, like the octopus, the children could easily discriminate ⌐ from ⌊ , but few learned to discriminate ⌐ from ⌐ . Rudel and Teuber suggested that this pattern of relative difficulty is related to the bilateral organization of the human body, and the direction of gravity. See chapter 12 for a further discussion of the relation between shape discrimination and pattern vision.

7.3 The judgment of eye level

Eye level is that horizontal plane which passes through the centre of the pupil. It may or may not contain the visual axis, depending on the direction of gaze. The horizon is the line at infinity to which all horizontal lines converge. The horizon at sea approximates to this line. The direction of any point at eye level is always in the same optical direction as the horizon; however, from the standpoint of the pointing arm, a point at eye level varies in its direction (relative to the horizon) as the point's distance from the subject varies. In other words, if a subject is asked to visually fixate a point on a wall at eye level, he should perform in the same way as when he is asked to visually fixate the horizon, but, if he is asked to point to a point at eye level on a wall, he will point in a different direction to the direction he would point in if asked to point to the horizon. It is no more, and no less legitimate to talk of eye level being the same as the horizon than it is to talk of toe level or arm level as being the same as the horizon. Eye level has a certain behavioural significance which planes level with other body parts have not, especially when we wish to represent the position of the horizon in a drawing. But this special significance of eye level must not lead us to necessarily equate it with the direction of the horizon.

Reduced to its simplest, the direction of the horizon is the direction of any horizontal surface at any height. Eye level is always a horizontal plane, but not all horizontal planes are at eye level. To study a man's ability to judge the direction of the horizon is merely to study his ability to judge the horizontal. The literature relevant to this problem has been discussed earlier in this chapter. Those studies which, according to their titles, are studies of the judgment of the horizon, are better described as studies of the judgment of eye level. It is under this heading that they are reviewed here. Where authors have referred to the horizon, we, in reviewing their work, have referred to eye level.

There has also been a tendency to confuse eye level with the transverse plane through the eye socket. Those two planes correspond when the person is erect, but if, for instance, he rotates his head upward, while keeping his pupil at the same level, his eye level remains the same, whereas the transverse plane through his eye socket is elevated. Figure 7.3 makes these relationships clear.

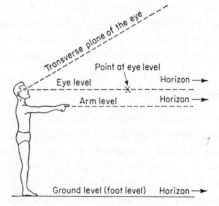

Figure 7.3 To demonstrate the relationship between eye level, the transverse plane of the eye, arm level, and the horizon

A further confusion has been to consider the horizon to be the horizontal analogue of the median plane. The direction in space of the horizon is not affected by the orientation of the observer, as the direction of the median plane is. The true horizontal analogue of the median plane would be a transverse plane at right angles to the body axis and, therefore, at right angles to the median plane. Since the human body is not symmetrical about any transverse plane, there is no transverse plane with a unique behavioural significance. If the body is upright, eye level coincides with a transverse plane of the body, otherwise, it does not. The direction of the horizon is independent of the position of the observer's body. The judgment of eye level, on the other hand, is not a purely objective judgment, since it demands a reference point (the pupil) on the body. Nor is it a purely egocentric judgment, for it also demands a reference system (gravity) outside the observer's body. We shall call such a judgment 'semi-egocentric'. Strictly speaking, it is not a purely directional judgment, for it involves, in addition to an angle (the horizontal), the linear position of a point in space (the pupil).

MacDougall (1903) did the first and, as yet, most comprehensive study of apparent eye level. He asked his subjects to position a disc on a large screen, 33 cm away, so that it appeared to be at the 'horizon' (at eye level). When the judgments were made in a lighted room the constant error was small. In a dark room the average and constant errors were greatly increased. The apparent eye level was set a few degrees below the real eye level for all 12 subjects. Hoppeler (1913) and Sharp (1934) also found that the subjective eye level was on average a few degrees below the objective eye level. Fitts (1947) asked blindfolded subjects to reach for targets which they had seen at various heights in front of them. The subjects undershot the targets above shoulder height. Similarly MacDougall described how people at sea commonly observe that lights on the horizon at night appear to be suspended in the sky.

MacDougall proposed explanations of the increased average and constant errors in the dark. He considered that the increased average error in the dark was due to the absence of a stabilizing visual frame. He suggested that convergence is normally accompanied by a depression of the eyes, and that this depression of the eyes during fixation causes the depression of the apparent horizon. In a further experiment in the dark, MacDougall asked the subject to close his eyes and direct his gaze to what he considered to be eye level. The subject was then asked to open his eyes and report the number on a vertical scale upon which his gaze was fixed at the moment his eyes opened. It was found that the subject's eyes were always set *above* the true eye level. It is known that the eyes tend to diverge and elevate when closed (see Fluur and Eriksson, 1961), and MacDougall thought that this tendency accounted for the eyes being set high.

H.S.O.—13

A related explanation of the depression of the apparent eye level with eyes open was suggested by Sandström (1951). He demonstrated that people have a preferred, most comfortable direction of gaze with eyes open. For men, this tends to be below eye level. In judging the position of eye level, there may be a tendency to deflect one's judgment in the direction of the most preferred direction of gaze.

We suggest a further but perhaps related explanation of the depression of the apparent eye level or visual horizon with eyes open. People tend naturally to judge the height of an object in relation to ground level. Except at an infinite distance, an object at eye level is above ground level and thus has the perceptual quality of being suspended. In spite of the subject's efforts to judge the position of the object in relation to eye level, this quality of being suspended will intrude and a compromise judgment will be made resulting in the apparent eye level being depressed. This mechanism will explain why objects at eye level nearer than the horizon will appear higher than they really are, but we need a second assumption to explain why objects on the horizon appear elevated. For this purpose it is only necessary to assume that objects on the horizon appear to be nearer than they really are. In this way we can explain why lights seen at night on the sea's horizon appear to be suspended above the sea.

Our assumption that ground level acts as a norm for judgments of above and below, even, to some extent, when an observer is attempting to make judgments in terms of eye level, leads to the following prediction. A shorter person or a person crouching down will have a less depressed apparent eye level. Women are, on average, shorter than men, and Sandström (1951) found that when asked to set a point 50 cm away to eye level, men set it about $0.8°$ lower than real eye level and women set it higher than true eye level by about the same amount. Nair (1958) found that taller men set the apparent eye level lower than short men, although no such difference could be found for women. Children have been found to set the apparent eye level higher than adults (Wapner and Werner, 1957, p. 33). The 6–7 year old group set apparent eye level higher than objective eye level; with increasing age the direction of errors was reversed, the cross-over point (no error) being at about age 10–11. One would expect very near objects to be set more accurately to eye level, for now the ground is not in view. Tschermak-Seysenegg (1952, p. 214) reports that this is the case. At a distance of 130 cm, the apparent eye level was on average three degrees below true eye level, and at 33 cm it was only one degree below true eye level. Thus the predictions from our theory are confirmed to some extent. But the finding that apparent eye level in women is actually above objective eye level lends support to the MacDougall–Sandström equation of apparent eye level with preferred direction of gaze.

MacDougall asked his subjects to strain their eyes upwards for a few seconds; when the eyes were restored to the normal position, the subjective eye-level position of a point of light seen in the dark was displaced upwards. Straining the eyes downwards had the opposite effect. MacDougall's subjects reported that the point of light appeared to float about in space in the manner of the autokinetic phenomenon; the direction of autokinetic movement is known to be influenced by the previous direction of eye strain and this could account for MacDougall's finding (Carr, 1910).

Sziklai (1961) and Comalli (1963) claimed that they were studying the effect of body tilt on the position of the apparent visual horizon, but in fact the position which they asked their subjects to judge was one above their eyes at right angles to their tilted body axis. This is, of course, not the horizon, nor even eye level, but is the position of the transverse body plane through the eyes (see figure 7.3). As far as we know these are the only studies of this type of judgment.

It has been found that, when the head is tilted backwards, the subjective eye level is higher than when the head is erect (MacDougall, 1903; Schubert and Brecher, 1934; Tschermak-Seysenegg, 1952, p. 214). MacDougall found that with the body tilted back 45° the apparent eye level rose 3° above the true eye level.

The shift of the apparent eye level with head or body tilt is presumably related to the concomitant changes in kinaesthetic or utricular stimulation. That kinaesthetic stimulation affects the position of the apparent eye level is suggested by two experiments. Sziklai (1961) found that loading the subject with a weighted vest caused a downward shift of the apparent eye level. Glick (1959) found that when the subject pressed down with his hands to force his head up against a spring, the apparent eye level was displaced upwards, and when the subject pressed up to force his chin down against a spring, the apparent eye level was displaced downwards. Glick interpreted these results in terms of the sensory–tonic theory. However, it is not clear how that theory can predict the results, for in both conditions of the experiment, the subject pushed one part of his body up and another part down. In terms of total body tonus, the situation was always symmetrical and no shift due to tonus asymmetry should have occurred. That utricular information is influential, is shown by the fact that changing the gravitational force acting on the body affects the apparent height of visible objects and therefore apparent eye level (see section 16.24).

MacDougall found that when the subject could see a cord or plane of wood stretching from his chin to the bottom of a screen, the subjective eye level dropped. This situation is analogous to the familiar experience of driving down a hill and overestimating the height of a hill on the other side of the valley. A cord or plane ascending from the subject's feet to the screen caused an elevation of the subjective eye level. Clearly, what is happening in this type of situation is that the subject tends to accept the ascending or descending plane as the horizontal frame of reference, in relation to which he judges the position of his eye level or visual horizon. MacDougall also found that a light put below objective eye level caused a lowering of the subjective eye level. A light put above had the opposite effect. Jaffe (1952) asked her subjects to set the top or bottom edge of a luminous square to eye level. The apparent visual horizon was found to shift in the direction of the asymmetrical extent. These effects are analogous to the effect of asymmetrical stimulation on the position of the apparent median plane. Bruell and Albee (1955a) suggested that their motor theory could account for both effects (see section 11.31). As in the case of the apparent median plane, Wapner and Werner (1955) found that the apparent horizon was shifted towards the half of the field of view containing a homogeneous pattern and away from the half containing a mixed pattern (see section 11.31).

A series of experiments done at Clark University, within the framework of the sensory–tonic theory, has demonstrated that extraneous stimuli and cognitive factors may affect the position of the apparent eye level (again referred to as the horizon). Kaden (1953) found that a hand pointing up, and words such as 'rising', depressed the apparent eye level; the opposite stimuli had the opposite effect. But Jaffe (1952) found that shapes having directional features did not affect the apparent eye level. Wapner, Werner, and Krus (1957) measured the position of the apparent eye level before and after telling their subjects the results of a mid-term examination. The subjects who failed showed a drop, and the successful students an upward shift.

Krus, Wapner, and Freeman (1958) found that a tranquilizing, depressant drug (reserpine) caused a downward shift of the apparent eye level. An energizing drug (iproniazid) had no significant effect. In trying to account for the negative effect of iproniazid, they presented evidence that this drug 'is neither consistently nor with high frequency accompanied by feelings of elation'. But if they knew this, why did they choose it to test their hypothesis that an energizing drug elevates the apparent horizon? One wonders whether the energizing properties of the drug would have been doubted if the expected shift of the apparent eye level had occurred.

Lysergic acid diethylamine (LSD-25) was found to elevate the apparent eye level, and Wapner and Krus (1959) interpreted this in terms of the 'primitivizing' effect of the drug which caused the subjects to behave like children. (Children had been found to set the apparent eye level higher than adults (Wapner and Werner, 1957, p. 33).) We have suggested that children set the apparent eye level higher than adults because they are smaller than adults. If this is so, Wapner and Krus would have to assume that LSD causes adults to imagine they are smaller than they really are.

Wapner and Werner claimed that the sensory–tonic theory predicts the results of these experiments on the effects of success, failure, and drugs, on the apparent eye level. Failure and depressant drugs are supposed to produce a downward vector. But what is supposed to be affected in a downward direction, the apparent position of the real eye level or the position of the apparent eye level? The theory provides no basis for deciding, and yet the two cases produce opposite outcomes. The theoretical confusion is increased when we read, in a paper by one of Werner and Wapner's students (Rosenblatt, 1956), that the sensory–tonic theory predicts that elated psychotics have an 'upward organismic vector', which causes an apparent elevation of the real eye level and a depression of the apparent eye level. Hence the same theory is used to predict the opposite result to that predicted by Wapner, Werner, and Krus, while it is not evident to an outsider how either result is implied by the theory. This is the same predicament which this theory encounters when used to predict the position of the apparent vertical (see section 7.45).

No one has studied the kinaesthetic–tactile judgment of the visual horizon, nor man's ability to set a point level with points on his body other than the eye, although a special case of the latter—the ability to maintain the arms in a forward horizontal position while blindfolded—is a test used by clinical neurologists (Wartenberg, 1953). A downward deviation of one or both arms in this 'arm deviation test' is said to indicate damage to the pyramidal system; an upward displacement is said to indicate damage to the cerebellum.

An ability related to the judgment of the horizon is the ability to judge the 'straight overhead'. This must not be confused with egocentric judgments relative to the body axis, in which the orientation of the observer is crucial. The 'straight overhead' direction would be indicated by the position of a rod which is loosely attached to the head and always remains vertical no matter what the head does; the body axis would be indicated by the position of a rod rigidly attached to the head, with the head held rigidly erect on the body. The straight-overhead type of judgment would be necessary if one wished to avoid being hit by a falling stone. As far as we know, there are no experimental studies of this type of judgment.

7.4 Body tilt and the judgment of the visual vertical

7.41 The Aubert and Müller effects

Aubert (1861) happened one day to be looking at a vertical streak of light in an otherwise dark room. He noticed that when he tilted his head to one side the streak of light appeared to tilt in the opposite direction. He found that the maximum apparent tilt was approximately 45° and occurred when his head was tilted at 135° to the vertical. Thereafter it decreased to zero when his head was upside down. When he moved his head quickly, there was a delay of a few seconds before the line appeared tilted. Even 'very small' head inclinations produced some effect. The room had to be completely dark; if the furniture became visible the effect disappeared. When darkness was restored, the effect returned after a few seconds delay. The effect was equally strong with a horizontal line of light and did not depend on constant fixation. When lying on his side, he noticed oscillations in the apparent tilt of the line; another subject noticed these oscillations when his head alone was tilted.

Aubert went on to consider possible explanations. First he tested the theory that the tilt of the head is underestimated. He set his head, with his eyes closed, to what he considered to be 90°. On opening his eyes and looking into a mirror which he had placed before himself, he saw that he had estimated his head inclination correctly. He concluded that one does not underestimate the tilt of one's head. He next considered the theory that the effect is due to eye torsion but rejected this idea on three counts; first, he could not see the torsion in the mirror; secondly, the optic nerve would not allow the eye to tort the 45° which was the amount of the effect he obtained; and finally, he got no evidence of eye torsion when he tilted his head using the after-image method of observing torsion. (It is now known that torsion usually does occur under these circumstances, see section 3.42.)

Aubert concluded that the effect was due to adaptation of those sensory impressions which indicate the position of the head, so that, while we do not underestimate the position of the head initially, we come to do so after some time in the tilted position.

Müller (1916) pointed out that with small tilts of the head, the apparent vertical is often displaced in a direction opposite to the tilt of the head, rather than the same direction, as in the Aubert phenomenon. Müller called this the E-effect.

In our further discussion, we shall refer to the Aubert-effect as the A-effect and we shall sometimes describe it as an apparent tilt of a truly vertical line in the opposite direction to the head tilt, and sometimes as a displacement of the apparent vertical in the same direction as the head tilt. The description we adopt will depend on the technique of measurement used in the particular experiment being described. Similarly, the E-effect will either be described as an apparent tilt of the true vertical in the same direction as the head or as a displacement of the apparent vertical in the opposite direction to the head.

7.42 The extent of the A- and E-effects

Müller found that most people experience the E-effect with small angles of head tilt and the A-effect with larger angles, while some people experience only the A-effect. Similar individual differences were reported by Passey and Ray (1950). Bourdon (1906a) found that the E-effect persisted with head tilts up to 50°; the A-effect occurred with larger degrees of head tilt up to a maximum at 160°. Bauermeister (1964) found a similar pattern of errors, a graph of which is shown in figure 7.4. Witkin and Asch (1948a) found the E-effect

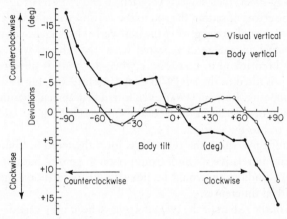

Figure 7.4 Results of Bauermeister (1964) showing the deviations of apparent from objective visual vertical and apparent from objective body tilt as a function of body tilt

to be maximal at a head tilt of 28°. They did not test for a possible A-effect at angles greater than 90°.

However, it has been shown (Sandström 1954, 1956) that people fall into more categories with respect to the two effects than Müller thought. With some subjects, the E-effect occurs for small degrees of head tilt and the A-effect for large, but with others the effects occur in the reverse order; some subjects report only the A-effect at all degrees of head tilt, as Müller found, but others report the E-effect throughout.

It has been claimed that as children grow up they progress from showing an A-effect to showing an E-effect (Wapner and Werner, 1957). Old people were found to show a return to the A-effect (Comalli, Wapner, and Werner, 1959). This developmental change was said to reflect a growing 'differentiation between object and self' away from a primitive state of 'egocentricity'. At the same time, adults were found to be more consistent and less influenced by the starting position of the line than were children. This was said to reflect a growth away from 'stimulus boundedness', when the subject is at the mercy of the changing and lingering effects of stimulus condition. Liebert, Wapner, and Werner (1957) hypothesized that the drug LSD-25 should induce a reversion to the primitive A-effect in normal adults and schizophrenics. However, the opposite effect was obtained for the normal adults, that is, there was an increased E-effect. The schizophrenics showed no effect of the drug.

Recently Davies and Leytham (1964) failed to confirm that older people revert to an A-effect; their subjects between 70 and 76 years of age showed an E-effect. The errors of setting the rod to the vertical with the body in the upright position were less the greater the non-verbal intelligence of the subject. This intellectual advantage disappeared when the subjects were tilted. The E-effect has been found to be stronger when the body is tilted to the right than when it is tilted to the left (Witkin and Asch 1948a), but Passey (1950b) found the opposite. Rosman (1960) even found that unseen asymmetries such as the position of curtains in the laboratory may affect the direction of error in setting a rod to the vertical.

The factors governing the two effects must therefore be complex; they evidently vary in relative strength from person to person, but in view of the contradictory findings, it would be pointless to speculate on the causes of these individual differences.

Reports of the extent of the two effects have been very varied. The maximum A-effect seems to be about 45° at a body tilt of about 160° to the vertical. The E-effect is never as large as this. Variability of estimates of the vertical also seems to increase with body tilt (Mann, Berthelot-Berry, and Dauterive, 1949). Nagel (1898), and recently Miller and Graybiel (1963) noted autokinesis-like fluctuations in apparent orientation of a luminous line.

There seems also to be an apparent displacement of the vertical in the direction of body tilt in the sagittal plane (Schubert and Brecher, 1934).

Effects analogous to the A- and E-phenomena have been demonstrated in the tactile–kinaesthetic modality. Sachs and Meller (1903) reported that the apparent tactile–kinaesthetic vertical was displaced to the same side as the tilt of the body. This is analogous to the Aubert effect in vision. All other investigators (Nagel, 1898; Sandström, 1952, 1954; Wapner and Werner, 1952; Bitterman and Worchel, 1953; Bauermeister, Werner, and Wapner, 1964) found that the apparent tactile–kinaesthetic vertical was displaced to the side opposite to the tilt of the body. This is analogous to the E-effect in vision. The effects reported vary in extent between 1° and 7° although body tilts of more than 90° do not seem to have been studied. The results of Bauermeister et al., using different hands for adjustment, are shown in figure 7.5.

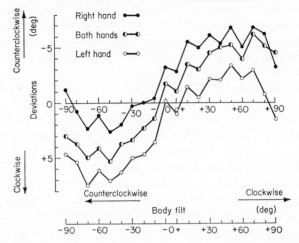

Figure 7.5 Deviations of apparent from objective tactile–kinaesthetic vertical as a function of the degree of body tilt. [From Bauermeister, Werner, and Wapner, 1964]

Thus judgments of the tactile–kinaesthetic vertical are affected by the same factors that affect judgments of the visual vertical although not always in the same way nor to the same extent.

7.43 Judgments during head movements

Nagel (1898) asked nineteen subjects to report their experiences while they were moving their heads from side to side and looking at a vertical line. Eleven of them reported that the line appeared to move in the opposite direction to the head and then, when the head was stopped in a tilted position, that the apparent tilt of the line increased. (This effect was also reported by Aubert and by Gloster, 1953.) However, Nagel himself and the remaining subjects saw the opposite of these effects, that is, the line appeared to move with the head and to return to the vertical when the head was held at an angle. This is the E-effect and it persisted for Nagel until his head was tilted beyond 60°, when suddenly the line appeared to tilt in the opposite direction to the head, that is, the A-effect. Sachs and Meller (1901) also noticed the apparent movement of the vertical line during the time the head was tilting.

7.44 Countertorsion and the A- and E-effects

There is general agreement that countertorsion cannot explain the A-effect, even though it may be a factor which modifies it. Nagel (1896) thought that countertorsion might be partly responsible for the A-effect. But, as Mulder had already pointed out (1874), it is difficult to see how this could be the case since countertorsion causes the retinal image to move less than it otherwise would. Meller, more plausibly, considered that torsion was the cause not of the A-effect but of the E-effect.

An additional criticism of Nagel's position is that he found the A-effect to be independent of the direction of gaze. He accounted for this by remarking that eye torsion is independent of the direction of gaze and that it is torsion, alone among eye movements, that affects the A-effect. According to Listing's law (see section 3.2) eye torsion (in the sense in which he defined it) is not affected by the angle of gaze. However, when defined in terms of the Helmholtz or Fick axis systems, torsion does alter with the angle of oblique gaze. It is arbitrary which definition of torsion is adopted. In any case Di Giorgi (1936) found that the extent of the A-effect *was* affected by the position of the eyes in the head, although the relationship was found not to be a simple one.

Fischer (1927, 1930a) took measurements of countertorsion and the A-effect from the same subjects under similar conditions. He found no parallel between the curves representing the two effects as a function of body tilt; there was not even a proportional relationship, although they were always in the same direction. Even when the two curves were reduced to the same scale, they were still very different. In a second paper Fischer (1930b) found that a patient with bilateral loss of the labyrinths, showed no torsion, yet did report a normal A-effect. Fischer concluded that there was no simple relationship between countertorsion and the A-effect.

7.45 Somaesthetic, kinaesthetic, and vestibular factors in the A- and E-effects

Aubert (1861) suggested that his effect was due to the subject underestimating the tilt of his head because of adaptation of the somaesthetic and vestibular senses. Helmholtz (1962) agreed with Aubert's interpretation. Nagel, on the other hand, disagreed. Lying on his side, he set a rod to the apparent vertical and found that it was in fact tilted in the same direction as his body (A-effect). In spite of this, his body felt as if it was tilted more than it was. He therefore dismissed Aubert's suggestion that the effect is due to underestimation of the tilt of the body.

Recently McFarland, Wapner, and Werner (1962) and Bauermeister (1964) have apparently confirmed Nagel's finding that people tend to exaggerate the displacement of their bodies from the vertical. They inferred this from the fact that when subjects are asked to set a luminous rod parallel to the mid-body axis, they in fact set it beyond the body tilt in the same direction. It is arguable whether it is legitimate to infer from this essentially visual judgment anything about the subject's apparent body position. Be that as it may, these workers also found that these same subjects showed an increasing E-effect as the angle of tilt was increased up to about 60°. For these angles of tilt, therefore, the apparent visual vertical was displaced in a direction which could be accounted for by the apparent shift in body position. However, the apparent body displacement was greater than the apparent displacement of the vertical. In view of the arbitrary nature of the apparent body vertical measure, this lack of quantitative correspondence between the two effects is not surprising. But beyond about 60° the direction of displacement of the apparent vertical changed to give the A-effect, whereas the apparent body position became increasingly exaggerated (see figure 7.4).

Nagel supported his view that the A-effect is not related to feelings arising from the musculature of the neck and trunk by hanging weights so that the head had to work against resistance when tilted. He also applied electric currents to the musculature of the neck. These procedures did not affect the extent of the A-effect. The results of more recent work conflict with Nagel's results. Kleint (1937) and Schneider and Bartley (1962), using counterweights and Wapner, Werner, and Chandler (1951) and Chandler (1961), using unilaterally applied noise and electrical stimulation of the sternocleidomastoid muscle, caused an increase in tonus on one side of the body. These procedures cause a shift of the apparent vertical to the opposite side of the body to the side of the increased tonus. Even though Werner and Wapner (1949), in their 'sensory–tonic field theory', seem to adopt the argument that the apparent vertical is displaced to the side opposite increased tonus, their own results on the effects of body tilt contradict their assumptions. Werner, Wapner, and Chandler (1951) tilted subjects from a sitting posture to 15° and 30°. The apparent vertical position of a rod was nearly always set in a direction away from the body tilt (E-effect). The effect was greater for the 30° body tilt. It was also greater when the body was unsupported. We interpret the results of this experiment as follows: when the body tilts, the side of the body which is convex takes the strain of supporting the body and will therefore be the side of increased tonus. The apparent vertical, therefore, was found to be displaced in the same direction as the increased tonus, whereas in their previous experiment with induced tonus, they had found a displacement away from the side of increased tonus.

There thus seems to be a contradiction in the results of the same investigators and yet Werner et al. claimed that the two results are analogous and that both support their sensory-tonic theory. They argued that, 'the degree of perceptual displacement depends upon the kind of support (amount of

muscular involvement) rather than simply on the angle of body tilt *per se*.'
It is thus the muscular involvement rather than eye torsion or labyrinthine
reflexes which is the crucial determinant of the E-effect according to this
theory.

Naylor (1963) could not duplicate the effects of unilateral tonus of the
sensory–tonic school. He found that auditory and muscular 'stress' produced
an apparent displacement of the vertical line to a particular side for a given
individual but that the direction of apparent displacement was not related to
the side upon which the stress stimulus was applied.

Recently Aarons and Goldenberg (1964) have shown that the effects
produced by asymmetrical Galvanic stimulation vary according to the location and polarity of the electrodes. Thus stimulation of the mastoid shifted
the apparent vertical away from the anode and towards the cathode, particularly so when the stimulus was applied unilaterally. In contrast, neck
stimulation produced shifts towards the anode. Aarons and Goldenberg
speculated that these differences result from the differential effects of the
stimulus on the muscular, vestibular, and oculomotor systems.

Nagel's view was that the A-effect is caused by vestibular reflex activity,
torsional eye movements, and strains in the eye muscles. He found that an
eight volt potential applied to the side of the head caused a vertical line to
appear to tilt by about 7° towards the cathode and at the same time gave rise
to feelings of dizziness and falling in the same direction. This evidence
suggests that it was the vestibular organ that was being stimulated,
and supports Nagel's view that this organ is important in producing the
A-effect.

In spite of Nagel's results with electrical stimulation of the labyrinths, the
A-effect has been reported in people lacking intact labyrinths. Mann (1951)
found that a patient with eighth-nerve paralysis experienced a larger A-effect
than a group of normal subjects. He concluded that the A-effect was en-
hanced either because of the absence of countertorsion arising from labyrinthine reflexes or because of a lack of compensating information regarding the
degree of head tilt arising from the labyrinths. It would be unwise to attach
much significance to Mann's result since this one subject in fact had an A-
effect the magnitude of which most investigators would regard as normal.
Mann's control group had an effect which was lower than the usually reported
A-effect. Fischer (1930b) showed that the labyrinths are not necessary for the
occurrence of the A- and E-effects. One of his subjects had unilateral loss of
vestibular function and experienced the E-effect on tilting his head. A subject
with bilateral vestibular loss experienced only the A-effect. Bárány (1921) and
Feilchenfeld (1903) also found that congenitally deaf subjects experienced the
A-effect.

7.46 The human centrifuge

The first human centrifuge was described by Erasmus Darwin in 1801. James Watt prepared a set of drawings for Darwin, but there is no record of the centrifuge having been constructed. Purkinje (1820) noticed that when he was riding on a merry-go-round, the platform seemed inclined. He regarded the effect as being due to the centrifugal force acting on the blood or semi-liquid contents of the cranium. In a general sense, Purkinje's explanation was correct: the endolymph of the vestibular system is a fluid in the cranium.

Spinning a human being in a centrifuge has four main effects on his sense organs. (1) It displaces the direction of the gravitational force acting on his body. (2) It increases the force acting on his body. (3) It rotates him about his own body axis on every cycle of the centrifuge. (4) It produces a gradient both in the direction and the magnitude of the force acting on his body. If he faces in the direction of motion his utricles will be unequally stimulated, and if he moves his head he will be subjected to Coriolis forces and cross-coupling effects (see sections 16.51 and 16.52).

The centrifuge has been used in many of the studies reported in the psychological literature solely as a means of studying the effects on the judgment of the vertical of a displacement of the direction of force acting on the body. The following argument shows that it is both an irrational and an inefficient method of studying the effects of a change in the direction of the force of gravity (Howard and Templeton, 1963).

Consider an enclosed room. There are two ways in which the direction of the force acting on the room may be altered. It may be rigidly attached to a centrifuge and spun so that the resultant of the centrifugal force and the earth's gravitational force makes a certain angle with the walls of the room, or it may be tilted so that the angle between the direction of the earth's gravity and the room is that same angle. These two procedures are identical in their effect on any object or person in the room so far as the direction of force is concerned. It follows that *a subject, blindfolded or in an enclosed room, cannot distinguish between the experience of the displaced direction of force when the room is centrifuged, and the experience he would have if the room were tilted appropriately.* The expense and trouble of making a centrifuge are unnecessary, and because of other factors this method introduces it gives results which are invalid as pure measures of the effect of a displaced direction of the force acting on the body.

There are purposes for which the use of a human centrifuge is ideally suited, for instance the study of the effects of increased gravity on human performance. When used for this purpose the cubicle would be allowed to swing out so as to keep the subject's body axis aligned with the resultant direction of force. This literature has been reviewed by Ham (1943) and White and Monty (1963). Rotating a subject about his own body axis is a sensible way of studying the vestibular reflexes. Wapner, Werner, and Morant (1951) and Holst and Grisebach (1951) used this method to study the effect of rotation on the judgment of the vertical. They found that a vertical rod appears to be tilted in the opposite direction to the direction in which the subject is accelerating. In the interpretation of their results, Wapner *et al.* were apparently unaware of the fact that Sacchi (1950) had shown that if a subject judges the position of a vertical line during nystagmic eye movements, the line is seen to tilt in one direction when its lower end is fixated and in the opposite direction when its top end is fixated. Sacchi concluded that this difference is due to the difference in the latency of the visual response between the centre and periphery of the retina.

The fallacy of using the centrifuge to study the effects of a changed direction of force seems to go back to Mach (1873, 1874, 1875). He formulated the hypothesis that when an individual is subjected to the resultant of centrifugal and gravitational forces he senses the direction of the resultant mass-acceleration and regards this as the vertical. Mach's hypothesis could be translated into the terms of the tilted room experience by saying that when a subject is tilted in the dark he can still set a line to the gravitational vertical. The A- and E-effects reveal that this is only approximately true. Mach was working in the nineteenth century and at that time not so much was known about the nature of gravitational or centrifugal forces, nor was much known about the sense organs involved in the judgment of the vertical. Mach's hypothesis could be understood as a (correct) statement that gravitational and centrifugal forces are equivalent in their action on the sense organs. Since Einstein we know that there is no way of distinguishing a gravitational field from a centrifugal field, so that it cannot matter whether we produce a change in the direction of the force on the body by tilting the subject or by rotating him. Hence Mach's hypothesis does not require experimental validation. Bourdon (1906b), and Breuer and Kreidl (1898) did experiments on a centrifuge similar to those done by Mach, and reached similar conclusions. Bourdon (1906b) stated that altering the direction of the force on the body was equivalent to tilting the subject, but this statement has gone unheeded. Tschermak-Seysenegg and Schubert (1931) suggested that the two processes are analogous, apparently not realizing that they are equivalent. In recent times Brandt (1962) in Sweden, Mann *et al.* in Pensacola and Tulane, and Witkin *et al.* in New York have used the human centrifuge as a means of altering the direction of the gravitational force acting on the body.

Noble (1949) and Clark and Graybiel (1951), working at Pensacola, had their subjects set a line to the horizontal in an otherwise dark cubicle rotated on a centrifuge. Their results fit Mach's hypothesis fairly well. Some of Noble's data departed from the hypothesis in the direction of the Aubert phenomenon. A subject in an enclosed chamber subjected to a displaced direction of gravity has no option (unless he reasons the situation out in a way that is not expected of him) but to adopt the new direction of gravity as his standard of reference. The Pensacola workers reported that a line which remains in line with the earth's gravity appears to rotate as the displacement of resultant gravity occurs. They called this effect the oculogravic illusion (Graybiel, 1952a). But it is *not an illusion*, the line *does rotate* relative to the direction of the subject's gravity, and that is what the subject was asked to report. It is no more an illusion than is the report that a person makes about the movement in relation to gravity of a line fixed with reference to his body as he is tilted. The only illusion is the extent to which the apparently vertical position of the line is *not* reported to be in line with the resultant gravity. Such an effect would be an Aubert or Müller illusion. The so-called oculogravic illusion is a fact of physics—not of psychology.

Other workers at Pensacola, including Woellner (1957), Graybiel (1956), Graybiel, Hupp, and Patterson (1946), and Wing and Passey (1950), also substantiated Mach's hypothesis. Their results would have had more significance had they simply tilted their subjects and concentrated on the deviations from Mach's hypothesis. Mann, Berthelot-Berry, and Dauterive (1949), who were also associated with the Pensacola unit, did in fact tilt their subjects in the dark, rather than centrifuge them. They evidently did not realize that the two experiments were materially equivalent; the one done at Tulane by Mann *et al.* was just a better way of doing what was attempted at Pensacola. Graybiel and Brown (1951) studied the delay in the subject's adjustment of a luminous line after he was subjected to a displaced direction of force on the Pensacola centrifuge. Clark and Graybiel (1962, 1963a) have studied the 'oculogravic illusion' as a function of the visual frame. These questions too would have been better studied by tilting the subject.

The second group, working in New York, did experiments both with a tilting room (Witkin and Asch, 1948b) and with a centrifuge (Witkin, 1950, 1952). The use of these two techniques was defended by the following statement: 'It should be noted that modification of postural factors by simply tilting the body—a technique employed in previous studies—is basically different from their modification by altering the direction of the force that acts on the body. Tilting the body may at worst make it more difficult to detect the direction of the gravitational vector and to use it as a basis for determining the upright. The direction of the gravitational pull, of course, remains unchanged and continues to be available as a proper basis for judgment. Changing the direction of the force on the body, on the other hand, directly alters the gravitational standard for judgment.' (Witkin, 1950, p. 93). Witkin (1964), in answer to Howard and Templeton (1963), defended this procedure by stating that he wished to know to what extent subjects could make allowance for the fact that they were in a centrifuge. The theoretical importance of such an apparently trivial question was not made clear. All efforts were in any case made to disguise from the subjects the fact that they were in a centrifuge, and it is not clear how they were expected to know.

It is remarkable that this fallacy has persisted for a hundred years, forming the basis of a great deal of elaborate experimental work and finding its way into the text books (Bartley, 1958, p. 328). There is one text book which does expose the fallacy (Tschermak-Seysenegg, 1952, p. 208).

Careful thought does not reveal any advantages in using the centrifuge for the study of the effects of changing the direction of the force acting on the body. The tilting room and tilting chair are less expensive and more easily and accurately adjustable, they do not vibrate as a centrifuge must and the results are not contaminated by side effects.

7.5 Visual versus postural factors

7.51 Basic facts

We have already emphasized that the judgment of the vertical may involve several sensory modalities acting alone or in various combinations. Even within one modality any one of a number of criteria may be used to judge the vertical. The full complexity of these possibilities has not impressed itself on many investigators. An oversimplified theoretical dichotomy has been the subject of dispute. The issue, as traditionally stated, is whether postural factors (vestibular, kinaesthetic, and tactile) or visual factors (the visual frame, egocentric features such as the shape of the nose and the orbital ridges, and the familiarity of shapes) are dominant in determining the apparent vertical.

Historically, the dispute began when Koffka (1935, p. 216) stated that the directions of the apparent vertical and horizontal are determined by the directions of the main lines of the field of view. In support of his argument Koffka cited an experiment by Wertheimer (1912) in which he looked through a tilting mirror at the reflection of the room in which he was standing. At first, people moving about looked as if they were walking on a tilted floor, and objects seemed to drop at an angle to gravity. But after a short time the mirror room 'righted' itself and things again looked normal.

Koffka also described an experience which he had when travelling up a steep slope on a mountain railway. He found, on looking out of the window, that the trees seemed to be growing at an angle to gravity. When he put his head out of the window, the trees looked vertical and when he withdrew his head, the trees still looked vertical and the window frame tilted. Koffka also described a building by Lake Cayaga which was on a wide slanting lawn, but looked as if it was leaning on a horizontal lawn. According to Koffka, in these last two examples there is an 'invariant' or constantly judged angle between the ground and the object. If a main sloping line in the field is accepted as level, then by this principle of invariance, any vertical object will be judged tilted. Koffka could also have cited the phenomenon of the 'haunted swing' (Wood, 1895) to support his case. The haunted swing was a fairground device in which people were enclosed. Artificial scenery was slowly swung backwards and forwards outside the windows and this gave the compelling illusion that the boat-like contrivance was rocking. So real was the experience that people felt all the kinaesthetic sensations and vertigo associated with real rocking.

Neal (1926) was the first to point out weaknesses in Koffka's theory as a complete account of the visual vertical. He showed that a line can be set to the vertical just as accurately when there is no frame present as when the frame is present. He asked four subjects to set a luminous line to the vertical in the dark. Neither the constant error nor the mean variation of the settings increased during one hour of repeated testing in the dark. Thus neither the visual frame, nor the immediate memory of it were necessary for the accurate judgment of the vertical. Neal found that a slight tilt of the head did affect the apparent vertical (Aubert phenomenon) a fact which Koffka's theory could not explain.

In contrast to Koffka, Gibson and Mowrer (1938) proposed ' . . . that both the visual and the postural vertical are determined by visual factors and gravitational factors acting jointly, with orientation to gravity, however, as the more decisive factor in cases of real conflict between the two types of sensory data, and the primary factor genetically' (p. 303). They pointed out that tilting an observer does not introduce a discrepancy between the visual and postural factors, for both are affected concomitantly and allowance can easily be made by a constancy mechanism. Gibson and Mowrer considered first the effect on the perception of the vertical when visual factors are eliminated. They claimed that the fact that pilots lose their orientation when flying in cloud demonstrates only that vision contributes to orientation rather than that postural factors do not. They reported an observation by Helmholtz (1962, vol. 3, p. 250) that on a ship the cabin initially appeared vertical and the suspended barometer seemed to sway, but that after a while the barometer appeared vertical and the cabin appeared to sway. This, thought Gibson and Mowrer, demonstrates that postural factors become dominant. They suggested an alternative explanation of Koffka's mountain railway experiences. They claimed that it has never been experimentally demonstrated whether the trees, etc. seem to tilt as a consequence of the apparent righting of the visual frame provided by the carriage window. They quoted evidence against this view. If a subject looks at a field of parallel inclined lines, there will be induced a simultaneous contrast effect on a single, objectively vertical line in this field; that is to say, the single line will look tilted in the opposite direction (the Hering illusion). The inclined lines continue to look inclined and so this is a contrast effect rather than a shift of the frame into alignment with the subjective vertical. It is difficult to see how this evidence is relevant to Koffka's example, since there the window appeared vertical, and the increase in apparent angle of separation produced by Gibson and Mowrer's contrast effect could not have brought this about. Similarly, in their example of the Hering illusion, the inclined lines of the visual field may come to look less tilted even though never completely vertical. Also Gibson and Mowrer cannot account for the reversal which occurred when Koffka accepted the trees as vertical and consequently the frame as tilted.

Gibson repeated Wertheimer's experiment, and noticed that, although the room looked more natural after a while, it never ceased to look tilted. Similarly, when wearing prisms which rotated the visual field by from 10° to 45°, Gibson's five subjects reported that the world came to look more natural but always looked tilted. The tilt-adaption effect which had been described by Gibson and Radner (1937) was, he said, only a small effect, compared with the Wertheimer effect.

Thus Gibson and Mowrer tried to show that the experiments which had been claimed to demonstrate the primacy of visual factors were not as conclusive as they appeared. They went on to cite evidence for the importance of postural factors, and finally reached the conclusion that, 'The visual stimuli can have specificity for either postural or phenomenal response-processes only if a fixed posture of the eyes is established. Visual lines are not in their own right stimuli for orientation. If the eyes rolled at random with the head, if the organism could not be oriented to gravity, a vertical line of stimulation on the retina would be neurologically meaningless' (p. 318). If Gibson and Mowrer meant to imply by this statement that there can be no direct visual cues to the vertical, they were surely wrong, for a plumb-line and the paths of falling objects provide direct visual information about the direction of gravity. A person whose postural muscles and vestibular apparatus had been completely paralysed from birth could still judge the vertical from plumb-lines, etc. The fact that he would be easily deceived is irrelevant, for any sensory cue may be deceptive. He would not of course be able to align his eye or body to the visual frame unless he could see his body at the same time.

Later Gibson (1952) modified his general view. The question, he wrote, was not whether the visual factor or the postural factor is prior but what interaction takes place between them. When the head tilts, they co-vary, that is, there is an 'invariant' relation between them. When the scene tilts, or when lenses are worn, or when a subject sits in a centrifuge, they do not co-vary, and two modes or choices are available to the subject. The choice actually made depends on attitude, sex, etc. Gibson implied that the study of verticality in these ambiguous situations is of little theoretical significance, although he admitted that it may be of practical importance, for example in flying (Gibson, 1950a).

Asch and Witkin (1948a) also repeated Wertheimer's tilting-mirror experiment but instead of relying on verbal descriptions, they asked the subjects to judge when a tilting line was 'set parallel with your body'. The mirror room was tilted 30° and was viewed both with and without a reduction tube. With the tube, the apparent vertical was 21·5° from the true upright; without the tube, the deviation was smaller (no average figure was reported). Thus the apparent vertical was closer to the visual frame than to the body axis, and Wertheimer and Koffka were supported rather than Gibson. Asch and Witkin suggested that Gibson may, by chance, have tested only subjects who responded in a particular way. In a further series of experiments Asch and Witkin (1948b) used a 22° tilting model room rather than a mirror. The subject stood outside the room and after four minutes judged when a rod was vertical or horizontal to the walls of the normal room in which he was standing. This was done (a) with a tube, when the subject was told about the tilt of the model room; (b) with a tube, when the subject was told that the model room was not tilted, and (c) without the tube. The mean constant error for the vertical judgments was 15·3° for condition (a), 14·9° for condition (b), and 8·5° for condition (c). The constant errors were all in the direction of the tilted room. The subject was then seated inside the 22° tilted room on a 24° tilted chair, both tilts being to the left. The mean error was now 19·4° in the direction of tilt. The differences between subjects were very large, but the variability of the readings for each subject was not given. When the chair was tilted 24° in the opposite direction to the room, the visual field was accepted as upright even more readily than before. In a further experiment, the tilting room was viewed while the subject sat in a tilting chair for an 'extended period of time', with full knowledge of the situation. Most of the twenty-four subjects deviated more in the direction of the visual frame after this period of time than at first, but some did the opposite.

Finally, Witkin and Asch (1948b) used a visual square frame with 40 inch sides which was tilted about its centre 28° to the left or right in the subject's frontal plane. A 39 inch rod was pivoted about the same centre and the subject had to judge when it was vertical. Nothing else was in view. Two frame positions (28° left and 28° right) and two body positions (upright and 28° left) were used in all combinations. The average constant error was again greatest when the body was tilted as well as the frame, especially when they were tilted in opposite directions. There were wide variations between the performances of the various subjects and these were discussed at length.

From all these experiments, Witkin and Asch concluded that the visual frame is more important than postural factors in judgments of verticality. With an upright visual frame, tilting the subject does not disturb judgments whereas even an upright observer is greatly influenced by a tilted frame. Witkin (1949) reviewed all the experiments which he and Asch had done and discussed the reported experiences of individual subjects. In a book written by Witkin, Lewis, Hertzman, Machover, Meissner, and Wapner (1954) an attempt was made to relate the individual differences found in the orientation tests to other perceptual tests and personality variables. A review of this work would be beyond the scope of our book.

A second team of experimenters, working at Tulane University, produced results which conflict with those reported by Witkin. One of these experimenters (Boring, 1952) had his subjects set a rod to the vertical. A visual frame, in the form of a window pattern, was tilted behind the rod. No differences were found in either the average error nor the constant error between the condition when the frame and body were tilted to the same side and the condition when they were tilted to opposite sides. Boring concluded that the visual frame had no effect on the apparent vertical.

Thus there are two conflicting sets of data. The following are some of the factors which may account for these differences.

(1) The relative strengths of the visual as opposed to the postural cues.
(2) The instructions and set given to the subjects.
(3) The effects of training in the use of the various cues.
(4) The duration of exposure of the tilted visual frame.

These factors will be considered in order.

7.52 The effect of the relative strengths of the visual and postural cues on the apparent vertical

Asch and Witkin (1948b) showed that the effect of the visual frame on the apparent vertical was stronger when it was more articulated. Mann (1952a), working at Tulane, suggested that Boring's visual frame may not have been strong enough to show any effect. He repeated Boring's experiment using a tilting room and tilting chair. The room was set at 30° and 10° left, 0°, 10°, and 30° right, and the tilting chair at 30° left, 0°, and 10° right. Like Boring, but unlike Asch and Witkin, Mann had the subject himself adjust the rod to the gravitational vertical. The results are set out in table 7.3. The apparent vertical was shifted about 10° to the same side as the room when the latter was tilted 30°; with 10° tilts the deviation was in the same direction but was not significant. Similarly, the variability increased with room tilt. Tilting the chair alone, on the other hand, had little effect on either the apparent vertical

Table 7.3 Mean constant errors and mean average errors in the judgment of the visual vertical obtained by Mann (1952a) when using a tilting chair in a tilting room

Chair position	Room 30°L	Room 10°L	Room 0°	Room 10°R	Room 30°R
		Mean constant errors			
30°L	2·58L	4·22L	0·45R	6·90R	16·35R
0°	9·61L	1·59L	0·08R	4·04R	11·71R
10°R	13·69L	1·29L	0·88L	2·91R	11·93R
		Mean average errors			
30°L	17·39	7·50	3·08	8·86	18·21
0°	12·27	4·95	0·72	5·37	13·74
10°R	15·32	6·90	1·75	5·63	14·50

or the variability of settings. This last result supports Gibson and Mowrer's hypothesis that there is constancy under these conditions. But the largest constant errors of all occurred when room and chair were tilted in opposite directions. This result is in agreement with that of Witkin and Asch, but unlike them, Mann found that the apparent vertical was always substantially less tilted than the visual frame.

An enquiry into the effects of different complexities of the visual stimulus was conducted by Weiner (1955a). Three stimuli of increasing complexity were used, a rod, a square and a cube. The stimulus was initially tilted 28° to the right or left. The subject was either erect or tilted 28° to the left, and had to set the stimulus object to the apparent vertical. There is a major difficulty in interpreting Weiner's results. The figures which he presents and on which he bases his conclusions are the deviations of the individual settings from the true upright, '*averaged without regard to sign*'. Thus they are, if any-thing, measures of dispersion. But Weiner interprets them throughout as constant errors, which would be correct only in the unlikely event of all the individual settings deviating from the vertical in the same direction. We shall, however, tentatively report his conclusions on the assumption that he did not base them solely on his published figures but also on at least a graphic inspection of his data.

He reported that with the subject erect the settings deviated from the vertical in the direction of the initial position of the stimulus—i.e. the usual tilt after-effect—and that this effect increased with the complexity of the stimulus. With the subject tilted to one side, on the other hand, the apparent vertical was displaced to the opposite side—i.e. Müller's E-effect. A measure of the E-effect is the difference in displacement between the condition in which rod and body are tilted to the same side—when the tilt after-effect and the E-effect oppose one another—and the condition in which they are tilted to opposite sides, and therefore the two effects reinforce one another. Weiner reported that the E-effect, unlike the tilt after-effect, *decreases* with increasing stimulus complexity.

Curran and Lane (1962) varied the illumination of the field, the degree of body tilt, and the amount by which the tilting body was supported by a counterweight. They thus varied the strength of the visual frame, of vestibular stimulation, and of somaesthetic stimulation. Significant interactions were found between each pair of variables. In general the results support Witkin's contention that visual factors contribute more than postural factors to the position of the apparent vertical, even when the visual cues are relatively few and dimly illuminated. When both the visual and the somaesthetic cues were minimized, the constant error became largely dependent on the degree of body tilt (vestibular cues).

One way to reduce the effectiveness of vestibular cues to the vertical is to lay the subject on his back and ask him to set a rod parallel to his body axis. Rock (1954) used this technique and found that his subjects were about as accurate in their settings as subjects are when they set a line to the vertical in the ordinary way. Rock concluded that, 'Egocentric orientation is perceived independently of postural cues of the direction of gravity.' This conclusion requires qualification. The subject's judgments in this situation are not independent of all postural stimulation; the subject must know where his head is in relation to his body, and for this purpose he can use only kinaesthetic cues from the neck muscles. If he were to tilt his head on his shoulders his judgment would probably be upset.

At the Holyoke Laboratories, Reese (1953, p. 24) found that the constant error of setting a rod to the apparent vertical increased with increasing tilt of the visual frame (a room) up to between five and ten degrees of tilt but after that there was a gradual reduction of error. They interpreted this reduction of error at larger tilts of the frame as due to an increasing dependence on postural cues.

Kleint (1936) studied the effects of having two visual frames present at the same time, one vertical and one tilted. He found that the visual frame which occupied the greater proportion of the field of view appeared vertical, and Kleint called this 'full-space'; the smaller frame appeared tilted and was called the 'part-space'. A typical situation is one where a person looks out of the window of a tilted room at an upright scene. The scene becomes the full-space when the subject is near the window but the room becomes the full-space when the subject steps back from the window. Kleint cited several examples of this type of situation and also related that subjects were very variable in their responses, even when the conditions were constant. He presented evidence to show that not only does the full-space affect the apparent orientation of the part-space but that the part-space also influences the full-space to some extent. Kleint called this mutual interaction 'induction' and cited an experiment by Jaensch (1911) in which it was shown that induction takes place also in the third dimension of space. A vertical line when put next to a line which was tilting away from the subject, appeared to tilt the other way. Such contrast or induction effects in the third dimension have also been demonstrated by Werner (1938), and by Howard and Templeton (1964a). Kleint also pointed out that damage to the labyrinths can cause permanent apparent tilt in the full-space (see section 5.6).

There is thus abundant evidence that the extent to which a tilted visual frame affects the apparent vertical depends on the complexity and size of the visual frame and also on the extent to which the labyrinthine and kinaesthetic modalities are stimulated.

7.53 The effect of instructions and set on the apparent vertical

Mann and Boring (1953) asked four naïve subjects to set a rod to the vertical without explaining to them what was meant by 'vertical'; and four sophisticated subjects, who were told to set the rod to the gravitational vertical. The naïve subjects produced larger constant and average errors, especially in conditions where the room was tilted. Mann and Boring suggested that such effects of instructions could account for the differences between Asch and Witkin's results and their own. Mann writes (private communication), 'In all our experiments, we trained our subjects carefully, giving them instructions and then a number of practice trials before the trials proper. We were interested in what a man *could* do under the maximum advantageous conditions, rather than what he *would* do given a fairly free choice within a framework of instructions.' In reply to this suggestion,

Witkin (1953) pointed out that the instructions which he and Asch had used corresponded to those given to the sophisticated group in Mann and Boring's study and that therefore the discrepancy between their two sets of results could not be due to differences in instructions.

The closely related problem of set has been studied by Gross (1959). He manipulated the subject's set in the rod and frame situation by interposing a sheet of glass between subject and stimulus; some subjects knew it was plain glass, others were told it was a lens which would introduce an unknown amount of distortion. The results showed that the introduction of the 'set for uncertainty' produced by the 'lens' gave more variability in the settings of the rod but only when the frame was present. The control 'glass' had no effect. Overall, the subjects showed less variability than Witkin's, and Gross explained this difference by suggesting that Witkin's subjects had more 'uncertainty set' as a result of doing a variety of verticality tests.

There is one difference in procedure which neither group of experimenters has considered: Asch and Witkin did not have their subjects set the rod themselves, whereas Boring and Mann had their subjects control the rod by pressing a control switch.

7.54 The effect of training on the apparent vertical

Bitterman and Worchel (1953) considered that the issue of visual versus postural determinants of the apparent vertical is not so 'fruitless' as Gibson (1952) maintained. They wrote, 'The key to a more satisfactory resolution of the problem is to separate the issues of genetic priority and dominance which have been hopelessly confounded in previous treatments.' Postural cues must be genetically prior, they thought, but visual cues may become more dominant by learning.

They tested this last statement by an experiment in which they used 22 subjects who had been blind since birth and a matched group of sighted but blindfolded subjects. The subjects stood and had to set a rod to the vertical and horizontal (defined with reference to the floor) using their hands. In a second condition the subjects were tilted alternately 42° to the left and 42° to the right. The two groups of subjects performed equally well when they were standing up, but the effect of the tilt of the body on the constant error was greater in the sighted subjects. This was presumably because they normally relied on vision and were therefore less practised in using postural cues.

Witkin (1948) set out to determine the effects of training and 'structural aids' on performance in three tests of spatial orientation. The three tests employed were (a) the tilting-room-tilting-chair test in which the subject had to set either the chair or the room to the vertical when these were tilted in various ways, (b) the tilting frame and rod test in which the subject had to set a rod to either the vertical or horizontal when the frame was tilted at various angles, and (c) the rotating room test in which the subject set a rod to the vertical in a room which was centrifuged at various speeds. Four groups of subjects were first given the tests. Then group I, the 'training group', was given training to 'furnish insight' into the problem of orientation and to afford further supervised training but only on the tilting-room-tilting-chair test. Group II, the 'structural-aids group', were retested on test (a) with a changed room in which 'the structure of the visual field was less compelling as a visual aid to orientation'. Group III had two hours of additional practice on test (a) without knowledge of results, and group IV were merely tested and retested.

The training procedures produced improvement in orientation in the situation in which the training was administered (test a) and also some transfer of training to the frame and rod test (test b). The structural-aids group performed even better than group I on retest, but only maintained this improved performance when the room had the reduced visual cues. Group III improved on retest but not so much as group I. The control group did not improve on retest.

In conclusion Witkin suggested that the most efficient way to improve spatial orientation ability is to provide 'structural aids', by which he meant a reduction in the conflict of visual and postural cues to the vertical. If this is impracticable, then training will improve performance. The way the subjects described their experiences led Witkin to consider that the improvement due to training resulted from 'a more valid interpretation of the sensory experiences', not to alterations in 'the perceptions themselves'.

Weiner (1955b) thought that the training which Witkin had given to his subjects put too much emphasis on intellectual knowledge. He suggested that if subjects were trained in the concrete procedures of using postural cues, then there might result, not merely a reinterpretation of sensory experiences, but a fundamental change in the precepts themselves. In order to test this suggestion, he used a tilting-frame-tilting-chair test in which the subject had to set either the frame or a rod to the vertical with various combinations of tilt of the subject and the frame. Interpolated training consisted of indicating to the subject the nature of bodily cues to the vertical and practical training with knowledge of results. The training significantly improved performance in the conditions where the body was tilted, and this improvement indicated a greater reliance on body cues. Most of the subjects reported that the rod or frame actually appeared upright in the retest, and that it was not just a matter of reinterpretation. Weiner concluded that, 'Subjects learned to perceptually reorganize the potency given postural and visual cues.' Elliott and Mc-Michael (1963) on the other hand, found the effects of two types of training on the rod-and-frame test to be either negligible or transient for a group selected for large errors. They concluded that, 'An adult's failure to have learned to use his body as a coordinate in judging up–down with accuracy is a stable and durable deficit.'

Perhaps also a result of training is the finding reported in the book by Witkin et al. (1954) that the influence of a tilted luminous frame on a rod decreases with age. However, Edgren (1953) in a replica of this experiment, found no such decrease with age over the years 8–16.

7.55 The effect of the duration of exposure of the tilted frame on the apparent vertical

Finally we shall consider the effect of the length of time that the tilted frame is in view before the subject is asked to make his judgment. Wertheimer, in his original experiment with the tilting mirror, noticed that it was some time before the mirror room looked upright. Kleint (1936) also noticed that as his subjects continued to look into a tilted room it gradually came to appear more vertical.

Cohen and Tepas (1958) used the Witkin rod and frame test to study this factor. A 25° tilting frame was exposed for 0, 4, 8, and 16 minutes before the rod was set. There were no significant differences in the constant errors obtained in the delay conditions but the overall constant error for the delay conditions was significantly greater than the error in the condition where the judgments were made immediately. A period of eight minutes' darkness before the rod-and-frame test or before the rod-alone test, produced similar constant errors to those obtained with immediate judgment. Therefore an increase in the duration of exposure of the tilted frame did increase the effect which the tilted frame had on the position of the apparent vertical. The results for the subjects under the various conditions did not correlate and Cohen and Tepas issued a warning against classifying people as 'frame-dependent' in the way Witkin has done.

Morant and Aronoff (in press) also studied the effect of long exposure of the stimulus in a tilted position. A two-minute exposure of either a rod or a frame before adjustment to the vertical increased the tilt after-effect by about a degree; the effects with the frame as stimulus (2·9° for immediate adjustment, 3·7° for delayed adjustment) were about a degree larger than those with the rod (1·5° and 2·5°). But the really potent factor was the presence of the frame during adjustment of the rod, which produced effects of about 7° irrespective of whether the frame had been inspected for two minutes.

This concludes our discussion of the effect of tilting the visual frame on the position of the apparent vertical. In view of all the factors which have been found to influence the effect which a tilting frame has, the differences between the results of Asch and Witkin and the investigators at Tulane are not surprising.

One final point, all Mann's subjects were naval men. It is possible that he sampled only one end of the individual-difference spectrum. It may not be a question of visual versus postural cues but of which is more important for whom under which conditions.

7.6 Brain damage and the judgment of the vertical

There are many reports in the clinical literature of apparent displacements of the visual vertical and horizontal resulting from cerebral injury. The most commonly implicated centre is the cerebellum (the effects of damage to the vestibular system have been discussed in section 5.6). Halpern (1949) reviewed the early literature. Damage to the cerebellum on one side has been found to cause vertical lines, houses, trees, etc. to appear to tilt in the same direction. Halpern describes how this symptom is commonly associated with other symptoms including deviation of walking to the affected side, distortions of visual shapes, slanting handwriting, deviation of the tactile–kinaesthetic vertical, and disturbances of comparative weight estimations between the two hands. Halpern called this collection of symptoms the 'sensorimotor induction syndrome'. He concluded that, 'The clinical phenomena in themselves permit the conclusion of the one fundamental physiological fact, that in some way the sensory perception of the external world is connected with the organization of the statokinetic system of the body.' This rather trite statement is derived from Schilder's (1942) and Goldstein's (1939) earlier formulation, as also is the similar 'sensory–tonic' formulation of Werner and Wapner (1952).

Both Schilder and Halpern cited evidence that damage to other centres besides the cerebellum may induce an apparent shift of the vertical; in particular they implicated the frontal lobes. Bender and Jung (1948) also reported an apparent displacement of the vertical to the side of a lesion in the frontal cortex. Occipital-lobe damage did not result in a disturbance of the apparent vertical, even when such damage was accompanied by hemianopia, which seems to be associated with apparent shifts of the vertical in some patients (Lenz, 1949).

Teuber and Mishkin (1954), although finding that patients with anterior cerebral lesions showed increased variability of verticality judgments, could not find evidence of constant errors in any of their patients. They suggested that the differences between their results and those of Bender and Jung may have been due to the fact that their own tests were done several years after the brain injury, whereas Bender and Jung tested their patients soon after their injury.

Bruell and Peszczynski (1958) found no evidence of constant errors in verticality judgments in a group of hemiplegic patients, although, like Teuber and Mishkin, they found an increased variability of judgments, especially when a rod's verticality was judged against the background of a tilted frame. Those patients with the largest variability benefited less from remedial training.

More recently Birch, Belmont, Reilly, and Belmont (1961) also failed to find any constant errors in visual verticality judgments in hemiplegics, although like the other investigators they found an increased variability. The introduction of a frame reduced this variability in the brain-damaged. In a later paper, these same authors (1962) found that the variability of the hemiplegics' judgments was increased by weighting the shoulder of the un-affected side, and decreased by weighting the affected side.

There is thus some conflict of clinical opinion about the effects of brain damage on verticality judgments. In view of the repeated qualitative clinical reports of very great displacements of the apparent vertical, complete in-version in some cases (Klopp, 1951; Schilder, 1942), it cannot be denied that such displacements occur. John Hunter, the famous clinician, had a disease of the nervous system, and found that verticals appeared to tilt 30° to 40° (Brain, 1952). His testimony cannot be doubted. That constant errors have not shown up in most of the quantitative studies, is presumably due to the fact that the chosen samples did not contain any patients manifesting these particular symptoms; the symptoms are clearly not an invariant, nor even a common accompaniment of brain damage.

8

Orientation to Gravity II

Adaptation to the vertical

8.1 Basic facts

In 1933 Gibson accidentally discovered a phenomenon during an experiment on the effects of wearing distorting prisms.

Prisms not only cause an apparent displacement of the visible world but also introduce an apparent curvature. Gibson found that the extent of the apparent curvature diminished as the subject continued to wear the prisms. When the prisms were removed, straight lines appeared to be curved in the opposite direction to the direction of apparent curvature induced by the prisms. This after-effect was produced whether or not the subject manipulated the environment and whether or not he moved his eyes, and is therefore not due to conflict between visual and kinaesthetic experiences. Even without prisms, curvature apparently diminished during inspection of a curved line, and a straight line seen subsequently in the same location appeared curved the other way, Verhoeff had reported this last effect in 1925. Gibson also noted that a straight line seen against a background of curved lines appeared to be curved the other way. This simultaneous effect had been known for some time, as Gibson realized.

Gibson conducted several experiments which demonstrated that the after-effect of seen curvature is restricted to the retinal locality stimulated by the inspection figure. For example, if a curved line was inspected for several minutes and then several straight lines were exposed together, only that straight test line which coincided with the position of the previous inspection line showed the apparent curvature. There was some evidence of a slight spread of the after-effect from one locality to another but Gibson concluded that most of the effect is limited to the position of the inspection line.

Gibson presented the inspection figure to one eye and the test figure to the other and found that the after-effect transferred to almost its full extent. This interocular transfer of the effect was said to demonstrate its origin beyond the level of the chiasma, a conclusion we shall presently question.

An analogous adaptation effect was later found for tilted lines (Gibson and Radner, 1937). Inspection lines which were off-vertical caused vertical lines seen subsequently to appear tilted in the opposite direction. Vernon (1934) had reported a similar effect and she interpreted Gibson's curvature adaptation effect as a normalization to the vertical of the parts of the curved line. Such an explanation would account only for curvature after-effects produced by vertically oriented curved lines. Gibson showed that the curvature after-effect is not dependent on the orientation of the inspection line, and thus disproved Vernon's suggestion.

The tilt after-effect was considered by Gibson and Radner to be analogous to the curvature after-effect. Both phenomena were explained in terms of adaptation processes in oppositional scales. Examples of oppositional scales are 'up and down' in relation to eye level, 'movement right and movement left' in relation to the stationary state, and 'tilt right and tilt left' in relation to the vertical. In each case there is a neutral point in the scale. So-called intensive scales, on the other hand, do not pass through a neutral value; examples are weight, distance, and loudness.

The neutral point in an oppositional scale is the norm, it is the point from which the intensities of the scale values increase in either direction. It is the most frequent value of the scale to be experienced. In many cases it is the point in the scale which is discriminated most acutely. All oppositional scales probably exhibit normalization, that is, stimuli which are off the norm come to be reported as being more like the norm as they continue to be inspected. Inspection of an off-norm stimulus produces an alteration over the whole scale in the correspondence between the physical values of the scale and the reported magnitudes, although this shift in correspondence may be maximal in the region of the inspected value. Such a shift persists for some time and manifests itself as an after-effect when subsequent judgments are made. Gibson wrote, 'If a sensory process which has an opposite is made to persist by a constant application of its appropriate stimulus-conditions the quality will diminish in the direction of becoming neutral, and therewith the quality evoked by any stimulus for the dimension in question will be shifted temporarily towards the opposite or complementary quality' (p. 223).

We are only concerned here with visual spatial dimensions. There are several spatial dimensions which are oppositional.

(a) Tilt or rotation of a line (or other figure) from the vertical or horizontal in the frontal or sagittal plane; rotation of a line in the horizontal plane from the pointing-straight-ahead position or from the frontal-parallel position (making three dimensions with two norms in each).

(b) Translation of a line (or other figure) from the median plane to left or right. Translation of a line from the horizontal plane up or down (making two dimensions with one norm each).

(c) Departure from straightness by curvature or bending in the frontal plane or in depth.

We shall be concerned largely with tilt in the frontal plane. When a tilted line gradually comes to appear less tilted, it is said to normalize to the vertical. The after-effect of inspecting an off-vertical line on a subsequently seen vertical line is called the tilt after-effect. It is not easy to measure normalization directly and it has often been assumed that the extent of the tilt after-effect is a measure of the normalization which the inspection figure has undergone. This would be true only if the shift of the subjective scale were homogeneous throughout the stimulus range, and if there were no other mechanisms which could account for, or influence the tilt after-effect. We shall see later that neither of these assumptions is justified.

Gibson (1937a, 1937b) and Gibson and Radner (1937) found the tilt after-effect to have the following properties. Like the curvature after-effect, it is limited to the location of the inspection figure, although it does transfer from one eye to the other. The amount of after-effect rapidly rises as the duration of the inspection period is increased, levelling off at 1·5° after between 45 and 90 sec inspection of a 5° tilted line. As the tilt of the inspection line is increased, the after-effect increases to a maximum for an inspection tilt of between 5° and 20°. For greater tilts, the after-effect falls off, reaching zero when the inspection line is about 45°. With an inspection line of more than 45°, the whole scale shifts towards the horizontal; a vertical test line is also apparently shifted, but now *towards* the position of the inspection line. In a similar way horizontal test lines are affected by inspection lines near the vertical. These reversed effects of inspection lines on test lines in neighbouring quadrants are known as *indirect effects*; they are not as marked as the direct effects. Table 8.1 shows the results which Gibson and Radner (1937) obtained for the effect on the vertical and horizontal of inspection lines tilted 5° from the vertical or the horizontal and inspected for 45 sec.

Table 8.1 The amount of the direct and indirect tilt after-effects obtained for a 5° tilted line inspected for 45 sec (Gibson and Radner, 1937)

Inspection line 5° from vertical		Inspection line 5° from horizontal	
Direct	Indirect	Direct	Indirect
1·09°	0·54°	1·42°	0·75°

These are the basic facts about tilt adaptation which were discovered by Gibson and Radner. It has been found that when subjects are asked to set a line to the vertical, they tend to set it to the side to which it was initially tilted (Werner and Wapner, 1952). The same effect has been reported when the body is set to the vertical. These effects are easily explained in terms of tilt adaptation.

McFarland (1962) has demonstrated that the tilt after-effect is accompanied by an apparent rotation of the body axis in the opposite direction. He suggested that a reflex tendency to set the body axis parallel with the tilted line contributes to the two perceptual changes.

Since Gibson and Radner's report, some workers have tried to demonstrate that the tilt after-effect can be explained in terms of other mechanisms, while others have tried to demonstrate that it is a distinct process. The following mechanisms could account for the tilt after-effect.

(1) The after-effects of Gibsonian normalization to the vertical.

(2) Adaptation to rotated visual frames in the manner of Wertheimer's tilted-mirror effect.

(3) Simultaneous-contrast effects of direction such as are seen in the Hering illusion.

(4) Figural after-effects.

Gibson's tilt adaptation will be compared and contrasted with each of the other processes in turn.

8.2 Tilt adaptation and shifts of the visual frame

Gibson realized that tilt adaptation resembles Wertheimer's reported experience that the reflection of a room seen through a 45° tilted mirror appears to straighten after some time. Witkin's visual-frame effects (see section 7.51) are akin to the Wertheimer effect. Gibson, Held, Morant, and others have given reasons why these two phenomena should not be considered the same. We shall refer to one as Gibson's adaptation and the other as a visual-frame shift. The suggested differences between them are listed below.

8.21 The magnitude of tilt adaptation and frame shifts

Gibson's adaptation is never more than about 3°. Frame shifts have been found by Wertheimer (1912), Witkin (1949) and Beller and Morant (1963) to be complete for angles of tilt up to about 25°.

8.22 Spatial transfer of tilt adaptation and frame shifts

Gibson stated that tilt adaptation is largely localized to the site of the inspection figure. On the other hand, it is generally stated that frame shifts transfer to all parts of the visual field. Both these statements may be challenged. Morant and Mikaelian (1960) questioned Gibson's reasons for believing that adaptation does not transfer. One of Gibson's experiments involved the inspection of three lines side by side, two vertical lines and a middle one which was tilted. Of three vertical test lines, only the middle line, corresponding in position to the tilted inspection line, appeared tilted. Morant and Mikaelian pointed out that this experiment demonstrated only that different inspection lines could produce differential effects in different parts of the field, and did not test whether the after-effect is restricted to parts of the field which correspond to the position of inspection lines. Gibson showed that no after-effect of a tilted line can be seen in a test field consisting of an ordinary room. He suggested that this is evidence that the effect does not transfer to all parts of the visual field. However, Morant and Mikaelian remarked that it demonstrates only that the tilt-adaptation effect does not manifest itself when a strong vertical–horizontal frame of reference is present. They reported their own experiment, in which a tilted inspection line and a vertical test line were either exposed in the same location or in different locations, 7° of visual angle apart. An after-effect of 1·52° was obtained when inspection and test lines coincided and of 1·09° when they were separated. There was thus considerable transfer of the after-effect at least over 7° of the visual field. This is not a large distance, and the experiment should be repeated for different distances.

Morant and Mikaelian's criticisms of Gibson's evidence against transfer do not apply to Gibson's 1933 experiments, which Morant and Mikaelian did not mention. These experiments were on curvature adaptation rather than tilt adaptation but otherwise involved the same procedure as the experiment by Morant and Mikaelian. Gibson used separations of 5·7° of visual angle between his test and inspection figures and obtained transfer effects about one-quarter as large as the effects with no separation between the figures. Thus Gibson did not deny that transfer of adaptation could take place; he insisted only that most of the effect is localized. More experiments are needed before anyone can say just how localized adaptation effects are.

We can find no experimental evidence to support the belief that visual-frame shifts transfer to all parts of the retina. If prism distortion were limited to half the retina while the other half was blanked out, it is not known whether adaptation would transfer to the blanked-out region of the retina. The distinction between Gibson's adaptation and frame shifts on the basis of transfer cannot therefore be accepted on these grounds as yet.

8.23 Passive and active inspection in tilt adaptation and frame shifts

Gibson found that tilt adaptation occurs whether or not the subject manipulates the inspection figure. It has been claimed that frame shifts depend on the active behaviour of the subject during the inspection period. Mikaelian and Held (1964) found a tilt-adaptation effect of a few degrees after wearing prisms which rotated the optical array. This effect occurred when the subjects were passively wheeled about in a hallway. This passively produced after-effect was thought to be a Gibson adaptation effect. When the inspection field consisted of luminous spheres providing no cue to the distortion introduced by the prisms, then passive movement of the subject did not produce any tilt after-effect.

When the subjects moved about actively during the inspection period, both inspection fields produced tilt after-effects. The normal inspection field produced after-effects nearly as large as the 20° tilt introduced by the prisms.

Mikaelian and Held also found that passive inspection of a prismatically tilted field produced a Gibsonian tilt after-effect but did not produce any distortion in the apparent position of single points of light in the egocentric median plane. Active inspection on the other hand not only produced larger after-effects of tilt but also apparent displacements of points of light from the median plane. However, the reported absence of a displacement of dots in the passive condition may only have arisen because of the difficulty of measuring small apparent displacements of dots from the median plane.

Hochberg (1963) objected that the after-effects consequent upon active movement which Mikaelian and Held described were not true visual after-effects, in that they did not involve an intravisual-field distortion. However, while Hochberg's paper was in press, Rekosh and Held (1963) and Held and Rekosh (1963) had produced evidence that active movement may induce curvature after-effects, which are certainly intravisual (Held, 1963b). The results of the Mikaelian and Held experiments suggest that active movement is necessary for adaptation to rotations of the optical array through large angles. The special case of prismatic inversion of the optical array in which there is no displacement of the main visual lines relative to the egocentric axes, is discussed in section 15.22.

Wertheimer, on the other hand, in the early experiment with a tilting mirror, did not report that active movement was necessary for the large apparent shifts of the field of view which he observed. Koffka and Witkin (see section 7.51) also reported almost full adaptations to large rotations of the field of view and yet did not mention the necessity for active movement.

Morant and Beller (in press) found that active movement doubled the effect of prismatic rotation obtained with a seated subject, provided the inspected field consisted of objects: active movement did not significantly change the after-effect when the field consisted of a series of parallel straight lines. With the object fields, active movement for 15 minutes produced a displacement in the apparent verticality of lines of almost 4° for a 15° tilt and almost 8° for a 75° tilt.

8.24 Tilt adaptation and frame shifts for 45° of tilt

The Gibson adaptation effect should be absent for inspection lines tilted at 45°. At this angle the opposed adaptation effects induced by the vertical and horizontal norms should cancel out. Gibson and Radner (1937) and Culbert (1954) found that this is the case, although Köhler and Wallach (1944) failed to substantiate this result. There is no reason why frame shifts should not occur for fields tilted at 45°. In fact Wertheimer obtained his effect with a field tilted at 45°.

Morant and Beller (in press) demonstrated that 45° tilts of a field consisting of objects affected the apparent verticality of a line whereas the same tilt of a field of parallel straight lines did not. Similarly the two fields when tilted to 15° produced congruent effects on the apparent verticality of a line whereas when tilted to 75° they had opposed effects: a field of lines adapts to the nearest main axis, whereas a field of normally upright objects always adapts to the vertical.

All this suggests that there are several factors which determine the extent of adaptation to a tilted visual frame.

(1) Active movement is necessary where the visual field itself gives no clue to the distortion, but even where it does, active movement will increase the effect provided that,

(2) the field of view contains familiar objects, and particularly when

(3) both the inspection and the test fields contain familiar objects.

These suggestions are not all proved by the foregoing evidence; further experimental work is necessary.

8.3 Tilt adaptation and simultaneous tilt contrast

Gibson was emphatic in his belief that the tilt after-effect is not the same process as simultaneous tilt contrast. A tilt-contrast effect is shown in figure 8.1. These effects were first described by Hoffmann and Bielschowsky (1909)

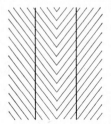

Figure 8.1 A simultaneous tilt-contrast effect

and later by Krantz (1930) and Kleint (1936). Gibson wrote, 'Although the simultaneous contrast phenomenon bears an intriguing resemblance to the after-effect phenomenon, it is far from being the same thing and requires some hypothesis of its own' (p. 568). All the experimental evidence which Gibson reported showed that the simultaneous and successive effects behave alike. The operational basis for making a distinction is therefore not clear in Gibson's account. The successive effect takes time to develop, whereas the simultaneous effect does not. But this does not provide a good basis for distinguishing between them, for if the after-effect is due to an after-image persisting from the inspection line, one would expect the successive effect to increase in strength as the after-image is strengthened by a longer exposure of the inspection line. One would also expect that the simultaneous effect should always be greater than the successive effect. Interocular transfer of the successive effect is no evidence that it is not dependent on after-images, for after-images persist when an eye is closed and may still affect the appearance of stimuli seen with the other eye.

8.4 Tilt adaptation and figural after-effects

Köhler and Wallach (1944) considered that Gibson's adaptation effects were a special case of a broader class of effects based on a mechanism which they called 'satiation'. According to satiation theory, Gibson's tilt after-effect is due to 'electrotonic' spread of the striate-cortex processes produced by the inspection line, which shift the site of the subsequent test-line processes and hence produce an apparent repulsion of the test line away from the location of the inspection line. The magnitude of the repulsion depends on the distance between the locations of inspection and test lines; this means that the size of the *tilt* after-effect should depend on the angular separation of the two lines rather than, as Gibson thought, their relationship to the main visual axes.

There are several operational distinctions between Gibson's tilt after-effect and Köhler's figural after-effect. These are listed below.

8.41 Normalization

Köhler's theory cannot account for normalization itself, that is, the progressive decrease in the apparent tilt of an off-vertical line. A figural after-effect cannot have any effect on the apparent position of the inspection figure itself. Normalization of a tilted line is a commonly reported effect (e.g. Gibson and Radner, 1937; Morant and Mistovich, 1960). We have already commented on the difficulty of measuring normalization directly. There seem to be three procedures by which this can be done.

The most obvious method is to ask the subject to make absolute estimates of the tilt of a line on first sight, and again after a period of inspection. Templeton and Howard (to be published) conducted an experiment of this type, and found a significant adaptation of a 5° line to the vertical. Magnitude estimations of a series of lines, including one at 5°, were separated by periods of inspection of the 5° line.

The second procedure for measuring normalization is one first used by Prentice and Beardslee (1950). A 3 in inspection line, tilted 10°, was exposed on one side of the fixation point. A 3 in test line was then exposed at an equal distance on the other side of the fixation point. The subject had to report whether the test line was tilted more or less than the inspection line had been. Conditions were used in which the inspection line was surrounded (a) by an upright square with 4 in side, (b) by a square with 8 in side, (c) by an aperture in which the sides were parallel with the inspection line, and (d) by a plain dark field. Neither the variations in the frame nor its absence had much effect on the normalization indicated by the method, which was about 2°. On Köhler's theory the inspection line should have tended to line up with the sides of the frame. But the fact that the different shapes and sizes of frame had no effect is evidence that this was not occurring.

These experiments were criticized by Heinemann and Marill (1954). They suggested that there were possibilities for figural after-effects even in the condition where the sides of the frame were parallel with the inspection line. This is because the frame had acute angles in two corners and obtuse angles in the other corners. Satiation is supposed to be denser in acute angles. They repeated the experiments with modifications. In one condition, the inspection line was vertical but the frame (not just the sides) was tilted 10°. In another condition the inspection line and the whole frame were tilted 10°. In the first conditon, the vertical line appeared to align with the edges of the frame. In the other condition, there was no significant tendency for the line to appear to turn towards the vertical, when the alignment effect was excluded. Thus the only effect found was one predictable from Köhler's theory.

Held (1963c) adopted a similar procedure for measuring normalization. The inspection figure was a 10° tilted line. The test figure consisted of the two 10° tilted lines, A and B, one of which (A) coincided with the inspection line. The subject fixated midway between the centres of the two lines and was first asked to set the comparison line parallel to the inspection line; this served as a control setting of parallelility. The inspection line alone was then exposed for 60 sec, after which the subject had to report which way line B had to be turned to be parallel with line A. Most of the reports were consistent with the presence of local tilt normalization to the vertical. There is a point of criticism to be made about this experiment. The geometrical arrangement of the two lines was either as shown in figure 8.2 (a) or as shown in figure 8.2(b). The lines themselves were tilted clockwise and anticlockwise from both the vertical and the horizontal, but this does not affect our argument. In figure (a), the top end of the line B is nearer to line A than is the bottom end of line B. B should therefore appear tilted towards the vertical as compared with line A. This is in conflict with the prediction from Gibson's normalization. If the two opposed effects are of equal strength then half the subjects would give judgments in favour of Gibson's hypothesis and half in

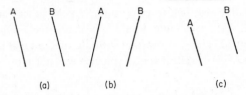

Figure 8.2 Arrangement of lines used in the experiment by Held (1963c) to demonstrate tilt adaptation (a and b) and suggested improvement in the arrangement (c)

favour of Köhler's. In the arrangement shown in figure (b) the bottom of line B is nearer the inspection line A than is the top of line B. Line B will therefore appear tilted further from the vertical than line A. This effect is in the same direction as the Gibson effect, and therefore all subjects should report in favour of Gibson's hypothesis. In total therefore about three-quarters of the responses should favour Gibson's hypothesis and one-quarter Köhler's. These are roughly the proportions of responses which Held reported. The geometrical arrangement which would have overcome this intrusion of a Köhler effect is shown in figure 8.2(c). This pattern has a symmetrical relation between the two lines.

Morant (private communication) could not reproduce Held's effect and attributes it to the fact that Held had his subjects set the comparison line parallel to the inspection line prior to the inspection period. It was always the inspection line which was adjusted, and Morant claims that this would lead to an 'error of the standard' which would provide a distorted control measure from which to measure the main effect.

Held's procedure has in any case a basic weakness, which he recognized: it measures only that part of normalization which does not transfer to the second test line. Held does not state the angular separation between his two lines, but if we assume that it was similar to the separation between the lines in Morant and Mikaelian's study, viz. 7° (see section 8.22), then at least two-thirds of the normalization effect transfers according to the results of that study. The procedure would therefore record only a fraction of the normalization.

The third procedure for measuring normalization directly is one proposed by Templeton. The inspection figure consists of two lines tilted symmetrically about the vertical. The test figure consists of the same lines as the inspection figure, with an extension of the two lines to form a symmetrical cross (see figure 8.3). If the two inspection lines normalize, the angle between them should appear to shrink. Thus, after inspection the top angle in the test cross would appear to be *smaller* than the bottom angle, as compared with its apparent relative size before inspection. On the other hand, if a figural after-effect occurs, the top angle should appear relatively *larger* after inspection, than the bottom angle. A constant stimulus method was used to measure the actual effect. The net effect for all subjects was not quite significantly in

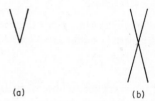

(a)   (b)

Figure 8.3 The arrangement used by Templeton to measure tilt normalization: (a) Inspection figure; (b) Test figure

favour of a Gibson effect. The situation is not simple. The simultaneous normalization of two lines in opposite directions suggests a complex deformation of the scale of inclination, with no actual shift of the norm itself—a phenomenon which would not be easily integrated into Gibson's theory. Presumably, complex transfer effects would also operate.

In an experiment by Prentice and Beardslee (1950) the subjects tilted their heads so that the tilted inspection line fell on the normally vertical meridian of the eye; this was ensured by having them align the inspection figure with the after-image of a vertical line induced when the head was erect. The inspection figure, when compared with an objectively parallel line had clearly normalized to the gravitational vertical. Prentice and Beardslee concluded that normalization is to a 'psychological' rather than a retinal axis and hence even the postulation of permanent satiation gradients from top to bottom of the cortical projection of the retina would not enable Köhler's theory to encompass normalization.

8.42 The symmetry of figural after-effects

Köhler and Wallach (1944) supported their argument that the Gibson effect was a case of figural after-effects by the following experiment. They measured the tilt after-effect produced on a vertical line by inspection of a 10° tilted line and compared this with the after-effect produced on a 10° tilted line by inspection of a vertical line. The two after-effects were similar, which fits the figural after-effect hypothesis but not Gibson's hypothesis, which predicts no after-effect of a vertical inspection line.

Templeton, Howard, and Easting (in press) repeated this experiment. They argued that Köhler and Wallach's result could have been produced by a faulty measuring technique which Templeton *et al.* corrected. They found significant after-effect from vertical line to tilted line, but it was significantly smaller than the after-effect produced by the tilted line on the vertical line. This result suggests that both Gibson and Köhler-type processes are operating.

8.43 Relative shifts of different parts of the subjective scale of tilt

A related study was conducted by Templeton and Howard (to be published). A line tilted 5° was inspected for one minute and then a test line was briefly exposed at one of ten angles between 9° clockwise and 9° anticlockwise to the vertical. The subject had to estimate the inclination of the test line using whatever numerical categories he wished. The test lines were exposed, one at a time, interspersed with five-second 'topping-up' exposures of the inspection line. In the control condition, the inspection line was replaced by an empty field. It was thus possible to assess the effect of an inspection line simultaneously on several different test lines. The predicted scale shift on Köhler's hypothesis is depicted in figure 8.4(a) and that predicted on

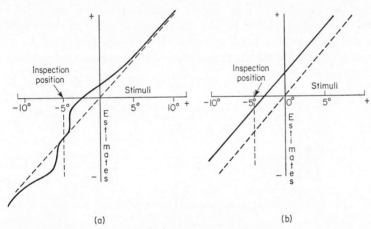

(a)   (b)

Figure 8.4 The predicted scale shifts in absolute judgments of inclination after inspection of a line tilted to —5° according to (a) Köhler and (b) Gibson

Gibson's hypothesis in figure 8.4(b). The results again suggest that both mechanisms are operating.

All displacements, including those of lines more tilted than the inspection figure, were in the direction predicted on Gibson's model, but the displacements fell to zero for the most distant lines i.e. those tilted more than 5° in the opposite direction to the inspection figure.

8.44 The indirect effect

Gibson and Radner (1937) reported the indirect effect which we have described in section 8.1. Briefly it is that exposure to a tilt off one axis produces an after-effect on the other axis. Köhler's theory cannot account for the indirect effect, but Köhler and Wallach (1944) and Prentice and Beardslee (1950) failed to confirm it experimentally. Morant and Mistovich (1960) reported findings which are in essential agreement with Gibson and Radner's results. The indirect effect was found to be approximately half the direct effect. Gibson had put this difference down to 'play' between the axes. The greater distance apart of the test and inspection lines in the indirect condition as compared with the direct condition could explain this 'play'. Morant and Mistovich, on the other hand, interpreted the difference between the two effects as due to the summation of Gibson's tilt after-effect and Köhler's figural after-effect. Whichever view one takes, the evidence suggests that there is a Gibson effect.

Morant and Harris (1965) made predictions about the after-effects on a vertical test line produced by inspection lines at various angles between vertical and horizontal. The predictions were made assuming only a Gibson-type process on the one hand, and only a Köhler-type process on the other. Figures 8.5 and 8.6 show the shapes of the two predicted functions. Figure

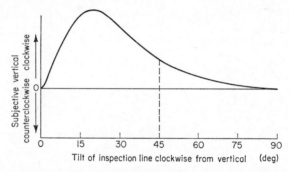

Figure 8.5 Hypothesized effects of 'satiation' process. [From Morant and Harris, 1965]

8.7 shows the probable function assuming that both processes are operating and figure 8.8 shows the empirical function which they in fact found. The results are a good fit to the summated function in figure 8.7. Contrary to the satiation hypothesis there is a cross-over point at which the effect is zero, but it occurs at about 60°, not at 45° as a purely Gibsonian hypothesis would predict.

This argument depends on the assumption that the vertical and horizontal norms are of equal strength. If the vertical norm is stronger than the horizontal norm then one would expect the null point to be displaced towards the horizontal, and satiation would not have to be invoked in order to explain

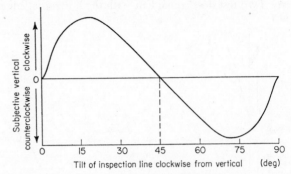

Figure 8.6 Hypothesized effects of 'adaptation' process. [From Morant and Harris, 1965]

the results. Gibson reported that the horizontal norm was only slightly stronger than the vertical norm; Morant and Mistovich (1960) that they are equally strong. Thus the assumption which Morant and Harris make seems justified. However, their interpretation also depends to some extent on the

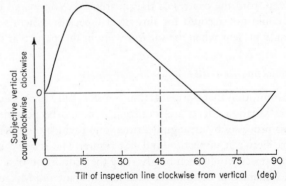

Figure 8.7 Algebraic summation of 'satiation' and 'adaptation' effects. [From Morant and Harris, 1965]

assumption that the Gibson effect transfers fully over all angular positions. If there were partial transfer only, this could account for the indirect effect being less than the direct effect. In so far as the cross-over point is significantly different from 45°, their experiment supplies further evidence that there are both Gibson and Köhler processes.

This view is supported by results reported by Fox (1951). In this study the inspection figure consisted of two squares; the bottom edge of one square and the top edge of the other were in a horizontal line. Fixation was between them. Two test dots coincident with the horizontal edges appeared

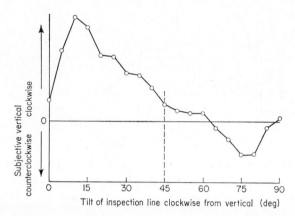

Figure 8.8 Measured amount of tilt after-effect for increasing amounts of tilt of the inspection line. [From Morant and Harris, 1965]

displaced away from the centres of the squares. Fox considered that figural after-effects could not account for this effect especially when it was found that it was only present when the squares were in this particular orientation.

8.45 Differential transfer of tilt and figural after-effects

On the assumption that normalization transfers fully (discussed in section 8.22) whereas satiation effects are localized, it should be possible to distinguish the two processes by arranging a situation in which there is a relatively large distance between inspection and test figure. The relative importance of the two processes would then be given by the proportion of a contiguous effect which remained in the transfer situation. Morant and Mikaelian (1960) found that two-thirds of a contiguous tilt after-effect transferred over 7° of visual angle. Morant and Harris (1965) had their subjects adjust a line to be parallel with a vertical line 14° away. A tilted inspection line had previously been exposed in the same position as one of these test lines and the constant error in setting the test lines to parallel was taken as a measure of the satiation effect alone, on the assumption that the Gibson effect would transfer fully and thus affect both test lines equally whereas the satiation effect would be restricted to the contiguous test line. The obtained function of magnitude of effect against inspection line tilt was a good fit to the predicted curve for the Köhler effect.

Finally, the fact that visual inspection of a tilted line appears to produce a negative after-effect on the tactile–kinaesthetic vertical (Morant and Mistovich, in press; Silver and Morant, 1962) suggests that a psychophysical theory is more likely to encompass all the facts than a model tied to specific neurological processes.

It seems reasonable to conclude, from all the evidence cited, that there are at least four perceptual mechanisms which can induce an apparent change in the tilt of the field of view. These are: (a) Gibson-type adaptation in which the inspection of lines off the main axes causes a local shift in the whole subjective dimension of tilt of at most a few degrees. (b) Perceptual accommodation to even large displacements of the visual frame of reference. This mechanism may be of two kinds, one dependent on active learning and the other not. (c) Simultaneous contrast of direction of a few degrees, seen when a line is superimposed on a background of lines running in a different direction. (d) A figural after-effect in which acute angles tend to look larger by a few degrees after one of their arms has been inspected.

Apart from all these mechanisms, there is a further obvious possible cause of normalization. Ogle (1950) suggested that it could be due to the eyes rotating about the visual axis (torsion) so as to keep the normally vertical retinal meridian parallel to the main lines of the field of view. This possibility will be discussed in the next section.

8.5 Tilt adaptation and eye torsion

Howard and Templeton (1964b) tested Ogle's suggestion that tilt adaptation may be due to optically induced eye torsion by photographically measuring the torsional position of the eye before and after the subject inspected a line for 10 sec at 10° of tilt. Nothing was in view but the line of light, which had a small fixation point at its centre. The measuring technique could reliably record torsional movements of 0·2°, yet no significant mean change of the torsional position of the eye was detected which could be related to the angular position of the stimulus line. Under the same conditions of viewing, tilt after-effects were recorded of approximately 2° in response to 10 sec inspection of the same line tilted to 10°.

It has been known for some time that visual objects rotating in the frontal plane about the visual axis induce eye torsion (Noji, 1929; Brecher, 1934). Howard and Templeton investigated whether rotation of a line from the vertical position has a different effect to rotation towards the vertical. The subject inspected the centre of a line of light in otherwise dark surroundings while it rotated in the frontal plane at various speeds and amplitudes both towards and away from the vertical. A speed of 3°/sec was found to be most effective; the mean amplitude of optically induced torsion increased as a function of the amplitude of rotation of the line up to a maximum for one subject of about 1·3°. However, there were no differences in induced torsion between rotations towards the vertical and rotations away from the vertical. It thus seems that the vertical orientation of a line has no significance for eye movements, and that tilt adaptation cannot be due to eye torsion, at least with a single line stimulus.

Perhaps other, fuller figures may induce torsion when tilted. Greenberg (1960) reported that eye torsion is induced by a frame tilted 28°. He used a moving line of light in his measuring procedure, and this would to some extent contaminate his results, although he claimed that the moving line alone did not have the same effect as when a stationary tilted frame was added. Whether or not torsion is induced by tilting frames, Howard and Templeton's results demonstrate that tilt adaptation may occur in the absence of eye torsion.

8.6 Tactile–kinaesthetic tilt adaptation

It seems that no direct comparison has been made between visual and tactile–kinaesthetic judgments of the vertical position of a rod. Sandström (1959) asked 10 subjects for tactile–kinaesthetic judgments of the position of a fixed vertical rod ten times in succession. He treated the resulting scores as a single sample of 100 judgments and so the measures of variability he gives confound inter- and intra-individual variation. But single estimates were as much as 30° in error, suggesting a much poorer level of discrimination than that usually obtained in a comparable visual task. However, the method of repeated presentation of a single stimulus may artificially inflate the variance to some extent, through subjects' unwillingness to repeat the same response. Other groups made similar estimates of the position of lines fixed at 30°, 45°, 60°, and 90°, and these produced similar, or even larger maximum errors; for example, estimates of the position of a 30° rod ranged from 5° to 75°.

Sandström's most interesting finding was that the distributions of these errors were in all cases skewed towards the middle of the quadrant: all rods tended to be judged closer to 45° than they actually were. These shifts were thus in the opposite direction to the normalization effects reported in vision; Sandström had no explanation to offer. The effect is particularly mystifying in the case of the vertical and horizontal rods since there would seem to be no reason to expect these to show a constant error in one direction rather than the other. It is possible that these constant errors were associated with the fact that all but one of the subjects used the right hand; their opposed directions for the vertical and horizontal may have resulted from a reversed orientation of the hand with respect to the rod in the two tasks, in which case a consistent tendency, for example, to misjudge the position of the rod in the direction of the back of the hand would explain the results.

In the case of the 30° and 60° rods the skewness may have been an artefact of a linguistic tendency to judge lines as being at the closest natural anchoring point, in this case 45°. This proximity to 45° would also decrease the size of the expected normalization effect, which should reach zero near 45°. For both these reasons, normalization might have been demonstrated had Sandström used positions closer to the vertical and horizontal, for example 15° and 75°. Indeed, the results of Silver and Morant (1962) imply normalization with kinaesthetically sensed rods in these positions (see below). A further difference between the studies is that the Brandeis workers had their subjects inspect the rod for some time before the judgments were made whereas Sandström's subjects were exposed for only the, presumably short, periods required to make the judgments.

In his original paper on visual curvative adaptation, Gibson (1933) reported that if a blindfolded subject feels along a curved edge for a few minutes, a straight edge then feels curved the other way. Even a curve with as little as 6 mm depth of concavity in a length of 30 cm gave a measurable after-effect. And several studies have demonstrated kinaesthetic figural after-effects (Köhler and Dinnerstein, 1947; McEwen, 1958).

Sandström (1959), in the second part of the study referred to above, confirmed the occurrence of these kinaesthetic after-effects. Subjects who had judged the 30°, 45°, and 90° rods, immediately afterwards estimated the position of a vertical rod; subjects who had judged the 0°, 45°, and 60° rods estimated the position of a horizontal rod. Both rods suffered an apparent displacement away from the position of the rods to which the subjects had previously been exposed. This finding, which is analogous to the tilt after-effect in vision is surprising in view of Sandström's failure to observe an initial normalization of the tilted lines.

In the third part of Sandström's experiment the subjects were asked to reproduce the stimulus to which they had been exposed in the first part of the experiment. It is difficult to see what this task can have meant to the subjects since it is clear from the results of the first part that the stimulus had a wide range of appearances, and apparently none of the subjects realized that only a single stimulus was involved. Sandström argued that the constant errors should be the same as in the first part when the subjects were asked to estimate the position of the rod, but 'with signs reversed because of the different psycho-physical methods used'. The logic of this argument is surely wrong.

If, for example, the subject had estimated the 30° rod to be 35°, in order to reproduce this impression he must now adjust the rod to 30° and not, as Sandström argued, to 25°. But Sandström's prediction was borne out, at least in the cases of the 30° and 60° positions. The 30° rod, initially estimated as 35°, was reproduced as 26°. However, our argument that the method of reproduction should not yield constant errors holds only when no factor which could alter the appearance of the stimulus is interpolated between exposure and reproduction. In this case Sandström neglects to take account of the effect of the middle stage of the experiment when the subjects who had estimated the 30° rod were exposed to a vertical line. The figural after-effect resulting from this vertical line might well make 26°, rather than 30°, give the impression of 35°. A similar argument holds for the effect of the interpolated horizontal rod on the reproduction of the 60° rod. This interpretation is supported by the fact that, contrary to Sandström's prediction, the vertical and horizontal positions, which would be little affected by the interpolated stimulation, were reproduced, on average, without error.

Morant and Mistovich (in press) demonstrated a small but significant tactile–kinaesthetic effect analogous to the negative after-effect of tilt in vision. After running the fingers along a tilted rod for a period the apparent vertical or horizontal (whichever was closer) was displaced towards the position of the 'inspected' rod. An attempt was made by Silver and Morant (1962) to separate the tactile and kinaesthetic components in this sort of inspection. In the purely tactile condition the subject placed his finger in a harness and a raised edge set at various angles (15°, 30°, 45°, 60°, and 75° off-vertical) was moved continuously across his finger tip. In the kinaesthetic–tactile condition the subject was allowed to feel the same edge with free hand and arm movements. The measure of the after-effect was the angle at which the edge felt vertical or horizontal. With tactile inspection the after-effect on the vertical increased with the tilt of the inspection line, reaching a maximum of about 7° with an inspection angle of 30°. Thereafter it fell off to zero with 75°. There was no indirect effect (see section 8.44). With kinaesthetic inspection, the after-effect on the vertical reached a maximum of 2° for an inspection angle of 30°, fell off to zero at about 50° and reached a negative value of 2.5° at 74° (indirect effect). The curve for kinaesthetic inspection is thus the one which Gibson's theory of tilt adaptation would predict, on the principle that tilted lines appear to move towards the nearest main axis (vertical or horizontal) and carry with them the whole dimension including both axes; tactile inspection, on the other hand, yielded a function analogous to that of the figural after-effect. Silver and Morant offered no further explanation of their findings.

Zacks and Freedman (1963) also compared the after-effects of active and passive tactile–kinaesthetic inspection of a tilted rod. In the active condition the subject moved his arm actively up and down the rod tilted to 20°, and in the passive condition his relaxed arm was moved by a carriage over the same path. Before and after each exposure the subject set a rod by feel to the apparent vertical. The active condition produced more after-effect (no figures given) than the passive condition and Zacks and Freedman interpreted the results in terms of reafference theory (see section 15.24). These results conflict with those of Silver and Morant who it will be remembered found a greater effect with purely tactile stimulation at about the angle of tilt used by Zacks and Freedman. Clearly more experimental work is called for.

Kinaesthetic tilt after-effects produced by the visual inspection of tilted lines have been reported by Morant and Mistovich (in press). They argued that this intersensory effect tends to rule out an explanation of the tilt after-effect in terms of satiation processes in the primary sensory cortex but rather demands the concept of central norms common to all modalities.

9

Orientation to Gravity III

The orientation of the body

9.1 Postural reflexes

9.11 Introduction

Postural reflexes are concerned with two broad functions; the first of these is the control of body attitude, that is, the positions of the parts of the body in relation to each other. The reflexes involved in the control of attitude are not necessarily related to the direction in which gravity acts on the body. The other function of postural reflexes is to maintain the body in a constant position in relation to gravity.

The eyes, the touch and pressure receptors of the skin, the receptors in muscle, tendons, and joints, and the vestibular apparatus, all contribute afferent signals which initiate component reflexes in the total pattern of postural-reflex behaviour. Central neural structures involved include the spinal cord, cerebellum, upper brain-stem nuclei, diencephalic nuclei, and the cerebral cortex. The segmental reflexes, such as the stretch reflex and crossed extensor reflex, are postural reflexes which have already been discussed. This section will deal with the suprasegmental postural reflexes.

Investigation of postural-reflex mechanisms began in 1824 when Flourens observed the disturbances of movement and posture in a pigeon when its vestibular canals were destroyed. In 1924 Magnus published his classic work *Körperstellung*, which contains an account of experiments on body posture which he, Rademaker, de Kleyn, and others had carried out in Utrecht. This work had its origin in some accidental observations which Magnus made while working in Sherrington's laboratory in Liverpool. He noticed that the distribution of tonus in the body of a decerebrate cat was affected when its head was passively moved about. He devoted the next fourteen years to the study of postural reflexes. An English summary of this work is contained in the Cameron Prize Lectures (1926). In man, postural reflexes are overlaid by complex motor mechanisms, although Fukuda (1961) has claimed that these reflexes may still be seen in the dynamic postures of gymnasts and other sportsmen. The young child does not possess a functional cerebral cortex, and therefore these reflexes may be seen in the child in their primitive form. This work has been thoroughly reviewed by Peiper (1963). Recent physiological studies are reviewed in Hess (1957). The following account relies mainly on these authorities, and for further details and bibliography the reader is referred to them.

9.12 Tonic reflexes of the decerebrate animal

A striking manifestation of postural-reflex mechanisms is produced when the brain stem is sectioned just above the vestibular nuclei. The extensor muscles throughout the body go into continuous spasm, resulting in a rigid extension of the limbs. This postural pattern is known as *decerebrate rigidity*. In the same decerebrate preparation, with or without the cerebellum, the distribution of tonus in the whole body musculature is changed when the head is placed in different positions. Every change in the position of the head induces two reflexes; (1) a *tonic-neck reflex* resulting from stimulation of neck-muscle receptors, and (2) a *tonic-labyrinthine reflex* resulting from stimulation of the utricles as the position of the head is moved in relation to gravity.

Tonic-neck reflexes can be studied only when the labyrinths are removed. When this is done, rotation of the head causes extension of the fore- and hind-limbs on that side towards which the jaw is rotated ('jaw limbs'), and relaxation of the limbs on the side towards which the back of the head is rotated ('skull limbs'). Inclination of the head towards one shoulder causes extension of the jaw limbs, and relaxation of the skull limbs. Elevation of the head causes an extension of the fore-limbs and relaxation of the hind-limbs. Lowering of the head causes flexion of the fore-limbs and extension of the hind-limbs. The centres for these neck-tonic reflexes were localized by Magnus in the first and second cervical segments of the spinal cord, although it will be shown later that centres in the diencephalon are also concerned.

Tonic-neck reflexes occur in many newborn or premature human infants. Figure 9.1 shows a typical reflex pattern induced by a sideways head position in a newborn infant. This pattern is known as the 'fencing position'

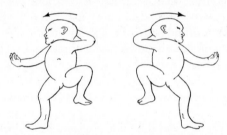

Figure 9.1 Asymmetrical neck-tonic reflex (fencing position) in an infant girl age 2 months 9 days. [Drawn from a photograph in Peiper, 1963]

for obvious reasons. These reflexes are less obvious beyond the first half year of life, when the cerebral cortex gains control over the lower reflex centres (Riesen and Kinder, 1952).

Related to the tonic-neck reflexes is the reflex tendency to keep the vertebral column straight. Rademaker called this the 'vertebral column reflex'. It may be seen in infant humans. It occurs in the dark, so that it is not of visual origin, and its exact mechanism is not known.

Tonic-labyrinthine reflexes may be studied in the decerebrate preparation when the head is immobilized in relation to the body by a plaster jacket, or when the tonic-neck reflex outflow is interrupted by cutting the first three cervical roots. If such a preparation is moved into a different position, the extensor tonus of all four limbs changes in the same way at the same time.

According to Magnus the tonus is maximal when the animal is in the supine position with its head held in such a way that the otoliths are pulling down on the macular epithelium; tonus is minimal when the animal is in the prone position and the otoliths are pressing on the macular epithelium. In other positions, extensor tone is intermediate.

Each utricular macula sends impulses to the limbs on both sides of the body but only to the contralateral neck muscles. As a consequence, unilateral labyrinthine loss entails no change in tonic-labyrinthine reflexes in the limbs, but produces a turning of the neck which in turn causes secondary tonic reflexes in the limbs.

If both neck and labyrinthine reflexes are present, the pattern of tonus in the body represents the algebraic sum of both reflexes. For example, if the head of a prone decerebrate cat is flexed ventrally, the utricular reflex is minimally elicited and all four limbs tend to relax. The neck influences cause the fore-limbs to relax also, but cause the hind-limbs to extend. The fore-limbs will therefore relax under the influence of both reflexes, but the hind-limbs may not change, as they are influenced in opposite directions by the two reflexes.

These attitudinal reflexes are called tonic because they last as long as the head is held in a certain position. They may be seen in the active behaviour of intact animals. For example, a cat, when reaching to food on the ground, lowers its head, and this causes the fore-limbs to relax. When a cat reaches up, the head is elevated and the fore-limbs extend, but the hind-limbs do not change markedly. These reflex tonic attitudes are not easy to detect in intact primates, but may be seen in decerebrate preparations, and in clinical conditions in humans. Magnus's early claim that they are present in some normal infants has never been confirmed (Peiper, 1963).

9.13 Righting reflexes

The reflexes discussed so far can be elicited in a decerebrate animal where the section is made just rostral to the vestibular nuclei. If the section is even more rostral, leaving the mid-brain and thalamus intact, the animal is known as a *thalamic preparation*. Such an animal no longer manifests the extensor contracture of decerebrate rigidity, and is able to restore itself to an upright posture when disturbed.

Magnus identified four groups of reflexes which cooperate in righting responses. In order to demonstrate any one of these components, the animal must first be placed in such a state that none of them is active. This so-called 'zero condition' is fulfilled if a thalamic animal, after bilateral labyrinthectomy, is suspended freely out of contact with any surface. In lower animals, which do not have optic righting reflexes, it is not necessary to cover the eyes; in higher mammals, this is necessary.

a. The labyrinthine righting reflexes All blindfolded thalamic mammals with intact labyrinths show the labyrinthine righting reflexes. If the animal is held by the pelvis, its head remains in the upright position, as far as possible no matter how the pelvis is moved. These reflex head movements depend upon the utricle and perhaps also the sacculus (see figure 9.2). According to

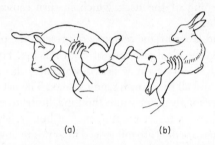

(a)   (b)

Figure 9.2 (a) Rabbit without labyrinths; (b) Intact rabbit in suspended
   dorsal position. In the animal without labyrinths the head falls. In the
   intact animal the labyrinthine righting reflex maintains the head in the
   normal relation to gravity. [Sketch by Peiper, 1963, after Rademaker,
   1926]

Magnus and Rademaker, they depend also upon the red nucleus, although Mussen (1927) found that vestibular righting reflexes survive the destruction of the red nucleus.

These reflexes are only faintly demonstrable in the neonate human, but develop during the first year of life. They enable the growing infant to lift his head and later to sit up and to stand.

b. The neck righting reflexes The neck righting reflexes orientate the body in relation to the head. If the body is tilted, the head regains the upright position by the action of the vestibular righting reflexes. This involves a twisting of the neck, which evokes the neck righting reflexes which in turn cause the thorax and then the lower parts of the body to be brought back into line with the upright head.

c. Body righting reflexes These reflexes may be demonstrated by holding a labyrinthectomized animal freely in the lateral position. If the animal is now placed upon a surface, it immediately rotates its head until it is in a normal position with regard to the surface. This reflex is evoked by the asymmetric stimulation of the touch receptors in the skin. If a board is pushed against the animal so that the tactile stimulation on each side of the body is symmetrical, the head will return to the lateral position. If an animal is held in the air in a lateral position and again lowered on to a board, but this time with its head held firm, its body will right itself. Again the asymmetrical stimulation of the skin induces this reflex, in spite of a tendency for the body to remain in line with the laterally placed head in response to the neck-tonic reflex.

d. Optic righting reflexes In intact higher mammals, such as cats, dogs, and primates, the orientation of the head is controlled largely by vision. If such an animal with labyrinths removed is freely suspended in the air, its head remains disoriented until the eyes are opened and the animal fixates on something in the environment.

All these reflexes normally work together to maintain the upright posture of the unconstrained intact animal. The head always leads; if the animal is disoriented, the head is first restored to the vertical position through the mediation of visual, vestibular, and tactile righting reflexes. The thorax is then brought into line with the head through the mediation of neck righting reflexes and tactile body righting reflexes. Finally the hind quarters and legs are brought into line by spinal and tactile righting reflexes. This sequence of events is called a chain reflex, and may be seen in the way a cat rights its body when falling. This chain reflex may also be demonstrated in infant humans.

9.14 The central control of postural reflexes

Hess and his coworkers in Zürich have contributed to the understanding of the way in which postural motor patterns are organized by the central nervous system. Hess worked exclusively on the cat, centring his attention on the diencephalon. Fine electrodes were embedded in the diencephalic region in the otherwise intact animal. For any one site and type of stimulation, the cat executed reproduceable attitudinal responses of the head or head and body. Figure 9.3 (a) shows the head-lowering-legs-flexing response to stimulation of the posterior commissure. Figure 9.3 (b) shows the opposite response to stimulation in a medial, narrow zone over the posterior hypo-thalamus. Figure 9.3 (c) shows a head-rotation response to stimulation of the thalamus or sub thalamus; the direction of turning depends on the exact site of stimulation. A turning response is shown in figure 9.3 (d). This is in re-sponse to stimulation of the thalamus lateral to the tract of Maynert.

All except this last response show rhythmic activity synchronous with low-frequency stimulation. The general rule is that the intermittence be-comes more accentuated the farther posterior and ventral the stimulation lies. This fact is related to the histological evidence that the posterior ventral regions are further from the fibres—mainly the rubrospinal and central tegmental tracts—which are responsible for carrying the motor impulses to the spinal cord.

Hess noted that the exact counterparts of the various head responses produced by diencephalic stimulation are the post-rotational, vestibular-reflex head movements induced by the different vestibular canals. He conclu-

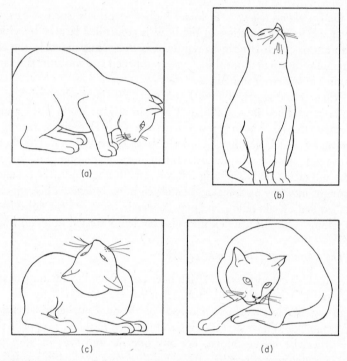

Figure 9.3 Some of the postural responses of the cat to stimulation of various parts of the diencephalon. Tracings from photographs by Hess (1957). (a) Lowering of the head and foretrunk; (b) Raising of the head and foretrunk; (c) Rotation of the head in the frontal plane; (d) Turning of the body in the horizontal plane

ded that the normal mode of stimulation of these diencephalic centres was from the vestibular canals, via the cerebellum and brachium conjunctivum. He also traced routes from spino-thalamic tracts and trigeminal tracts, which carry information regarding the relative position of body parts to these diencephalic centres.

A further set of diencephalic responses was observed, which involved lifting of the fore-limbs and perhaps a whole side of the body. That these were not related to nociceptive or pain reflexes was evident from the calm demeanour of the animal. Hess concluded that they are related to postural reflexes under the control of proprioception, such as the crossed extensor reflex.

Hess has thus shown how postural reflexes are organized by central nuclei and do not merely represent the interplay of separate, peripherally determined reflexes, as Magnus was prone to think.

Even a general treatment of the neural structures involved in postural control would be beyond the scope of this book. For a discussion of spinal structures and functions see Sherrington (1947), Denny-Brown, Eccles, Liddell, and Sherrington (1938), Lloyd (1960); for a discussion on the extrapyramidal system see Hassler (1960); and for a discussion of the cerebellum see Brookhart (1960). For a general review of the motor system see Howard (1966).

9.2 The judgment of the postural vertical

9.21 Introduction

It has been known for some time that under normal circumstances a person is able to set his body to the vertical to within a degree without the aid of visual information (Gemelli, Tessier, and Galli, 1920). The position of the apparent postural vertical is modified by many factors, some of which we shall consider in this section. Unless otherwise stated, subjects in these experiments were blindfolded and seated in a mechanically tilting chair; they were invariably moved passively into the tilted position but usually controlled their own return.

One of the disturbing features of research in this field is the lack of consistency in the statistics used by different workers to summarize their data. The two most useful measures are the constant error, which is the algebraic mean of the deviations from the true vertical, and the variable error (standard deviations appear to be rarely used), which is the mean of the unsigned deviations from the constant error. These two statistics are independent of one another and reflect, respectively, the accuracy (or bias) and the consistency (or variability) of a series of judgments. A third statistic used by several workers is the mean of the unsigned deviations from the true vertical. This measure inextricably confounds bias and variability and, while giving an overall measure of error, is much less informative than separate measures of these two factors. Most results involve one or two of these three statistics but it is not always clear which ones; the term 'average error' is particularly ambiguous. Passey (1950a) and Mann and Passey (1951) for example use the constant error and a 'crude average error'. They do not specify how this latter statistic is calculated. But out of 48 mean constant errors (in a 6 × 8 factorial design) three are the same size as their corresponding 'average error' and none is larger. We suspect that the measure used is not the variable error, as defined above, but the mean of unsigned deviations from the vertical, since this latter measure provides a maximum limit for the constant error (when all judgments deviate from the vertical in the same direction the two measures are identical). This suspicion is strengthened by the fact that it is even clearer that this was the measure used by Passey and Guedry (1949). Passey, and Mann and Passey analyse separately the data from their two measures and find that they both vary in the same way with each of the independent variables. This is scarcely surprising since, if their 'average error' is indeed the mean of unsigned deviations, then it will be largely, and in some cases wholly, dependent on the constant error.

Fleishman actually argues in favour of using the unsigned deviations from the vertical because 'primary interest in the present study is in precision with respect to a standard, the "true" upright position'. In conjunction with this average error he uses the constant error to give 'an indication of the direction of the obtained error'. Using the true variable error together with the constant error, Fleishman could have obtained independent estimates of two types of information he required.

9.22 The degree of initial body tilt

Several investigators have studied the effect of the degree of initial tilt of the body on the constant and variable errors of setting the body to the vertical (Clegg 1954; Clegg and Dunfield, 1954a, 1954b; Fleishman, 1953; Mann and Passey, 1951; Mann, Passey, and Ambler, 1950; Mann and Ray, 1956a). It is agreed that the constant errors increase as the degree of initial tilt is increased, and that these errors are always in the direction of initial tilt.

Mann and Passey (1951), using initial tilts up to 55°, found a maximum constant error of 1·4° at about 35°, the initial body tilt being maintained for periods ranging from 0–65 sec (see figures 9.4 and 9.5). Clegg and Dunfield, using passive movement, found rather larger effects over a narrow range of initial tilts, again in the lateral plane. Their effect increased from ½° at 6° of initial tilt to 2° at 15°. Similarly, Fleishman (1953), using 90 naïve subjects, in contrast to Mann and Passey's three sophisticated subjects, obtained effects ranging from just over one degree at 15° of initial tilt to just over two degrees at 25°, the tilted position being maintained for five seconds on each trial. The crude average error from the true vertical was of similar magnitude to the constant error for each amount of body tilt, suggesting that few judgments deviated from the mean by more than the amount of the constant error.

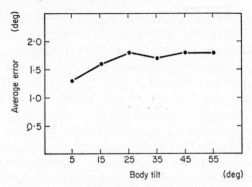

Figure 9.4 Average error of adjustment to gravitational vertical for various amounts of initial body tilt. [From Mann and Passey, 1951]

Experiments using larger angles of tilt need to be done. It may be that at angles larger than 55° (the maximum studied so far) the direction of the constant error changes, just as the direction of the constant error for the visual vertical changes, at about this angle of body tilt (see section 7.42).

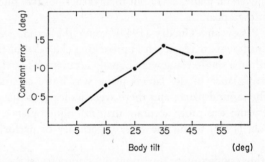

Figure 9.5 Mean constant error in direction of initial tilt for adjustments to the gravitational vertical for various amounts of initial body tilt. [From Mann and Passey, 1951]

9.23 The direction of the body tilt

A subject may be tilted in the lateral plane, to left or right, or in a sagittal plane, forwards or backwards, or in an oblique direction.

Clegg and Dunfield (1954a and 1954b) compared the accuracy with which subjects could judge when they had reached the vertical when passively returned from each of the four primary directions. These results were compared by Clegg (1954) with the errors arising from tilts in diagonal planes. The average constant error was found to be greater when the subjects were returned from backward or from right tilt (2°) as compared with forward or left tilt ($\frac{1}{2}$°). Correspondingly, the right-backward diagonal direction gave a larger effect than the left-forward, while there was no difference between left-backward and right-forward, although whether the effects on these two diagonals were intermediate between the effects on the other two, as would be expected, is not made clear. Clegg and Dunfield could offer no explanation of the pattern of errors for the various quadrants. They suggested that instrumental inaccuracies may have been the cause but pointed out that Fleishman (1953) had obtained similar results for lateral tilts using different apparatus. The weight of evidence would of course have been greater if Clegg and Dunfield had independently validated their own method.

Mann, Passey, and Ambler (1950) had earlier found the same difference as Fleishman, and Clegg and Dunfield, in the constant errors between the two lateral directions. But the Tulane group redesigned their tilting chair and in a series of experiments (Mann and Passey, 1951; Mann and Ray, 1956a and 1956b) reported that there were no differences between either the constant or the 'crude average errors' attributable to the direction in which the subject was tilted in the lateral plane. They put their earlier positive finding down to inaccuracies in the apparatus.

Similarly, Passey and Guedry (1949), using the 'crude average error', found that adjustments made when approaching the vertical from the two directions of tilt in a single plane were equally accurate. They did find, however, that performance in the lateral plane was more accurate than performance in the sagittal plane, and there were indications that performance in the sagittal plane was more accurate than in oblique planes. Burtt (1918) and Kleinknecht (1922) found the same superiority of performance in the lateral plane.

There are thus conflicting results about the symmetry of the effect of body tilt in the two directions of a single plane. Apart from Clegg and Dunfield there is general agreement that performance in the lateral plane is superior to performance in the sagittal plane. One could account for this by assuming that the vestibular apparatus is more sensitive to lateral tilts.

9.24 The speed of return from the tilted position

Burtt (1918) reported that the ability to detect small displacements of the body from the vertical improves as the speed of displacement is increased, but Mann and Ray (1956a) were unable to substantiate this finding.

Clegg and Dunfield, keeping their subjects tilted 15° in the right lateral direction for 15 sec, found that the constant error in the direction of initial tilt increased fairly consistently from 0·3° to 3·5° as the speed of return dropped from 0·57°/sec to 0·06°/sec. This narrow range demonstrates the extreme sensitivity of the constant error to even minute changes in return speed. All the other investigators used greater speeds of return. Mann and Ray (1956a and 1956b) used speeds of from 1·2°/sec to 2·4°/sec, and Fleishman (1953) used speeds of from 4°/sec to 6°/sec. The other conditions of these various experiments were not the same and so the results are not, in any case, comparable. However, they all showed that the constant errors of body settings were greater for slower speeds of return.

9.25 The duration of the delay in the tilted position

Passey and Guedry (1949) first reported that holding the body at an angle for some time decreases the accuracy with which it can be returned to the vertical. They used one angle of tilt (10°) and two delay periods (0 and 60 sec). Both the 'crude average error' and the number of errors in the direction of initial tilt were found to be greater for the longer period. Further experiments at Tulane University extended these findings for periods of delay up to 65 sec, and angles of initial tilt up to 55° (Mann, Passey, and Ambler, 1950; Mann and Passey, 1951; Mann and Ray, 1956b). The same tilting chair was used in all these experiments and the results were all in substantial agreement (see figures 9.6 and 9.7). The apparent vertical was increasingly displaced in

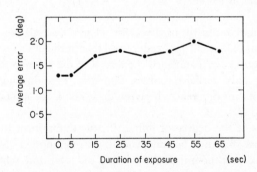

Figure 9.6 Average error of adjustment to gravitational vertical for various durations of exposure to body tilt. [From Mann and Passey, 1951]

the direction of the initial tilt of the body as the duration of the initial tilt was prolonged. In the study by Mann and Passey (1951) the effect reached a maximum of 1·5° for a duration of 45–55 sec and was somewhat lower at 65 sec,

the longest duration used. The effects were averaged over tilts ranging from
5° to 55°. These workers collected data on their three subjects in a factorial
arrangement of the two variables, magnitude and duration of tilt, but unfortunately in their analysis they did not evaluate any possible interaction
between the two factors, choosing instead to analyse the results for each factor
separately. However, an examination of the published data summary suggests that any systematic interaction would not be substantial.

Results which conflict with those from Tulane were reported by Clegg
(1954) and by Clegg and Dunfield (1954). They found that delays of up to
105 sec did not increase the constant errors in settings of the body to the

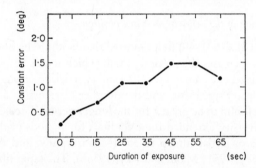

Duration of exposure   (sec)

Figure 9.7 Mean constant error in direction of initial tilt for adjustment to
the gravitational vertical for various durations of exposure to body tilt.
[From Mann and Passey, 1951]

vertical. The maximum tilt used was 15°. The only apparent difference between Clegg and Dunfield's procedure and that of the others was that in their
work the experimenter controlled the return of the chair to the vertical, the
subject giving only verbal responses. Similarly, Pearson and Hauty (1960)
found no significant differences between delays of 0, 30, and 60 sec for initial
tilts of 10° and 30°.

The effects of the degree of initial tilt, the duration of the tilt, and the
speed of return may not be independent of one another. Mann and Ray
(1956a) claimed that the important factor is the total time which the subject
is out of the vertical position. It is this total time which governs the amount
of adaptation which occurs and hence the extent of the error in setting the
body to the vertical. Obviously, the three variables which have been studied
would all contribute to this total time spent away from the vertical position.
However, if Mann and Ray's claims were true, then the speed of initial movement into the tilted position should have a similar effect to the speed of
return (cf. Mann and Ray, 1956b). Also, there may be some doubt about the

overall effect of the delay variable (Clegg, 1954; Clegg and Dunfield, 1954a, 1954b).

9.26 The sensory modalities involved in setting the body to the vertical

The main non-visual sensory modalities which could be used for setting the body to the vertical are the labyrinths, touch, and kinaesthesis. We shall consider first the case where the subject rights himself in a tilting chair in the dark.

Bourdon (1904) varied the somaesthetic cues available to the subject and the position of the head on the body and concluded from the results that proprioceptive cues are at least as important as vestibular. Garten (1920) tested subjects with defective inner ears and found that they could accurately set their bodies to the vertical in a tilting chair. He concluded that the labyrinths are not important for this ability. He found also that the performance of normal subjects was affected by complete immersion in water, although anaesthetizing the skin areas which were in contact with the chair (by cooling the buttocks) had no effect on performance. He concluded that kinaesthesis must therefore be the crucial modality for this ability.

The unimportance of the sense of touch in judging the vertical position of the body was confirmed by Arndts (1924) who found performance to be unaffected by local anaesthesia. However, Mann, Berthelot-Berry, and Dauterive (1949) found that the average error was greater when tactile stimulation was reduced by padding the chair. This result could have occurred because the subjects relaxed more in the padded seat and thus reduced the information available from the movements of the body which an unpadded and less well-supported subject probably makes as the chair tilts.

On balance it seems that tactile stimulation of the skin is not an essential factor in the ability to set the body to the vertical, at least for the seated person. Under ordinary conditions of life, the tactile sense is used actively. In the restrictive conditions of the tilting-chair experiments, this active, exploratory role of touch was denied the subjects.

Garten's suggestion that the labyrinths are not essential for body orientation had already been made by Cattell in 1895, but it was not until quite recently that supporting evidence began to appear. Mann (1951) studied a subject with VIIIth nerve paralysis on the tilting chair. There was a larger than normal constant error in the *opposite* direction to the initial body tilt, but Mann suggested that the damage may not have been complete on one side. The variable error was, if anything, less than the normal average. It would be unwise to place much reliance on results from one defective subject, especially when the precise extent of his defect was not known. More recently, Clark and Graybiel (1963b) found that 10 men with labyrinthine defects performed almost as well as normal subjects. Thetford and Guedry (1952a, 1952b) studied five subjects with unilateral labyrinth loss, under a variety of conditions on the tilting chair. They performed just as well as normal subjects. This was probably because the subjects had become adapted to the asymmetrical vestibular input (see discussion of this topic in section 5.6). One cannot conclude from these experiments that vestibular stimulation is unimportant for setting the body to the vertical.

Errors have been found to be greater when the head is free to move than when it is fixed in the median plane of the body (Fleishman, 1953). In the latter condition the inputs which tell us when the head is vertical also tell us when the body is vertical. The difference was particularly marked in the more difficult tasks (e.g. right tilt or slow return speed). Some support for the effect of head position is provided by Solley (1956, 1960) who reported experiments in which the subject was tilted 30° to right or left while his head was independently tilted 30° right or left relative to the body, or remained upright on the body. He found that errors were always greater when the body was tilted and the head held upright than when the head was held in line with the body. The errors (average unsigned deviations from the true vertical) fell off considerably with practice in both these conditions. But in the third condition, in which the head was tilted in the same direction as the body but twice as far, the fall in errors was much less marked. In fact, this condition had initially the lowest error rate and, after practice, the highest. This interaction with practice resulted from the comparison of the results of the two experiments and was therefore not tested for significance. If significant it might indicate that learning can modify the relative importance of different postural inputs. For example, the deviant condition was the only one in which the head was never at any stage gravitationally upright.

The influence of the visual frame on the setting of the body to the vertical has been studied by Passey (1950a). The subjects adjusted themselves to the vertical in the tilting chair from an initial tilt of 45°, with the frame tilted to various angles up to 20° to either side. The constant error in the direction of the body tilt was found to increase as the tilt of the frame was increased, particularly when the frame was tilted to the same side as the body. However the maximum effect of the tilted frame on the constant error was only 2°. The subjects at all times set their bodies much nearer to the true vertical than to the position of the visual frame. Passey suggested that these results conflict with those of Witkin's experiments on the influence of the visual frame on the visual vertical (see section 7.51). Such comparisons are, however, not valid for the tasks in the two cases were quite different. Witkin himself stated that the effect of a visual frame on a visual rod is greater than on the body vertical.

9.27 The effects of training on the setting of the body to the vertical

Klein and Schilder (1929) have stressed that when vision is excluded the sense of position, and especially of the static position of the body, is vague. A more adequate sense of position is built up only as we make differential responses to reality which are correlated with changing sensory consequences. There is considerable evidence that practice can lead to an improvement in the ability to orient the body in space.

Garten (1920), Gellhorn (1921), Kleinknecht (1922), Kleinknecht and Lueg (1924), Moore and Cramer (1962), and Clark and Graybiel (1963b) have demonstrated substantial effects of practice on the accuracy of postural orientation, both to the vertical and to other positions. Kleinknecht and Lueg found that the effect of practice was more marked when the subjects were blindfolded than when they were allowed to see. Performance with vision was initially superior to performance without it. This suggests that we normally set our bodies to the vertical by reference to the visual frame and that we operate at our maximum capability under these circumstances. When vision is denied us, we have to rely on the less used, non-visual modalities, and it is because these are not normally used that we show rapid improvement in their use. Effects of practice were still found by Kleinknecht and Lueg (1924) when the subjects were retested after a lapse of two years.

Solley (1956, 1960) enquired further into the nature of this improvement with practice. The subjects had to restore themselves to the vertical from an initial tilt of 30° in the Tulane tilting chair. Some subjects were tilted to the left, some to the right. Figure 9.8 shows that there was improvement over the

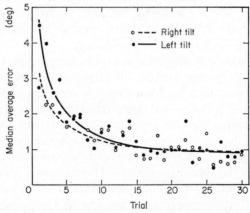

Figure 9.8 Changes in median average error (*E*) of adjustment to the postural vertical as a function of trials practice. [From Solley, 1956]

H.S.O.—17

30 trials, most of it in the first 15. No doubt the error-reduction resulted from the subject being returned to the true vertical after each trial, although, because they were returned by 'random' movements, Solley argued that this did not constitute knowledge of results. Fleishman, on the other hand, did not correct his subject's judgments and obtained very little error reduction with practice. Some of Solley's subjects said that they used the 'weight-on-the-buttocks' cue, others the leg-and-arm balance cue. Those who continued throughout the thirty trials with either one of these cues did not improve, but those who first used the leg-and-arm balance cue and then changed to the weight-on-buttocks cue, did improve. None of the subjects changed from the buttocks cue to the leg-and-arm cue. We question the validity of verbal reports of this kind from subjects. The only valid way of deciding what sensory information subjects are using is to manipulate that information.

Solley also found that training had a differential effect on performance under different experimental conditions (see discussion in section 9.26), suggesting that its effect might be to modify the relative importance of different sensory modalities.

Pearson and Hauty (1959) attempted to analyse the effect of practice on the accuracy of postural orientation. In their first experiment the subjects had to return themselves to the vertical from an initial tilt of 30° in a tilting chair Half the subjects were tilted only to the left, the other half were tilted alternately left and right. Knowledge of results was presented either visually (on a dial) or posturally (by putting the subject upright after each trial) or was absent. Both alternating and non-alternating subjects showed a significant reduction in average error during the first few trials. In the alternating condition, improvement occurred whether or not there was knowledge of results, whereas in the non-alternating condition, improvement occurred only with knowledge of results, either visual or postural. Also, the performance of the alternating group was superior throughout.

Two hypotheses were suggested to explain these results. One hypothesis stated that the alternating subjects, 'in *passing through the vertical*, enjoy a unique experience in that they learn what it is like to be on the other side of true vertical' (p. 370). Pearson and Hauty called this 'proprioceptive learning'. The other hypothesis was that alternation cancels out the effects of adaptation. In view of their interest in the directional adaptation effect it seems odd that their main published analysis should be of the crude average errors, which do not give any directional information. However, they state that they repeated the analysis using the constant errors and achieved similar results.

In a second experiment (Pearson and Hauty, 1960) designed to decide between the two hypotheses, they had half the subjects return themselves from 10° left, the other half from 30° left. Between each of these scored trials was interpolated an unscored trial on which half the subjects returned themselves from 10° right, the others from the position used for their scored trials. In this experiment they analysed only the crude average error despite the fact that at least one of their alternative hypotheses predicts specific directional errors. In order to make much sense of their results one must therefore assume that, as in their previous experiment, the constant errors followed the same pattern as the average errors.

The 30° condition produced larger errors than the 10° condition, and the subjects with interpolated experience of 10° in the opposite direction had smaller errors than those with experience of tilt in only one direction. However, there was no interaction between these two factors: the experience of 10° right reduced the errors in the 10° and the 30° condition by a similar amount. Pearson and Hauty argued that this supports the 'proprioceptive learning' hypothesis against the adaptation hypothesis, but we cannot see why this result could not be equally well predicted from adaptation theory. If the 10° right stimulus cancels wholly the adaptation effect of the 10° left stimulus then surely it will cancel the same *amount* of the adaptation effect of the 30° left stimulus. Pearson and Hauty used as an additional independent factor the delay at the tilted position, and argued that the adaptation hypothesis would require that the different delays should differentially affect the difference between the alternation and the control group. It is difficult to see how this should be so, since they themselves found, and quoted Clegg and Dunfield's confirmatory finding, that delay has no effect on the judgment of the postural vertical, even in the control condition. Thus Pearson and Hauty's experiment does not seem to have distinguished between their two hypotheses. In any case, we find it difficult to understand the distinction they make between adaptation and 'proprioceptive learning'; they seem to be merely different ways of expressing the same thing. Their description of proprioceptive learning, 'knowing what it is like to be on the other side of the vertical', could equally well be a description of the way that adaptation in one direction is cancelled out by adaptation in the other.

The reliable conclusions which we can make from all this experimental work is that when a tilted, seated subject is asked to return himself to the vertical, he is likely to show evidence of adaptation in the direction of the initial tilt; the degree of this adaptation depends to some extent on the degree and duration of the tilt; with knowledge of results, and perhaps with practice without knowledge of results, the effects of this adaptation on the position of the apparent vertical may be overcome. It is possible that the improvement results only from a change in the sensory modality used. Little can be said about the consistency or precision, as opposed to the accuracy, of performance, owing to the variety and ambiguity of the measures used.

The method of using a passive, seated subject for studying the ability to set the body to the vertical has little relevance to man's capacity to maintain a vertical posture in conditions where he is free to move actively. The fact that the seated subjects usually controlled the movement of the chair themselves is not important, as this involved only the pressing of a switch; the subjects were essentially passive.

In a real life situation, the usual task is that of maintaining body balance while standing or moving about. The interesting and important problems can only be studied under such dynamic conditions.

9.3 Vertical posture

9.31 Introduction

Man, alone among the primates, has adopted an exclusively biped posture. It is often argued that man's anatomy and physiology have not yet fully adapted to his upright posture, and that a variety of malfunctions, such as respiratory deficiency, visceral prolapse, indigestion, varicose veins, arthritis, lumbago, etc. result from bad postural habit. However, few of these etiological associations are based on fact, and Hellebrandt and Franseen (1943), in their review of the evidence, conclude that postural habit has little effect on general body functions. People are interested in posture for a great variety of reasons: comparative anatomists are interested in the evolution of the biped posture in the ancestors of man (Keith, 1933); reflexologists are interested in postural reflexes; militarists have been interested in the effects of the army pack on posture (Hellebrandt, Fries, Larsen, and Kelso, 1944); physiotherapists are interested in the rehabilitation of postural control (Hellebrandt, 1944); hypnotists are interested in postural stability as a test of suggestibility (Furneaux, 1946); industrial psychologists are interested in the problems of postural fatigue and efficiency, and athletes have an obvious practical interest in the subject.

Many methods for measuring body attitude and movements have been devised. Reviews of these techniques are contained in Schäfer (1900), Hellebrandt and Franseen (1943), and Smith and Smith (1962). A procedure in common use for studying postural stability is the sway test, in which the sway of a standing person is continuously recorded in any desired plane by leading a thread from the body to a recording lever. A second procedure for studying postural stability is to use the 'stabilometer'. This is a device designed by Travis (1944) and consists of a platform mounted on a universal joint with springs under each corner. The subject stands as steadily as possible on the platform and his movements are recorded by a writing lever. One must guard against the assumption that the various techniques necessarily measure the same aspects of performance.

Attempts have been made to determine the location of the vertical projection of the body's centre of gravity in normal standing. Braune and Fischer (1885–1904) defined normal standing (*Stellung*) as the alignment of the body when the axes of rotation of the legs and the lobe of the ear are vertically in line. This was an arbitrary assumption however, and more recent determinations have revealed that the mean position of the centre of gravity of adults is usually directly above a point slightly to the left of and behind the geometric centre of the total supporting base (Hellebrandt, Nelson, Larsen, 1943). Hellebrandt accounted for this asymmetry in terms of a difference in weight between the left and right sides of the body. The centre of gravity of the body and its determination are discussed further in section 16.31.

9.32 Body sway

When a person stands with feet together in a relaxed posture, the body sways slightly particularly in the anterior–posterior plane. Men sway somewhat more than women, and this may be due to the greater average height and weight of men. However, these two factors of body build have been found to have very little effect unless the feet are in a splayed position (Fearing, 1924; Liebert, 1940; Travis, 1945; Wapner and Witkin, 1950). Other factors which have been found to increase sway include alcohol, muscle tension, attention, fatigue, and music (Edwards, 1942; Fearing, 1925; Husband, 1934). It has been found possible to condition the body sway induced by electrical stimulation of the vestibular apparatus, to a tone.

The amplitude of body sway with eyes closed is notoriously affected by suggestions to the subject that he is falling. Hull (1933) first used the amplitude of postural sway as a test of suggestibility and hypnotizability. Subsequently Eysenck and Furneaux have shown high correlations between the extent to which the suggestion, 'you are falling forward' affects body sway, and susceptibility to trance-inducing suggestions (Eysenck and Furneaux, 1945; Eysenck, 1947; Furneaux, 1946, 1952). These effects of suggestion on sway were found to correlate specifically with other measures of the motor effects which hypnotic suggestion may induce, rather than with sensory effects of hypnosis. De Rivera (1959) interpreted the trait of susceptibility to sway suggestion as a willingness to obey instructions, and suggested that such people are more readily taught skills such as flying.

The effect of suggestion on sway has also been found to relate to neuroticism and extroversion (Furneaux, 1961), although even without suggestion neurotics have been found to sway more than normal subjects (Ingham, 1954).

The effect of suggestion on sway has also been related to various forms of psychosis (Williams, 1932; Bartlett, 1936, 1944; Freeman and Rodnick, 1942).

9.33 The sensory basis of postural stability

Man has four sources of sensory information which could serve to preserve postural stability: vision, vestibular inputs, proprioception, and touch.

Vision is of obvious importance to man. Edwards (1946) found that people sway about 50% less with eyes open than with eyes closed. Witkin and Wapner (1950) and Wapner and Witkin (1950) compared the ability of subjects to stand steadily on a sprung platform (ataxiameter) under four visual conditions: (a) room lights on (b) room lights off, leaving in view only a cube with one side horizontal (c) nothing in view and (d) an unstable rocking cube in view. Steadiness decreased progressively from condition (a) to condition (d).

The last condition in Wapner and Witkin's experiment demonstrates that deceptive visual impressions can induce body sway, even to the point of falling. People often fall in the 'haunted swing' (see section 7.51). Edwards (1943, 1946) found that people sway much more when looking at a pendulum, or at a picture hung 15° askew. Strongly illuminating one eye has also been found to increase sway to the same side (Stein, 1910). Cantrell (1963) studied the effect of visual figures presented tachistoscopically to subjects on the stabilometer. Stability was increased in conditions where figures were reported to be stationary, relative to conditions in which either the figures were perceived as in motion or no figures were presented. The direction of movement of the figures (e.g. the direction in which a car was pointing) was not related to the subject's direction of movement.

Even when other systems are defective, vision can serve to stabilize posture. However, it is clearly not essential: blind people have no trouble in maintaining steady posture (Edwards, 1946).

There can be no doubt that labyrinthine stimulation can affect postural steadiness dramatically. Patients with recent unilateral labyrinthine or cerebellar damage are prone to fall to the damaged side. They may compensate to some extent by holding their heads on one side, and when they do this there is improvement not only in their balance but also in associated sensory defects which together constitute the 'induction syndrome' (Halpern, 1954a, 1954b, 1956; Halpern and Kidson, 1954). On the other hand, people with bilateral labyrinthine loss are just as capable as normal people of maintaining a steady posture in the Romberg position, that is with eyes closed and feet together (Birren, 1945). Rademaker (1935) found that such people in the Romberg position can adjust their stance to compensate for small inclinations of the platform upon which they are standing but with large inclinations they lose their balance whereas a normal subject would still compensate. Labyrinth-defective patients are less well able to stand on one leg with closed eyes (Worchel and Dallenbach, 1948). Even a normal person in this position sways a good deal—beyond the maximum point from which labyrinth-defective subjects can restore themselves. Defective subjects have one advantage over normal subjects: they are not affected by post-rotational dizziness (James, 1882).

It would seem therefore that the labyrinths do not provide the crucial information for the maintenance of the normal standing posture. Birren (1945) deduced that this is so by considering the vestibular threshold. Dodge had reported that only movements having a sudden onset and a terminal velocity of 4°/sec or more produce reflex eye movements, and if eye movements are used as a criterion of the vestibular threshold, a body sway must reach this velocity to trigger-off vestibular responses. Even at only half this threshold, a 5 ft 10 in man would have to sway at 2·4 in/sec to stimulate the labyrinths. Sway movements are normally much slower than this. Goldscheider (1898) found that the sensitivity of the hip joint is between a third and one degree per second which is more like the value required for postural adjustments. The proximal hip joint is more sensitive than the more distal knee and ankle joints.

The basic physiological mechanism of static upright posture in man would therefore seem to be proprioceptive control, from the hip joint and spine, of the bilateral balance of body tonus. The receptors involved are probably the muscle spindles as well as joint receptors in the ligaments. The inputs trigger-off myotatic reflexes and also integrate with the tonus-controlling mechanisms of the cerebellum, vestibular nuclei, and basal ganglia. The erect body is never still, but sways from side to side, constantly invoking corrective responses. In this way the sensory systems are prevented from adapting. Only minimal amounts of muscular contraction are normally involved, giving little or no electromyographic evidence of their presence (Beevor, 1903; Eldred, 1960). It is not surprising that a tabetic patient, in whom the proprioceptive tracts are affected, tends to fall into the washstand when washing his face.

10

Geographical orientation

10.1 Introduction

The geographical orientation of a person is the way that person is facing with respect to objects on the earth's surface. A person's orientation is always changed by rotations about his own body axis; whether it is also changed by linear movements depends on the direction of movement and on whether the distance moved constitutes a significant fraction of the distance of the object.

The phrase 'a person's orientation' is sometimes used to refer, not to the actual orientation he may have, but to his ability to behave according to his actual orientation. If that behaviour is tolerably correct, we say the person is well oriented; if it is not, he is said to be disoriented. Then again, the term 'orientation' is sometimes used to describe the actual movements made in setting the body to a particular direction. It would be pedantic to coin new terms for each of these usages; the meaning is usually apparent from the context.

Geographical orientation ability takes many forms. There is the ability to walk in a straight line, the ability to maintain a sense of direction when one is rotated or moved, the ability to draw a map or point to distant places, etc. Each of these abilities involves a different complex of modalities, movements, and conceptual skills. To what extent these various abilities are correlated is not known. Witkin (1946) is apparently the only worker who has attempted to find out. Although he found positive correlations, the study was on a small scale and firm conclusions could not be drawn.

Geographical orientation skills fall naturally into two classes. On the one hand are those tasks which involve the ability of a person to maintain a sense of direction when moving about in strange surroundings. Such tasks do not require any prior intellectual knowledge of the spatial position of particular objects. On the other hand, there are those tasks, such as drawing a map or pointing to the north, which do require intellectual knowledge. These two classes of orientation skills will be dealt with in turn.

10.2 The ability to maintain a sense of orientation when moving about

It is essential for success in this type of task that the subject obtains some information regarding his change of position in space, and also that he correctly interprets this information. Vision is clearly man's most important modality for orientation. In order to study the other modalities, it is necessary to blindfold the subject.

10.21 The role of vestibular and kinaesthetic factors in geographical orientation

The simplest way to study the role of kinaesthesis in geographical orientation is to set up a situation in which the kinaesthetic modality alone can provide the required sensory information. The ability to walk in a straight line with the eyes closed approximates to such a task.

People lost in a mist commonly find that they have walked in a complete circle. Animals, too, have been reported to show this behaviour (Guldberg, 1897). The fact that animals and men tend to circle when deprived of practically all sensory communication with the environment is not surprising. Indeed, it would be surprising if they could walk straight for long. However, the consistent individual differences in the direction of circling, which all investigators report, require an explanation.

Several investigators have found that most people veer to the right rather than to the left (Szymanski, 1913; Blumenthal, 1928; Lund, 1930; Brigden, 1935; Claparède, 1943). Abderhalden (1919) found that the majority of his subjects descended by the right staircase of a twin symmetrical stairway. Szymanski (1913) found that girls veer to a greater extent than boys.

Lenkner (1934) is the only investigator to report a preponderance of left veering in his subjects.

There have been two types of explanation put forward to account for these consistent trends. The first is that there is some fundamental circling mechanism in all animals. The second is that circling is due to physical asymmetries in the body.

Schaeffer (1928) was the strongest proponent of the first type of theory. He observed veering tendencies in many species and explained them by postulating a 'spiralling mechanism' which impels animals to turn in spirals when ordinary sensory control is absent. This mechanism was supposed to reside in the brain but to be independent of handedness and all structural asymmetries of the body. He found that the particular veering tendency of a person was constant, whether the person walked, swam, or drove a car. Schaeffer did not report any measurements of body symmetry, and therefore his denial of such causes of the veering tendency is unwarranted. His theory was unclearly formulated and has fallen into disrepute.

Other investigators have sought to discover the basis for consistent veering tendencies in asymmetries of the body (Abderhalden, 1919; Guldberg, 1897; Lund, 1930). Lund carried out the most systematic study of this kind. He asked his subjects to walk blindfolded in a straight line across a football field. Their actual course was plotted, and consistent veering was found, predominantly to the right. They were also asked to walk backwards. The geographical direction of veering was now reversed; and this, Lund claimed, is consistent with a structural theory. He recorded various indices of body symmetry: handedness, eyedness, the lengths of the arms and legs, and the verticality of the body mid-line. Most subjects had a longer left leg, and most of these veered to the right. In fact 80% of his subjects showed a correspondence between leg length and veering tendency. The difference in leg length was on average about 5 mm. One would like to be certain that Lund's method of measuring the length of a leg to such fine limits was reliable.

Apparently no one has considered the possibility that asymmetries in the vestibular apparatus may cause veering. It is well known that after spinning about the body axis a person will veer in the same direction as the spin when attempting to walk straight (see section 5.12). Slight persistent asymmetries in vestibular 'tonus' could account for the consistency of the veering tendency. Such a cause might account for Schaeffer's finding that the mode of locomotion does not affect the direction of veering, and would fit in with his claim that the direction of veering is independent of structural asymmetries of the body.

It cannot be said that the study of veering tendency has yet thrown much light on the role of kinaesthetic and vestibular mechanisms in orientation. Subjects with deficient physiological mechanisms should be studied. Also, shoes with soles of different thickness could be used to control the effect of leg length.

Apparently no one has studied a person's ability to rotate his body through a given angle or a given number of turns. This ability should be studied with self-produced movement and also passive movement.

One of the best ways to study the role of vestibular and kinaesthetic cues in geographical orientation, is to compare the performance of blindfolded subjects on orientation tasks when they are moved passively, with their performance when they are allowed to move themselves. In the first case vestibular cues are predominant (assuming that auditory cues have been eliminated), and in the second case vestibular and kinaesthetic cues are present, as well as information from the motor outflow.

Liebig (1933) showed his subjects a light in an otherwise dark room. The light was then put out, and the subjects were either led about or wheeled passively on a cart, in paths of varying complexity. They then had to point to, and return to, the position of the light. The subjects who walked about performed with much greater accuracy than those who were passively wheeled about. It is difficult to see how these results could have been otherwise. A subject on a smoothly running cart could only be expected to detect rotary or linear accelerations. If the cart were rotated or translated with a steady velocity, he could have no sense of the velocity except by extrapolating from the terminal point of acceleration. To know the distance moved, he would have to estimate the time spent at that particular velocity. However, in walking he would have continuous information about the distance moved in terms of the length of his own step.

The ability to maintain a sense of objective orientation when the body if self-rotated, has been studied by Piercy (1957). Subjects were shown a luminous arrow, pointing to one of the eight points of the compass. The subjects then rotated themselves through 180°, in the dark, and placed a second arrow in the same direction in space as the first arrow. They made many mistakes. This was not a test of the subject's ability to rotate himself through 180° because the second arrow indicated the correct way in which they had to face. The task was a test of the ability to dissociate egocentric from objective spatial reference.

George and McIntosh (1960) repeated the experiment and found that their subjects performed faultlessly. They suggested that Piercy's results were due to the fact that only five of his 28 subjects were free from neurological and psychiatric disorder, and these five may have been of low intelligence. George and McIntosh used a similar test under four conditions, all in the dark. In condition 1 the subject rotated himself through 180° and then set a second arrow to the same direction in space as the first. In condition 2 the subject was rotated passively through three or four complete rotations, and reset the first arrow. Condition 3 was the same as condition 2, except that the experimenter moved about and it was stressed that the arrow might not remain in its initial position. In condition 4 the subject was rotated passively, sometimes to finish facing the inspection arrow and sometimes facing the second arrow; the experimenter again moved about. Practically no errors were made in condition 1, where the subject's movement was self-produced. Only a few mistakes were made in condition 2; the subject's success in this condition must have been due to the fixed position of the experimenter for when his position was varied in condition 3, the subjects made more mistakes. Just how the subject sensed the presence of the experimenter was not stated. Condition 4 produced the highest error rate.

It is not clear what issues George and McIntosh were investigating; the study appears to have been designed to show how much confusion of several different types has to be introduced before a subject becomes disoriented; there was no attempt to isolate the effect of any one variable and little light was thrown on the question of which cues enable a person to maintain a sense of direction when rotated.

Witkin (1946) tested the ability of blindfolded people to maintain a sense of orientation to the walls of a room after being passively subjected to one or more turns in a rotating chair. Most of the subjects did poorly, although there were wide individual differences. Witkin made no attempt to relate these differences to differences in vestibular sensitivity.

Persons with a more sensitive vestibular mechanism should perform better on a test, like the one Witkin used, where the subject is passively moved. One would also expect that such people would do better in an orientation task where they had to move actively. According to Worchel (1952) this is not so. In one test, his blindfolded subjects were led along two sides of a triangle and had to return to the start by themselves. In a second test they were led along the hypotenuse of an isosceles right-angled triangle and had to walk unaided to complete the triangle. The subjects were given a number of tests of vestibular sensitivity. The results showed that the subjects with deficient vestibular function, especially those whose semi-circular canals were not functioning, did better than the subjects with high vestibular sensitivity, on the first orientation test. The degree of vestibular sensitivity did not affect performance on the second test. Worchel concluded that persons with defective vestibular functions compensate by developing their kinaesthetic sensitivity. The tasks which Worchel used required knowledge of distance walked, which could only be given by kinaesthesis, and knowledge of angle turned, which would be more precisely given by kinaesthesis than by the vestibular system. Worchel's study should be repeated, using tasks where vestibular-defective and normal subjects are actively and passively rotated, that is, tasks where the vestibular information could be important.

10.22 Visual experience and geographical orientation

The role of visual experience in geographical orientation is best studied by comparing the performance of sighted subjects with that of subjects who have been blind for varying periods of time. The two main questions on which attention has been focused are (1) the relative performance of blind and blindfolded sighted subjects on orientation tasks, and (2) the effect of the age at which blindness occurs. The work on the first question has produced contradictory results. Using human maze-learning tasks, Koch and Ufkess (1926) and Duncan (1934) found that sighted subjects were superior, whereas Knotts and Miles (1929) found sighted subjects inferior on a stylus maze though just as good as blind subjects on a finger relief maze. Similarly, Worchel (1951) using his triangle completion task (see above) found sighted subjects superior, whereas they were inferior on a peg-board task in which they had to replace sets of pegs in an orientation which they had tactually inspected earlier (Drever, 1955). Those workers who found blind subjects superior concluded that the blind learn to make more efficient use of their remaining modalities, while those who found the opposite concluded that the availability of visual imagery facilitates the symbolization of the patterns involved in the task, a suggestion made earlier by Fernald (1913).

Some support for the latter conclusion arises from the work on the second question, which tends to show that some visual experience before blinding assists in later orientation tasks. Duncan found that those blind subjects who had had a period of sightedness were less inferior to sighted subjects, Koch and Ufkess found that those blinded after up to 17 years of at least partial vision were as good as sighted subjects, while those of Drever's subjects who had been blind before the age of four were as poor as sighted subjects. Similarly Sylvester (1913), using a form-board test, found late-blinded subjects superior to early-blinded.

Worchel (1951), on the other hand, concluded that blindness was incapacitating irrespective of when it occurred, and McReynolds and Worchel (1954) found that neither age, sex, I.Q., degree of blindness, etiology of blindness, nor age at blindness, affected performance when subjects were asked to point to geographical locations both near and far.

Maze learning, form-board tests, and Worchel's tests are all rather complex. There is need for a series of studies comparing blind subjects, vestibular-deficient subjects, and normal subjects, under conditions of active and passive movement, on a variety of very simple orientation tasks, such as estimating a distance moved or an angle turned, etc. Only when such analytic, detailed, and comprehensive studies have been done will we be able to assess the role of the various modalities in different types of orientation behaviour.

10.3 The ability to point in a given direction and draw maps

Trowbridge (1913) first used the technique of asking subjects to indicate direction by placing marks on a circular piece of paper. They were asked to indicate in this way the direction of New York, the North Pole, London, San Francisco, and Panama, relative to the centre of the paper. More than half of the 27 subjects were said to have revealed by their performance that they had more or less adequate imaginary maps. The scoring procedure was not indicated, and the subjects were apparently not asked whether they knew of these places.

Trowbridge distinguished between egocentric orientation, which is based on the directions of the compass or other conventional coordinate system and is present only in civilized man, and domicentric orientation, which is centred on the dwelling-place and is typical of animals and primitive man. A better name for egocentric orientation is geocentric orientation (Gregg, 1939) or conventional orientation (Claparède, 1903), that is, orientation according to a conventional coordinate system.

Angyal (1930) used a method similar to that of Trowbridge. The subjects were seated in a particular orientation and had to draw the way from one place to another in Turin. They were given twelve such tasks. Angyal used only subjects who were well acquainted with the town. He gave them a drawing of one of the routes depicted at an angle of 90° or 180° to the orientation in which they had drawn it. Individuals differed in the ease with which they recognized these routes, and this was taken to be a measure of the stability of the individual manner of representation. He divided the subjects into two groups according to the way they performed the drawing tasks: (a) Those who drew their routes in an alignment with the actual route from the point of view of their own position, and (b) those who oriented their routes without reference to their own position in space. Most people belonged to the second group, many of them appearing to use the main streets of the town as their axes of reference.

Claparède (1903, 1924, 1943) used similar methods. His subjects had to indicate the directions of certain large towns in relation to Geneva, where the study was carried out. They were also given a circular map of Geneva without compass reference marks and asked to place it in front of themselves in the most natural way, when seated in various orientations. He distinguished four types of person according to their performance. (1) The realistic type, who aligns the directions of streets, rivers, etc. in the map with their counterparts in reality. This type corresponds to Angyal's group (a) and to Trowbridge's domicentric type. (2) The egocentric type who orients the map in a constant relation to his own body. This type corresponds to Angyal's group (b) and Trowbridge's egocentric type. (3) The conventional type, who always places the north of the map furthest from himself and the east to the right. This seems to be a special case of type (b); it was found to be rare. (4) The indifferent or variable type, who do not use a consistent method. They also were few in number.

Ryan and Ryan (1940) asked subjects a variety of questions about the way they thought about spatial orientation. The subjects were also blindfolded and rotated slowly in a chair. After being stopped they were asked to indicate the direction of a given object in the room or an object outside. They were also asked to point in the direction of distant cities. The behaviour of the subjects was minutely described, but Ryan and Ryan drew no general conclusions from their study. Binet (1894) and Peterson (1916) have also written general accounts of the problem of geographical orientation in man. Baumgarten (1927) described how we use fixed reference points when we visit a new city, and are at first lost if we later approach the city by an unfamiliar route.

McReynolds and Worchel (1954) studied local and geographical orientation in the blind. The blind subjects were asked to point to local and distant places. Neither sex, age, I.Q., nor etiology of blindness were found to affect performance.

The most significant conclusion to be drawn from all these studies of the ability to draw maps is that there are consistent individual differences in mode of representing geographical directions. Claparède's classification of types into realistic and egocentric seems to be the most logical and aptly descriptive. The fundamental questions, however, remain to be studied. We suggest that the following two questions would be worth studying.

Are those people who choose one mode of map drawing incapable of using other modes if asked, or does their consistency in performance merely reflect their preference to use one of several methods of which they are equally capable? If people do differ in their ability to use one or other mode, do these differences reflect fundamental differences in spatial intelligence, or do they merely reflect differences in the way the people have been taught?

10.4 Human maze learning

We shall make no attempt to review the literature on human maze learning. However, there are a series of studies concerned with the effects of the orientation of a maze on the ability of a subject to learn it. These studies are the most relevant to the theme of this book.

The results of an early study by Perrin (1914) suggest that a subject who has learned a maze in one orientation makes few errors when asked to perform with the maze turned through 90° or 180°. Perrin's subjects could also go through the maze backwards without much trouble.

Subsequent work has confirmed that there is a good deal of transfer of learning from one orientation of a maze to another. For instance, Higginson (1936) found that 33 trials were needed to learn a maze in one position; it took a further 25 trials to learn it in a 90° rotated position, then 18 trials in a 180° position, and a further 18 in a 270° position.

Whereas Higginson's subjects learned all four positions in one session, Langhorne (1948) spread the learning over four days. The gain was consistently positive from position to position, and when, on the fifth day, the original position was relearnt the gain was greater than that shown by subjects who merely relearned the original position after either one or four days without learning any other position. The men in Langhorne's sample were superior to the women and were less disturbed by rotation of the maze.

Worchel and Rockett (1955) found that a maze in a fixed orientation was more easily learned than one which was placed in several orientations during the learning period. The difference in difficulty was not due to differences in difficulty for particular positions, for all positions were found to be equally difficult when presented without alternation with other positions. Sato (1960) has presented evidence which conflicts with Worchel and Rockett's, in that he found that a rotating maze was as easy to learn as a stationary one. Perhaps the level of difficulty of Sato's maze was too low to discriminate between the two methods of learning.

Performance on a 180° rotated maze has been found to present different levels of difficulty for different subjects depending on the amount of visual imagery or systematic verbalizations of the choice points (Davis, 1933).

Du Mas and Worchel (1956) used two kinds of 180° rotation: on the one hand, rotation of the maze and on the other, rotation of the subject, leaving the maze stationary (i.e. the subject and experimenter changed places). Both types of rotation disrupted relearning. Some subjects were more affected by one type, some more affected by the other, but group means showed that subject rotation was overall more deleterious than maze rotation. This difference was significant for only one of the two mazes used, an irregular rambling maze, and not for the other, a regular T maze. The experimenters suggested that the latter may be learned in a predominantly verbal manner, relatively independent of the spatial context (i.e. the room, which the subjects could see), so that under either type of rotation all that would be required is a reversal of directions, 'left' becoming 'right' and 'towards me' becoming 'away from me'; whereas verbalization would be of little value in the learning of the irregular maze, which would depend on a pattern of motor activity related to the visible context, and would therefore be especially disrupted by a change in the relationship between subject and context.

10.5 The development of geographical orientation

The points of the compass provide an objective reference system for directions in a horizontal plane. This system is geometrically analogous to the vertical reference system, that is, to the direction of gravity. But, whereas the direction of gravity can be directly sensed, there is no evidence that animals possess any special sense for directions of the compass.

There have been those who were convinced that man has a separate modality for geographical direction, which gives a direct awareness of the earth's magnetism (Viguier, 1882; Hudson, 1922; Lucannas, 1924; review by Jaccard, 1931) and a popular belief persists that primitive people and children possess an innate sense of direction. Darwin (1859) speculated on the possibility of an instinct of orientation, but omitted such speculation from later editions of his book. No good experimental evidence has been produced in support of this hypothesis.

There are many accounts given by travellers of the remarkable abilities of primitive peoples to find their way about in unknown terrain when the sun is not visible (see Claparède, 1943 for review). All these accounts are anecdotal; the abilities of the primitive peoples probably rest on such factors as the use of landmarks, and dead reckoning. Jaccard pointed out that Arabs in the Sahara proceed in single file, so that those at the end immediately notice any deviations of the leader from a straight path. Pechuel-Loescher (1907) found that bushmen soon became lost in a heavy mist. There is no good evidence to suggest that primitive people have an orientation ability which a civilized man could not match, given training in the use of natural landmarks, dead reckoning, and other skills.

A popular belief persists that children possess an innate, vestigial sense of geographical orientation. Warren (1908) wrote, 'If such a sense has been developed in the phylogenetic scale (as suggested by the migration of birds) it may still appear in a rudimentary form in man, and distinct traces may be discovered in childhood which are lost in later life' (p. 377). Smith (1933) tested children between the ages of four and eleven years. Each child sat facing north and was given a circular card. Starting at the centre, they had to move a stylus in line with each of the eight principal points of the compass in turn. The extent of any error greater than two degrees was noted, as well as the time taken. Both time and errors decreased with age, and Smith concluded that there was no evidence for Warren's suggestion of a sense of direction in children which declined with age. However, Smith's task was more a test of the ability of the children to attach verbal labels to particular directions than of a magnetic sense of direction. Because they were facing north, the children had only to use the normal cartographic convention to get the directions right; a real test of a magnetic sense must involve performance when facing in different directions. Smith's results would also be contaminated by the varying ability of the children to draw straight lines and judge angles.

Warren (1908) described a boy with what he called a 'magnetic sense of direction'. He attempted to disorient him but was not successful. Twenty-two years later De Silva (1931) located this person who disclaimed ever having had any special magnetic sense. De Silva described the case of another boy, twelve years old, who had a well developed sense of direction. His ability was found to depend on a correct initial orientation which the boy could then maintain without effort. The boy's mother had been in the habit of using geographical directions when she indicated directions in the home. De Silva thought this accounted for the boy's abilities.

In the absence of any good evidence for a special direction sense, we will assume that a man can orient himself to the points of the compass only when he can see some familiar landmark or a compass. Of course there may still be inherited differences in orientation aptitude. The only study on this question was done by Malán (1940). He employed Liebig's method in which the subjects (40 fraternal and 40 identical twins) were shown a luminous point and then blindfolded. After being led on foot about the room in different directions for a while, the subjects had to indicate the position of the point of light. The identical twins were more alike in their ability than the fraternal twins. Malán concluded that the ability to orient is to some extent inherited. This does not of course mean that there is a special modality for orientation, it may mean only that some people are more readily able to learn to orient themselves than others, or it may mean only that twins are likely to be taught to orient themselves in the same way. Sandström has pointed out that the very limited test procedure which Malán used does not provide a valid basis for generalizing about the role of inherited factors in orientation abilities in general.

Finally we shall discuss the teaching of geographical orientation to children. Most young children have been shown to have difficulty in indicating the directions of the compass, even in a familiar environment (Howe, 1931). Most teachers have been found to have difficulties too (Ridgley 1922). Gulliver (1908) found that even when children were told where the directions of the compass lay, they could not correctly orient a simple map of streets which they knew well. Howe (1932) made recommendations for improving the teaching of geographical orientation. He described a programme of teaching which he gave to children in the first three grades of school. The children were told that the sun rises in the east and sets in the west, and is in the south at midday, and other such facts. Tests showed that this training improved the children's sense of direction. Before training, many of the children had used such phrases as, 'Santa Claus lives over there', and, 'The wind blows that way', when justifying a judgment about the direction of a point of the compass.

Gregg (1940) also made recommendations about how to teach compass orientation. He claimed that most people, when asked to indicate a compass direction, make small movements of the head or body. He recommended that training consist of spending some time every now and again in standing in a given orientation and deliberately making the small body movements which are characteristic of one's self. He gave no evidence that such a procedure improves orientation ability, and several children whom he asked to do this thought it was silly, which is scarcely surprising.

Lord (1941) has conducted the most thorough study of geographical orientation in children, using 173 boys and 144 girls. She tested their ability (a) to point to cardinal compass points and distant localities, (b) to indicate the directions of local features in the town, (c) to draw maps, and (d) to maintain a sense of direction when travelling about. This last test was conducted by driving the children at 20 miles per hour round a two mile course in the city of Ann Arbor, stopping now and again to test the subjects' ability to indicate north and the directions of the previous stopping places. Half the children were 'lost' before the first stop. Boys performed better than girls on all the tests. Children who normally sat facing north in school performed better on the tests than children who sat facing other directions. Lord stressed the need for better teaching of geographical orientation.

10.6 Clinical disturbances of geographical orientation

Geographical disorientation is a commonly reported symptom of brain damage. The parietal lobes are most commonly implicated (Critchley, 1953). The symptoms of geographical disorientation cannot be considered as

separate from disturbances in the more basic spatial abilities, which are discussed in sections 2.4 and 11.4. For instance, unilateral visual inattention, in
which objects in one side of the visual field are ignored, produces a tendency
to turn persistently in one direction, even when this is inappropriate. Brain
(1941b) described several patients showing this kind of behaviour; they had
lesions in the right parieto-occipital region causing left hemianopia and
neglect of the left half of visual space. They always tended to turn to the
right, although they showed good topographical memory and realized their
mistakes soon after they were made. Such patients, when asked to draw a
map of a familiar place, tend to omit things to one side, or shift them over
towards the 'good' side (see figures 10.1 and 10.2).

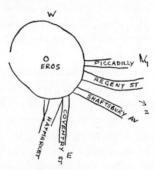

Figure 10.1 Plan of Piccadilly Circus drawn by a patient with a right
parietal lesion. Note the neglect of left-hand landmarks. [From Critchley,
1953]

On the other hand, geographical disorientation may result from an inability to recognize or remember familiar landmarks ('loss of topographical
memory') rather than from any deficiency of spatial ability as such. Zangwill
(1951) reported three cases of this kind. One patient complained that when
walking in places well known to him he often felt that he did not know what
was round the next corner and that the scenery unfolded as though he were
in a strange country.

Another typical symptom of parietal disease is losing oneself. Zangwill
has proposed the term 'topographical agnosia' for a particular form of this
defect in which patients have great difficulty in finding one particular object
when there are several similar objects in a row. In such a case, recognition
of the particular object depends on memory for position. For example
Critchley reports cases of patients who could not locate their own bed in the
ward unless some familiar object were placed upon it. One patient tended to
pass his home without knowing it, and asked his wife to leave a light on so

that he could recognize the house more easily. In another case, the patient, when faced with two or three doors or passages, was unable to choose the correct one.

A second form of losing oneself occurs when, despite the fact that a varied array of familiar objects is present, a patient with a topographical disorder is unable to relate them into one coherent pattern (Meyer, 1900; Hartmann, 1902). For example, Paterson and Zangwill (1945) reported the case of a patient who could recognize the main buildings of his home town, Edinburgh, although he could not find his way about. Critchley (1953) described many other such cases. The degree of topographical loss depends on the familiarity of the setting. For instance, Zangwill (1951) described

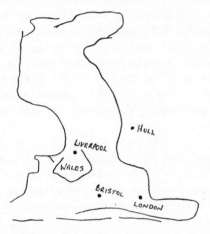

Figure 10.2 Map of England drawn by a patient with a right parietal lesion. Note the shift of topographical detail towards the right. [From Critchley, 1953]

how a Londoner could always find his way about in the vicinity of his own home, but was apt to get lost in other parts of London well known to him.

On a larger scale, patients with defective topographical ability may become confused about which town they are in. Paterson and Zangwill (1944) described a patient who said that he was in his home town, Grimsby, although at the same time admitting that he was in Scotland. He gradually became clearer about his location, correctly saying that Grimsby was 300 miles away, and yet insisted that it was just around the corner. He realized he was wrong when he went for a walk, and finally fully recovered his sense of orientation. An affective element was probably involved; the patient wished to get home to Grimsby.

Spatial disorientation may also result from aphasia (Head 1926); in this case the patient may have difficulty in describing his location or the location of places, although able to find his way about in practice.

Attempts have been made to distinguish between different patterns of spatial disability, according to whether the dominant or the non-dominant hemisphere is damaged, and according to the site of the damage within the hemisphere. Zangwill (1951) associated loss of bearings in familiar surroundings with parietal lesions of the major hemisphere; loss of topographical memory, such as is involved in route finding, with lesions in either parietal lobe. The basis for the distinction between loss of bearing and route finding is not clear in Zangwill's account, especially since McFie, Piercy, and Zangwill (1950) had previously associated difficulties in route finding and map reading with damage in the parietal lobe of the minor hemisphere.

Critchley concluded that spatial disorders are more likely to result from minor lobe damage than from major lobe damage. As regards localization within the parietal lobe, Critchley concluded that, 'The clinical occurrence of marked disorder of spatial thought should, at the bedside, lead to the strong suspicion of a lesion of the hinder part of the brain, and more precisely of the territory linking the parietal, occipital, and temporal lobes' (Critchley, 1953, p. 355).

Marie and Béhague (1919) and Pollock (1938) reported disorientation symptoms associated with injury to the frontal lobes, although the scores which Marie and Béhague's patients obtained on their orientation tests were no worse than Ferraro (1921) obtained from normal subjects.

The pitfalls of analysis of dysfunction based upon selected clinical cases have been stressed by Semmes, Weinstein, Ghent, and Teuber (1955). The frequency of cases with a given lesion but without given symptoms is not assayed; when lesions are widespread the symptoms may be falsely ascribed to some part of the total lesion; performance on tests is alleged to be subnormal without reference to the performance of matched normals.

In the same paper Semmes et al. presented evidence that geographical disorientation is transmodal. The test they used required the subject to follow, by locomotion, routes represented on maps. Five path diagrams were presented visually, and ten tactually, five to each hand. The tactual maps were rotations and mirror images of the visual ones. The test was given to 62 brain-injured subjects and 17 controls. The mean score of those subjects with parietal-lobe damage was less than that of the other brain-injured and the control subjects. The mode of presentation of the test had no effect. These results were interpreted as being contrary to the idea that disorders of route finding reflect a basic disorder in any one modality. In a later paper (Weinstein, Semmes, Ghent, and Teuber, 1956) they concluded that general intellectual deterioration and visual or tactile agnosia, while sometimes accompanying spatial disorientation, cannot entirely explain it. In this paper they also modified their earlier conclusion regarding the site of the lesion. Parietal lesions produced greater disorientation than non-parietal only when accompanied by somaesthetic defect (two-point discrimination); without somaesthetic defect, patients with parietal lesions were as good as those with non-parietal lesions, or normal controls.

In a more recent paper (Semmes, Weinstein, Ghent, and Teuber, 1963) they showed that impairment on their route-finding task was about equal to that on a personal-orientation task in which the subject was required to touch parts of his own body as indicated on a diagram of the body. Both tasks were impaired by left-posterior lesions, whereas only route finding was impaired by right-posterior lesions. This paper also reinforces their earlier conclusion that vision as such has no role in long-term spatial disorientation and, on the other hand, that disorientation rarely occurs without somaesthetic defect, although the converse is common. Whether this latter relationship reflects partial coincidence of lesion site or a true functional relationship is not known. They suggested that disorientation may involve a pathological inattention to backgrounds, since performance on the route-finding task was correlated with performance on a conditional-reaction task in which the background of the stimuli had to be taken into account.

The clinical literature as a whole is characterized by a tendency to 'symptom naming', which produces a welter of named disorders with little attempt at a theoretical or experimental analysis. The answers in this field are not simple; man's skills of geographical orientation are very complex and very idiosyncratic.

11

Egocentric orientation

11.1 Introduction

Egocentric orientation implies the positioning of an object or of a part of the body with respect to some axis or plane defined entirely with respect to the body or some part of the body of the observer. There is no reference to any other point or plane outside the observer.

The eyes, the head, and the trunk may each be regarded as having three principal planes according to figure 1.3 and figure 3.7. Egocentric judgments may be considered with reference to each of these planes for each of the three body parts specified.

Consider first the planes of the eye. The vertical meridional (median) plane of an eye may be defined as that vertical plane containing the visual axis when the eye is in its primary position and the body and head are upright. As the fixation point is always on the visual axis, an observer's ability to set a point in the eye's median plane will only be limited by the steadiness of his fixation. If he were to attempt to align a rod with the median plane of an eye it might be expected that he would succeed to the extent of his ability to discriminate a lack of visual alignment, that is by his visual acuity. This is not so, however, for normally a rod on the visual axis (median plane) of an eye does not appear as if it is pointing directly at the eye, but rather it appears to point to the egocentre (see section 2.2). In order to succeed, a person would therefore have to consciously use the criterion of visual alignment which would not be difficult once the task had been explained.

Whether an observer can align rods with the frontal plane or with the intersections of the frontal with the median and transverse planes (i.e. the normally vertical and horizontal meridians) is a difficult question to answer. When he stands erect with his eyes in their primary position, then in so far as he can set a line to the vertical or horizontal, he can set the line to the normally vertical and horizontal meridians. But if his head is on one side and his eyes tort, then it is very doubtful whether he would understand an instruction to set a line in the normally vertical or horizontal meridional plane of the eye, even if the terms were explained to him. In other words, these planes or their corresponding retinal meridians do not normally have any psychophysical counterpart. That is not to say that the position of these visual planes does not enter into spatial judgments (this topic has already been discussed in section 7.44). There are ways of bringing particular retinal meridians to the notice of a subject, for instance by impressing on them an after-image; and this is what is done when one wishes to study their relation to spatial judgments. It follows that the study of visual meridians is not subject to experiment except in special circumstances; and therefore this topic will not be discussed further in this section.

There are three head and body planes as shown in figure 1.3. The median plane and coronal plane are uniquely specifiable with reference to the mid-vertical head or body axis. The coronal plane of the trunk and of the head has behavioural significance in acts such as setting the body squarely in front of a surface; however, such behaviour has not been studied experimentally. Behaviour associated with the median planes of trunk and head has been studied, and will be discussed in the next section. There is no horizontal or transverse plane in the trunk which has a unique judgmental significance.

Man's bilateral symmetry imposes on him the difficult task of discriminating between the two halves of his body and identifying them by name. These problems will be discussed in the final section of this chapter. This topic is closely related to that of the body schema, but this subject is not discussed in this book.

11.2 The egocentre

Fundamental to the problem of egocentric localization is the concept of the egocentre. This concept is implicit in the idea of the centre of projection or cyclopean eye which was discussed in section 2.2. The term 'egocentre' was introduced by Roelofs (1959) to describe that centre, fixed with reference to the body, from which absolute directions are judged, such as straight ahead, to the left, to the right, upwards and downwards.

The egocentre is an ambiguous concept. Its simplest meaning is that location in the head towards which rods point when they are judged to be pointing directly at the self. We shall call this egocentre (if indeed it is a single centre common to all visual directions) the *direct egocentre*. The direct egocentre may be determined in the following manner.

A 20 cm rod about 0·5 cm in diameter is held at a specified distance from the bridge of the nose with its front end pointing roughly towards that point at a slight downward inclination to the visual axes when fixation is maintained on the front of the rod. With binocular fixation so maintained, the subject is asked to rotate the rod in a horizontal plane about its front end until he judges the rod to be pointing directly towards him. In so far as the egocentre has any behavioural significance it should not be necessary to explain to the subject what is meant by the instruction 'pointing directly towards you', and in fact this is not necessary. The procedure is repeated for at least three positions of the rod in the horizontal plane of the subject's eyes, and for other planes if the vertical position of the egocentre is being determined. The position of the outline of the subject's head is recorded together with the judged angular settings of the rod. The mean point of intersection of the extensions of the rod's axis in its various positions is the direct pointing egocentre for that fixation distance. The experiment may be repeated for different distances.

We shall now consider the relation of this egocentre to Hering's laws of visual direction and to Hering's projection centre or cyclopian eye.

When a person is asked to point a rod directly at himself using two eyes he does so by positioning the rod so that he is apparently sighting along it. In other words, *when a person is asked to point a rod directly at himself the position he chooses is one which he would have chosen had he been asked to sight along the rod*, with both eyes. Anyone can verify this statement in a few moments with aid of a pencil. The egocentre is defined as above by the point where such binocular apparent sighting lines meet. If the subject habitually uses one eye for sighting then the sighting lines will converge on that eye and that will be his direct egocentre (Roelofs, 1959). Most people when sighting binocularly do not use either visual axis but make a compromise sighting, usually more towards one eye than the other, and people are not necessarily consistent.

Consider now what happens when one eye is closed. *The subject will behave as if both eyes are open and when asked to point the rod directly at himself will again sight down it.* But unless this eye was his binocular sighting eye, the position in his head to which the rod is objectively pointing will no longer be his previously determined egocentre. *He judges the situation to be the same as it was when both eyes were open* and will therefore judge that the rod is directed towards the same egocentre as before and not towards his eye, as it really is. The fundamental rule still holds, that directing a rod to the egocentre is the same judgment as sighting along it, but the direction of the direct egocentre cannot be the same for both eyes.

The direct binocular egocentre is only in the median plane of the head for a completely balanced visual system. Each monocular egocentre is at the centre of rotation of the eye. However, the subject will probably judge each monocular egocentre to be in the median plane, for that is where he would normally suppose he would have directed a rod when asked to point it directly at himself. In other words, the position of the direct binocular egocentre will probably correspond to the position of the point which the subject would judge to be his egocentre, but the monocular direct egocentres can never both correspond to that point, and probably neither of them will do so.

One may ask what point does a person judge to be his egocentre. We shall call this the *judged egocentre*. The geometry of the procedure for determining the judged egocentre is outlined in figure 11.1. The subject fixates the front end of the rod monocularly and adjusts it until it is on his visual axis. He then states towards which point on his face the rod appears to be directed. This point is plotted on a scale plan of his head and the procedure repeated for three positions of the rod. The point where the three apparent sighting lines intersect is the judged egocentre. The procedure may then be repeated for the other eye and for two eyes. The positions of the three judged egocentres may then be compared. According to Hering's law of identical visual directions the two judged monocular egocentres should coincide. According to our principle that when we sight with one eye we judge the situation to be the same as it is when we sight with two, the monocular egocentres should coincide with the binocular egocentre. If the judged binocular egocentre is midway between the two eyes, the above principle becomes Hering's law of cyclopean projection, that is, monocular visual lines are judged to be directed towards a point midway between the eyes.

The experiments which would establish the above predictions have yet to be done adequately. When they have been done, the position of the direct

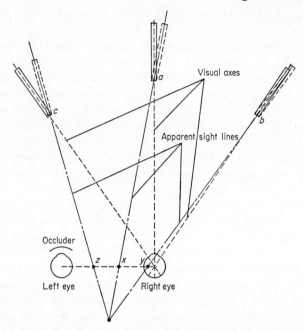

Figure 11.1 Demonstrating a procedure for determining the 'monocular', apparent-alignment or 'judged egocentre'. The subject sights along the rod while fixating its front edge in each of three positions *a*, *b*, and *c*. He then indicates, in each case, the point on his face towards which the rod appears to point, *x*, *y*, and *z*. The apparent-alignment egocentre is then given by the point of intersection of the three apparent lines of sight. It is assumed that the points *a*, *b*, and *c* are judged to be in their true position

and judged egocentres will have been established but the relation between objective and judged directions from those egocentres will not have been established. It has been implicitly assumed in the above discussion that the judged direction of fixated objects corresponds to their objective direction. If this assumption were not true, the method we have outlined for determining the direct egocentre by the procedure for determining the judged egocentre would be invalid. This can best be understood by inspecting figure 11.1. The egocentre is determined by extending the apparent sight lines *ax*, *by*, and *cz*—but if the objective direction of these lines does not correspond to their judged direction the justification for this geometrical procedure collapses. We would have to know the apparent positions of *a*, *b*, and *c*, in order to construct the correct apparent sight lines and the position of the egocentre would vary with every apparent change in the directions of a, b, and c. The only direction for which a check can readily be made of the correspondence between objective and subjective directions is the median plane of the head. If the objective and subjective median planes are found to correspond at the monocular fixation point (whether they correspond outside this point is not relevant) then at least the plane containing the monocular egocentres could be specified with certainty. Satisfactory procedures for removing the ambiguity in the position of judged monocular egocentres within this plane have never been proposed. Bailey (1959) has attempted to remove the ambiguity by suggesting that the egocentre always lies on the interocular axis—an unsatisfactory assumption. He further proposed (1958) that the apparent position of visual objects may be indicated by asking the subject to point to them with a hidden hand. But this procedure only adds the further uncertainty of intersensory spatial coordination, and as used by him did not remove the ambiguity of which we have spoken, for his procedure still depended on the assumption that the apparent directions of objects correspond to their true direction.

What is needed is an independent measure of the accuracy of directional judgments. The Holyoke team (Corbin, Reese, Reese, and Volkmann, 1956) have approached this problem by asking subjects to estimate the position of a point of light at various azimuth angles and displayed against a white background 15 ft distant, concentric with the observer—the so-called cyclorama. The subjects classified directions on a 41-point scale, either with the position on the far left called '1', or running from -20 through 0 in the centre to $+20$ on the right. Fixation was either in the centre or on the last appearing stimulus. The mean constant errors were less than two category steps of $5°$ each. The two scales gave different results; all positions tended to be underestimated on the 1–41 scale, but no such trend was apparent on the centre-zero scale (see figure 11.2). The lack of any anchor effect in the centre-zero scale and its presence in the end-zero scale suggests that the limit of the field of view rather than the median plane served as a norm in these azimuth judgments. The variability was unaffected by the type of scale. The two types of fixation had no differential effect on either the constant or variable error. The tolerable variable errors and even distribution of constant errors revealed by these experiments is reassuring to those who wish to assume, for the purposes of plotting the egocentre, that objects are judged to be where they really are, although the relative crudeness of the category scaling procedure leaves much to be desired.

It has commonly been reported that the judged egocentre lies on the vertical axis of rotation of the head (Funaishi, 1927; Roelofs, 1959). Directional judgments made in relation to such a centre would not be affected by rotations of the head on a vertical axis as they would be if the egocentre were

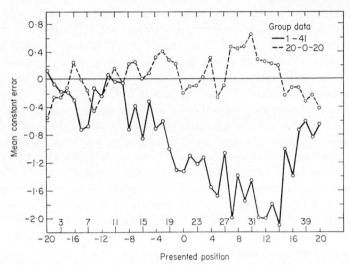

Figure 11.2 Mean constant error of bearing estimation as a function of presented position in the cyclorama for two systems of responding: a scale from 1 to 41 and a scale from minus 20 to plus 20. Group data. [From Corbin *et al.*, 1956]

situated outside this axis. Similar procedures may be used to determine the vertical position of the egocentres. One would expect them to lie on the same horizontal plane as the interocular axis. The position of the judged egocentres is affected by squint, phoria, and faulty convergence of the eyes. Roelofs (1959) has analysed the effects of these conditions and the reader is referred to him for details.

Charnwood (1949) and Francis and Charnwood (1951) used a binocular sighting procedure similar to the one we have outlined to determine the direct binocular egocentre. They reported that the egocentre shifted over towards the eye which was most strongly illuminated. Certainly the point towards which the objective sighting lines converged would move over, and when one eye only was illuminated would centre on that eye. Their results do not indicate whether the judged egocentre is affected by a difference of illumination between the eyes and it is doubtful whether they were aware of this distinction.

The direct and judged egocentres as defined above do not exhaust the possible meanings of the concept. We shall conclude this section by referring to another type of egocentre. The methods described so far for determining egocentres involve constant fixation with the alignment of points both in and outside the fixation point. This is a somewhat artificial situation; we usually scan our fixation along an object when judging its direction. If the subject is allowed to scan his fixation along a rod when setting it to point to himself he is less likely to be influenced by eye dominance, but for symmetrical convergence will probably set the rod so that each point along it falls on the line bisecting the angle of convergence. It is more likely that this *successive fixation egocentre* will fall on the true median plane of the head. A hypothetical relationship between the two types of egocentre is depicted in figure 11.3. It can be seen from that figure that not only may the position of

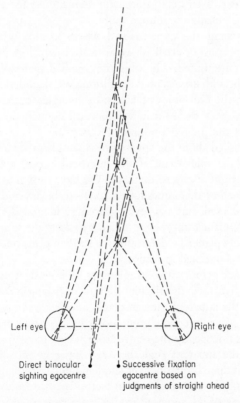

Left eye   Right eye

Direct binocular   Successive fixation
sighting egocentre   egocentre based on
                        judgments of straight ahead

Figure 11.3 Demonstrating how the egocentre derived from settings of points to the apparent straight ahead position for three convergence points *a*, *b*, and *c* may be in a different position to the egocentre determined by asking a subject to point a rod directly at himself. The position of the apparent median plane can also be seen to vary depending upon the method of determination. It is assumed throughout that the positions of the points *a*, *b*, and *c* are correctly judged

the two egocentres differ but also the position of the apparent median plane, although the apparent straight ahead is common to both procedures.

11.3 The localization of straight ahead

11.31 Visual factors

The question to be discussed under this heading is whether the apparent straight ahead corresponds to the objective median plane of the head. The type of judgment is entirely egocentric, demanding for its definition no reference system outside the human body.

Before discussing the experimental work on this topic certain geometrical concepts must be clarified, a clarification which it seems no previous investigator has attempted. The objective median plane of the head is an arbitrary concept with no accepted definition. We shall define it as the plane passing through the mid-point of, and at right angles to, the line joining the corneal surfaces, with the eyes in symmetrical convergence. The apparent median plane is the judged position of this plane. There are two distinct questions to be asked about the apparent median plane, the first is whether it passes through the mid-point of the interocular axis, and the second is whether it is at right angles to that axis. We have shown in section 2.2 that the answer to each of these questions is likely to be affected by the psychophysical method used, but whatever procedure is used the position of the apparent median plane cannot be specified by asking the subject to position a single point in that plane. To determine the median plane one must adopt one of the procedures outlined in section 2.2.

In spite of these geometrical complexities, all investigators of the apparent median plane have used the simple method of asking a subject to align a single point to the apparent median plane. *This procedure does not specify the apparent median plane*, but merely one point in it for that particular fixation distance. It does not specify the centre from which median plane judgments are made, nor the apparent angle between apparent and objective median plane. In spite of these limitations the single point determination may be useful for comparing the effects of various factors on visual judgments of direction and, as many of the reported studies were concerned with such effects, their results are probably valid as a basis of generalization at least for the fixation distance used. It is not legitimate to describe the judgments as median-plane judgments, a better description is 'straight-ahead judgments'.

Several investigators have reported that people have consistent constant errors in judging the straight ahead when the external stimulus conditions are symmetrical. Adults are usually found to set the straight ahead to the right of its true position (Akishige, 1951; Bruell and Albee, 1955a; Werner, Wapner, and Bruell, 1953). Akishige found that children are predominantly left-setters.

Several possible explanations of the consistent constant errors suggest themselves. Werner et al. had their subjects indicate the position of the straight ahead by pointing, and as the subjects used only their right hands, this may have accounted for the directional bias in their results.

Eyedness is certainly related to the direction of the constant errors. Fischer (reported in Tschermak-Seysenegg, 1952, p. 213) found that the apparent straight ahead with monocular viewing shifts towards the eye which is used, a result consistent with Hering's analysis of monocular visual direction (see section 2.2). This result suggests that if people use their sighting eye for aligning an object to the median plane when both eyes are open, they will show an apparent rotation of the apparent median plane to that side. This too is confirmed by studies on the egocentre described in section 11.2. Eyedness may not, however, affect the apparent straight ahead position of a fixated point, but only the apparent alignment of a rod to the median plane. It is to be expected that amblyopic people would show an apparent rotation of the median plane towards their functioning eye, even if no displacement of the apparent straight ahead for a fixated point.

No one, it seems, has made a direct study of the relationship between handedness and the position of the apparent median plane. Hall and Hartwell (1884) reported that, 'To binocular vision, a line at right angles to the median plane seems a little longer to the left than to the right of it, if the observer is right handed.'

One possibly important factor which could account for consistent constant errors in judging the straight ahead is the bilateral symmetry of the binocular visual field. It may be that if the orbits allow the visual field to extend more to one side than the other, the apparent straight ahead would be shifted towards that side. This factor has never been studied; however, there is abundant evidence that asymmetrical visual stimulation does affect the position of the apparent straight ahead. We shall now discuss this evidence.

Dietzel (1924) found that if the left-hand edge of a luminous figure, seen in the dark, is placed so that it is in the objective median plane, it is judged to be displaced to the left. Roelofs (1935) discovered this phenomenon independently, and so apparently did Akishige (1951) who found that the apparent straight-ahead position of a spot of light shifts in the direction of a second light.

A series of experiments confirming the Dietzel–Roelofs effect was conducted by Werner, Wapner, and Bruell (1953). In their first experiment they asked each subject to mark a point straight ahead on a wall. The subject could

not see his hand but could see a square which was placed straight ahead or 15°
to left or right. The apparent straight ahead was shifted as much as 5 cm in the
direction of the off-centre square.

Werner, *et al.* did not distinguish between the visual and kinaesthetic
straight ahead. It was the kinaesthetic straight ahead which they were studying,
and one must be cautious when relating the results of their experiments to
experiments in which the visually judged straight ahead was determined.

In a second paper, Wapner, Werner, Bruell, and Goldstein (1953) reported an experiment similar to Akishige's, in which the subject was asked to
centre the left- or right-hand dot in a horizontal row of three dots. Their
results were similar to Akishige's, that is, the apparent straight ahead was
shifted towards the other dots.

Bruell and Albee (1955a) also extended the study of the Dietzel–Roelofs
effect, using rectangles of various widths. The subject had to report when the
fixated part of the figure was straight ahead. The apparent straight ahead was
found to be shifted towards the centre of the figure when the subject fixated
one edge, and the size of the effect was found to be a function of the width of
the figures (see figure 11.4). In order to account for these and similar results,
Bruell and Albee (1955b) developed a motor theory, which we shall describe
later.

Wapner, Werner, Bruell, and Goldstein (1953) repeated Dietzel's and
Roelof's experiment with a luminous solid square and also with a luminous

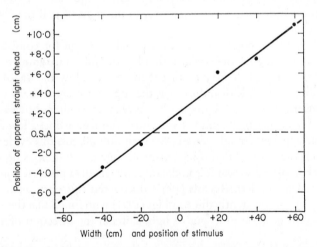

Figure 11.4 Results from Bruell and Albee (1955a) showing the position of
the apparent straight ahead as a function of the width of the stimulus
rectangle left and right of the fixation point

outline square. Both stimuli produced a similar shift of the apparent straight ahead towards the position of the square, demonstrating that the shift was a function of the asymmetry of shape rather than of the asymmetry of the light flux. They did not ask whether asymmetry of light flux by itself could have an effect on the apparent straight ahead, but Giannitrapani (1953), working in the same laboratory, did approach this problem. Luminous rectangles were used, one with a brightness gradient extending from left to right, one with a gradient from right to left, and one with uniform average brightness. Each of these was placed symmetrically about the subject's fixation point, and the subject had to set a small pointer to the apparent straight ahead. The apparent straight ahead was found to be displaced in the direction of highest brightness, that is, towards that edge of the figure where the contrast between figure and dark background was highest. Giannitrapani suggested that it was probably not light-flux asymmetry itself which caused the shift in the apparent straight ahead but rather the asymmetry of figure–ground contrast. In order to study flux asymmetry alone one would need to remove the figure–ground contrast by gradually fading the rectangle into darkness in all directions. As one would predict from these findings, the visual straight ahead of hemianopics is displaced towards their 'good' side (Fuchs, 1920). It would be interesting to investigate whether the kinaesthetic straight ahead of hemianopics is similarly displaced.

It seems that the apparent straight ahead is affected, not only by an imbalance in the amount of contour, but also by asymmetry in the directions of the contours. Wapner and Werner (1955) used a display of three squares, each containing parallel lines; two adjacent squares with the lines running in the same direction, the third square with lines running at right angles to the lines in the other two (see figure 11.5). The subject fixated the centre of the middle

Figure 11.5 The test pattern used by Wapner and Werner (1955) to demonstrate the effect of visual asymmetry on the judgment of the straight ahead

square and moved the whole display until it appeared centred. When the third square was to the right of the two similar ones, the display was set further to the left than when the third square was to the left. The fact that in both conditions the display was moved to the right from the initial starting position, which was claimed to be symmetrical about the objective median plane, suggests that this difficult measurement was not done accurately; the experimenters did not give details of how the measurement was made. However, this is not a crucial point as the true median plane was not used as a baseline in the results. More important was the apparent omission of a fixation point at the true centre of the figure. This would have the effect of adding an additional component to the subject's task: he would have to select a point as the centre of the figure and then shift this point until it was straight ahead. Either or both of these components could be affected by the nature of the visual display, and Wapner and Werner's conclusion that only the second component was so affected may be unwarranted.

Werner and Wapner used the language of 'organismic theory' to discuss the displacement of the apparent straight ahead with asymmetric stimulation. They assumed that, 'Asymmetric stimulation arouses a tendency in the organism so to change its state that a more harmonious (symmetric) stimulus–organism relationship ensues.' This is merely to redescribe the actual findings in their own terminology. Such a description gives no insight into the mechanisms involved.

A precise mechanism has, however, been postulated by Bruell and Albee (1955b) in their motor theory of egocentric localization. They formulated two hypotheses. The first states that a fixated object is seen to one's right if fixation is maintained by voluntary innervation of the dextro-rotators: similarly, a fixated object is seen to one's left if fixation requires voluntary innervation of the laevo-rotators. The second hypothesis states that a fixated object is seen as straight ahead if fixation does not require voluntary innervation. They suggested that the pattern of voluntary oculomotor innervation at any time can be determined if certain assumptions are made. The first of these assumptions is that the fixation reflex causes eye turning towards objects in the periphery of the field of view. The second assumption is that when the eyes are turned out of the primary position, reflexes tend to restore them (see end of section 3.43). These hypotheses and assumptions were then applied to the analysis of the experimental results. With a stimulus extending into the left periphery of vision, there exists a reflex tendency to turn the eyes to the left, which the subject has to overcome voluntarily in order to maintain his central fixation. According to the first hypothesis, such voluntary innervation of the dextro-rotators results in the judgment that the fixated edge of the stimulus is to the right. The fixated part of the figure has to be moved to the left in order to be judged straight ahead, but this causes the eyes to move out of the primary position. Restoring reflexes become increasingly active until they cancel out the fixation reflex. At this point of 'reflex equilibrium', fixation of the right edge of the stimulus can be maintained without voluntary control and therefore, according to the second hypothesis, the fixated edge will be

judged straight ahead. The fact that the shift of the apparent straight ahead
was greater when the rectangle was wider, was explained by the assumption
that the strength of the fixation reflex is greater for more peripheral stimuli.
A further test of the theory would involve the use of intermittent flashes as
the interfering stimulus; these would presumably produce a stronger fixation
reflex, and therefore a larger displacement of the judged straight ahead.

11.32 Prismatic displacement of the visual straight ahead

We shall now consider the effects of wearing prisms which displace the
field of view to one side. Bossom and Held (1957) used prisms which displaced the field by 12° left or right. One set of subjects walked along a road
for 60 minutes. The other set of subjects were pushed along passively in a
wheelchair. Thus, while the visual stimulation was the same for both groups
of subjects, in the former case the sequence of visual stimulation was contingent upon self-produced motion, while in the latter case it was not. In
neither case were the subjects allowed to view their own bodies. All subjects
were asked to position a pointer to the straight-ahead position with the prisms
on. The prisms, of course, caused a 12° apparent shift of the field of view when
the prisms were first put on. The walking subjects showed about two degrees
of adaptation towards the true median plane after their 60 minutes experience
with the prisms. The passive group showed no adaptation. These results were
interpreted as supporting Held's theory that recovery of coordination following visual–motor disarrangement requires stimulation contingent upon
the self-produced movement of the subject. This viewpoint is derived from
von Holst's reafference principle (section 15.24). Excitation that is not contingent upon the voluntary movement of the subject is called exafference.
Held affirmed that, 'Reafference is necessary for the genesis and maintenance
of visual–motor coordination.'

It seems to us that Bossom and Held unwittingly biased their experimental situation in favour of their hypothesis. They provided little or no
possibility for exafferent information. They should have concluded that reafference is sufficient rather than necessary for visual–motor coordination.
There are three types of exafferent information which could indicate to a
subject that he is wearing displacing optical devices. Bossom and Held provided their subjects with none of these.

a. Intermodal discordance The first type of exafferent information is
provided when a person wearing an optical displacing device does not collide
with those objects which appear to him to lie directly in his path, while, on
the other hand, he does collide with objects which are objectively ahead but
appear off to one side. The road along which Bossom and Held wheeled their

subjects did not, it seems, provide opportunities for these discordant experiences. But even if it had, the prisms which were worn might not have given rise to such experiences. These prisms introduce an angular displacement: as an object approaches the subject, the linear difference between judged and actual position becomes reduced and is nil where the object touches the skin. Any discordant intermodal stimulation that results would depend on the remembered apparent position of the object when it was still some distance away. The discordant information which was available to Bossom and Held's subjects was the unusual progressive change in the apparent position of objects as they were approached.

If one wanted to study the role of this type of exafferent information in visual–motor adaptation, it would be necessary to introduce a parallel displacement of the visual axis; this may be done by using two parallel mirrors (see figure 15.5). Howard, Craske, and Templeton (1965) have conducted such an experiment, which is described in section 15.26. It was found that discordant exafferent information does produce some adaptation of pointing to the position of displaced targets.

b. Discordance between felt and seen body position The second type of exafferent information would be provided by allowing the subject to look at his own body or part of his body, which would appear to be displaced compared with its felt position. Bossom and Held deliberately excluded this information by not allowing the subjects to view their own bodies. See section 15.26 for a fuller discussion of this topic.

c. Visual-frame asymmetry The third possibility for exafferent information in this situation would be provided if a symmetrically placed viewing window were attached to the head. Such a window, seen through the parallel-mirror device or even through prisms, would appear asymmetrical. We have already cited evidence that the position of the apparent straight ahead is displaced by an asymmetrical figure in the field of view, thus suggesting that such a source of exafferent information could induce visual adaptation to displacing prisms. It is not known whether visual–motor adaptation results from such a source of information. This source of information is analogous to the apparent tilt of vertical lines seen through prisms which rotate the optical array. Failing to use such a window is analogous to wearing tilting prisms and looking at a world which is tilted so as to appear upright through the prisms. Bossom and Held did not provide such a window.

11.33 Figural properties of the stimulus and the apparent straight ahead

Werner and Wapner (1954) and Morant (1958) stressed the importance of what they called the 'dynamic vectorial quality' of the stimulus as a determinant of the apparent straight ahead. When a subject had to set the apex of a triangle to straight ahead with the apex pointing left, it was moved to the right of the true median plane. That is, the apparent straight ahead was displaced to the right, and this shift was found to be greater than the shift produced by a rectangular stimulus. Morant concluded that the apparent straight ahead is shifted in a direction opposite to that of the 'dynamic vectorial quality' of the figure.

Werner and Wapner (1954) admitted that their results were ambiguous. The triangles differed from the rectangle in shape as well as 'vector quality', and it may be that the results were a function of the shape differences, rather than any difference in perceived vectorial quality. Werner and Wapner overcame this ambiguity in a second experiment. They used as stimulus the following pattern,

which was judged to be either an aircraft or a bird, depending on which end of the pattern the subject was told to regard as the front. According to the dynamic vector quality hypothesis the expectation was, for example, that under 'bird' set, with the bird flying to the right, the apparent straight ahead would shift to the left. This prediction was supported by the evidence.

11.34 Non-visual stimulation and the apparent straight ahead

Labyrinthine stimulation, induced by a rotary acceleration of the body about its vertical axis, has been found to displace the apparent straight ahead in a direction opposite to the direction of acceleration. Deceleration from rotation in one direction is equivalent to acceleration in the opposite direction (Morant, 1958, 1959b; Graybiel and Hupp, 1946). Graybiel's opinion is that this apparent displacement is due to the apparent movement of the visible surroundings induced by the slow phase of the vestibular nystagmus. Morant argued that phenomenal displacement and phenomenal movement are two distinct effects and that nystagmus may be a sufficient but not a necessary condition for either. In support of this argument he reported that his subjects did not judge the visual target to be moving back and forth as he would have expected had nystagmus occurred. But we suggest that such a back-and-forth movement may not be what one would expect to result from nystagmus. The slow and quick phases of nystagmus are controlled by different neural centres, and it may be that there is compensatory stabilization for one phase but not for the other (see section 3.5). In further support of his contention

Morant cited an experiment by Christian (1939) in which an illusory movement was produced by rotary acceleration, but where it was demonstrated by
means of an acuity test that nystagmus did not occur. We suggest that if and
when apparent visual displacements occur in the absence of nystagmus, they
may be induced by the voluntary muscular activity which keeps the eye
steady against the nystagmic tendency. We have discussed these problems at
greater length in section 5.4.

Morant used a head rest, but not a bite. If his subjects moved their heads
to one side when being accelerated, this may have contributed to the apparent
displacement of the straight ahead. Chandler (1953) found that objects seen
moving induce head turning about a vertical axis in the same direction. There
is also evidence that head turning causes an apparent shift of straight ahead.
Werner, Wapner, and Bruell (1953) found that the apparent kinaesthetic
straight ahead shifted in the opposite direction to a turn of the head, with the
eyes kept straight in the head. The angle of head turning was not specified,
nor was there any mention of the method used to ensure that the eyes were
kept straight.

Akishige (1951) briefly reported that tilting the head in the sagittal plane
affected the variability of straight-ahead judgments.

Tilting the head or head and body to the side has been reported to shift
the apparent straight ahead in the opposite direction (McFarland, Werner,
and Wapner, 1962). In this experiment, the subject set a rod by hand to the
median plane with eyes closed. It is known that body tilt causes an apparent
tilting of a vertical rod; the top of the rod going to one side of the median
plane, the bottom to the other side. Perhaps the apparent shift of the straight
ahead in the above experiment was a function of the point of contact between
subject and rod. It was not stated what this point of contact was.

The position of the eyes has been found to affect the apparent position of
the visual straight ahead. With eyes to the right the apparent straight ahead is
shifted to the right (Fischer, 1915; Kiss, 1921; Goldstein and Riese, 1923;
Werner, Wapner, and Bruell, 1953). Werner et al. refer in their summing-up
to the results of an experiment which is not reported in the body of their
paper. These results showed that when the eyes were closed, the apparent
kinaesthetic median plane was shifted in the opposite direction to that in which
the eyes were turned. The first effect could result from a tendency to accept
the mid-point of the field of view as being straight ahead; the second effect
would be more difficult to explain.

Finally, it has been suggested that increased muscular tonus influences the
precision with which straight ahead is judged. Freilicher (1963) induced
symmetrical muscular strain or tonus in three ways: two base-out, 4° prisms
were worn so that the subject had to converge more than usual to maintain

binocular vision; the subject was given a seven pound weight in each hand; and finally he was subjected to a binaural tone. All three agents caused a reduction in the variability of settings of a vertical line to straight ahead. The symmetrically heightened tonus was interpreted as increasing the strength of the kinaesthetic cues to straight ahead. But it is possible that the increased tonus produced a general arousal of the subject via the reticular activating system.

The position of the apparent straight ahead has been found to be shifted towards the affected side in hemiplegic patients (Birch, Proctor, Bortner, and Lowenthal, 1960).

To sum up, judgments of the position of the straight ahead, whether made visually or manually, are influenced by a great many factors which may be grouped into two broad categories: visual asymmetry and proprioceptive asymmetry. However, experiments which have been done to reveal the influence of any one factor have usually been contaminated by unrecognized factors and by the ever-present problem of ambiguous instructions.

A special case of judgments of straight ahead is the judgment of the position of the vertical mid-body axis. It is of practical importance in several skills to be able to judge the position of the extension of the mid-body axis. For example, in diving one must aim the body axis at a particular point in space, or when putting on a hat, one must judge where the top of the head is. Any parent is familiar with the difficulty an infant has when first attempting to sit unaided on a stool—his difficulty stems from not having learned where his unseen posterior is pointing. As far as we know, no experimental work has been reported on this topic in the psychological literature.

11.4 The discrimination of right from left

11.41 Right–left discrimination in children

The ability to discriminate right from left is reflected in several diverse types of skill. A child may be said to have the capacity to discriminate right from left as soon as he can reach out with the appropriate hand to the side where there is a desired object. A hand preference for a particular task implies right–left discrimination. At a more complex level is the ability to copy the movements of another person who is facing the same way, and more difficult still is the task of copying the movements of a person who is facing the subject. Then there is the range of verbal skills associated with right–left discrimination. There is the ability to move or point to a named side of the body, and the related ability to name a touched part of one's own body or of the body of another person. An essential component of all these skills, especially the verbal ones, is the dissociation of the concept of right–left, which has an egocentric reference, from other spatial concepts, such as north and south, which have absolute spatial reference.

The five year old child of one of the authors could present her left hand when requested, but insisted that objects which had been on her left when she was facing one way, were still on her left when she was turned through 180°, and she became distressed when asked to reconcile this with the new position of her left hand. Here there was a confusion between the ego-reference concept, and the concept of a stable world. The child could not fit the two together. Very little work has been done on the development of right–left discrimination. Piaget (1926) reported that children learn to discriminate right from left on their own bodies by the time they are six years old, but it is not until they are eight years old that they are able to discriminate left from right on the bodies of other people. Piaget interprets this development as a growth away from egocentric thought, but the order of development surely follows from the fact that one has always the same relation to one's own body, but not to the bodies of other people. His findings were confirmed by Swanson and Benton (1955) who gave a test battery to 158 normal children between the ages of $5\frac{1}{2}$ and $9\frac{1}{2}$ years. The mean I.Q. of each age group was fairly constant. The child had to identify parts of his body with eyes open and with eyes closed; identify, with eyes open, parts on the front-view drawing of a boy; and carry out various 'crossed' commands with eyes open and with eyes closed. An example of a crossed command was, 'touch your right ear with your left hand'. The answers were scored according to the number of correct responses made, and also according to the consistency of discriminations disregarding the correctness of the response. If a child consistently pointed to the left of his body when asked to point to his right and vice versa, he was given an incorrect verbal score but a correct discrimination score. Such errors reflect only a verbal confusion and not any inability to discriminate. The six year olds scored just above chance, so that some learning must have occurred at an earlier age. Nearly perfect scores were obtained by the nine year olds. Both types of score showed the same age trend. There was no difference in performance between the eyes-open items and the eyes-closed items, but the own-body score was significantly superior to the pictured-body score. Swanson and Benton reported that some preliminary results from adult subjects indicate that performance in these tasks goes on improving after the age of nine.

The ability to make discriminatory movements in response to seen left–right asymmetries must surely develop before the ability to point to a given side in accordance with a verbal command or the ability to name a given side. Presumably the verbal learning requires that a good deal of operant learning has preceded it. If this is the case, then an operant training procedure should help in the development of correct verbal behaviour. Jeffrey (1958) put this idea to experimental test. One group of four year old children were shown two stick figures, one with its left arm raised and the other its right. The children had to learn to name one figure Jack and the other Jill. If they were correct, they were allowed to hear some pleasant music. A second group were given sandwiched training on pushing a button to indicate the direction of the raised arm of each doll. The second group showed evidence of positive transfer from the operant training to the labelling task. However, the results were not very striking, for the tasks were very easily learned in any case. A repeat of this kind of study, using more difficult tasks, would be worth while.

11.42 Right–left disorientation

Confusion between right and left occurs as a clinical symptom. It is most commonly reported in cases of damage to the parietal lobes (Rosenberg, 1912; Brain, 1941b). The confusions take one of two forms. In one form, the patient may display confusion when asked to indicate the right or left hand, or other part of his body, or of the body of another person, or of a drawing of a human body. Performance tends towards the level of chance, irrespective of the position of the stimulus. This form of confusion will be referred to as right–left disorientation. The other form of right–left confusion is known as allochiria. The patient will consistently report that a touch, applied to one particular side of the body, is located on the other side. Allochiria is a form of the more general condition known as allaesthesia or allacaesthesia in which a tactile stimulus is reported as being remote from its actual location. The term 'sensory displacement' has also been used to describe these conditions (Bender, 1952). We shall consider each of these forms of right–left confusion in turn.

Gerstmann (1927, 1930, 1940) and others before him (see Critchley, 1953) noticed that finger agnosia (inability to name or point to particular fingers), acalculia (deficiency in numerical ability), agraphia and right–left disorientation tend to occur together. This cluster of symptoms has become known as Gerstmann's syndrome. He regarded the finger agnosia and agraphia as the core symptoms, the others being described as 'bordering' symptoms which may not be present. These four symptoms seem to arise most commonly as a result of damage to the parietal lobe of the dominant cerebral hemisphere, which is usually the left hemisphere (Neilson, 1938), although right–left disorientation has been found associated with a frontal-lobe tumour (Pollock 1938).

That right–left disorientation is not a general verbal effect is suggested by the fact that it is specific to 'right' and 'left' and does not apply to 'up' and 'down' or 'behind' and 'in front'. Critchley argued further that it is not even a total inability to use the words 'left' and 'right', for in mild cases there is doubt as to the sidedness of external objects or persons but not as to the sidedness of parts of the self. The Gerstmann syndrome has been interpreted as a fundamental disorder of spatial ability and, more specifically, as a breakdown in the distinction between personal and extrapersonal space and in the ability to organize spatial experiences (Stengel 1944).

Strauss and Werner (1938) have studied the association of right–left discrimination and arithmetic ability in high-grade defective boys. They used a test battery which assessed both finger localization and right–left discrimination, and found a relationship between performance on this test battery and arithmetic achievement.

The suggestion that these four symptoms form a syndrome was challenged by Benton, Hutcheon, and Seymour (1951) and Benton (1955). They reviewed the literature and found reports of cases where each of the four component symptoms occurred without the others, and pointed out that the relative frequency of occurrence in adult cases of one, two, or three of these symptoms as compared with the frequency of all four together is not known. Until these relative frequencies are known, they argued, it cannot be claimed that the occurrence of the four together in some patients is due to anything other than chance. They also re-analysed Strauss and Werner's data and found that it did not in fact indicate any evidence of a strong association between arithmetic ability, left–right discrimination, and finger localization. The only significant relations which their own study of deficient children revealed were between agraphia and acalculia, and between right–left discrimination and finger localizing ability. They explained these associations by assuming a close proximity between the cortical centres responsible for the control of the various abilities, which increases the probability that they will be simultaneously affected by cerebral damage or disease. Critchley criticized this 'rather statistical conclusion'; he considered that negative cases 'only too often indicate inadequate examination, or even ignorance of what to look for'. However, Critchley must admit that clinicians may 'find' the symptoms they expect to find.

Juba (1948) and Benton and Abramson (1952) found that Gerstmann's syndrome tends to occur immediately after electro-shock therapy, and it is certainly a common experience that a trauma of any kind produces disorientation.

11.43 Allochiria

This condition is often associated with spinal pathology, usually of tabetic origin (Obersteiner, 1881). Where the cause is damage to the brain, a lesion in the parietal lobe is usually implicated. In such cases, there is no gross loss of somatic sensitivity and the general opinion is that allochiria results from a defect of the body-image, and is associated with unilateral neglect. Clinical observations reveal that tactile stimuli applied to the side of the body contra-lateral to the brain damage are felt as if they are on the normal side (Critchley, 1953). Sometimes voluntary movements in localizing a stimulus are affected, whereas reflex movements, such as are involved in scratching, are not.

An illustrative clinical case is provided by Bender, Shapiro, and Teuber (1949). The patient was a 52 year old man who manifested symptoms of progressive mental deterioration. Stimuli applied to the right side of the body were reported on the left for all cutaneous modalities, and sometimes in vision and audition. These symptoms cleared up for the head and legs, but remained for the arms and trunk. A strong painful stimulus was correctly localized but not a weak one. These differences reveal that the trouble was not basically a conceptual one, although he was unable to use the terms 'left' and 'right'; sodium amytal injected intravenously caused the allochiria to spread over the whole body. The patient showed a left-turning tendency in his motor be-haviour; his head was tilted to the left, he veered left in walking, and his writing was cramped to the left side of the paper. He was unable to point to any body structures on one side, and was unable to orient things in space, for instance his clothes when dressing (dressing apraxia).

We suggest the following neurological explanation of allochiria. Most sensory fibres decussate and terminate in the contralateral cerebral hemi-sphere, but it is known that not all sensory fibres decussate (Dusser de Bar-enne, 1913, 1935; Ray and Wolff, 1945); a proportion terminate in the ip-silateral hemisphere. If the brain is damaged on the left side, a stimulus applied to the right side of the body may produce more activity in the right, un-damaged hemisphere than in the left hemisphere. If we assume that a stimulus is localized according to which side of the brain registers the most activity, then it is clear that the above considerations will explain allochiria. One might expect, in rare cases, that there would be an even balance of ipsilateral and contralateral central activity engendered by an unilaterally applied stimulus. Such a stimulus would be felt as if it had been applied to both sides simultan-eously. Such cases have been reported; the condition has been called synchiria (Jones, 1907). If the fibres from one modality decussate more than those from another, allochiria may affect stimuli arising in the one modality but not the other. Halbrook and de Guitérrez-Mahoney (1947) reported a case of this kind in which pain stimuli were subject to allochiria and touch stimuli were not.

12

Orientation and shape I

12.1 Introduction

In this chapter we shall use the term 'shape' to mean the internal relations within a pattern which remain constant for different positions or orientations. There are two main questions to be distinguished, (a) the effects of shape on perceived orientation and (b) the effects of orientation on perceived shape.

With regard to the first question many things, such as trees, people, chairs, and words, and many geometric shapes, such as squares and pyramids tend to appear upright when they are in a particular orientation (i.e. are more or less strongly mono-oriented); while other objects such as scissors, match-boxes, and hands, do not have a logically favoured orientation (i.e. are polyoriented). Section 12.2 is concerned with the intrinsic features of shapes which determine their judged orientation.

Sections 12.3 and 12.4 explore the second main issue, the discrimination of shape as a function of its orientation, assuming that the observer and the visual frame are always upright. We shall consider the case where the task is to discriminate between a standard shape and a comparison shape. There are three ways in which orientation may be altered, and each may have a different effect on the responses of the subject. These three ways are (1) changes in the relative position of the two shapes in the visual field of the observer, in other words, changes in the direction of the line joining the centres of the two shapes (section 12.3), (2) changes in the absolute orientation of the standard and comparison shapes, the orientation of the shapes relative to one another being held constant, (3) changes in the orientation of the standard shape relative to the comparison shape (section 12.4).

If the discriminability of a shape is affected by its orientation we would want to know the relative contributions of disorienting the shape relative to, (1) the observer, (2) gravity, and (3) the visual frame. Section 12.5 is devoted to this problem. The developmental aspects of shape perception and orientation are considered in chapter 13.

12.2 Intrinsic axes used in the judgment of a shape's orientation

Before a shape can be reported as having a particular orientation there must be some recognizable axis in the pattern itself. There are three possible types of axis which could serve this purpose. We shall call them intrinsic axes, they are: (1) axes of symmetry or of greatest symmetry, (2) the directions of the main lines of the pattern, called here 'the main-line axes', and (3) axes between pairs of significant landmarks in a pattern, which will be called 'polar axes'. There has been no previous systematic attempt to isolate and compare these three types of axis. What literature there is will now be reviewed.

12.21 Axes of symmetry and main-line axes

A shape may have any number of axes of symmetry: an arrow has one, a square four, a circle an infinite number. Most solid objects have one plane of symmetry, that is, they are bilaterally symmetrical. It is difficult to find an object in an ordinary room which is not bilaterally symmetrical, and it is even more difficult to find a bilaterally symmetrical mono-oriented object which does not normally have its plane of symmetry upright. The principal reason for this is probably that objects designed in this way are most easily balanced.

Main-line axes are defined by the direction of the predominant lines in a pattern. They may be present in asymmetrical patterns. Where there is an axis of symmetry the main lines are usually parallel with it, but this is not always the case. For example, in figure 12.1 the axis of symmetry is at right angles to the main-line axis.

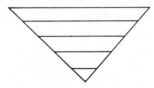

Figure 12.1 Illustrating how the main lines of a pattern may be at right angles to the axis of symmetry

Mach (1886) noted that a square looks like a diamond when stood on one corner. Here there are two distinct axes of symmetry to choose from, although in the 'square' position the impression of verticality is reinforced by the vertical–horizontal directions of the main lines.

The importance of bilateral symmetry as a stimulus variable has been stressed by Zusne and Michels (1962). It was by far the most important factor determining judgments of the geometricity, regularity, and familiarity of a large group of systematic distortions of a square. The forms of bilateral symmetry in decreasing order of potency were, symmetry along two axes with two pairs of equal angles (right angles), symmetry along two axes with two pairs of equal angles (any size) and, finally, symmetry along one axis with one pair of equal angles.

Goldmeier (1937) reported that shapes which were symmetrical about a vertical axis were judged more similar than shapes which were symmetrical about a horizontal axis. The Goldmeier effect was further investigated by Rock and Leaman (1963). They showed that the greater saliency of symmetry about the vertical axis obtains only when the axis is 'phenomenally' vertical and not necessarily retinally or even geographically vertical. There was a strong effect of symmetry about an axis which was judged vertical even when it was not vertical on the retina or not vertical relative to gravity. The effect disappeared when the axis of symmetry was an axis designated diagonal, by instructions, even though it was upright on the retina and, most strikingly, even when the axis of symmetry was both gravitationally vertical and vertical on the retina.

12.22 Polar axes

Many objects have features which distinguish one end from another. For instance, a tree has roots at one end and tapers towards the other, a person has a head and feet, and a knife has a blade and a handle. Such asymmetrical features will be called polar features and the axis joining a pair of them a polar axis. Some object, such as a tree or an arrow, have one main polar axis; a man and a car have two (top–bottom and front–back). An object can have no recognizable upside-down position, and cannot therefore be a mono-oriented object, unless it has at least one polar axis. For example, a square has no polar axis and, although it may appear tilted, it cannot appear upside-down. If a pattern has a single axis of symmetry and an important polar axis they will normally be coincident.

The basic question to be asked about polar axes is non-behavioural, viz. whether there are any general features of objects which have a consistent relationship to the directions 'up' and 'down'. 'Taper' is an example of such a polar feature, there are probably more objects which taper upwards than there are objects which taper downwards. Assuming there are such consistent relationships between general polar features and 'up' and 'down', a second question is whether people are influenced by them in their judgments of the orientation of shapes. If they are so influenced, a third question is to what extent this behaviour has to be learned.

There is some general evidence which suggests an affirmative answer to the first two questions. Arnheim (1954, p. 17) reported that adults judge the intended orientation of abstract paintings with significant consistency. Chou (1935) asked 142 Americans to judge the orientation of Chinese characters presented in several positions. About half of 312 abnormally oriented charac-ters were detected as being rotated. He suggested that his subjects were responding to constructional details which tend to be universally seen as upright.

Ghent (1961) independently arrived at a similar conclusion. Children between the ages of four and eight were presented with the 16 pairs of 'non-realistic shapes' shown in figure 12.2. The children had to say which member of each pair was upright. There was more agreement among the younger children than among the older ones. The preferred orientation for some of the forms changed with age, in some cases clearly because the older children recognized them as letters, for example V and Y. Ghent's description of the shapes as 'non-realistic' does not seem to be justified, several of the shapes were letters and others may have suggested particular objects to the children. Ghent appears to have made no attempt to find out whether this was so, although Antonovsky and Ghent (1964) found that other similar abstract

H.S.O.—20

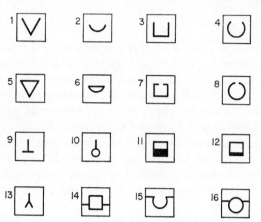

Figure 12.2 The 16 abstract shapes used by Ghent (1961) to study children's orientation preferences

shapes were consistently oriented by children in Iran in the same way as by children in America.

There has been no systematic attempt to indicate what general polar features of objects may be related to 'up' and 'down'. Some possibilities will now be considered.

a. Taper Many objects taper upwards. Objects which have a narrow base and a broad top often look top-heavy, unstable and upside-down. Goldstein and Andrews (1962) found that when asked to put abstract shapes upright, subjects tend to place the longest straight side horizontal and at the base, although some subjects balanced the shapes on a point.

b. The distribution of visual mass This factor is related to the factor of taper, but not invariably, since some objects, for example tables and water towers, are not tapered and yet have an uneven distribution of visual (and actual) mass. In these particular examples the main mass is at the top and yet they do not look unstable or upside-down when placed in their usual orientation. There may be a tendency for objects to be, and to look upside-down when their visual mass is predominantly high, but there are many exceptions to any such rule.

c. The light-intensity gradient Gradients of light intensity may be associated in a particular way with the experience of up and down. The way to test this would be to ask subjects to place in the upright position a rectangle of paper graded along its length from black to white.

d. The texture gradient. Under ordinary circumstances, objects can extend only about five feet below eye level. It follows that the apparent texture gradient due to perspective is often more extensive in the upward direction. This would tend to make a pattern with a real texture gradient look upright only when the smaller detail is at the top.

However, if one considers a visual scene as a whole, the lower part is usually crowded with objects while the upper part is mainly sky and relatively devoid of objects. The relation between the direction of texture gradients and the directions of up and down is therefore not a simple one.

e. Points of attachment If an object is attached at one end to a surface, then usually that end is lowest. In other words there are more objects which stick-up than there are objects which hang down.

f. Relative movement An object which is attached to its base is obviously more free to move at its top end than at its bottom end. A hanging object, on the other hand, is more free to move at its bottom end.

g. Reflex eye-movement tendencies Ghent (1961) suggested that the eye naturally first fixates the top of a picture, and also that fixation is attracted to centres of dominant detail. When the dominant detail is in the top of the picture, these two eye-movement tendencies are in harmony and the picture looks upright. When the dominant detail is in the bottom of the picture, the eye-movement tendencies are opposed and the picture looks upside-down. Ghent supported her suggestion that the eye scans from top to bottom, by pointing out that all written languages are read from top to bottom even though varying in all other respects.

In order to give experimental support to her theory Ghent presented children with 24 pairs of non-realistic shapes and asked them to choose the member of each pair which appeared upright. She found that if there was a focal point, such as a dot at one end of the pattern, then this end was chosen as the top. In another experiment Ghent, Bernstein, and Goldweber (1960) tested whether preferences still appear when eye movements are eliminated by exposing the figures for 1/25 sec. The preferred orientations were unaffected by this procedure. The authors concluded that the postulated eye-movement tendencies must involve 'an internal motor process facilitating perceptual activity in a particular sequence'. It would be more parsimonious to account for the fact that children prefer dominant detail in the top of a pattern by reference to the many common objects which have dominant detail at the top. Children would generalize from their experience with the familiar shapes to the meaningless shapes. However, without additional assumptions neither theory can account for Ghent's finding that these preferences decline and alter with age.

It may be concluded that axes of symmetry, the directions of the main lines, and the polar features of patterns serve as indices for judgments or the orientation of shapes. If a shape is not vertical with respect to these axes the evidence suggests that it will be recalled or reproduced as more vertical than it was (see section 12.24).

We shall conclude this section with a short discussion of the problem of right–left polarity in art.

12.23 Right–left polarity in art

Claims have been repeatedly made that the mirror-images of many pictures do not look as artistically correct as their originals. Faistauer (1926) stressed the symbolic qualities of the left and right sides of a picture. The left side was said to be the near, 'home-side'; the right side the far, 'foreign-side'. Schlosser (1930) related differences between the left and right halves of a picture to laterality.

Wölfflin (1941) suggested that in looking at a picture, the eye scans from left to right and that therefore most important detail should be in the right-hand part of the picture. Keller (1942) supported Wölfflin's theory and claimed that in European art, moving objects enter from the left. She at first put these differences down to the preponderance of right-eyedness but later discovered that in Eastern art moving objects usually enter from the right.

Gaffron (1950) pointed out that all previous theorists had ignored the three-dimensional aspect of pictures. She suggested that the 'glance curve' starts at the near left, then goes to the back of the 'space' in the picture and at the same time moves over to the right. A change to the mirror-image arrangement of a picture was said to apparently shift the position of the spectator relative to the centre of the picture. This was said to be because the spectator tends to locate himself at the starting point of the glance curve. Objects in the path of the glance curve were said to stand out. Objects in other positions have to be sought out by secondary eye movements. Other 'deductions' of a similar kind were made from the direction of the glance curve with illustrated examples provided. It is impossible to view these illustrations without bias once one has read Gaffron's theories, yet before one has read the theories one does not know what to look for. No experimental data are provided by any of the writers in this field and until such evidence is given the theories remain merely interesting speculations.

12.24 The uniqueness of the vertical orientation

The vertical position of an abstract object seems to have a special significance in perception when the object has an axis of symmetry. Bakay and

Schiller (1948) asked 100 adult subjects to examine a row of 65 cards upon each of which was mounted a figure. Some of these were single patterns, others consisted of two parts which could be put together to give a single symmetrical figure. The subjects were asked to adjust each figure in any way they wished. It was found that the figures with an axis of symmetry were usually arranged with this axis vertical. When two parts of a figure were united into a symmetrical pattern there was a conflict between the direction of the axis of symmetry and the direction of the join between the two parts which consituted a main-line axis. Two-thirds of the subjects righted the axis of symmetry and one-third the join. On the other hand, Zusne and Michels (1962) showed that judgments of the geometricity, regularity, or familiarity of a large group of shapes were unaffected by rotations in the frontal plane.

We shall show in section 12.41 that shapes which are vertically symmetrical, are attended to in preference to shapes which are not.

There is considerable evidence to show that shapes which have their main axes tilted tend to be reproduced in a vertical orientation. When abstract shapes are exposed in a tilted position they tend to be recalled as upright (Perkins, 1932; Hanfmann, 1933). Similarly, horizontally symmetrical shapes are sometimes reproduced in a vertically symmetrical position whereas vertically symmetrical figures are always recalled in their correct position (Takala, 1951b). Radner and Gibson (1935) also reported a verticalizing effect using squares and nonsense shapes, but they discovered that when the subjects were instructed to note the tilt the reproductions were even more tilted than the originals. It was suggested that, with respect to orientation, a percept tends to occur at its 'perceptual centre', but that when a percept is experienced as being off-centre, the eccentricity tends to be exaggerated. Gibson and Radner must have meant by 'perceptual centre' the vertical–horizontal orientation of the main lines of the pattern, as most of their shapes had no symmetry (see figure 12.3).

A tendency to symmetry in children's drawings was shown by Hanfmann (1933) when she asked children to put a chimney on a drawing of a house. They usually placed it symmetrically on the apex of the roof.

12.3 The discrimination of shapes and their relative position in the field of view

12.31 Basic facts

It has been shown that an English word is more easily recognized in tachistoscopic presentation when it is to the right rather than to the left of the fixation point (Mishkin and Forgays, 1952). Jewish subjects who normally

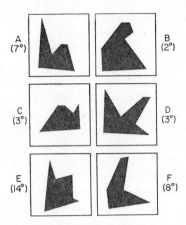

Figure 12.3 The abstract shapes used by Radner and Gibson (1935) to study the effect of tilt on the reproduction of shapes

read Hebrew, which is written from right to left, recognize words which are on the left more easily. Bilingual subjects recognize English words best when they are on the right and Hebrew words when they are on the left, although Orbach (1952) reported that bilingual subjects show this response pattern only when they have learned Hebrew first and English later.

These facts led Mishkin and Forgays to conclude that training establishes a more efficient neural organization in the visual area of one hemisphere. They realized that any such localized learning in the cortex contradicts Lashley's theory of equipotentiality. They admitted that in normal reading the right side of the eye does not 'see' more words than the left side and that it is therefore necessary to postulate a complex attention mechanism to account for the difference which they postulated. This theory amounts to saying that the attention span for a given fixation is asymmetrical about the fixation point for certain material.

Heron (1957) further stressed these difficulties in Mishkin and Forgay's theory and cited a number of experiments in which single letters were more easily recognized, not on the right, but on the left (Glanville and Dallenbach 1929; Crosland, 1931; and several German studies, discussed by Woodworth, 1938, p. 742 f). Similarly, in apparent contrast to the findings of Mishkin and Forgays, Anderson (1946) had reported that bilingual subjects recognize more English letters to the left, and more Hebrew letters to the right of the fixation point. In this latter study there were letters simultaneously on both sides of the fixation point, whereas Mishkin and Forgays had shown letters on only one side at a time. Heron realized that this was the key to the apparent contradiction and demonstrated in an experiment of his own that single letters or words are recognized more easily on the left when there are letters simultaneously on both sides of the fixation point (a law confirmed by L'Abate, 1960), but that when letters or words are presented on only one side then those on the right are more easily recognized. In addition Forgays (1953) found no significant hemifield differences with successive presentation of letters to right or left, a result later to be confirmed by Dyer and Harcum (1961) for simultaneous presentation of binary patterns of filled and unfilled ellipses.

All this evidence suggests that this dependence of recognition on position may be closely connected with the behaviour patterns utilized in reading. Anderson and Crosland (1933) and Harcum (1957a, 1957b) proposed such an explanation which is supported by Heron's finding that when letters are arranged in the form of a square the frequency of recognition decreases from the top-left position, through top-right, bottom-left, to bottom-right.

Lincoln and Averbach (1956) and Mudd and McCormick (1960) found that in searching an array of dials for one which showed a deviant reading, subjects showed progressively increasing errors as the target was varied from the upper-left, through upper-right and lower-left to the lower-right quadrant. This represents the scanning sequence using actual eye movements which is analogous to the post-exposure scanning sequences discussed in this section.

In the tachistoscopic experiments discussed here, there is not sufficient time for actual eye movements to occur. Heron accordingly assumed that the subject attends to the material sequentially. This attentional scanning process was said to take place in the period during which the after-image is visible when the exposure is brief. It was said to proceed from left to right in response to English verbal material. He deduced that when there is verbal material on both sides of the fixation point more letters are seen on the left than on the right, in the brief period before the after-image fades. When there is a word or letter on the left side only, the subject has to take his attention to the left before he starts to scan the word or letter from left to right. But when there is a word or letter on the right side only, he can scan it directly. Thus single letters or words are more easily seen on the right. When the subject is told on which side the stimulus will be shown, recognition of words or letters on the left is facilitated, whereas those on the right are unaffected. The subject attending to the centre of his field is already in the optimal position for scanning material on his right, but if he knows the material will be on the left he can adjust his attention to the left.

Terrace (1959) suggested that the subjects in Heron's experiment were set to perceive verbal material and that this factor should be controlled before it could be concluded that the results are due to sequential attention activity in the after-image period rather than to differences in preparatory set. He therefore used a series in which words were mixed at random with an equal number of nonsense geometric forms. These stimuli were presented singly to either left or right at random. Twenty-nine out of his 30 subjects recognized the words more readily on the right and Terrace concluded that Heron's theory was upheld.

It is difficult to see why Terrace expected his procedure to destroy the set for verbal material, since the subjects still had a 50% expectancy of verbal material. It seems, however, that the procedure did have the desired effect, for it is clear from Terrace's results that the nonsense material was not more easily recognized on the right, which it presumably would have been had the subjects been set to perceive verbal material.

Kimura (1959) reported the same order of recognizability for geometric forms arranged in a square, as Heron had reported for letters: top-left, top-right, bottom-left, bottom-right. So it is clear that under some conditions at least, the scanning habits of reading are applied to non-verbal material and hence, presumably, Heron's thesis that the first element in the process is identification of the type of material presented, does not hold.

The most recent restatement of the post-exposure scanning hypothesis (Harcum, 1964) is based on the earlier work already discussed, together with a long series of experiments carried out by Harcum and his colleagues, using for the most part linear binary sequences composed of filled and unfilled circles. This theory postulates two hypothetical constructs to explain the typical error distributions found, a sensitivity factor and perceptual scan factor.

12.32 The sensitivity factor

Harcum's sensitivity factor, which tends to produce a maximum of errors for the north–south meridian and a minimum for the east–west meridian (Harcum, 1958a), is related to, but not identical with, retinal sensitivity as usually measured: errors tend to increase with distance from the fixation point but are even more affected by the position of an element relative to other elements in the pattern (Harcum and Rabe, 1958b). In this connection it is interesting that in the same study it was found that patterns produce fewer errors when they are perpendicular to a retinal radius, a finding which confirms the visual acuity results of Higgins and Stultz (1948) (see section 2.61).

The sensitivity may also depend on which eye, which side of the retina, and which hemisphere is stimulated. The differences in vividness of stimuli in the right and left halves of the visual field demonstrated by Dallenbach (1923), Burke and Dallenbach (1924), and White and Dallenbach (1932) were related to handedness, stimuli presented to the non-dominant cerebral hemisphere being more vivid. Harcum and Dyer (1962) used ten-element binary patterns bisected by the fixation point, and showed that with monocular viewing there was an effect of viewing eye only for the few subjects who did not show a marked left-superiority in the binocular-viewing condition: for these subjects the left eye showed a left-superiority and the right eye a right-superiority, in line with Sloan's (1947) demonstration of a greater sensitivity of the nasal retina.

The other variable studied by Harcum and Dyer was a reduction of the black–white contrast on one side of the fixation point. Such a reduction on the right enhances the original left-superiority whereas a similar reduction of the left largely nullifies it and even, in the case of subjects without an original left-superiority, produces a right-superiority.

For right-handed subjects the alleged superiority of the non-dominant hemisphere is of course confounded with a learned left-field primacy based on the directionality of written English, and Harcum and Dyer conclude that this latter effect, if well established, can overcome other factors such as eye or hemisphere dominance, which may otherwise be important.

Harcum and Rabe (1958c) used eight-element patterns of filled circles and squares, instead of the usual filled and unfilled circles. In this case the east–west meridian had the lowest error rate, but there were no consistent differences between the left and right halves of the field. It was thought that this lack of hemifield differences might obscure true hemifield differences which were in opposite directions for different subjects, and that these differences might depend on varying sensitivities of the nasal and temporal halves of the dominant eye. This suggestion was not, however, confirmed in an experiment using the circles and squares and presenting them to each eye alone (Harcum, 1958f).

Bryden (1964) summarized the results of several experiments in which material was randomly presented in either the left or the right visual field and performance was related to the subjects' handedness. The data showed a tendency for single letters to be more readily analysed in the hemisphere in which speech is represented. With multiple-letter stimuli, however, the effect of cerebral dominance is overridden by highly learned directional reading habits.

The question of cerebral differences in recognition has been most intensively studied by Wyke and Ettlinger (1961) who found that outline drawings of familiar objects had a higher recognition threshold when presented on the left of the fixation point, irrespective of whether the right and left figures were presented successively or simultaneously. This result appears to conflict with those of Heron and Bryden but Wyke and Ettlinger point out that the earlier workers were using exposures well above threshold, and were presenting *series* of letters, words or figures rather than single objects; these differences could have facilitated the operation of left–right reading habits which would otherwise be absent.

Wyke and Ettlinger ruled out attention differences as an explanation of their results since, with simultaneous presentation, even after the right-hand object had been identified it often took many more exposures for recognition of the left-hand one. They concluded that the results probably indicate a better visual acuity in the right half of the binocular field, an hypothesis which has apparently never been directly investigated but which is opposed by the implications of the results discussed above. They point out that such a difference need not be retinal but could arise from a greater activation of the left (dominant) cerebral cortex. Hubel and Wiesel (1959) showed that contralateral (nasal) afferent projections activate more striate cortical units than do ipsilateral (temporal) projections. Nor are the two eyes usually equally effective in producing cortical arousal. Hence greater arousal in the left hemisphere could result from a combination of dominance of the right eye and dominance of nasal over temporal projection.

That this differential modulation of transmission may be sited in the geniculate body is suggested by the results in Wyke and Ettlinger's experiment of a patient with a right-anterior temporal lesion impinging on the geniculo-calcarine tract. The normal right–left difference in recognition shown by this patient was greatly inflated in the case of simultaneous presentation: the left-hand pictures required exposures 200 times longer with simultaneous bilateral presentation than when they were presented alone. In this case a marked preponderance of left-occipital activation during bilateral stimulation could be accounted for if the lesion interfered with geniculate transmission on the right side.

12.33 The perceptual scan factor

The other factor postulated by Harcum is the perceptual mechanism which 'reads' the trace while it is decaying. This factor, unlike the sensitivity factor, would not produce any net effect on whole meridians, but if the scanning is laterally sequential then hemifield differences in recognizability would be expected on all meridians except the null, north–south meridian (Harcum, 1957a, 1958c, 1958h)—indeed, if there was a tendency to scan downwards rather than upwards we might expect even a north–south difference and it has occurred in some experiments (e.g. Harcum, 1957b).

Whether or not such a sequential analysis is required may depend on certain characteristics of the task, such as length of pattern, difficulty, and the degree of practice of the subjects. In the case of difficulty, there is an obvious interaction with the sensitivity factor. As already reported, Harcum and Rabe (1958c) used eight-element patterns of filled circles and squares instead of the usual filled and unfilled circles. In this case the east–west meridian had, as usual, the lowest error rate, but there were no consistent differences between the left and right halves of the field. This last result may have been due to decreased difficulty of the task because of greater discriminability of the elements from their background.

A further experiment by these authors (1958a) suggested that the half-meridional differences might be reduced by practice. That this may have been due to redundancy in the patterns is suggested by the failure to confirm the decrease of differences in a later experiment (Harcum, Filion, and Dyer, 1962) in which the binary pattern for each exposure was selected at random. If recognition of one half of the pattern were sufficient to delimit the pattern, then on later trials performance in both hemifields would depend on the acuity of the superior field. Such an interpretation would imply that the perceptual scanning process involves the use of redundancy. In order to test this interpretation Miller and Harcum (1963) presented ten-element binary patterns with the two five-element halves identical, and fixation at the midpoint of the pattern. When subjects were switched from this task to one in which the redundancy was eliminated by having the two halves of the targets different, there was no increase in error rate, despite the fact that the instructions led the subjects to expect redundancy. This discrepancy remains a puzzle and Harcum is at present unable to account for it (private communication).

Harcum (1958d) found that the primary difference between the left and right halves of the field could be ironed out if the length of pattern was reduced from ten to eight, suggesting that when more than eight elements are exposed, selective aspects of the perceptual mechanism first come into play. That this effect was truly dependent on number of elements, and not on angular size of display was confirmed in a later experiment (Harcum, 1958e).

If a pattern is long enough or difficult enough to require the involvement of Harcum's scanning factor, then the direction of scanning will be largely determined by the reading habits and other characteristics of the subject, by set, and by directional characteristics of the stimuli.

Harcum (1958g) hypothesized that if the typical pattern of differences in error rate was produced by the reading history of the subject, then it should become more marked if the binary sequences were composed of letters rather than meaningless shapes. Accordingly, patterns composed of the letters 'H' and 'O' were used. The expected difference in error rate between the north–south and east–west meridians occurred, but no half-meridian was different from the opposite half-meridian. Harcum accounted for this failure to confirm his hypothesis by presenting evidence that the subjects saw the stimuli merely as patterns and not as letters.

On the other hand, the assumption that the directionality of the post-exposure scanning process is partly determined by the inherent directionality of the stimuli was confirmed by Bromleigh (1961). He used eight-letter nonsense words presented symmetrically about the fixation point and consisting of either symmetrical letters (H, M, T, V, W, X, Y) or asymmetrical letters (B, G, J, K, N, R, S). Although all words produced a left-superiority of reproduction, the differential was greater in the case of the words consisting of asymmetrical letters. This assumed facilitation of the left–right scanning process by the inherent directionality of the stimulus elements also resulted in an overall reduction of errors at each letter position.

An obviously related question is whether scanning is from left to right as such or is from the beginning to the end of the word. In an extension of Mishkin and Forgay's work, Finkel and Harcum (1962) found that the mirror images of words were more easily recognized when presented on the *left* of the fixation point. In this case the primary scanning away from the fixation point corresponds with scanning from beginning to end of the word. Harcum and Filion (1963) and Harcum and Smith (1963) found similar effects of reversing the orientation of individual letters or the sequence of letters in a word; the effects were most marked when subjects had prior knowledge of the nature of the patterns to be reproduced. Like Bromleigh's these results suggest that the scanning depends on the directional characteristics of the stimuli.

Bryden (1960) suggested that the order of recognizability of letters and other shapes results from subjects' reporting of the items in a row from left to right. By the time the items on the right are reported, the memory trace has faded somewhat and so those items will be less accurately recalled. The results of his experiments show that subjects do in fact report rows of items from left to right. This theory has the advantage of being more closely tied to observable events.

Bryden asked subjects to report a row of items from right to left instead of from left to right. When the subjects did this, the order of recognizability for non-verbal shapes was the reverse of what it had been with left-to-right reporting. The order for the letters, however, remained unchanged. Bryden explained this result with letters by assuming that the visual memory trace for letters is 'polarized' and that before a subject can report from right to left he must create an auditory image of the letters by repeating them to himself in the usual order. During this process letters on the right tend, as usual, to be forgotten first. The auditory image for letters is not polarized and may thus be reported either way. The introspective evidence supported this interpretation.

Harcum (1962) found that the hemifield differences persisted to some extent, even when the task was one of recognition rather than recall and the effects of direction of reproduction were therefore precluded. Ayres and Harcum (1962) investigated more fully the effects of forcing the subjects to report the material in various sequences. They concluded that although differential recall contributes to hemifield differences, there is also an effect due to differences in the strength of the memory trace between the two halves of the field. They had their subjects reproduce in different conditions the ten-element binary patterns either from left to right or from right to left or from the centre out, or, finally, in any manner they chose; instruction as to required mode of reproduction was given simultaneously with the exposure. The obtained correlation between chosen direction of reproduction and the distribution of errors (almost all subjects *chose* to reproduce from left to right) was attributed to the sequential perceptual mechanism, which caused left elements to be more accurately perceived and also to be reproduced first.

It is still possible, however, that even when they did not know the required direction of reproduction the subjects may have had a consistent set to reproduce in one direction and this might facilitate actual reproduction in that direction and conflict with reproduction in the other direction. Harcum, Hartman, and Smith (1963) controlled for this possibility by comparing performance with and without pre-exposure knowledge of the required direction of reproduction. Like Ayres and Harcum they found that although error distribution was affected by required reproduction direction, right–left reproduction was not sufficient to produce a right-superiority though it tended to cancel the left-superiority of other conditions. Prior knowledge of the required direction tended to strengthen the effect of the direction itself and, in the case of right-to-left reproduction, was strong enough to create an actual right-superiority. They concluded that the effects of responding sequence cannot alone account for the hemifield differences.

Another possible weakness not only in the Ayres and Harcum study but also in most others in this area is the assumption that the subjects are fixating on the fixation point at the moment of exposure. Harcum, Hartman, and Smith attempted to control fixation more tightly by having a small faint light which alternated on and off, and the subject could produce the next exposure only when it was on. This did not affect the results and they themselves admitted that it is not a very satisfactory method of controlling fixation. In any case, by systematically varying the position of the fixation point in the series, Camp (1961) has shown that it can be moved at least one element position without affecting the error distribution. A similar conclusion is reached by Harcum (1958b) and Harcum and Rabe (1958b).

We have already noted Anderson's (1946) study in which he showed that bilinguals recognize more Hebrew letters on the right of fixation and more English letters on the left when letters from a single language are presented simultaneously on both sides of fixation. Harcum and Friedman (1963) criticized Anderson's study on the grounds that when material from languages of different directionality is presented to bilingual observers, it is difficult to extricate the directional perceptual tendencies of the subject from the intrinsic directionality of the languages. They presented subjects whose first language was Hebrew with non-linguistic sequences of open and closed circles and compared the results with those of similar experiments by Ayres and Harcum (1962) and Harcum, Hartman, and Smith (1963) carried out on American subjects. In this experiment the subjects did not know until the actual moment of exposure whether they had to reproduce the elements from right to left, from left to right or whether they had a free choice. In a comparable situation, American subjects, when given a free choice, reproduced predominantly from left to right whereas the Israelis chose in general to reproduce from right to left. The Israelis also showed predominant right-superiority irrespective of the specified direction, just as the Americans had shown a left-superiority even when reproducing from right to left. Hence, Harcum and Friedman arrive at the same conclusion as Anderson, viz. that the directionality typically imposed on visual material is culturally determined, as is the preferred direction of reproduction of such material.

Harcum (1958e) and Camp (1960) found consistent error patterns in reproducing ten-element binary displays associated with fixation at either extreme (i.e. successive presentation) or in the middle (i.e. simultaneous presentation). With fixation on the extreme left there were fewer errors in the left half of the pattern and this distribution was maintained to a less marked degree for central fixation. With fixation on the extreme right, on the other hand, errors were fewer on the right half of the pattern. Accordingly Camp (1961) predicted that with fixation at some point between centre and extreme right there should be an error distribution symmetrical about the centre of the pattern. When the subjects had to reproduce the patterns by filling in appropriate circles in a series of ten outline circles without reference to the fixation point, the fixation position giving a symmetrical distribution of errors about the centre of the pattern was on the extreme right. When the response templates consisted of twenty outline circles, which subjects had to fill in the correct position relative to a centrally marked fixation point, the point of symmetry actually occurred at central fixation. Both these results contradict the pattern shown in previous work and Camp concluded that the two conditions used bracket the situation in which confirmation would be obtained for his hypothesis of a symmetrical distribution for a fixation somewhere between centre and extreme right. This experiment demonstrates that this sort of behaviour is closely dependent on the details of the reproduction procedure and not only on the required direction of reproduction.

Another aspect of the situation was altered by Harcum and Blackwell (1958) who changed the task from one of reproducing a pattern to one of estimating the number of filled circles in eight-element binary patterns, one of which was presented on each side of the fixation point. They found that this had little effect on the distribution of errors; the north–south meridian still had the highest error rate, and, although differences between opposing half-meridians were not significant, there was a tendency for errors to be greater in the right half of the field. There was also an unexplained tendency to overestimate the number of filled circles in patterns lying in southeast, south, or southwest directions, but to underestimate in all other directions.

12.34 Conclusion

Harcum suggests that most of the results in this area can be interpreted as the effect of the balance between the two hypothesized mechanisms, the sensitivity factor and the perceptual scanning mechanism. That this latter mechanism may be similar to the one which produces the typical serial rote-learning curve is suggested by Harcum and Hartman (1961). They found that the error distribution was different depending on whether a particular space contained a filled or an unfilled circle. This was presumably due to the relative dominance of the sensitivity factor and when this was removed the distribution showed good agreement with the serial rote-learning curve.

Some results suggest that recency as well as primacy may be an important factor which ought to appear in any comprehensive theory. For example, Dyer and Harcum (1961) found that in children the hemifield difference which appeared with reading experience consisted of a *right* superiority in the recognition of binary patterns presented simultaneously to right and left. This unexpected result they attributed to a dominance of recency over primacy in young children. This point is further strengthened by the work of Friedman (1961) who presented ten-element binary patterns symmetrically about the fixation point. The elements of the pattern were presented either simultaneously or in one of various spatio-temporal sequences. The exposure time for the whole pattern or for a single element was 1/8 sec. Inspection of the data suggested that the subjects were left-to-right scanners—when all a pattern's elements were exposed simultaneously errors fell progressively from right to left across the pattern. However, when the elements were successively presented one by one from right to left there were no more errors than when they were presented from left to right, suggesting that the primacy effect does not dominate over a recency effect. The fact that simultaneous presentation of all elements for 1/8 sec produces fewer errors than successive presentation suggests that the sequential scanning process operates more rapidly than the presentation rate of this experiment. The difference in error rate between right and left sides was greatly reduced when the elements were presented one by one in random order.

Any interpretation of these results is dependent on the assumption that central fixation was maintained throughout ten successive 1/8 sec exposures during which the fixation point was not shown; an eighth of a second is ample time for the fixation reflexes which would be induced by the exposure of the single target elements. In addition, no statistical analysis of the data was presented.

The relationship between eye movements and hemifield differences in recognizability has been studied by Bryden (1961). He found no relationship between the direction and extent of eye movements and individual differences in the order of recognizability for rows of items. Nor was there any relationship over subjects between eye movements in the immediate post-exposure period and the order of recognizability. However, Bryden did find that intra-individual differences in recognizability did correlate with eye movements. Such a relationship was also found by Crovitz and Daves (1962). Using an electro-oculographic eye-movement recording technique, they found that the first post-exposure eye movements tended to be to the side where numbers were reported most accurately. The latency of the eye movements was about 150 msec. Crovitz and Daves could not say whether the eye movements caused the differences in recognizability or whether they were the result of such differences.

12.4 The discrimination of shapes and their orientation with respect to an upright observer

In this section we shall be concerned with the problem of how the ability to compare two shapes is affected by the absolute and relative orientations of the shapes. The problem can be analysed into several logically distinct questions although these questions have not in general been distinguished in the literature.

(a) With no difference in orientation between the shapes, what is the effect of their absolute orientation? (Section 12.41.)

(b) With a fixed difference in orientation between the shapes, what is the effect of their absolute orientation? (Section 12.42.)

(c) How is discrimination affected by changes in the orientation of the shapes relative to each other? (Section 12.43.)

(d) Does the effect of relative disorientation depend on the absolute orientation of a particular one of the stimuli? For example, if the answer to question (a) shows a particular favoured absolute orientation, does this apply to the comparison or the standard stimulus, or both? (See p. 316.)

(e) Do the answers to the previous questions depend on the type of shape used? (Section 12.44.)

(f) Do the answers to the previous questions depend on whether 'orientation' refers to gravitational, egocentric, or visual-frame axes? (Section 12.5.)

We shall now consider the available evidence within the framework of these questions.

12.41 Absolute orientation

Question (a) asks, with no difference in orientation between the shapes, what is the effect of their absolute orientation? Two studies have been reported which, while they do not fall easily into the framework of our series of questions, nevertheless serve to underline the importance of certain absolute orientations. Superior detection of vertically symmetrical components of complex figures was reported by Takala (1951b). The subjects were shown a simple shape and asked to locate it in a complex pattern. Figure 12.4 shows one example of such a model and complex pattern. The model was always presented at 45° to the vertical. There were in fact four sub-figures in each pattern which were congruent with the model, two symmetrical about a vertical axis and two symmetrical about a horizontal axis. Takala found that his subjects were able to find more figures which were vertically symmetrical than figures which were horizontally symmetrical. On the basis of the single published stimulus figure, it could be argued that the results could equally well demonstrate a preference for horizontal over vertical main-line axes or for figures at the top and bottom, rather than the sides of a picture. The first possibility was eliminated in a subsidiary experiment; the second remains a possibility. We cannot therefore accept without reservation Takala's conclusion that his results were due to differences between vertical and horizontal symmetry.

Goldhamer (1934) found that the plus cross in the ambiguous pattern of a Rubin cross was the one which stood out as the figure most of the time.

Since both alternatives had vertical axes of symmetry, this study seems to demonstrate a superior discrimination of patterns with horizontal and vertical main-line axes.

Several studies have confirmed a suggestion by Bühler (1913) that differences between shapes are more readily reproduced when the shapes are

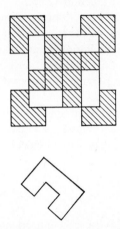

Figure 12.4 One of the embedded-figure patterns used by Takala (1951b). The model is embedded in the complex pattern in four positions

vertically oriented. Hanfmann (1933) found that children between the ages of four and eight copied equilateral triangles most accurately when they were presented in a vertically symmetrical orientation i.e. with base horizontal. There were more errors when the triangles had one side vertical. When the base was at 45° the error rate was highest of all and the triangles tended to be reproduced in the vertically symmetrical position. Similarly, it has been shown that subjects can detect deviations from isoscelesity with greater sensitivity when the base of the triangle is horizontal, although this effect appears only in conditions of brief exposure (Takala, 1951b, p. 66).

Fitts, Weinstein, Rapaport, Anderson, and Leonard (1956) generated patterns by selecting random numbers and filling in columns of an eight by eight matrix. Each of the patterns so generated had one continuous straight side and the lines were all at right angles to each other. Some of the patterns were duplicated in mirror-image form and the two parts made into a single symmetrical pattern. Figure 12.5 shows one such symmetrical pattern. They had their axis of symmetry vertical or horizontal. Other patterns were asymmetrical. The subjects had to pick out as quickly as possible, from an array of 48 patterns, those which were identical, both in shape and orientation, to a test pattern which had been exposed for two seconds. It was found that patterns which were symmetrical about a vertical axis were more quickly recognized than either asymmetrical patterns or patterns symmetrical about a horizontal axis. This result was explained by reference to the predominant daily occurrence of shapes which have a vertical axis of symmetry.

Figure 12.5 One of the randomly generated patterns used by Fitts *et al.* (1956) to study the influence of the orientation of the axis of symmetry on the discriminability of a pattern

Ghent and Bernstein (1961) presented children aged between three and five years with an array of abstract shapes such as the one shown in figure 12.6. Those shapes not marked with a cross were briefly exposed, one at a time, on the circle in the centre of the array. On each trial the stimulus figure was either upright or inverted. (The criterion for choosing the figures to be used was that they were selected as upright when in a particular orientation

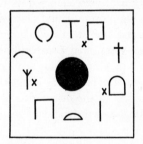

Figure 12.6 One of the arrays of multiple-choice figures used by Ghent and Bernstein (1961) to study the influence of orientation on recognition. The figures are shown here in their 'upright' orientation

by at least 80% of children in an earlier experiment.) The exposure was too brief to allow the children to recognize the shapes correctly on every occasion. They had to identify the shape which had been exposed, from among the array, taking as much time as they wished. The experiment was thus focused on the registration of the image rather than the actual recognition. It was found that performance was better when both the stimulus figure and the comparison figure were upright than when they were both inverted. This suggests an effect of absolute orientation but when we pass to question (d) we find that the orientation of the comparison figure is irrelevant; perform- ance was always better when the first-presented, standard figure was up- right than when it was inverted, irrespective of the orientation of the com- parison figure. This ineffectiveness of the comparison figure's orientation presumably stemmed from the fact that the children had been set in a training session to expect the figures to be in different orientations, and the fact that they had unlimited time to make the judgment.

Thus it seems that the upright figures were more adequately registered. Ghent and Bernstein pointed out that the focal area of a figure was invariably at the top and, if scanning is predominantly downwards from the focal area (see our discussion of Ghent's eye-movement theory in section 12.22) then the upright figures will be more adequately scanned. The children had not seen the shapes before and Ghent claimed that it would be unreasonable to suggest that these results could be due to learning. We have already suggested that children may generalize habits which have been built up from experience with meaningful shapes to meaningless shapes, and we consider that a learn- ing theory of Ghent's results is not so unreasonable as Ghent suggests; although the decline of the effect with age suggested by her data would be a stumbling block.

The absolute orientation of two shapes does therefore appear to affect their discriminability though presumably only when the shapes have a recognizable axis. Ghent and Bernstein's work suggests that when subjects are prevented from making repeated comparisons of the two shapes and instead have to compare a present stimulus with a memory image, then it may be only the orientation of the memory image that is crucial. Under their conditions there was no effect of the orientation of the comparison shape in relation to the memory image of the standard shape.

12.42 Absolute orientation with a fixed difference

Question (b) asks, with a fixed difference in orientation between the shapes, what is the effect of their absolute orientation? It seems that no one has investigated this question directly. However, Rudel and Teuber (1963) have studied whether the discrimination of a difference in position between identical shapes is affected by the absolute orientation of the pair of shapes. They attempted to train children aged between $3\frac{1}{2}$ and $8\frac{1}{2}$ years to discrimin- ate between pairs of identical shapes (either a straight line or a U-shaped figure consisting of three sides of a square) by designating one member of each pair 'correct' and the other 'incorrect'. They found that whereas the youngest children could almost always learn to discriminate vertical from horizontal lines, the discrimination of two opposed obliques ($\diagup$ vs. $\diagdown$) was almost impossible. They could easily discriminate $\sqcup$ from $\sqcap$, but found $\sqsupset$ vs. $\sqsubset$ almost impossible. These results corresponded with the behaviour of octopus studied by Sutherland (1957) using the same figures, and the findings on the U-shaped figures, at least, can be explained on the basis of the relative importance of reversals and inversions to animals who strive to maintain a constant orientation of their sense organs relative to gravity. Even the eight year olds showed the same differential abilities, though in reduced form. In the case of the single straight lines, the discrimination between obliques and vertical or horizontal was just as easy as that between vertical and horizontal, though obliques were more easily discriminated from horizontals than from verticals.

12.43 *Relative orientation*

Question (c) asks, how is discrimination affected by changes in the orientation of the shapes relative to each other? We shall now consider a series of studies which bear on this problem of the effect on shape discrimination of the relative orientation of comparison shapes to standard shapes or to the memory traces of standard shapes.

Brown, Hitchcock, and Michels (1962) used oddity problems involving plane shapes differing on one or more of several dimensions—sidedness. axial rotation, elongation, compactness, and areal symmetry. They found that figures matched on axial rotation were consistently difficult to discriminate irrespective of differences on other dimensions.

Deese and Grindley (1947) found that after subjects had been taught to respond differentially to meaningless dot patterns, there was an increase in reaction time, though not in error rate, when the patterns were turned through 90°. This was presumably due to the disorientation of the patterns in relation to the traces with which the responses had been associated. It had already been shown in a much earlier study (Dearborn, 1899) that recognition could be differentially affected by different degrees of relative disorientation. Comparison of pairs of ink-blots was poorest when the blots were set at 270° to one another and was least affected by separations of 180°. Dearborn's results are summarized in table 12.1.

Accuracy was also found to be highest at 180° when subjects were asked to copy an abstract line drawing in different orientations to the original (Sato, 1960). Performance was not so good at an orientation of 90° and was poorest when mirror-image reproductions were required. Sato's subjects were faster though less accurate when working from memory than when copying; they thought it was easier to imagine the rotation when working

Table 12.1 Results of Dearborn (1899) showing the percentage
of correct shape recognitions for different relative orientations

Relative orientation angle	Percentage of correct recognitions
0°	70
90°	43
180°	51
270°	33
Mirror	46
Inverted mirror	32

from memory. No relationship was found between the ease of tachistoscopic recognition of the patterns and accuracy in making rotated drawings.
This situation was as much a test of visual imagery, memory, and motor
skill as of discrimination or recognition.

Arnoult (1954) reported an elaborate study in which 256 subjects compared pairs of identical ink-blots presented in differing relative orientations
from 0° to 360°. Error rate and latency both varied with angular separation
up to a maximum at 180°.

12.44 The type of shape

Question (e) asks, do the answers to the previous questions depend on
the type of shape used? The apparent contradiction between Arnoult's results
where errors were maximal at 180°, and the results of Dearborn and Sato
where errors were maximal at 270° may have occurred because different
shapes are affected in different ways by disorientation. Indeed Arnoult
found that his shapes were not equally affected by the same changes in relative orientation. He illustrated this point by referring to the groups of letters:
o and x; p, d, b, and q; and a, e, and g, which are clearly not affected in the
same way by changes in their orientation.

Support for the shape-specificity of these effects had been provided
earlier by French (1953) with another large-scale experiment. Here it was
shown that discrimination of pairs of five-dot patterns was affected in a
similar way to discrimination of Arnoult's ink-blots, being most disrupted
when the patterns were presented at 180° to each other; whereas with three-
dot patterns, discrimination was most disrupted by separations of 108° to
144° and least affected at 180°.

These last two studies disclosed anomalous differences between trials in
which the two patterns had the same shape (S trials) and those in which they

had different shapes (D trials). In Arnoult's study the tendency for errors to increase with the angular separation of the patterns manifested itself only on S trials. On D trials, on the other hand, which comprised three-quarters of the experiment, there was no tendency for errors to vary with orientation. Arnoult explained this difference by suggesting that there are two distinct effects of introducing an angular separation between compared shapes: a tendency for the shapes to appear different and a tendency for their comparison to be more difficult. In the case of identical shapes (S trials) both these factors would operate to increase errors with increasing angular separation. In the case of different shapes, while the increasing difficulty of the comparison would still increase the error rate, the tendency for the shapes to appear different would lower the error rate, and the two factors would tend to cancel out. This is a neat explanation but unfortunately French found an equally consistent but different pattern of differences between S trials and D trials, and moreover this pattern of errors varied according to the type of shape used. However, like Arnoult, he found that errors on the two sets of trials did tend to vary inversely, suggesting that pairs of shapes appear the same at certain relative orientations (especially 0°) and different at others. The difference between Arnoult's results and French's might be explained on the basis of variations in difficulty among the shapes used.

12.45 Theoretical interpretation

The main conclusions so far are the following. Two shapes are best discriminated when they are vertical (question a). If two shapes are observed successively, once only, Ghent and Bernstein showed that under certain circumstances it is the uprightness of the first which is crucial (question d). Whether or not the shapes are vertical, they are best discriminated when they both have the same orientation, although Ghent's results are an exception to this rule (question c). The effects produced by disorienting two shapes relative to each other depend on the type of shape used and the type of discrimination required (question e).

We shall now propose a theory to account for these facts. We shall suppose that when a shape is inspected it is scanned, either by eye movements or some internalized scanning mechanism, and that a sequential signal is produced containing all the information of both the shape and orientation of the stimulus. This information is processed and stored at various levels of abstraction. At the first level, a complete 'memory-image' of the shape in the particular orientation in which it was seen is stored. At another level, the 'shape' information is abstracted from the directional information and coded in terms of conceptual (linguistic) criteria. When abstract shapes are being discriminated, we shall assume that it is the first level of processing and storage which is used, we shall refer to it as the memory-image. In discriminating two unfamiliar shapes, the observer first looks at one shape and forms a memory-image of that shape which he carries over as he attends to the second shape. If the two shapes are in a similar orientation then the main outlines of the memory-image and the second shape will match, and minor differences will be easily detected. If the shapes are differently oriented, then the image and the second shape will not even approximately match unless some internal operation takes place equivalent to rotating the memory-image. In terms of sequential codes, this would be equivalent to bringing the two sequences into a correct 'phase' relationship. We shall assume that even when a rough match is established in this way, there is a tendency to compare the shapes in terms of the original position of the memory-image, and that this interferes with performance. There is some evidence that some people have more 'control' over the 'orientation' of memory images than others. A standard test of this ability is the letter square test (Woodworth and Schlosberg, 1955, p. 721). In this test the subject learns a square of 9, 16, or 25 letters or digits, reading by rows, and has to recall them by columns (see also the experiment by Rauth and Sinnott, section 12.5).

If the shape is repeatedly seen in several orientations, the observer will build up a series of related memory images and the detrimental effects of differences in relative orientation will diminish. On the other hand, if a particular shape is seen repeatedly in one orientation, the effects of relative disorientation on discrimination should increase. There are many everyday objects which are seen in many orientations (polyoriented) and there are many which are normally seen in only one orientation (mono-oriented). The study of these types of material should provide a way of testing the above predictions.

A study by Gibson and Robinson (1935) is directly relevant. They presented their subjects with four pictures of mono-oriented objects, a cat, a toy camera, a rabbit, and a bonnet, along with twelve contours of continents, countries, and states, and also a group of polyoriented objects. As expected, the percentage of the polyoriented forms recognized was not influenced by their orientation. On the other hand, the mono-oriented forms were more often correctly recognized in their usual orientation. Gibson and Robinson concluded that experience was the only factor which could account for this difference between the two groups of shapes; the maps had no structural features, such as the direction of main lines, which could explain why one orientation should be favoured. These results suggest that our description of the way in which memory images are oriented and compared with stimulus shapes may be correct.

Further evidence for the role of experience in recognition was advanced by Henle (1942). She showed that letters and numbers in their normal orientations are more readily recognized than their mirror-images. The subjects were set to see nonsense shapes and the critical figures were embedded in a context of such shapes; nevertheless, in order to demonstrate that the difference was not produced by an expectation of letters rather than their mirror-images, Henle repeated the experiment with different groups of subjects set to see either normal letters or reversed letters. In both cases recognition of the reversed letters improved to the level of that of the normal letters. This suggests not only that the initial difference was due to long-term experiential, rather than short-term attitudinal factors, but also that there is unlikely to be any significant structural difference between letters and their mirror-images, since they have been shown to be equivalent in recognizability under certain conditions.

That there are no structural differences between letters and their mirror-images would have to be established independently to make Henle's hypothesis watertight, but since it would be impossible to disentangle the structural from the semantic aspects of letters, her evidence is inevitably of an indirect nature. This evidence is that nonsense figures designed to resemble letters in structure but not in appearance were seen no more readily than their mirror-images, suggesting that the pairs of figures are structurally equivalent and that therefore the letters and *their* mirror-images may also be structurally equivalent. This is an inconclusive experiment because of the difficulty of selecting nonsense shapes which resemble letters but do not resemble reversed letters, and the consequent difficulty of deciding which of a pair of nonsense shapes should be regarded as normal and which reversed. Henle also found that Chinese and Arabic characters were no more readily recognized in obverse than in reverse orientation by subjects who were unfamiliar with them. Henle concluded from this evidence that it is unlikely that upright Latin letters are better inherent structures than their reversed forms. It is not clear how Henle scored the drawings and descriptions which her subjects made; it is not clear whether they were required to recognize the letters as letters or merely to be accurate in drawing and describing their shapes in the orientation in which they were presented. If she was inconsistent in applying scoring criteria to the different types of stimuli, her results would be invalid.

Both these studies, and particularly the one by Gibson and Robinson, demonstrate the important role which experience plays in the discrimination of shapes in different orientations; however, they do not tell us whether there are any unlearned preferences for particular relative or absolute orientations of shapes.

We shall assume in the first place that there is some unlearned ability to discriminate shapes when they are not in the same orientation. The results with the nonsense shapes show that performance is not equally good in all orientations and so the innate ability cannot be entirely independent of relative orientation. If it is true that polyoriented, meaningful shapes are discriminated equally well in all orientations, this is presumably because we learn to overcome the innately determined disadvantage of a difference in relative orientation. The relative lack of ability to discriminate mono-oriented shapes in different orientations would be due to the absence of this learning for these shapes. The assumption of at least some unlearned ability therefore fits all the facts.

If we now assume instead that there must be learning before any ability to recognize a shape in different orientations can develop, then there are two possibilities; either the learning is specific to shapes which have been experienced in many orientations or it transfers to all shapes. If there is transfer of learning, it cannot be complete, otherwise mono-oriented shapes would be as easily recognized in different orientations as polyoriented shapes are. If there is no transfer then we would not be able to discriminate between nonsense shapes in various orientations. Therefore, provided we assume that there is partial transfer, the assumption that the ability must be learned also fits all the facts.

Whether or not the basic ability to recognize shapes independently of orientation is unlearned, there is no doubt that conventional and linguistic (and therefore learned) habits come to play a decisive role in many responses to shapes in various orientations. For example, many objects have a 'top' which is defined by conventional usage, and part of our ability to recognize such objects depends on our correct choice of the part of the shape which is the 'top'. Some things, for example, the letters 'b' and 'p', are ambiguous in this respect. Discussion of these matters will be deferred until later in this chapter.

We have now completed our review of the ability of the upright observer to discriminate patterns in various orientations and positions. The experimental work has been very piecemeal. What is needed is a study which combines, in one design, the three variables of absolute and relative orientation and relative position. Only then could the interactions between these variables be studied; and it is almost certain that important interactions exist, at least between the first two of these variables.

12.5 The discrimination of shapes and the orientation of the observer and the visual frame

We shall define as extrinsic axes those axes outside a shape by means of which the orientation of the shape may be judged. They are:

(a) The egocentric axes. These are axes which are defined by reference to the body of the observer. The three significant egocentric axes are a meridian of the eye, an axis of the head, and an axis of the body.

(b) The direction of gravity.

(c) The visual frame. There may be one or more visual frames in view at the same time, and they need not have the same orientation.

We have shown in section 12.4 that the discriminability of shapes may be affected by changes in their orientation. But none of the extrinsic axes was varied, so that we do not yet know the effects of disorienting a shape relative to each of these axes separately.

Over the last fifty years repeated attempts have been made to decide whether it is more important for the correct identification of a pattern, to have it normally oriented with respect to gravity or to the egocentric axes. In none of these studies were distinctions made between the various egocentric axes. It has often been assumed that the head axis always coincides with the same retinal meridian. But this assumption is invalid, for when the head tilts there is countertorsion of the eye (see section 3.42). Several procedures have been used, often without consideration of the ways in which they may affect the results. For example, stimuli have been presented simultaneously or successively and subjects have been asked to respond either to differences or to similarities between shapes or even to reproduce the shapes by drawing. It will emerge in the following discussion how such differences in procedure may be crucial. Care has not always been taken to ensure that the subjects were responding to the required aspect of the situation, and in some cases it can only be concluded that the experimenter himself did not know what question he was investigating.

Köhler (1940, p. 15), using himself as subject, observed photographs of faces when looking through his legs backwards, that is, with his head upside-down. He observed that the expression on the faces looked normal only when the faces were normally oriented with respect to his head and eyes. On the other hand, the judgment as to whether the faces were upside-down depended on their relation to gravity. Köhler assumed that his own observations would apply to the general population.

Thouless (1947) repeated Köhler's experiment using fourteen adults and thirteen children between the ages of five and eight years. He used the ambiguous picture shown in figure 12.7. With head upright, all the subjects saw the 'Jew' when this picture was one way up, and the 'sailor' when it was the other way up. The subjects now looked backwards through their legs and were asked whether they saw the 'Jew' or the 'sailor'. If they saw the one which was upright in relation to gravity they were said to have made a geographical response, otherwise they were said to have made a head response. They had also to report whether or not the one they saw appeared to be upside-down.

Almost all the subjects, whether adults or children, gave the head response. Over half the subjects reported the figure they saw as being upside-down, some were doubtful, and others described it as upright. Thouless did

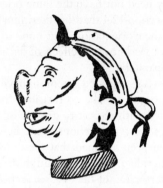

Figure 12.7 The ambiguous shape used by Thouless (1947). The shape is of a sailor when viewed in one position and a Jew when inverted

not state how he defined 'upside-down' to his subjects; perhaps some of them were undecided, not about what they saw, but about how to describe it (cf. the consistency of response of the children in the study by Ghent and Bernstein, 1961). He did not discuss the significance of the background against which the ambiguous picture was seen. It will be shown later that this question is crucial in this type of experiment. Thouless did show, however, that judgments of upside-downness are not as clear-cut as Köhler's behaviour would suggest.

Oetjen (1915) tested his subjects' ability to recognize nonsense syllables and shapes when the subjects, the stimuli, or both, were rotated through 90°. Recognition was good only when the stimuli were in line with the normally vertical meridian of the eye, but there was also some deterioration due to displacement of the pictures relative to gravity. Oetjen overlooked the fact that the eye may tort 6° or more when the head is tilted 90°. Therefore, he should not have assumed that when the stimulus and the head were tilted through the same angle the stimulus would be in line with the vertical meridian of the retina. This, rather than gravitational tilt, may have accounted for the slight deterioration in recognition found in this condition; if this were true, Oetjen's results would even more clearly underline the dominance of the retinal factor.

Studies of the effects of looking backwards through the legs (the so-called Matanozoki posture) were reported by Miyakawa (1944, 1950). It was found that rotation of the field of view through 180° did not affect size-constancy judgments, whereas looking through the legs backwards did. Miyakawa concluded that the inversion of the image relative to the retina was not the crucial factor in the effect produced by looking through the legs. He also found that tilting the whole body through 180° had no effect on the constancy judgments and concluded that the effect produced by the Matanozoki posture is due to the bending of the body rather than the disorientation of the head.

The importance of the direction of the visual framework for the recognition of patterns was demonstrated by Kopfermann (1930). He showed that a square looks like a diamond if it is tilted 45°. It also looks like a diamond if, when level, it is surrounded by a frame tilted at 45° (figure 12.8a). Similarly a diamond looks square when surrounded by a frame tilted at 45° (figure 12.8b).

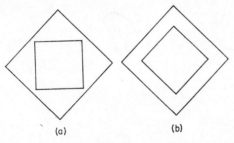

(a)   (b)

Figure 12.8 Figures illustrating the influence of the surrounding frame on the apparent shape of an enclosed square

An observation made by Rauth and Sinnott (1937) provides a further striking demonstration of the importance of the orientation of the visual frame in picture recognition. They asked eidetic imagers to 'project' a visual eidetic image on to a screen which was then inverted. The subject reported that the image too seemed to turn upside-down. In a further experiment they showed an upside-down picture to eidetic subjects. After a time the picture was removed and the subjects were asked to 'project' the image of it on to a screen. They reported that the meaning of the pictures became clear only in the eidetic phase and after the screen had been rotated 180°. It is not clear from the account of the two experiments whether the subjects reported that the image rotated with the screen or whether it was merely a case of the image being reported to have an upside-down or upright appearance as the screen rotated. In any case, confirmation of these striking results is needed.

Rock (1956), and Rock and Heimer (1957) have reported what is by far the most systematic and penetrating study of the relationship of pattern recognition to the egocentric, gravitational, and visual axes of reference. Their experiments were carefully designed and there was an adequate number of subjects to form a basis for generalization. The chi-squared test was erroneously applied to correlated observations; however, an examination of the data suggests that the 'significant' differences are in most cases probably real.

One series of experiments involved nonsense shapes (Rock, 1956, experiments III to VIII). The task was to select from a briefly exposed circular array of six shapes, that one which most resembled a training shape shown earlier. Two of the six shapes were identical to the training shape but at different orientations to each other. The other four shapes were similar but not identical to the training shape. There were three such arrays, each mounted on a square card and each corresponding to a particular training figure (see figure 12.9). The room was always in view.

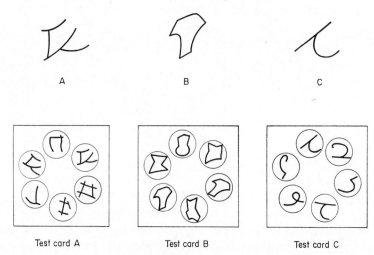

Figure 12.9 Nonsense shapes used by Rock and Heimer (1957) to study the relationship of pattern recognition to spatial axes of reference

It was found that when one of the two critical patterns in the selection had the same orientation as the standard (referred to as upright) relative to gravity and the visual frames (card and room) and the other had the same orientation relative to the retina (see figure 12.10a) the former was more often chosen as being most similar to the training pattern. When the critical patterns differed in orientation by 45° and the whole scene was tilted 45° by means of a prism, so that one pattern was upright on the retina and relative to gravity, the other upright relative to the visual frames (figure 12.10b), the latter had the highest frequency of selection. That this was not merely due to its being lined up with the card on which it was mounted was shown in a control experiment in which the card alone was tilted 45° (figure 12.10c); the pattern which was upright in relation to gravity and to the room was preferred to the alternative, which was upright on the card. Even when all lines which could serve as a frame of reference were eliminated (figure 12.10d) the only situation in which the retinal factor was as strong as the

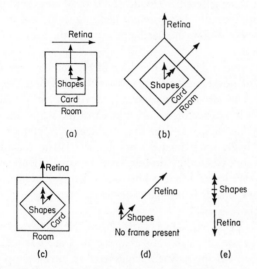

Figure 12.10 Summary of the experimental conditions and results of experiments III to VIII carried out by Rock (1956). (a) Gravity and frames stronger than retina; (b) Frames stronger than gravity and retina; (c) Gravity, room, and retina stronger than card and retina; (d) Gravity stronger than retina; (e) Gravity and retina equal

gravitational factor was one in which the two patterns differed in orientation by 180°, and the observer inverted his head by looking backwards between his legs (figure 12.10e). In this case the two versions were selected with about equal frequency.

These findings were confirmed in a further series of experiments (Rock and Heimer 1957, experiments I to III) using a slightly different technique. Three critical patterns were inspected and then the eighteen stimuli contained in the three arrays were combined into a single series. They were presented one at a time tachistoscopically, and the subjects were asked to respond to those that appeared familiar. An additional finding with this technique was that the frequency of choice of the gravitationally upright pattern was not appreciably affected by whether or not it was also upright on the retina. This result further demonstrated that retinal orientation is not important in this situation. Similar results were obtained with the head tilted during the training exposure and upright during the test trials.

In a final experiment involving nonsense shapes, Rock and Heimer (experiment VII) placed the stimuli on the floor and had the subjects look down at them, thereby eliminating the gravitational reference. The retinally upright figures were selected as frequently as those in previous experiments which were both retinally and gravitationally upright, and it was suggested that under these conditions the head axis assumes the function of the gravitational reference.

Thus the relative order of importance of the three extrinsic axes for the discrimination of nonsense shapes was shown to be, first the visual frame, second gravity, and last the egocentric (retinal) axis. In the absence of any intrinsic features indicative of the orientation of the shape, the observer will tend to assume that the part of the shape which is gravitationally 'up' is the top. Unless he overcomes this tendency he will fail to recognize that two shapes are the same when they do not have the same orientation to gravity. When the observer looks down at horizontal shapes, he will assume that the part of the shape which is retinally 'up' is the top and will make his discriminations accordingly.

A further series of experiments (Rock and Heimer, experiments IV to VI) involved the use of meaningful shapes which are normally seen in one orientation (mono-oriented). Such shapes have an intrinsic top which should be recognized whatever the orientation of the shape relative to gravity or the visual frame. The figures used were eight fragmented pictures which had been made difficult to recognize even when upright. The pictures were of a car, a typewriter, a ship, a piano, a boy on a bicycle, a horse and carriage, an elephant, and a bull. They were presented for a maximum of 20 sec.

The results are summarized in figure 12.11. When the figures were both retinally and gravitationally upright (figure 12.11a) they were recognized 66% of the time. This percentage dropped to 12 when the figures were tilted 90° (figure 12.11b). The experimenters were able to separate the gravitational and retinal contributions to this drop in performance by tilting the subject's head also. In this way it was shown that gravitational tilt alone accounted for more than half of the total drop; the percentage recognized was now 37 (figure 12.11c). However, they found that this decrement due to gravitational tilt (66% to 37%) could be totally eradicated by telling the subjects that the pattern would be tilted 90° in the same direction as the head. Thus only with the proper set were the subjects able to recognize quickly the true top of the pictures in different orientations to gravity; otherwise the natural set to see the gravitationally 'up' part of the picture as the top was still effective for meaningful familiar shapes, though less so than for meaningless shapes. When the effect of retinal tilt alone was measured directly by having the subject look at an upright figure with head tilted 90° (figure 12.11d) it was found that the percentage recognized dropped from 66 to 51.

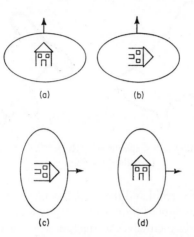

(a)   (b)

(c)   (d)

Figure 12.11 Showing the relationships between the shapes, the retina (the oval), and gravity in Rock and Heimer's experiments IV to VI. (a) Recognized 66% of the time. Figure upright to gravity and retina; (b) Recognized 12% of the time. Figure at 90° to gravity and retina; (c) Recognized 37% of the time. Figure at 90° to gravity, upright on the retina; (d) Recognized 51% of the time. Figure upright to gravity, at 90° to retina

This difference is significant and larger than the corresponding effect for nonsense figures. In contrast to the effect of gravitational tilt this one was not diminished at all by telling the subjects beforehand that the figure would be upright.

The finding that retinal disorientation has a disruptive effect when meaningless shapes are shown in a horizontal plane and the subject views them with his head horizontal, was confirmed for meaningful shapes (experiment VIII).

Another part of the investigation (Rock, experiments I and II) concerned ambiguous (bi-oriented) shapes similar to those used by Thouless. The two stimuli used are shown in figure 12.12); one is seen as 'dog' or 'chef', the other as 'face' or 'map', depending on which edge of the figure is seen as top.

The two interpretations are 90° apart. The results were similar to those obtained with meaningless figures. The gravitationally upright interpretation was favoured even when the alternative was made upright on the retina by tilting the head 90°. The only condition in which the retinally normal alternative was chosen was one in which the interpretations were both tilted

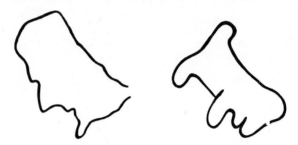

Figure 12.12 Ambiguous shapes used by Rock (1956). One is a face or a map, the other is a dog or chef

45° to either side of vertical and the head also tilted 45° to line up with one of them. In these ambiguous figures there are two intrinsic tops. As there is nothing in the figures themselves to suggest which is to be selected at any one time we suggest that, as with nonsense shapes, the position of the shapes relative to the extrinsic axes will be decisive.

Rock and Heimer suggested that Oetjen's finding of a stronger effect of retinal than of gravitational disorientation was due to the fact that his subjects served over a period of twelve days and may have become sophisticated about the fact that the stimuli were presented in varying orientations; also they had unlimited time to inspect each figure and search for its top. Rock and Heimer had shown that such factors are likely to lessen the effect of gravitational but not retinal disorientation. Köhler also was shown to be wrong in his claim that the effects of disorientation are wholly due to changes of retinal orientation. It is not therefore necessary to assume, as Köhler did, that there is a permanent direction gradient in the tissues of the visual centre. But Rock and Heimer suggested that the retinal effect they established may be based on a maintenance by the trace of its retinal orientation, and that disorientation had the effect of disrupting communication between the trace and current inputs. This view is similar to the one we have put forward in section 12.45.

Rock and Heimer finally concluded that the crucial step in shape recognition is the identification of the top of a shape. This may be supplied by an intrinsic top or by a verbally induced set. In the absence of such factors the gravitationally 'up' indicates the top, unless a strong visual frame intrudes or the gravitational factor is eliminated by exposing the shape in a horizontal plane. In our theoretical discussion we also emphasized the importance of selecting the 'top' of an object in adult behaviour towards shapes in various orientations. Whether the part selected as top is ever innately determined in the case of unfamiliar objects is not known.

These results for adults have been contrasted with the behaviour of 4–5 year old children by Ghent, Bernstein, and Goldweber (1960). These authors used ten realistic figures together with the abstract shapes for which children had been found to have orientation preference (see section 12.22). They claimed that most pre-school children selected as upside-down those abstract shapes and realistic shapes which were inverted with respect to the eye rather than with respect to gravity.

Rock may have biased his own results by using only 45° and 90° of displacement between his standard and comparison shapes. Ghent *et al.* used 180° of displacement. We suspect that retinal orientation is more significant for larger displacement angles. For instance, it is not difficult to read print which is at 90° to the retina or to gravity, although at this angle disorientation of the print relative to gravity is probably more disruptive than disorientation relative to the retina; however, it is difficult to read print which is at 180° to the retina whatever its orientation to gravity, whereas print which is disoriented 180° to gravity but upright on the retina is easily read. In other words, Rock's conclusions probably hold for displacements of up to 90°, and Ghent's conclusions hold for larger displacements.

But the results of these two investigators are not strictly comparable, for the two studies were not concerned with the same question. Rock studied the relation between extrinsic axes and shape discrimination whereas Ghent *et al.* studied the relation between these axes and judged orientation, although in fairness to Ghent *et al.* it must be pointed out that Rock interpreted his results as showing that phenomenal orientation is the most relevant variable for discrimination, and that apparent orientation is determined by the environmental framework rather than intrinsic axes. We prefer to keep the question of discrimination and recognition of top distinct from that of apparent orientation; they are separate issues, as Thouless realized. This theme is discussed further in section 15.3.

13

Orientation and shape II
Developmental aspects

13.1 Introduction

Anyone familiar with young children will have noticed that they are indifferent to the way in which a picture is oriented. They make no attempt to right a picture if it is upside-down, and seem to be capable of recognizing objects in the picture however it is oriented. This observation was confirmed in experiments by Burckhardt (1933). Stern (1909b) gave an account of a report by Pechuel-Loescher (1907) that members of the Loango tribe were indifferent to the position of pictures. Wyndham (1936) reported similar behaviour among the Dinka tribe of the Sudan.

It seems to be well established that brain damage tends to produce rotations in the reproductions of shapes (Bender and Teuber, 1948; Hanvik and Anderson, 1950). Shapiro (1952), in a more detailed study, had his patients reproduce a block design, the orientation of the design and of the card which formed its background being varied. Brain-damaged patients produced more rotations than non-brain-damaged controls, especially when the ground appeared diamond-shaped rather than square. Both groups showed more rotation when the main axis (of symmetry) of the design itself was not vertical on the retina. The orientation of the line of symmetry was a more powerful factor than the orientation of the ground. However, Halpin (1955) warned that these errors of rotation could not be predicted from one visual–motor task to another, and Fuller and Laird (1963) in a methodological critique, pointed out that there is little agreement on the degree of rotation required to indicate pathology.

Critchley (1953), in his review of spatial disorders associated with parietal-lobe damage, notes that such patients show some confusions which are also shown by semi-literates, such as N and И, S and Ƨ, but in addition some which are not, such as E, Ǝ, ꟼ, ꟺ. Parietal patients may also be unable to hold a stick in a vertical or horizontal orientation, and are confused about the meaning of spatial words such as 'up' and 'down', 'right' and 'left'.

It should, however, be noted that a more recent study by Hermelin and O'Connor (1961) throws doubt on the whole tendency of subnormals to show reversals and rotations. They found no such tendency on the part of mongols or of imbeciles, groups which generally have some organic damage.

This peculiar behaviour of children, primitive people, and defectives, suggests three fundamental questions:

(a) Are children indifferent to the orientation of pictures? If so, does their indifference extend to objects as well?

(b) Is the speed and accuracy with which children respond to the shape of objects affected by the orientation of the objects?

(c) Are children able to recognize or to match the orientation of things?

There is very little experimental evidence relevant to the first (see page 341) and third questions. However, there have been several attempts to answer the second question though most of them have been unsuccessful because of methodological failings. We shall now consider these attempts.

13.2 The ability of children to discriminate shapes in different orientations

Rice (1930) seems to have been the first to study whether disorienting a familiar pattern affects the ability of children to recognize it. The children were first shown an elongated diamond with its long axis vertical. They were then asked to identify this diamond from among several different arrays, each array consisting of identically shaped diamonds, which were either vertically or horizontally oriented, and nonsense shapes. The children below the age of five often ignored differences of orientation when choosing the same shape but most of the children over six years old chose only those diamonds which were oriented the same way as the one they had been shown. The children were also given a second test which was similar to the first but in which they had to recognize a spoon from among arrays of other familiar objects. The results of this test were similar to those of the first one. These results are difficult to assess, for Rice did not make it clear whether the children were asked to choose only those diamonds and spoons which matched the model in orientation or whether they were to choose diamonds and spoons irrespective of orientation. Wohlwill (1960, p. 270) made a similar criticism of Rice's experiments on the ground that they only demonstrated a lack of spontaneous verbalization about the orientation of a figure and did not prove a lack of ability to discriminate differences of orientation.

Tanaka (1960, 1962) conducted experiments similar to those of Rice. The subjects were shown a standard abstract shape for ten seconds; this was followed by the same shape arrayed in seven orientations, 45°, 90°, 135°, 180°, 225°, 270°, and 315° relative to the standard. The subjects had to choose the one which had 'the greatest similarity' to the standard. Most of the kindergarten children chose the 180° rotated figure. Adults chose the figures which were nearest in position to the standard. The transition from the childhood to the adult form of behaviour occurred between the ages of

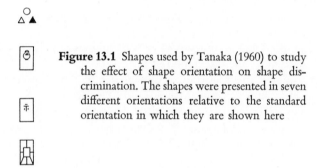

Figure 13.1 Shapes used by Tanaka (1960) to study the effect of shape orientation on shape discrimination. The shapes were presented in seven different orientations relative to the standard orientation in which they are shown here

six and eight. These differences in performance may have hinged on differences in interpretation of the words 'greatest similarity'. This is the same problem that we met in discussing Rice's results. Tanaka's shapes (shown in figure 13.1) show that in most cases the 180° shape matches the standard but for the relative position of detail inside the rectangular outline. The children were obviously ignoring this slight difference. On the other hand, the adults must have had more regard for the position of the detail within the pattern for they chose the one in which the detail was least displaced relative to the standard.

An inconclusive experiment was reported by Newhall (1937). His subjects, aged between three and five years, were shown one of eight pictures of familiar objects hung on the wall. They then had to select the same picture from an array of about five cut-out figures on an inclined tray in front of them. One of the figures was the same as the picture on the wall and was either in the same orientation, inverted, or laterally reversed. Performance was just as good on the disoriented figures as on the normal ones and New-hall claimed that this is evidence for the indifference of children to the orientation of pictures. However, his data suggest that scores were close to the maximum throughout, and the ease of the task may thus have masked any possible superiority of the normally oriented figures. After making their selection the subjects had to return the shapes to the tray by hand. They tended to replace them in an upright position. Newhall concluded that this was evidence that the children could perceive differences of orientation. No age trends were apparent in these effects but Newhall admitted that the age range of his subjects was rather narrow. One factor which may have influenced the results was that the training picture was always placed vertic-ally in front of the children and thus had a clear gravitational reference, whereas the selection pictures were tilted away from the children and did not have such a clear gravitational reference. It is not clear how the children held the shapes when they were allowed to handle them and their performance under this condition may not have been comparable to their performance when the shapes were on the tray.

If these studies by Rice, Tanaka, and Newhall indicate anything, it is only that, on the one hand, young children pay little attention to differences of orientation when matching shapes and, on the other hand, that young children can identify shapes when they are rotated. In view of their method-ological shortcomings they do not tell us whether children can recognize objects and patterns equally well irrespective of orientation.

Ling (1941) used a discrimination-learning technique in an attempt to circumvent the ambiguities of verbal instructions and to extend the study of shape discrimination to the pre-verbal stage of development. She used sugar-coated objects in the shape of circles, squares, triangles, and crosses. Two shapes were shown at a time and if the child selected the correct one he was rewarded by being allowed to lick it. Fifty infants between the ages of six and twelve months were first trained to select the circle and reject the other shapes. When this was accomplished, the non-reinforced shapes were ro-tated through various angles. This was found not to affect the selections. Similarly, when the circle was the only non-reinforced shape, reversing the other shapes did not affect the selections. Ling concluded that changing the orientation of the shapes had no effect on the ability of the children to dis-criminate them. This conclusion is very misleading. At all times the child had to discriminate a circle from other shapes which were 'not circle'. There is nothing to suggest that the children discriminated any other aspect of the non-circular shapes. This being so, it is irrelevant what orientation they had; they still remained 'not circle'. Ling's experiment proves nothing about the ability of these children to discriminate shapes in various orientations.

A similar technique was used by Gellermann (1933) who trained two two year old children and two chimpanzees to choose a triangle from among several other shapes. Rotation of the triangle through 30° or 60° did not affect the performance of either the children or the chimpanzees but they were all seen to tilt their heads, apparently to keep the image upright on the retina. This suggests that the subjects could not discriminate the shapes when they were in different retinal orientations. Deutsch (1960) suggested that the subjects must have recognized the shapes when their heads were erect, as otherwise they would not have known to which forms to tilt their heads. This interpretation is suspect, for it would not be necessary for the subjects to recognize the shape of a triangle before tilting their heads but only to see that there was no straight line at the base of the figure. The subjects were sometimes seen to tilt their heads to non-triangular shapes when these were the non-reinforced shapes, which suggests that the tilting was to some extent a trial and error process. This interpretation is supported by the verbalization of one of the children, from which it is clear that recognition of the familiar figure occurred only after the head was tilted.

Deutsch (1960) discussed the case of his young son who confused the letter 'V' with the letter 'A' and wrote letters rotated at various angles. He assumed that these 'confusions' were the result of the child's ability to recognize the common shape of the letters independently of orientation, and concluded, on the basis of these observations and his reinterpretation of Gellermann's results, that children are able to recognize shapes independently of their orientation. We have already pointed out that Deutsch's reinterpretation of Gellermann's results is suspect and the observations on his own child do not prove whether shapes are recognized in different orientations without the necessity of learning. Deutsch was interested in giving support to his theory of shape recognition as opposed to the rival theory of Dodwell. The reader is referred to chapter 10 of Deutsch's book for the details of this dispute.

With meaningful, pictorial material there is another methodological problem. We have already pointed out in section 12.45 that recognition can involve different levels of abstraction. For instance, the same object may be identified as a living thing, as a human being, or as a particular person, and in each case a variety of cues may be used. This point is illustrated in a study by Hunton (1955) in which she distinguished three indices of recognition of pictures in children from one to 14 years of age, (1) the naming of objects (substantive responses), (2) the naming of actions, and (3) the naming of functions and relations (such as the point of a joke) in the pictures.

The young children made predominantly substantive responses. When the pictures were inverted they made even more substantive responses and also more errors. The older children made more responses in terms of actions and relations, and their accuracy and consistency were little affected by inversion. All the children, even the two year olds, revealed by the way they handled and talked about the pictures that they could discriminate between the normal and inverted orientations.

Hunton concluded that we initially learn to recognize objects in the conventional orientation and until this ability is generalized to other orientations our recognition behaviour is likely to be influenced by disorienting the objects. These conclusions are in marked contrast to the suggestion made by Rice (1930) that children below the age of five are not influenced by the orientation of objects. Hunton's is the better based conclusion and is in agreement with the results of a well-conducted experiment by Ghent (1960). Using a tachistoscope, Ghent showed children pictures of a boat, a clown, a horse, and a wagon. The pictures were upright, 90° to the left, 90° to the right, or upside-down. The subjects named the figures or pointed to similar ones in an array of twelve forms. The 3 to 4 year olds recognized more upright figures than disoriented figures. The 5 to 7 year olds recognized them all equally well.

Tampieri (1963) attempted to solve the problem of ambiguous instructions by having the subject say whether a particular pattern would go through a standard hole after making it clear by example that the patterns could be rotated. The three standard holes consisted of upright geometrical figures, and each one was matched with a series of patterns which consisted of slight variations in shape on the 'hole' pattern, and which were presented either in the same upright orientation or at 45° to it. For two of the standard patterns he found that 5 to 7 year old children were very poor at the task whatever the relative orientation of the pattern and the hole, whereas adults were almost equally poor when the pattern was tilted relative to the hole but improved greatly when the pattern also was upright. This result may suggest support for the hypothesis of children's indifference to changes in orientation, but the third standard pattern yielded very little improvement with age, even when pattern and hole were in the same orientation. It looks as if the task was too difficult for the children, so that any orientation preferences were probably masked.

Further support for Ghent's scanning theory (see section 12.22) was provided by Wohlwill and Wiener (1964). Four year old children were shown a standard nonsense shape and two comparison shapes which were identical with the standard except that one of them was either a left–right reversal or an inversion of it. The children had thus to select on the basis of orientation alone which of the comparison figures was identical with the standard. The fact that less than a fifth of all selections were errors shows that they could do this very well, and were therefore not indifferent to orientation.

It was further deduced from Ghent's theory that inversions should be more readily discriminable than left–right reversals, and that discrimination should also be facilitated by a high degree of directionality (i.e. pointedness), by openness as against closedness of contour, and by asymmetrically placed detail. The error scores confirmed only that inversions were more discriminable than reversals, and a latency measure confirmed only an effect of the directionality variable. The closure and detail variables did not show a significant effect on either measure. Wohlwill and Wiener concluded that the difficulty children have in mastering the alphabet and learning to read cannot be due to insensitivity to orientation differences. They suggested that it lies rather in the learning of differential responses to the stimuli: children typically respond to stimuli as equivalent over a broad range of variation, and generalization between stimuli differing only in orientation may be assumed to be considerable. It is difficult to see how this interpretation differs from insensitivity to orientation differences. A sensible suggestion, however, which these workers put forward is that pre-differentiation training of the type used in this experiment should facilitate the learning of subsequent differential responses e.g. letter names.

During pre-training, Wohlwill and Wiener had to reject a 3 year old group because not enough of them could do the task even with meaningful shapes. They suggested that a different method of presentation and/or more potent reinforcement may be required with such children, and that this and well-known related phenomena, such as very young children looking at pictures upside-down, may result from an identification of objects by means of specific salient cues such as the tail of a dog, and from the failure of amused adults to correct such behaviour, rather than from an inability to appreciate orientation differences.

In a further experiment in the same study (Wohlwill and Wiener, 1964) children aged between 4 and 6 years were trained to discriminate orientations either by the perceptual 'matching-from-sample' method used in the main experiment, or by means of a motor method whereby the child actively indicated the direction of the figure in various orientations. Although both methods were efficacious in producing responses to orientation alone, neither showed a significant degree of transfer to a task in which the child had to learn to differentially attach verbal labels to another set of similar figures according to their orientation. In considering the child's alleged insensitivity to orientation it is therefore essential to consider the degree of transfer involved in the task, on both the stimulus and the response sides. There is evidence, for example, that if the same set of stimuli had been used in both training and transfer tasks, there would have been facilitation, at least in the case of the motor pre-training (Hendrickson and Muehl, 1962; Jeffrey, 1958).

Gibson, Gibson, Pick, and Osser (1962) designed a group of standard letter-like forms and had young children select forms 'identical' to a standard from a series of systematic transformations of the standard. The errors were classified according to the type and degree of transformation erroneously identified with the standard. With children aged 4 through 8, overall errors decreased with age.

Gibson *et al.* related the error patterns for a particular type of transformation to the question of whether the dimension transformed is critical for discriminating real objects or letters, or, on the other hand, is one in which changes have to be discounted since they do not involve changes of the letter or object. The child must learn to tolerate perspective changes in objects and in letters and, accordingly, projections of the standard forms slanted backwards from top to bottom or from right to left were, of all the transformations, the least accurately discriminated from the standards. Opening or closing a gap in a contour, on the other hand, is critical for distinguishing letters (e.g. C and O), and these topological transformations were discriminated with very few errors, even by the 4 year olds. The third type of transformation involved changing one, two, or three lines of the standard from straight lines to curves or vice versa. The 4 year olds, whose previous experience involved objects rather than letters, often neglected such changes and, indeed, certain objects such as faces and soft toys do remain invariant under such transformations, while other, rigid objects do not. Such differences are, however, critical in distinguishing letters (e.g. U and V) and with increasing age, errors on such transformations dropped to near zero. The same age trend was evident in the case of left–right and up–down reversals, and rotations through 45°, 90°, or 180°; again, such transformations are often not critical for discriminating objects but are of great importance for distinguishing between letters (e.g. M and W, U and C, d and b, p and q). These transformations are of most direct relevance to our present theme. Although Gibson *et al.* did not present an analysis of this aspect of their data there appear to have been no marked differences between the 45°, 90° and 180° rotations nor between up–down and right–left reversals, but reversals in general were apparently more disruptive than rotations.

Gibson *et al.* concluded that it is the distinctive features or invariants of 'grapheme patterns' which are responded to in the discrimination of letter-like forms, and that the detection of these invariants improves during the period from 4 to 8 years. A supplementary study of 5 year olds, using real letters, yielded a similar pattern of errors over the same range of transformations as had been used for the letter-like forms. These workers recommended that the set of such invariants should be found and used, instead of pictures of objects, in visual 'reading readiness' tests.

The conclusion therefore seems clear that young children are more affected than older children by changes of orientation. It has been falsely assumed by many, for example Stern (1909b), that because children show a lack of concern for orientation when drawing or looking at pictures, as they get older their ability to recognize an object therefore becomes more dependent on its being in a familiar orientation. The situation appears to be the reverse, *the familiar orientation is more necessary for recognition in the young than in the older child*. Ghent explained this developing independence of orientation as children mature, by suggesting that the older children become less dependent upon particular eye-scanning habits and can in any case recognize an object from one small part more easily than can young children.

We pointed out in section 12.45 that whether or not the basic ability to recognize shapes in various orientations has to be learned, conventional and linguistic habits become decisive in our responses to shapes in different orientations. Letters such as d, b, p, and q present a special problem, for their identity depends, not only on their shape, but also on their orientation. Here is a case where the growing child, having perhaps learnt to recognize that shapes are the same in different orientations, is presented with a class of shapes which it must learn to recognize as different in different orientations. Furthermore, the representation of spatial relationships in drawing present special difficulties for children. These two issues will be discussed in the following sections.

The answer to our third question, whether identical shapes can be discriminated by children on the basis of orientation alone appears to be that they can. However, in section 12.42 evidence is discussed which suggests that at least one of the shapes must either be vertical or horizontal, and that inversions are much more easily discriminated than reversals.

13.3 The representation of direction in children's drawing

In our society there are certain techniques and conventions in drawing: (1) the drawing should be a projective transformation of the thing drawn, (that is, straight lines should be represented by straight lines), (2) the proportions of the original should be kept (as we are not concerned with the representation of depth we shall ignore the problem of perspective), and (3) that which is gravitationally 'up' should be placed towards the edge of the paper farthest away from the drawer.

All the evidence suggests that children must learn these techniques of drawing. With regard to the representation of straight lines, Piaget and Inhelder

(1956, chapter 6) demonstrated that the average child under three years of age cannot draw a straight line or arrange matches in a line except coincident with a line already provided. On the other hand, such a child can distinguish a straight line from a curved line. At a later stage the child is able to draw lines parallel to a model and at some distance from it but is not able to draw lines at right angles to the model. At this stage the child's performance is said to be governed by 'intuitive internalized imitations or mental images'. Only at a later stage is drawing based upon what Piaget calls 'operations', when the child can free itself from the influence of the visual frame. The crucial 'operation' here is that of 'sighting' along the line of regard. For details the reader is referred to Piaget and Inhelder.

Having mastered the drawing of lines and other shapes, children must learn other techniques of drawing such as the representation of perspective and the spatial orientation of objects. Children often seem indifferent to the spatial orientation of what they are drawing. Kirschensteiner (1905) asked nearly 3,000 children to draw a boy presented to them in profile. Nearly half the children drew the front view of a boy and quite a few drew the mirror-image profile. However, one must be cautious in interpreting such findings which could be due to the use of different conventions rather than an in-difference to spatial position. For example, the child may imagine the model brought round on the paper in the same way that a person facing another person would have to be brought round in order for them to be facing in the same direction. The child meets the need to imagine parts of the body brought round in this way when, for example, he has to point to another person's left hand when he is facing that person.

Meyer (1913) found a consistent tendency for children to introduce reversals and inversions when drawing things from memory. The incidence of such changes of orientation appears to decrease sharply between the ages of five and six years (Rice, 1930) or six and eight years (Burckhardt 1925). Katsui (1962) also reported confusions of orientation, particularly for left–right positions, when children between the ages of four and eight were asked to recall the position of a radius in a circle. He did not notice any decline of this tendency with age, however.

Stern (1909b) noticed that his young son could draw a boat equally well in any of four orientations. He discussed various possible explanations of the indifference which children have to the orientation of their drawings. One possibility is merely that they have not learned the convention of putting that part of the drawing which they know to be the top at the farthest edge of the paper. But Stern pointed out that children's drawings are still disoriented in cases where this convention does not apply, for example, when they draw on a vertical paper.

Stern considered the possible importance of motor disability as opposed to perceptual factors but argued that as the children did not notice that their pictures were disoriented, the perceptual factor was predominant. Many of the investigators since Stern would not agree that young children do not notice when two pictures are differently oriented. We must therefore reserve judgment about the role of motor factors in the orientation of children's drawings.

What Stern called the 'empirical eye-movement theory of shape recognition' was dismissed because his own observations showed that altering the pattern of eye movements by rotating the shape did not affect the child's ability to recognize it. But the type of eye-movement theory to which Stern's criticism would apply would be a very naïve one. An adequate eye-movement theory would suppose that there is a central mechanism capable of taking out the information, specific to the shape scanned, from the total information supplied by the eye-movement centres. A shape-scanning device capable of such a performance would not be difficult to design. Stern favoured a nativistic, Gestalt theory of shape perception in which recognition is independent of orientation or position.

Stern's simple antithesis between the empiricism of the eye-movement theory and the nativism of the Gestalt theory of shape recognition is misleading. The essential point about the eye-movement theory is that the signal from the retina is said to trigger-off eye movements and that reflex or learned discriminatory responses to shapes are mediated by signals from the eye-movement centres rather than from the retina direct. The theory need not stipulate whether the original eye-movement tendencies are innate or learned. The Gestalt theory, on the other hand, stipulates that the patterned stimulus from the retina is available to the response mechanisms. Some Gestalt theorists make the further but unnecessary assumption that shape discrimination is innate. To say that shape discrimination is innate can only mean that humans have innate abilities to respond differentially to shapes. Clearly, some general response tendencies must be present before any learning is possible, otherwise the initial responses necessary for differential reinforcement would never be made. But in order to account for the development of shape discrimination, it is only necessary to assume that there is a tendency to attend to and reach towards objects in the field of view. Shape discrimination itself could arise as the result of differential reinforcements contingent upon the occurrence of particular shapes, once the general ability to reach accurately towards any shape had been learned or had matured. The apparently indiscriminate reaching for and exploration of objects by the young child certainly seems to support this view, although Spitz and Wolfe (1946) and Fantz (1958) claimed to have demonstrated unlearned differential response tendencies to specific shapes (faces).

Thus, the extent to which shape discrimination is innate is one question; whether it is mediated by eye movements or by the retinal image directly is another question. Stern confused these two issues.

For the recognition of orientation as distinct from shape, Stern proposed an empirical theory, suggesting that the 'psychic dimensions' of up and down, left and right, do not have a purely visual meaning, but are in fact, visual–motor relations. He went on to argue that these visual–motor relations are learned, by referring to Stratton's experiments on inverted vision (see section 15.22) and the fact that people have to learn to recognize the correct orientation of letters. But these facts do not support Stern's view. Stratton's experiment proved nothing about the origin of the initial spatial coordination of vision and movement, and the fact that children must learn to recognize the correct orientation of letters is irrelevant to this issue because (as we shall show in section 13.4) this skill depends wholly upon an arbitrary convention. We suggested in fact that many visual–motor relationships, for example the fixation reflex, are independent of post-natal learning.

We suggest that shape recognition involves complex behaviour which is largely learned, but that visual–motor spatial coordination involves much simpler relationships many of which are probably independent of learning. This is the reverse of Stern's view.

A child may correctly orient his drawing as a whole on the paper and yet not use the same spatial frame of reference for all parts of the drawing. Stern (1909b) gave an example of a child's drawing of people on a river bank (see figure 13.2). He also cited a report by Levinstein (1905) that Indian and

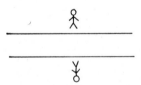

Figure 13.2 A child's drawing of a river with people on the bank. [After Stern, 1909b]

Egyptian drawings lack a consistent relationship between up and down and the top and bottom of the paper even within a single drawing. For instance the drawing of trees round a pond would look like figure 13.3. Piaget gave several examples of the way in which children use the local main lines of a drawing for gravitational reference. One of these examples is shown in figure 13.4. A further example is his account of a child who, when asked to draw the water-level in an inclined jar, drew it at right angles to the inclined sides of the jar

(Piaget and Inhelder, 1956; Smedslund, 1963). Apparently adults also tend to do this (Rebelsky, 1964).

Hanfmann (1933) found that when children were asked to draw a second chimney on a roof, they usually drew it out at right angles to the line of the

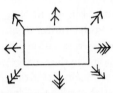

Figure 13.3 A drawing of trees round a pond, typical of the drawings made by primitive Indian and Egyptian artists. [After Levinstein, 1905, cited by Stern, 1909b]

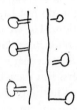

Figure 13.4 A child's drawing of trees along the side of a road. [After Piaget and Inhelder, 1956)

sloping roof (see figure 13.5). In the case of the second chimney they were clearly taking the roof line as the horizontal reference line. Hanfmann gave another example of the tendency of children to draw lines at right angles to each other. Children were asked to copy the two forms of figure 13.6 (a) and (b). The angles in (a) were usually drawn correctly but those in (b) were usually nearer to being right angles. The frontispiece of this book is a reproduction

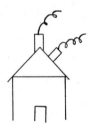

Figure 13.5 Showing how a child uses the line of the roof as horizontal reference in placing the second chimney. [After Hanfmann, 1933]

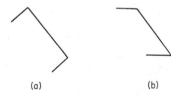

(a)   (b)

Figure 13.6 Children copy (a) correctly, but copy (b) with the short arms tending to make a right angle with the main line. [After Hanfmann, 1933]

of a drawing by the four year old daughter of the senior author; it shows how two horizontal frames of reference may be used in the same picture.

Again we must be cautious in our interpretation. The children and primitive artists do not represent relative directions at random but have their own consistent and logical conventions. In the examples which we have given, the sides of the paper have been used for orienting the main part of the picture but this frame has not been applied to every part of the picture. In each locality of the drawing the horizontal or ground reference has been taken from the local main line, for example, the banks of the river or the sides of the pond. In the real world, the trees and the people *are* perpendicular to these ground lines and therefore, within the logic of this system of drawing, they are drawn at right angles to that ground line which is nearest to them. If one were to consider these drawings in relation to ordinary conventions they would be approximately correct if they were drawings from a bird's eye view. It is possible that some children draw from this viewpoint but this is a most unlikely explanation of the general tendency for children to draw in this way.

Piaget and Inhelder (1956) outlined the steps of learning through which the child progresses before it is able to use an overall, consistent, spatial reference system, external to a drawing. The first stage is the topological stage in which the non-metric aspects of spatial relationships, such as order, proximity, and enclosure are understood by the child. These concepts are related to the 'mathematically primitive' concepts of topological geometry. In investigating this stage, Piaget gave children tasks involving drawing, haptic perception, knots, and the linear ordering of beads on a string. In the second stage, the child develops an understanding of projective concepts, that is, those concepts involved in the understanding of perspective. The tasks used to study these concepts included the drawing of figures in perspective, asking questions about the projection of shadows, and the relations between objects seen from different points of view. The development of the third stage, the understanding of Euclidian concepts, was studied by the use of tasks involving 'affine transformations', that is, transformations preserving parallels. The children were asked about the similarity of proportions in such figures as the rectangle and triangle, and about horizontal and vertical axes of reference. The order of these stages of development has been confirmed by Dodwell (1963) who tested 194 children between the ages of five and eleven years on a battery of tests similar to those used by Piaget.

We have seen that children may be indifferent to the way in which they place their drawings on paper and they have to learn to represent spatial relations within a picture according to adult techniques and conventions. It does not follow from these facts that children cannot discriminate different orientations of objects or drawings nor that they can recognize objects equally well in all orientations. In fact there is no evidence to show that the ability to discriminate differences in the orientation of objects develops later than any other visual ability, but there is evidence that the ability to discriminate shapes is affected by orientation (see section 13.2).

H.S.O.—23

13.4 Orientation in children's reading and writing

Many children have difficulty in learning the correct orientation of letters. Mirror-image and upside-down mistakes are common in early attempts at writing, and confusions between such letters as 'p', 'q', 'd', and 'b' are common in early reading. We shall first consider reversals in reading.

Orton was the best-known advocate of the view that reversals in reading are due to a failure to develop dominance of the major lobe. He suggested that mnemonic records exist in mirror-image pairs, one in each hemisphere, and that the child must suppress the image in the non-dominant hemisphere in learning to write and read correctly. Davidson (1935) pointed out that this theory would account only for mirror-image confusions, which are not the only type of confusion to occur.

In her own study, Davidson experimented with 48 kindergarten and 111 first-grade children. A training letter was first shown to the children who had then to select this letter from an array of 40 letters. The array contained five copies of the training letter and five of each of a number of other letters likely to be confused with it. Nearly all the children below the age of seven and a half years confused d, b, q, and p. These confusions persisted longer than confusions between other letters. When pressed, several of the children admitted that the letters which they had checked off as being the same as the model were facing different ways. They were apparently unconcerned by this fact.

This led Davidson to hypothesize that the 'confusions' which the children showed in responding to the letters d, b, q, and p were the result of their ability to recognize the shape independently of orientation, and the fact that they ignored the orientation. The number of confusions for each combination of these letters is set out in table 13.1.

Table 13.1 Results of Davidson (1935) showing the percentage of kindergarten and 1st grade children making each type of error in confusing the letters d, b, q, and p

	N	d–b	d–p	d–q	b–p	b–q	q–p	q–b	q–d	b–d
Kindergarten	48	93	50	35	40	42	96	43	27	87
Grade 1	111	65	19	13	19	15	62	11	13	60

It can be seen that the confusions between mirror-image pairs were the most numerous. This would be expected in a world where the left–right position of objects has little significance. Davidson's explanation of children's behaviour towards letters seems to be the most reasonable yet given. In an earlier paper, Davidson (1934) had presented other evidence in favour of her theory and reviewed other literature.

Hendrickson and Muehl (1962) succeeded in training $5\frac{1}{2}$–7 year old children to discriminate 'b' from 'd' visually, without using the words 'left' or 'right' nor the names of these letters during either training or testing. The test consisted of a visual paired-associate task in which a different picture followed the presentation of 'b' and 'd' The training consisted of selecting which of two opposed arrows pointed in the same direction as the round part of the letter, and designating the selected arrow by means of a motor response to either the left or the right. For one group the required response was consistent throughout, right movement for 'b', left for 'd'; for the other group the left response was required on half the 'b' trials and the right response on half the 'd' trials, in order to designate the correct arrow. There was no significant difference between the groups on the paired-associate task but both were superior to a control group which received no training involving 'b' and 'd'. This indicates that the attention-directing aspect of the training was effective but the motor aspect was not. The study also demonstrates that a right–left inversion can be learned considerably before Davidson's (1935) normative age of $7\frac{1}{2}$, a conclusion supported by Jeffrey's (1958) study of even younger children.

It has sometimes been assumed that because children's reading ability is often unaffected by the orientation of the print, they are therefore better than adults at reading inverted print. This, of course, does not follow, and no one seems to have made the direct comparison. It may be that people do not deteriorate in the ability to read inverted print but merely improve in conventional reading.

We shall now consider briefly the orientation of children's writing. Preyer (1895) seems to have been the first to report mirror-writing. Stern (1909b) cited Petrie to the effect that the ancient Egyptians and Phoenicians were indifferent to spatial orientation in writing. Mirror-writing had been regarded as an abnormality until Stern (1909a) pointed out that it was very common among apparently normal children. He suggested that in some cases it may be due to the child copying the writing movements of another person facing him across a table. However, one of his own children, aged nearly 5 years, wrote numbers in all orientations.

It has frequently been reported that mirror-writing is more common among left-handed than among right-handed children (Beeley, 1918; Burt, 1921; Carmichael and Cashman, 1932; Gordon, 1920). It has been suggested that this difference may be related to discrepancies between the handedness of the teacher and that of the child (Kirk, 1934). The child may copy the movements of the teacher's hand rather than the shape of the actual letters; if the teacher moves his right hand out from the body, the left-handed child would produce a mirror-image outward movement with his left hand. Kirk and Kirk (1935) put this suggestion to experimental test, but found that the hand used by the experimenter did not affect the number of reversals made by children of the opposite hand preference. These results do not support an explanation of mirror-writing in terms of child–teacher handedness differences.

Stern (1909a) noticed that in a left-handed child mirror-writing usually occurred when the child started writing on the right of the page. Left-handed children are more likely than right-handed children to start writing on the right side of the page, probably because in this way they can see what they have written and the pen does not dig into the paper. Leonardo da Vinci began mirror writing, apparently when his right hand became paralysed (Ireland, 1881).

Stern's son at first wrote mirror-writing but later improved; he still lapsed into mirror writing when asked to draw a figure using a series of small rings instead of lines. The movements were not now the usual ones and the child could not utilize the motor and kinaesthetic cues associated with correct writing. This emphasizes the role of the motor factors in learning to write in correct orientation. A fuller account of children's writing is given in Vernon (1957).

14

Sensorimotor and intersensory localization

14.1 The accuracy of pointing to visual targets

The earliest attack on this topic seems to have been made by Bowditch and Southard (1880) who studied the accuracy with which a target could be hit using one hand after its position had been sensed with either the same hand, or the other hand, or by vision. Location by vision was even more accurate than location by the hand which was used for pointing; the lowest accuracy occurred in the intermanual condition. Additional findings were that as the interval between position-sensing and pointing increased so the accuracy increased and then decreased, the optimum interval being two seconds, and that accuracy was facilitated by free movement of the head.

Szafran (1951) had his subjects point with a stylus to the mid-point of one of ten large targets ranged in various orientations about them. He measured the time taken for each of several components of the task, but, paradoxically, 'no mention of speed or any other criterion of efficiency was made' to the subjects. He found that without vision search time increased with the age of the subjects so that those in their fifties took more than twice as long as those in their twenties. The older subjects tended also to turn their heads, and even their bodies, in the direction of the target, even though this resulted in a loss of efficiency in another component of the task. Many of them could not perform the task at all without prior practice with the aid of vision, even though they had been shown the target arrangement before the experiment started.

Fitts (1947) and Fitts and Crannell (1949) found that in reaching for visible objects at shoulder level without visual guidance, performance was affected by the starting point, target positions, and by the distance of the target. When the movements were initiated from a median plane position somewhat below shoulder height, targets forward of the shoulder, below shoulder height, and closer to the starting position were more accurately localized. When the starting position was at the side of the body the more detailed error pattern between different areas was modified, although targets forward of the shoulder remained the most accurately localized. The most obvious of the constant error patterns was a tendency to reach too low. When the distance of the targets from the shoulder was reduced from 28 to 21 in, there was an increase in accuracy though not enough to keep the angular error constant. Fitts recommends that where such tasks are involved in machine operations, objects should be located at least six to eight inches apart (i.e. three or four times the average localization error).

The apparatus used in a study by Loemker (1930) consisted of a horizontal screen which prevented the subject from seeing his own arms. Above the screen, a downward pointing arrow could be moved in a horizontal arc. The subject, seated in front of the apparatus, had to extend his arm under the screen and point to the tip of the arrow, which he could see. The visual field of each eye was limited by a tube worn on the subject's head. The point of the arrow was always fixated in the centre of the tube. The median plane of the head was straight forward, 12° to the left, or 12° to the right. The pointer was directly in front of the subject, 40° to the left, or 40° to the right. Readings were taken for all combinations of these variables. The results showed that when the median plane of the head was to the left, the finger was set to the left of the arrow and when the head was to the right, the finger was set to the right of the arrow.

In a second experiment, the tubes were off-centred relative to the visual axis, so that the target was to the left or to the right of the centre of the circular visual field. The results showed that when the target was on the left of the visual field, the finger was set to the left of the target and when the target was to the right, the finger was set to the right of the target.

Edgington (1953) conducted an experiment with apparatus similar to Loemker's, but in addition to testing the ability to point where one is looking, he also studied the ability to look where one is pointing. The apparatus is shown in figure 14.1. The subject wore a tube which restricted the field of vision to a small circular area. In the first experiment, there were two tasks. The first of these was called the 'arm-to-head' task in which the subject had to turn his head till he saw the arrow, and then point to the arrow (a) by moving his hand straight away from his body beneath the partition, (b) by swinging

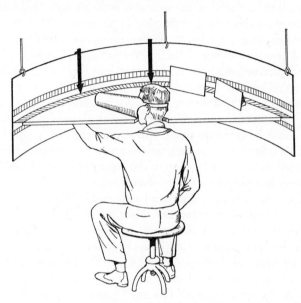

Figure 14.1 Schematic representation of the apparatus used by Edgington (1953) to study the accuracy of pointing to a visual target

his horizontal arm out from the straight-ahead position, and (c) by swinging it in from an 85° lateral position. The arrow was placed in various positions on either side of the straight-ahead position. The left arm was used for pointing to the left and the right arm for pointing to the right. The second task was the head-to-arm task, in which the subject's finger was placed in position by the experimenter, and the subject had to turn his head until his gaze was centred on the position of his finger-tip. The head was either swung out from the straight-ahead position or swung in from an 85° lateral position. The actual centre of gaze was read off on a lettered scale (revealed to the subject only when he had settled on his final position).

The results for the head-to-arm tests showed greater variability than those for the arm-to-head tests. The variances for the lateral positions of the pointer were greater than for the straight-ahead position in the head-to-arm test. All positions gave the same variance for the arm-to-head test. In all cases, the organ which was being swung was stopped short of the true equivalent position. Thus when the subjects swung their heads or arms in, they placed them more laterally than the correct position, and when they swung them out, they placed them on the straight-ahead side of the correct position. When the arm was brought straight out from the body, there was some tendency for it to be placed on the same side as the straight-ahead. Edgington did not discuss any theoretical or practical implications of these findings, and it is indeed difficult to see what theoretical importance they have.

In a book entitled 'Orientation in the Present Space', Sandström (1951) was principally concerned with analysing what he called 'the luminous point phenomenon'. This was described as follows:

'A luminous point that does not give any guiding light in an otherwise completely dark room, and which is given at a convenient distance for pointing, cannot be correctly pointed to and touched by a direct pointing movement. Another feature of the phenomenon is that the individual usually feels quite convinced of the location of the point of impact in relation to the target, and yet in reality he is nearly always wrong' (p. 14).

The subjects were requested to stand at a comfortable distance, some 45–55 cm, from the luminous point, and while holding a short 'mapping pin' firmly between thumb and forefinger, to point to the luminous point, and then let the pin remain sticking in the board at the point of impact. The mean average error was 15·5 mm for men and 22·3 for women. Sandström suggested that the effect was due either to changes in the visual mechanism or to the fact that the hand could not be seen. A series of supplementary experiments were carried out, among them the following:

(1) Pointing to a luminous point.
(2) Fixating a point in ordinary lighting, then shutting the eyes and pointing to it.
(3) Pointing to a luminous point with dark-adaptation.
(4) Pointing to a luminous point without dark-adaptation.
(5) Pointing to a point on a table top with the finger under the table.

In the first three experiments, the subjects stood 50 cm from an upright screen and used a pin for the actual pointing. The results for the left hand are presented in table 14.1 (the right-hand results were similar).

The luminous point and pointing from below gave similar results, the pointing with eyes shut gave the largest average errors. The state of dark adaptation of the eyes had no effect on the average error. It can be seen that women were less accurate than men. The pattern of the mean constant errors is shown in figure 14.2. Both vertical and sideways errors are depicted. Constant errors to the left were obtained with the left hand, and errors to the right with the right. The constant errors were above the target in the luminous-

Table 14.1 Results from Sandström (1951) showing the mean average errors in mm for the various pointing experiments

	Men	Women
Luminous point	15·0	24·8
Pointing with shut eyes	24·8	33·4
Pointing from below	17·9	25·1
With dark-adaptation	15·3	16·2
Without dark-adaptation	15·0	19·5

point experiment, beyond the target in the pointing-from-below experiment and below the target in the pointing-with-shut-eyes experiment. Women had larger constant errors than men. Sandström did not attempt to explain the

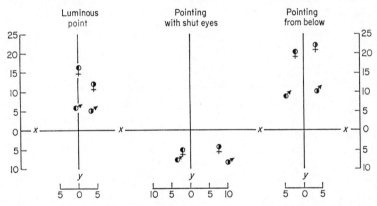

Figure 14.2 Graphical representation of the mean positions of pointing in the various conditions of the experiment by Sandström (1951)

direction of the constant errors but concluded that the inability to hit the target in the dark is due to the absence of visual–motor coordination.

14.2 Intersensory localization

The theoretical barrenness of this area has been relieved by an interesting set of theoretical predictions made by Howarth which formed the basis of the work of one of his students, Fisher (1960a, 1960b, 1962b). Howarth postulated a spatial framework in the CNS to which all the spatial modalities are referred. The following predictions were made from the 'framework hypothesis'.

14.21 Constant errors of intersensory localization

If stimuli are referred to the hypothesized localization framework and if there are constant errors characteristic of each pair of modalities, then the constant errors for the three intersensory localization situations concerned should be interrelated. For example, if a light is localized to the left of a tactile–kinaesthetic stimulus and a tactile–kinaesthetic stimulus is localized to the left of a sound, the sound should now be judged to be to the right of the light. It should, in fact, be possible to predict the direction and magnitude of the constant error for localization of any one of the three intersensory pairs from the direction and magnitudes of the other two pairs.

Expressing this in a way rather more convenient for calculation; the vector sum of the constant errors should be zero. Another way of putting this is to say that intersensory constant errors are transitive, or that the system is linear in this respect.

14.22 Variable errors of intersensory localization

The variable errors of localizations should also be interrelated on the framework hypothesis. For example, the variance of visual–tactile–kinaesthetic localizations should equal the sum of the variances with which visual and tactile–kinaesthetic stimuli are localized separately on the hypothetical framework.

Hence, if SD^2_{VK}, SD^2_{KA} and SD^2_{AV}, are the observed variances for the three intersensory localization conditions, and SD^2_V, SD^2_K and SD^2_A are the hypothetical variances with which each single modality is referred to the framework then:

$$SD^2_{VK} = SD^2_V + SD^2_K$$
$$SD^2_{KA} = SD^2_K + SD^2_A \qquad (2)$$
$$SD^2_{AV} = SD^2_A + SD^2_V$$

Since values for SD^2_{VK}, SD^2_{KA}, and SD^2_{AV} may be estimated, SD^2_V, SD^2_K and SD^2_A may be deduced by solving the three simultaneous equations. One would then expect, for example, SD^2_V to be related to the accuracy with which two visual stimuli can be localized, one with respect to the other, if the additive-variances model is appropriate. Merton (1961) made a similar prediction.

The apparatus used for presenting the stimuli to subjects is shown in figure 14.3. The stimuli, visual, auditory, and tactile–kinaesthetic, were

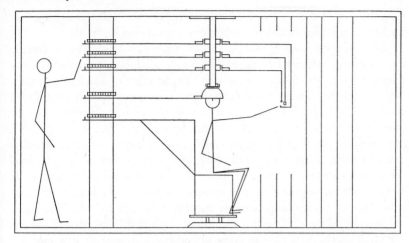

Figure 14.3 Schematic representation of the apparatus used by Fisher to study intersensory localization

mounted on the ends of L-shaped arms which were capable of being rotated independently about a rigid bearing system. A set of five identical fixed scales was used for each modality. Scale C was placed centrally, scales B and A were displaced by five degrees and ten degrees to the left respectively, and scales D and E were displaced by five degrees and ten degrees to the right respectively. Using these scales, the stimulus positions were set up for each localization trial from a table in which the letters A to E had been randomized. The subject had to run the index finger of his preferred hand down a wire guide until he touched a button. The subject was presented with pairs of stimuli in various positions and had to report which of the two was to the left of the other. Light, sound, and touch stimuli were presented in all possible pairs over a wide range of positions.

Fisher's experimental results were inconclusive. The intersensory constant errors were found to fluctuate over time. In fact, Fisher concluded that an 'autokinetic movement' was occurring in each of the modalities (Fisher, 1961). Consequently many of the vector sums of intersensory constant errors differed significantly from zero. Furthermore, the method of constant stimuli did not reveal the majority of intersensory constant errors. However, when adequate time samples of data were taken and a suitable psychophysical method used, it was found that the majority of sums of constant errors were not significantly different from zero. It was also found that many intersensory constant errors were significant.

Secondly, it was predicted that there should be a relationship between the variances of intersensory localization judgments. Unfortunately, the variances were too variable for reliable conclusions to be drawn.

There are two features of these ideas which we consider to be in error. In the first place, we think that the hypothetical spatial framework for the three modalities is a superfluous assumption, like the ether of nineteenth century physics and the sensory–tonic substratum of sensory–tonic theory. Fisher considers the 'variances with which each single modality is referred to the framework'; he admits that these cannot be measured, but we suggest that they have no meaning. For instance, it is meaningless to talk of the localization of a point of light, seen in the dark, except in relation to another visual stimulus or another modality. All localizations must be either intrasensory or intersensory. We agree that it is meaningful to ask whether the constant errors of intersensory judgments are transitive; this tells us something about the linearity of the system. But we do not think that Howarth and Fisher's statement of the additive-variances hypothesis is meaningful. In practice, Fisher interpreted the unimodal variances of localization as the accuracy with which two visual stimuli are localized with respect to each other. He thus implicitly abandoned the hypothetical framework as he had to do if the unimodal variances were to be measured. But now, the unimodal variances become simply the spatial acuities of the various senses, and the additive-variances prediction simply states that the acuity of intermodal localizations is limited only by the separate unimodal acuities. Methods of measuring these acuities could probably be selected so that the unimodal variances did sum to the intermodal variances, but this would prove nothing. In order to give any meaning to the additive-variances prediction, the unimodal and intermodal acuities must be measured by identical psychophysical methods. In Fisher's study this condition was satisfied; he used a successive visual localization task and a successive intersensory task in this part of his work.

Howarth's concept of unimodal acuities is too restrictive. It is not realistic to suppose that the only factors which limit the ability to localize a felt point with respect to a seen point are visual acuity and the tactile–kinaesthetic acuity of the arm. The intersensory judgment also demands that the subject has information about the position of his eyes in his head and his head on his body. The intersensory variance will therefore be a function of at least four variances: visual acuity and eye-position acuity (these are not entirely separable), head-position acuity and limb-position acuity. It may be a worthwhile experimental task to enquire into these relationships, and once again, the answer will tell us something about the linearity of the system.

The second misleading feature of the work of Howarth and Fisher and the other investigators we have reviewed in this section is their use of the terms 'visual localization' and 'kinaesthetic localization'. In all the studies, the visual stimulus was fixated, and we can assume that this would be done accurately and constantly to within a fraction of a degree. Even in a visual–visual successive localization experiment, a visual judgment of direction must depend on and be limited by the accuracy with which the subject can maintain a fixed eye and body position (if the successive positions of the lights are the same) or be aware of movements of the eye and body (if the second light is not in the same location as the first). Our point, therefore, is that the so-called visual localizations are primarily kinaesthetic and/or motor-innervation dependent. In the 'visual' case, one uses the fovea as the equivalent of the finger tip in the 'kinaesthetic' case. In both cases this 'centring' is not the factor which limits the accuracy of the performance. The information from the so-called visual stimulus is purely visual only in a task where the subject has to match a distance between two lights with a distance between two other lights, with a single fixation. For this task it does not matter whether the subject knows where his eyes or head are, for he is no longer judging direction relative to his body but only relative distance between external points, i.e. oculocentric directions. Such studies have of course been done, but are beyond the scope of this book (Abel, 1936; Budkiewicz, 1926; Jastrow, 1889; Kelvin and Mulik, 1958; Raffel, 1936).

The so-called 'kinaesthetic' localizations in Fisher's study were not purely kinaesthetic; the subject held his own arm in position between two guides. Muscular innervation information was therefore available to the subject. For the task to have been purely kinaesthetic, the subject's arm should have been supported on a horizontal surface.

14.23 Intersensory localization and the egocentre

The third of the Howarth–Fisher predictions was concerned with the consequences of assuming that all localizations in all spatial modalities are referred to a common 'centre of projection'. The assumption was made that, if two stimuli are aligned one behind the other, the subject's central reference point must be at some point on an extension of the line joining the two stimuli. If these two stimuli are again aligned when in a different direction; the central reference point for that modality should be at the point of intersection of the two extrapolated lines.

Consider visual–tactile–kinaesthetic localizations; suppose subjects with their heads held in a fixed position are required to make intersensory localization judgments of visual stimuli with respect to tactile–kinaesthetic stimuli presented in the horizontal plane, at two different distances. If the centres of the sensory spaces associated with each modality are different then the mean angular constant errors should not be the same at the different distances.

However, if the centres for all modalities are on the same vertical axis, then the angular intersensory constant errors at all distances should be the same, both in magnitude and direction.

If the centre for visual space is in front of the centre for tactile–kinaesthetic space, then the mean constant errors for intersensory localizations should be different depending upon whether the stimuli are presented to the left or right of centre. Suppose the centre for visual space is in front of the centre for tactile–kinaesthetic space. If visual and tactile–kinaesthetic stimuli are presented together at an angle of 45 degrees to the left of the centre of a subject's body then the tactile–kinaesthetic stimulus should appear to be to the right of the visual stimulus. However, if the stimuli are now presented at an angle of 45 degrees to the right, the tactile–kinaesthetic stimulus should appear to be to the left of the visual stimulus (see figure 14.4). If both centres are in the same

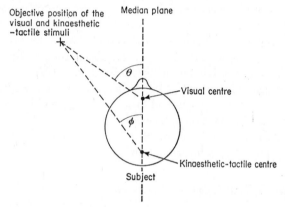

Figure 14.4 Showing how the apparent directions of visual and kinaesthetic-tactile stimuli vary according to the centre in the body from which they are judged

place, the two constant errors for presentation to the left and right should be the same. The above argument may be further elucidated by considering figure 14.4. The angle θ is larger than angle ϕ. This is the only criterion of leftness or rightness and as the angle for the visual centre (θ) is larger than that for the kinaesthetic centre (ϕ), the visual stimulus will be judged to be to the left of the tactile–kinaesthetic when the stimuli are on the left. This analysis is not the same as that given by Fisher; he predicted the opposite result, erroneously we think.

This is a very neat formulation, but perhaps artificial. A person is surely able to judge the alignment of objects with respect to any specified 'centre' according to the instructions he is given. If, for instance, one is pointing at objects at different distances, they may be judged to be in line with the extended arm or with the mid-body axis. If a subject were asked to align stimuli with reference to the mid-body axis using several modalities, Howarth and Fisher's formula could be applied to reveal whether or not the subject was successful and consistent, but in such an experiment the experimenter would have imposed the idea of a common centre of reference on the subject. If, on the other hand, the instructions are left vague, the results will reveal only the way in which the subject has chosen to interpret them. Apparently in Howarth and Fisher's experiment, the subjects tended to make the localizations in the different modalities in relation to a common centre, for the constant errors at different distances and in different directions were similar, but the procedure by which they showed this is very unclearly stated.

Fisher (1964) found that, contrary to common belief, the localization ability of blind subjects in audition and tactile–kinaesthesis was no better than that of sighted subjects, at least when spatial frames of reference were absent. Similarly in intersensory localization the blind have significant constant errors for localizing the source of auditory and tactile–kinaesthetic stimuli presented in the same place.

Apart from a paper by Wertheimer (1961) there appears to have been no work done on the development of intersensory localization. Wertheimer sounded clicks next to the left or right ear of a human infant before the age of ten minutes. Of 52 trials, 18 produced eye movement towards the side of the click and only 4 movement in the opposite direction.

Work has of course been done on the development of reaching behaviour (e.g. Baruk, Leroy, Lauray, and Vallancien, 1953), but it is not relevant to the present discussion since the reaching hand was always visible.

14.3 The resolution of conflicting intersensory information

When the different modalities signal conflicting information, vision usually predominates. For example, if one cuts wood when looking at it in a microscope, it feels as if one is cutting cheese. By converging the eyes, Schilder (1942) produced a double image of a key held upright by the fingers. His impression was that he not only saw but felt two keys. In a more recent experiment Rock and Victor (1963) asked subjects to hold an object while viewing it through distorting spectacles. They were subsequently asked to draw the object and to match its shape with another shape. The results revealed that vision was strongly dominant: the subjects drew and matched the distorted visual shape, often without being aware of the conflict.

Similarly, Stratton (1896) reported while wearing prisms that after a while his feet and other visible body parts came to look normal and feel the way they looked. He obviously resolved the spatial conflict by ignoring it. However, the unseen parts of the body, such as the head, could not come under the direct influence of vision and because the visual scene was accepted as upright he felt that his head and shoulders were inverted, as if he were viewing objects from between his legs. More recently Nielsen (1963) reported that while drawing along a straight line subjects could be induced to accept as their own the mirrored image of the hand of another person drawing along the same line. While both hands followed the straight line the subject reported the observed movement as the result of his own volition, but deviations of the seen hand from the straight line were interpreted as involuntary movements.

Most work on intersensory conflict has been concerned with visual–auditory spatial conflict. Klemm (1909) found that when a visible spark and a sound were presented together, the sound was apparently displaced in the direction of the spark. The sound caused a similar but much smaller apparent displacement of the spark. Allers and Schmiedek (1925) reported similar findings in which sounds were apparently displaced towards the direction of an after-image or even of an imagined visible object. Thomas (1941) also reported an apparent displacement of a sound towards a light, particularly towards a flickering light 'in-rhythm' with the sound. Young (1928) reported that when wearing his pseudophone, which reversed the auditory field through 180°, sounds were localized correctly when the sources of sounds could be seen. In such experiments it is important that the subjects are not asked to indicate the direction of the sound by pointing, for then the results may be due, not to an interaction between vision and sound, but rather to an effect of asymmetrical visual or auditory stimuli on the apparent position of the arm. Furthermore one must distinguish between effects due to visual–auditory spatial conflict and effects due to asymmetrical gaze. These latter effects were discussed in section 11.3.

Both Witkin, Wapner, and Leventhal (1952) and Jackson (1953) have conducted quantitative experiments in which subjects were required to make judgments about the position of an apparent-single source when light and sound stimuli were conflicting. Jackson, for example, used specially prepared steam kettles and compressed-air whistles arranged in such a way that the puffs of steam from the kettles and the whistles were able to be presented independently. He found that there was no apparent conflict in this experimental situation until the puffs of steam and the whistles were presented at angular separations exceeding 30 degrees. Witkin allowed his subjects to observe a person reading through the window of a sound-proofed room. The sound from the room was led to the subjects' ears along tubes of variable length in order that the time relationships of the sound source reaching the ears, and thus the angle of presentation, could be manipulated. In this experiment there was no apparent conflict until the angular separation of the visual and auditory sources was between 28 and 38 degrees.

Stratton (1897b), with reversed vision, reported that sounds of objects out of sight, for instance of stones thrown out of sight, seemed to come from the opposite direction to where they had been seen to pass out of sight. However, when the source of sound was in sight the sound seemed to originate in the visible object responsible for the sound. In this case, therefore, vision dominated.

Thus, when spatial information in light and sound is made conflicting there is no apparent conflict until the separation of the sources becomes very large. Separations of this order indicate clearly that we are concerned here not with a simple problem of acuity, but rather with a mechanism, or mechanisms, which operate in such a way that, when spatial information in two sensory modalities is available, the information in one of the modalities is partly or wholly discarded in favour of that in the other. This phenomenon has been called the 'ventriloquism' effect. It is the same mechanism which operates when we watch the cinema or television, where very often the positions of the sound and vision sources are displaced by a considerable distance.

One mechanism by which spatial conflict could be resolved may be called 'stimulus dominance'. When sound and light stimuli are made conflicting, light is dominant over sound and thus the ventriloquism effect is one example of the stimulus dominance effect. It may be that ventriloquism is a special case of a more general stimulus dominance effect involving all the spatial senses. It may be expected that if spatial information in any particular modality is discarded then the information from the remaining modality is the more accurate.

Fisher (1962a) carried out a series of experiments in which subjects were told that two stimuli in two different modalities were in the same place. In fact their relative location was varied and the subject had to indicate by pointing, where the joint stimulus was. Vision was found to be completely dominant over audition, that is, judgments about position were made entirely on the apparent position of the light stimulus. However, with each of the other paired modalities dominance was incomplete. The pooled data for all subjects showed that visual stimuli were dominant over both tactile–kinaesthetic and auditory stimuli, and tactile–kinaesthetic stimuli were dominant over auditory stimuli. This is the order of dominance which Fisher predicted if dominance is related to the order of accuracy of localization of successive stimuli within each of the modalities. However, in the case of two subjects, tactile–kinaesthesis was dominant over vision. In the case of blind subjects tactile–kinaesthesis appears, as with sighted subjects, to be dominant over audition (Fisher, 1964).

14.4 Directional preferences in operator–control–display relationships

Such a variety of answers has been given in practice to the question of which direction a control requires to be moved in order to produce a movement in a particular direction on a display, that one is forced to the conclusion that for designers at least, it is a matter of indifference. There is considerable evidence that it is *not* a matter of indifference for operators. This evidence has already been adequately reviewed by Loveless (1962) and it will suffice here to summarize his conclusions. Display–control relationships which are expected by most of the population have been called 'population stereotypes' (Fitts, 1951). Some are quite obvious or 'natural' as when a pointer moves in the same direction as a control lever and movement of the lever is expected to produce pointer movement in the same sense. Others are more subtle and may depend on the conventions of a particular culture and may not be obvious until teased out by quite complex experimentation.

Although it appears that relationships contrary to expectation may take longer to learn to an accuracy criterion, particularly for older or less intelligent subjects, yet this difference may be of little practical importance. However, there is some evidence that even with extensive practice the new learning never really becomes as well established as the old. The inferiority may show up if a different criterion of performance, such as reaction time, is used, or after a period away from the task, or under stressful conditions, e.g. with the other hand, at a faster rate, or in an emergency. Such findings agree with Broadbent's (1958) predictions about the relative stability of short- and long-term memory.

Loveless warns that casual observation of a few operators is not likely to provide the answers in this area: culture group, sex, previous mechanical experience, age, intelligence, and handedness may all be relevant factors in determining which preferences an individual will display in a particular situation. Many of Holding's (1957a) subjects, even though in a minority on a particular response preference, were surprised that anyone would choose a different response to the one they had made.

With a linear indicator and translatory control, if the lines of movement of the two are parallel, the stereotype seems intuitively obvious. The little work done on this arrangement shows that when lines of movement are not parallel there is a marked tendency to expect upward indicator movement to be produced by forward control movement and possibly also by control movement to the right. Little is known of the arrangement in which a linear indicator is controlled by a lever or joystick and no consistent stereotypes have emerged except for the case when lever and indicator movements are parallel. More attention has been paid to the control of a linear indicator by means of a knob. A clockwise rotation of the knob is expected to displace an indicator upwards or to the right. The only exception appears to be in cases of conflict with a stronger expectation, viz. that when the axis of the knob is perpendicular to the line of indicator movement and passes to one side of it, the indicator is expected to move in the same direction as the part of the knob nearest to it. When the knob axis is parallel to the line of indicator movement there is some evidence, though it is not unequivocal, of an expectation that clockwise rotation will move the indicator away from the control.

Loveless warns against the use of circular indicators in conjunction with rotary controls. There is an expectation that clockwise control movement will produce clockwise pointer movement but also that it will produce pointer movement upwards or to the right. In the left and top quadrants of a dial these expectations are in agreement, but in the right and bottom quadrants they are opposed, and this conflict is reflected in performance. Similarly, translatory control is likely to lead to confusion as it will probably be expected to cause movement of a pointer in the same sense and will therefore have opposed effects on the two halves of a circular dial. It is not known whether such an arrangement carries also expectations of rotary movement, as, for example, a rack and pinion. Lever control of circular indicators involves a similar conflict, and Loveless recommends that such an arrangement be confined to the upper and left hand quadrants, and also that lever and pointer should extend in the same direction from their pivots, and that the lever should be mounted with its free end towards the display. In all the reported work, levers and dials have rotated in the same plane.

In support of Loveless's warning about the use of circular dials is the fact that subjects can check more accurately whether a dial reading is too high or too low when the normal position of the pointer is at 9 o'clock rather than at 3 o'clock (Warrick and Grether, 1948) presumably because in the latter case the spatial and numerical 'higher' are in conflict. Similarly Fitts and Simon (1949) found that pointers were more accurately maintained in the normal position when this was 9 o'clock or 12 o'clock rather than 3 o'clock or 6 o'clock. Verbal judgments of the direction of change represented by a particular pointer movement are also more accurate in the left and top quadrants (Connell and Grether, 1948; Long and Grether, 1949).

It also seems that a moving pointer is more satisfactory than a dial moving behind a stationary pointer (Long and Grether, 1949; Loucks, 1949).

Holding (1957a) found that most subjects chose to move a knob clockwise to produce upward movement of a pointer on a vertical scale, and anti-clockwise for a downward movement; but this tendency depended on the initial position of the pointer on the scale: predominant responses were 14% fewer at the extremes of the scale than in the middle. This confirmed an earlier finding of Bilodeau (1951). When control–display relationships are ambiguous there is a general tendency to turn knobs clockwise (Warrick, 1947). But the results of Holding (1957b) demand in addition a helical or screw-like tendency i.e. an expectation that clockwise rotation will produce motion away from the point of rotation along the axis of rotation. The sub-ject had to rotate a knob which appeared on the top, bottom, front or right-hand side of the apparatus, to produce movement of a pointer perpendicular to the plane of rotation. When the required movement was away from the knob, responses were predominantly clockwise, in accordance with both hypothesized tendencies. When movement was towards the knob the clock-wise tendency was predominant but the now opposed, helical tendency was shown to be operative by the higher proportion of anticlockwise responses which occurred in this case than in the case of movement away from the knob. When the knob was on the left side of the apparatus and the left hand was used there were no significant preferences, but left-handed subjects gave more anticlockwise responses, even when using the right hand, than right-handers.

Similarly Bradley (1957) found that whereas 90% of right-handed subjects, when asked to grasp and turn a control knob, turned it clockwise, left-handers showed no predominance either way.

Just as Holding had to hypothesize a helical tendency in addition to the clockwise-turning tendency so Bradley found that one of his results depended on a combination of a general clockwise tendency and clockwise-to-increase tendency. Asked to increase brightness, 86% turned the knob clockwise: asked to decrease brightness only 61% turned it anticlockwise.

One of the findings of Warrick (1947) confirmed the rather obvious con-clusion that performance is poor when stimuli arriving in rapid sequence demand different responses based on contradictory direction-of-motion principles. A response conforming to a stereotype appears to be more affected by this alternation than the contradictory response, presumably because the latter is carried out more deliberately in any case.

The importance of population stereotypes or direction of movement preferences is also stressed by Fitts and Seeger (1953). They used three sets of responses (stylus movement) and three sets of stimuli (lights); each response set was a direct spatial analogue of one of the stimulus sets. Different groups of subjects were trained on each of the nine possible combinations of a stimulus and a response set. The three 'compatible' S–R combinations yielded consistently lower time, error, and information-loss scores than the other combinations. When a separate group of subjects was given prolonged training on all three stimulus sets combined with only one of the response sets, differences between performance on the three stimulus sets showed no tendency to diminish, so indicating the relative impregnability of expectancies and habits based on a subject's general life experiences.

This ineffectiveness of short-term learning was confirmed in a further study (Fitts and Deininger, 1954) in which a single response set of stylus movements along radii of a circle was combined with two spatial stimulus sets (a circle and row of lights) and two symbolic sets (times of the day and first names). Pairing of stimuli and responses within each stimulus set was arranged to provide either normal or mirrored or random S–R correspondence, except that only random pairing was used with the set of first names. As well as the persistence of group differences over the training period it was found that with either normal or mirrored pairing, performance was best on the circular stimulus array; with random S–R pairing performance was generally poor, but better with the symbolic than with the spatial arrays.

Nystrom and Grant (1955) studied speed of key pressing as a function of the angular orientation of a row of lights relative to a row of keys. Only rotations as large as 135° or 180° produced a significant deterioration, although performance tended to fall off as separation increased, throughout the range.

Battig (1954) investigated various modes of training on a task in which the subject was required to use a control stick to switch on green lights matching in position a given display of red lights. The best learning resulted from practice on the actual task. Intermediate in achievement was the verbal-stimulus group, for whom the red lights were replaced by numbers and instructions were given verbally rather than visually, and the kinaesthetic-response group who could not see the red lights while they were actually making the adjustment. The verbal-response group, who merely described the movements they would carry out, and the verbal-stimulus-kinaesthetic-response group, who carried out movements in response to verbal instructions without the use of lights, were no better than a group which had no practice at all. These latter types of training might even produce interference rather than learning. Battig concluded that visual cues are most important in this type of task.

The operator's orientation to the display, as well as the control–display relationship, appears to be of importance. Shephard and Cook (1959) used the Toronto complex coordinator to study the effect of changing the subject's orientation to the display through 90° in 30° steps i.e. from facing the display to being side-on to it. The subject's body always faced the control lever directly. The subject could be moved as much as 60° from the straight-ahead position before there was appreciable deterioration in performance, but at 90° it was markedly poorer e.g. the subject still moved the lever directly away from him to raise the pointer, a response which had been correct when he was facing the display. This suggests that at some point a sudden transformation occurs in the subject's response to the spatial relationships.

Similar results were reported by Humphries (1958) using the same apparatus. The subject tended to refer display movements to his line of regard and control movements to his body, so that movement of the vertically mounted joystick away from his body was expected to produce upward display movement and movement to his right was expected to cause display movement to the right of his line of regard. These effects of body position disappeared entirely when the joystick was mounted horizontally so that its plane of movement was parallel to that of the display.

However, the operator's orientation to the controls, as opposed to the display, appears to be of little importance. Helson and Howe (1942) found that accuracy in their tracking task was not affected by the orientation of the hand-wheel, whether vertical, horizontal or oblique, and Reed (1949) reported that the maximum speed at which a crank could be rotated was little affected by its orientation. Jenkins (1947a and b) found that no direction of arm movement led to more accuracy than any other in applying force against *isometric controls*, and Grether's (1947) results suggest that the degree of arm flexion involved in positioning a control is not a significant factor, and within limits operators may, without loss of accuracy, adopt any comfortable position; fore-and-aft movements of a wheel or a stick control were more accurate than rotary or side-to-side movements. But Fletcher, Collins and Brown (1958) showed a tendency for tracking accuracy to be higher with a right-hand than with a central control stick.

15

The behavioural consequences of rotations and displacements of the optical array

15.1 Introduction

This chapter is concerned with the behavioural effects of laterally displacing or rotating the whole proximal optical array relative to the distal stimulus. It is not concerned with spatial distortions within the optical array itself (except for the special case of the visible limits of the field of view, e.g. spectacle frames, which may remain constant while the rest of the field of view is changed).

Ultimately, so-called perceptual problems are problems of behaviour. Normally, a visible object in a given location relative to the body of an observer evokes behaviour (including linguistic behaviour) which is appropriate to its position and to its orientation. If the proximal optical array arising from an object is displaced or rotated without the subject knowing, the behaviour associated with it is appropriate to that same object in a position or orientation where it would normally produce that proximal optical array.

Many aspects of behaviour related to a visible object are affected by a disturbance of the normal position and orientation of the proximal stimulus with respect to the distal stimulus; the behavioural consequences are more complex than many of the investigators in this field have realized.

The behaviour affected by such disturbances may be classified into four main categories: (1) visual–motor coordination of movements other than eye and head movements; (2) the coordination of visuo-spatial judgments with eye and head movements; (3) intersensory localizations; and (4) behaviour related to mono-oriented objects.

15.2 Visual–motor coordination

15.21 Introduction

The most obvious consequence of wearing displacing spectacles is the disturbance of visually guided behaviour, such as pointing. Movements towards objects will be directed towards that position in space whence the displaced optical array would normally emanate. If the pointing limb is in view, the person will correct his initial mistake and be able to guide it visually to the target. Therefore, in any experiment in which the effects of distorting spectacles are being studied, the subject must not be allowed to see the moving part of his own body, at least until he has completed the movement.

Human subjects, given time and knowledge of results are able to adapt their movements to simple visual displacements or rotations. There has apparently never been any disagreement about this fact since the experiments by Stratton in 1896.

Other mammals can apparently adapt their movements to some extent also. Foley (1940) found that monkeys adjust some of their movements after wearing an inverting lens for eight days and Bossom and Hamilton (1963) found that they could adapt to a 13° lateral visual displacement after two days. Cats have been shown to adapt to displaced vision (Bishop 1959). We shall discuss the case of submammalian species in section 15.25.

We shall consider first the effects of rotary distortions of vision.

15.22 Inversion and reversal of the optical array, and visual–motor coordination

Stratton (1897b) wore a lens system in front of one eye which inverted and reversed the optical array. He wore this device continuously for seven days and gave a full account of his visual–motor disturbances during that time. On the first day he reported that, 'Almost all movements performed under the direct guidance of sight were laborious and embarrassed.... The wrong hand was constantly used to seize anything that lay to one side.... Relief was sometimes sought by shutting out of consideration the actual visual data, and by depending solely on tactual or motor perception.... In order to write my notes, the formation of the letters and words had to be left to automatic muscular sequence, using sight only as a guide to the general position and direction on my paper' (p. 344). By the third day he reported that, 'I could watch my hands as I wrote, without hesitating or becoming embarrassed thereby.... Yet I often stretched out the wrong hand to grasp a visible object lying to one side; right and left were felt to be by far the most persistently troublesome relations when it came to translating visual into tactual or motor localizations' (p. 349). On the fourth day he reported, 'My hands, in washing, often moved to the soap or to the proper position in the basin, without premonition or any need of correcting the movement. At one time in the morning, I pictured the basin and its appurtenances before me in pre-experimental terms. But my actions were the opposite to those which would have been appropriate to this image' (p. 352). He was still having difficulty with left–right visual–motor coordination on the fifth day; however, he reported, 'But I found that the appropriate hand often came to the appropriate side of the visual field directly and without the thought (frequently necessary before) that *that* visual side meant the *other* side in motor or older visual terms' (p. 355). On that day also he reported, 'the most harmonious experiences were obtained during active operations on the scene before me. In rapid, complicated, yet practised movements, the harmony of the localization by sight and that by touch or motor perception— the actual identity of the positions reported in these various ways—came out with much greater force than when I sat down and passively observed the scene' (p. 356).

Stratton gave himself no systematic tests of visual–motor coordination, he merely reported on those common actions which occurred in his normal routine of life. American investigators since Stratton have used experimentally controlled visual–motor tasks.

Ewert (1930, 1936, 1937) asked his three subjects to sort cards and to point to visual targets, before, during, and after a one-hour period of inverted and reversed vision, on 14 consecutive days. Snyder and Pronko (1952) timed the performance of a single subject at a card sorting task, the Minnesota Rate of Manipulation Test, the Purdue Pegboard, and a mirror-tracing task, before, during, and after a 30-day period during which inverting-reversing spectacles were continuously worn. Both experimenters found that performance in the motor tasks steadily improved, provided there was knowledge of results. Performance was found to be disturbed for a while when the spectacles were removed. Snyder and Pronko used a control condition to investigate the effect of the constriction of the visual field which inverting spectacles necessarily impose. They found that this constriction of the field to 20° did not appreciably influence the quantitative or qualitative results.

Peterson and Peterson (1938) and Snyder and Pronko (1952) found that the visual–motor habits learned whilst wearing distorting spectacles were retained when the subjects were again tested with the spectacles after a period of several months of normal viewing.

Erisman began working on the problem of displaced vision in 1928 at the University of Innsbruck. His assistant Kohler published a series of papers (1951, 1953, 1955, 1956a, 1956b, 1962) and has, since Erisman's death, been the director of the laboratory (see Kottenhoff, 1957a, 1957b for an English summary of this work). Kohler's approach is phenomenological, relying on the introspective reports of his subjects, rather than on the application of controlled experimental tests. He used a variety of optical devices, inverting-reversing lenses, a mirror which inverted only, prisms which reversed left and right only, and displacing prisms.

He described various strategies which a subject may adopt in order to make movements conform with inverted or reversed vision. Certain movements are not disturbed. A hand moving quickly to a particular unseen part of the body successfully reaches the target, even when the hand crosses the field of view, and thus appears to run in reversed fashion. The displaced vision is not impelling enough to disturb the automatic character of such movements. Writing may be done correctly and without difficulty if done as a set of learned, automatic, kinaesthetic–motor movements, with vision as only a guide to the general position of the paper. A subject writing in this fashion, with left–right visual distortion, reported that the movements of his fingers ran off automatically, as if controlled by some external agent. Every attempt to affect them intentionally led to complete blockage.

This procedure of kinaesthetic–motor guidance does not succeed when the task is to reach to, or follow, a visual target, for the visual information is essential for the success of such tasks. Kohler distinguished between two types of task. The first is where the subject is required to initiate a rapidly executed reaching or aiming movement, such as kicking a ball, throwing a dart, or ordinary walking over rough ground. The second type of task is where the moving limb is in the field of view and may be guided continuously in relation to the visual target. The second type is not much disturbed by visual distortion.

For the difficult impulsive movements Kohler described various strategies. The first strategy which subjects adopt is deliberately to take the glasses into account and delay the motor response until the habitual movement may be inhibited and replaced by one which the subject predicts will hit the target. The method demands a fatiguing degree of concentration, and the reasoning is likely to fail when some unforeseen factor occurs which has been omitted from the calculation. When the situation is a potentially dangerous one, the subject becomes alarmed and all attempts to move in the direction which reasoning has decided are blocked.

The next strategy is the command to do the opposite of the habitual movement—to move the opposite ('wrong') foot or hand in the opposite ('wrong') direction. Here the point is not to decide first where objects really are and act accordingly, but merely to do the opposite of the first impulse. Mistakes are common with this method and movements are slow.

As time goes on, inappropriate movements become negatively reinforced by undesired outcomes, such as unintended impacts with objects or failure to hit targets. Gradually it becomes sufficient for such false moves to be only partially carried out for a 'warning' to result and the movement to be inhibited. At this stage the need for deliberate thinking diminishes, and correct movements begin to be carried out automatically. Kohler reported that for him the apparently inverted field of view passed in front of him, like the pictures on a cinema screen. He did not take them seriously, he achieved a 'liberation from the visual picture'. Eventually complex movements, such as skiing, climbing, cycling, and driving were correctly and smoothly executed. However, each new task had to be learned piecemeal; success at one skill did not transfer to other skills.

Kohler insisted that his introspective method revealed the essential 'inner experience' involved in what he called rehabilitation to visual distortion. He was critical of Ewert, Snyder and Pronko, and other American workers after Stratton for their 'one-sided behaviourism'.

The Americans may have elicited a narrow range of responses from their subjects, but this narrowness need not have stemmed from their behaviourism. We claim that all that is capable of becoming communal knowledge (scientific knowledge) may be derived from observing the behaviour of others. Kohler need not himself have been a subject to have gained the knowledge he has. Having been a subject probably helped him to formulate ideas, but the experience was in theory not essential. The facts or ideas which Kohler reported are only more 'inner' than any other facts of science in that they were derived from the verbal reports of his subjects. They are now 'outer' because they have become communicated, and therefore communal, facts and ideas.

Kohler was perhaps only attacking that form of behaviourism in which verbal reports are not allowed as evidence. Kohler's whole approach is otherwise a brave attempt to analyse the changes underlying rehabilitation in terms of visual–motor habits (see in particular Kohler, 1956b). He wrote '... the path to correct seeing ... can only be understood against the background of a theory of habits and their interweaving.' Again, 'It's clear that the goal of the subjects is to learn in some manner how to make correct movements. It is rather interesting to see how this happens, and how, gradually and unnoticed, behaviour transforms itself into seeing.' (Quotations from a translation by Gleitman of Kohler's 1953 paper.) Kohler used what we consider to be non-behaviouristic terminology but otherwise made what amounts to a behavouristic analysis with concepts which, for the most part, can be given operational definition.

Recently Taylor (1962), working in Innsbruck and South Africa, has presented what he claims to be a full behavioural account of the experiments on distorted vision. His theory uses a Hullian framework and a notation derived from set theory. He came to rely also on ideas derived from Ashby's theory of multistable systems (Ashby, 1957). In spite of Taylor's intention to give a behaviouristic account of this field of study, his language is often subjective; he talks as if his formulae describe 'perceptions', 'experiences', etc., rather than observable behaviour.

Papert, who collaborated with Taylor, wore left–right reversing spectacles each morning over an extended period. The prediction was that habits appropriate to the distortion would be built up but at the same time normal habits would be retained by being practised in the afternoons. A series of visual–motor tasks was administered to the subject while he wore the distorting prisms. These included reaching by command to particular objects, moving a hand or foot which was touched, executing complex commands to place particular objects in particular places, walking round a chair, riding a cycle, etc. It was found that training on one particular task did not transfer to others. It was this specificity of learning which led Taylor to talk of the visual–motor system as a complex, multistable system.

Rhule and Smith (1959a, 1959b) also stressed the specific nature of sensory–motor learning with inverted vision. Their studies are puzzling in several ways. The four groups of subjects were asked to write rows of a's, triangles, and dots under four conditions; normal vision and normal kinaesthetic feedback, normal vision with inverted kinaesthetic feedback, inverted vision with normal kinaesthetic feedback, and inverted vision with inverted kinaesthetic feedback. By 'inverted kinaesthetic feedback' was meant upside-down writing movements. How anyone can write a row of dots, or even a triangle, upside-down is not made clear. Nor is it clear why upside-down writing movements should be regarded as inverted kinaesthetic feedback, which properly would involve an anatomical reversal of the kinaesthetic nerves in relation to the motor supply and vision. All that is reversed in drawing something upside-down is the pattern of motor movements normally associated with the particular shape. The letter 'a' was the only one of Rhule and Smith's shapes which is obviously associated with a particular orientation of movements.

Their only measures of performance were the time during which the pen was in contact with the paper (manipulation time) and the time it was not in contact with the paper (travel time). No measures were taken of the quality of the shapes produced. It is well known in mirror-drawing experiments, that time can be 'traded' against errors. A measure of either alone is no indication of the rate of learning. We can see from an illustration in Smith and Smith's book (1962, p. 136) that the quality of performance was abysmal on the first day of the experiment. If the subjects were told to work as fast as possible, and we are not told what they were asked to do, their learning would not have been reflected at all in the time measures which were used.

Therefore we have no reason to trust any of the results which these authors present, and this applies to most of the results in the book by Smith and Smith, especially since many of their results contradict what we can find out from casual observation. For instance, they found that there was little if any difference in people's ability to draw 'a' and upside-down 'a'. Anyone trying these two tasks is immediately aware that it is much more difficult to draw an upside-down 'a', but one learns in a few minutes to become fairly proficient. The time-scale of averaged scores on each day for ten days which Rhule and Smith used, fails to disclose the learning which must take place here.

From the conditions where vision was inverted it was concluded that the effects of inversion were greater in tasks of increasing complexity. The triangle showed the most effect of inversion, the dots least. That the dots would show least effect should surely have been obvious before the experiment started, and to say that the triangle shows most effect, because it is the most complex shape, is meaningless in the absence of any independent measure of 'complexity'. Rhule and Smith concluded that learning was specific to each shape. Their conclusion would carry more weight if they had tested whether training on one letter improved the ability to write other letters under similar distorting conditions. However, they did find that training to read upside-down writing did not transfer to writing with visual inversion (Rhule and Smith, 1959a) but in view of the crude measure they used, even this finding cannot be accepted as a fact.

These experiments and others by Smith and Smith which we shall presently describe were repeated using a closed-circuit television camera and monitor. The subject saw his hand and the visual target in the monitor only. The hand was actually off to one side where it could be photographed by the camera (see figure 15.1). The sideways displacement of the hand was a con-

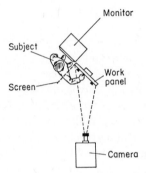

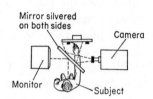

Figure 15.1 Arrangement used by Smith and Smith (1962) to study visual–motor disarrangement

Figure 15.2 Suggested improved arrangement for studying visual–motor disarrangement

tamination. A better technique would have been to arrange the camera and monitor as shown in figure 15.2. In spite of their vast technical resources, Smith and Smith apparently did not think of this simple device. Using the television system, Smith and Smith (1962, pp. 168–172) went on to analyse the relative disturbing effects on drawing dots, a's, and triangles, of inverted, reversed, and inverted–reversed vision. Performance speed was most affected by inverted viewing, next by inverted–reversed viewing, and least by reversed viewing. They concluded that this order reflects the order in which all skills are affected by these disturbances. This conclusion is completely unwarranted. Two of the shapes they used, dots and triangles ($\triangle$), are bilaterally symmetrical, so that reversal could not be expected to disrupt performance. It is not stated whether the order of drawing the rows of shapes was specified to the subjects, but in any case, inversion of the optical array would not disturb this aspect of performance, whereas reversal would.

Smith and Smith (pp. 180–183) also used a star-tracing task. This is the correct way to study the relative effects of the various types of distortion, for the figure is just as symmetrical one way as the other. They still found that inversion produced the greatest disturbance, and reversal least. They found, contrary to commonsense expectation, that movements in a particular dimension were not disturbed most by displacement in that dimension. For instance, those portions of the star figure which ran left to right were not most disturbed by left–right reversal of vision. This result is unacceptable for it is based on time measures only.

Smith and Smith (1962, pp. 185–210) also studied the effects of varying the position of the television camera in various planes relative to the hand executing given tasks. The tasks included assembly tasks, tapping a matrix of dots, drawing geometric shapes, writing, and maze tracing. For the details of these displacements and tasks, the reader is referred to the book by Smith and Smith. It was found that performance was not affected until the angular displacement of the seen hand reached about seven degrees, although the size of this 'break-down angle' varied for the different tasks: the assembly task was most affected by a 120° horizontal displacement; other tasks were affected most by other degrees of displacement. Displacements in planes other than the horizontal and displacements of the panels upon which the movements were executed had differential effects for the various tasks and components of those tasks.

These studies do not lead to any important theoretical conclusions, except that the effects of various types of distortion on various kinds of movement are highly specific, and one's faith in even this conclusion is shaken when one considers the crude measure used. Smith and Smith interpret their findings in terms of their neurogeometric theory, which we discuss in section 15.23.

In a recent paper, Smith and Greene (1963) report that children between nine and twelve years of age consistently failed to perform the drawing of dots, triangles and a's with inverted visual feedback. Children over twelve seldom failed to learn. But we are not told whether the younger children could write upside-down a's at all. If they could not, then it would be misleading to conclude that they cannot compensate for inverted vision in the case of this shape. Our assumption is that learning to adapt to distorted vision involves a high-level habit substitution mechanism; it is reasonable to suppose that this mechanism will be relatively late in maturing. We would, like Smith and Greene, predict that very young children are unable to compensate in the ordinary way for large optical distortions. Before we accept the critical age of twelve, we would like to see experiments done on children younger than nine and with a greater variety of tasks. We have found, for instance, that four year olds readily adapt their pointing, wearing 20 dioptre laterally displacing prisms. Anyone with a young child can verify our observation in a few minutes.

Visual–motor adaptation to disturbed visual input is most profitably studied using visual displacement, rather than inversion or reversal, for there is no contamination by the other disturbances which inversion and reversal entail. Furthermore, relearning is quicker, and therefore easier to study in a reasonable period of time, and also for this reason the experimental conditions are more easily controlled. The theoretically significant studies of visual–motor adaptation in recent years have involved the use of displacing prisms or mirrors.

15.23   The site of the recalibration involved in visual–motor adaptation

Helmholtz (1962, vol. 3, p. 252) noticed how quickly pointing is adjusted to a displaced visual input. He argued from this observation that visual–motor coordination is learned during the development of an animal. This is not a valid conclusion any more than would be the conclusion that visual–motor coordination is innate if it were the case that it could not be relearned by an adult.

Visual–motor adaptation involves a change in the control system which relates visual inputs to localizing motor responses. Harris (1963a, 1963b) has talked as if such a change was one of several possibilities: a change in visual perception; a reorientation of the axes of perceptual space; motor-response learning. But 'visual perception' and 'axes of perceptual space' are operationally definable only in terms of visual–motor behaviour. We fail to appreciate how all Harris's distinctions can be given operational significance. However, there are two apparently distinct possibilities.

These possibilities are that visual–motor adaptation may occur either on the afferent, or on the efferent side of the control system. Let us assume for the time being that this is a real distinction. There are no direct ways known for finding out on which side the change has occurred, but there are two indirect methods which might give some indication. The point of the first method is to discover whether a subject, who has adapted his visual–motor behaviour to a displaced optical array, reports a target to be in a new position, or whether he reports his arm to be in a new position. In order to give such questions any meaning, one must define an independent criterion of directionality. In the course of a person's lifetime the verbal label 'straight ahead' has become conditioned to a particular position of eyes, head, image on the retina, and to a particular position of the pointing finger in relation to the body. The procedure consists in using these conditioned verbal responses to indicate whether changes have occurred in the afferent or in the efferent part of the total system which coordinates movements of the arm with the position of a visual target relative to the observer. The observer is alternately asked to set a light to the median plane using vision alone and to point to the median plane, before and after adapting to the prisms.

There would appear to be three main possible results.

(1) In the first place, a subject may come to attach the verbal label 'straight ahead' to a new position in space relative to his body. In other words he may recalibrate the visual input side of the visual–motor control loop in relation to this criterion. Any recalibration of the visual median plane may involve a recalibration, not of retinal space values, but of the position of the eyes in relation to a given position of the visual target. When we call this a recalibration of the visual median plane, we are using the word 'visual' to include the position of the eyes as well as the spatial position of images on the retinae. It is reasonable to conclude that any recalibration of the position of the eyes would involve primarily the motor innervations to the eye muscles, rather than the kinaesthetic input from these muscles (see our discussion in section 3.5).

(2) The second possibility is that the subject will come to attach the verbal label 'straight ahead' to a new position of his arm. This could involve either the kinaesthetic inputs from the arm, or the motor innervations, or both. If the newly labelled straight-ahead position were displaced to the full extent of the experimentally produced displacement, it is reasonable to suppose that both kinaesthesis and motor innervation would have been relabelled. If the relabelling were limited to one system, the old labelling of the other system would conflict with the new labelling, and something less than a full change in the reported position of the arm would result. In either case, one would conclude that the visual–motor adaptation had involved a 'recalibration' of the motor–kinaesthetic output side of the visual–motor control loop.

(3) The third possibility is that the subject will relabel neither the visual median plane nor the kinaesthetic–motor median plane. After learning to hit the target, the subject will report that the light looks straight ahead but that he has to point to one side in order to touch it. One would conclude that he has not recalibrated any part of his visual–motor system. In ordinary language one would say that he has consciously made an allowance for the fact that the visual target although appearing straight ahead was in fact appreciably displaced to one side. This procedure and terminology appears to give us an operational behavioural definition of the term 'conscious adjustment'.

Although no details were given, Harris (1963b) apparently did an experiment of this kind. When subjects were asked to point straight ahead (presumably in the dark), after having adapted their motor behaviour to displacing prisms, their pointing deviated in the direction of the visual displacement. Judgments of the visual straight ahead were not required, but Harris found that the auditory straight ahead was not affected. Our own experiment along these lines (Howard and Craske) produced results with such wide intra- and inter-individual differences that a clear-cut conclusion was impossible. We suspect that the instructions, 'set the unseen finger to straight ahead' and 'set the light to the straight ahead' which were involved in the experiment, are essentially ambiguous. For instance, a light may be set either to the visual straight ahead, or to that position where it would be located if the hand were straight ahead and touching it. Part of the task of judging the visual straight ahead is knowing where the head and body are, and these are motor–kinaesthetic judgments which are also involved in the judgment of the motor straight ahead. We could find no way of overcoming this ambiguity. In other words, the judgment 'straight ahead' is perhaps not an independent criterion, and cannot therefore serve as an indicator of the site of recalibration.

The second procedure which could apparently serve to identify the site of recalibration is to investigate whether the effect transfers across hands and across eyes. Harris also argued that if the change involved in adaptation were visual, the subject would point in a similar way with either hand. However, he found that the learning did not transfer to the hand which had not been used in the training. Furthermore, the adaptation with the trained hand was the same whether the target was a light or a sound. Hamilton (1964) confirmed that adaptation does not transfer across hands; although he found a little transfer when the subject was allowed to move his head and body. It is well established that mirror-drawing performance transfers to some extent from one hand to the other (Ewert, 1926; Cook, 1933a, 1933b; Simon, 1948; Hauty, 1953). Although the distortion involved here is not the same as that involved in prismatic displacement, there is no obvious reason why bimanual transfer should occur in the one case and not in the other.

If the recalibration is of the proprioceptive–motor system, visual–motor adaptation learned with one eye open should transfer when tested with only the other eye open. Bossom and Hamilton (1963) have found that such transfer does occur in the monkey, and even in a monkey which has had both its corpus callosum and optic chiasma mid-line sectioned.

Helmholtz reported results which conflict with these recent findings: he found that adaptation to lateral displacement did transfer across hands but not across eyes. Whereas Harris concluded that the recalibration is on the kinaesthetic side, Helmholtz concluded that, '... it is not the muscular feeling of the hand which is at fault or the judgment of its position, but the judgment of the direction of the gaze ...' (Helmholtz, 1962, p. 246). Harris concluded that, 'When proprioception and vision provide conflicting information—when a person feels his hand in one place and sees it in another—proprioception gives way. The person comes to feel that his hand is where it looks as if it is.'

Harris's conclusion does not follow from either his evidence, nor the other evidence cited. In the first place Harris failed to consider the change in motor outflow which is probably involved in visual–motor adaptation. We shall discuss this issue later. Our main criticism of Harris's conclusion is that it is based on the results of one type of training procedure. In this procedure, the subject was asked to point to a visual target. His first attempt was out by the amount of optical displacement and he gradually and deliberately altered the direction of movement until he hit the target. His eyes did not have to modify their position, and the retinal image remained unaffected. Small wonder therefore that the recalibration affected the arm and not the eye. The subject had no option but to deliberately modify the position of his arm. Furthermore, it is not surprising that the effect of training transferred from one eye to the other, for there was no reason to suppose that anything had happened even to the eye which was open during training. In so far as the effect does not transfer from one arm to the other, one must assume that the visual–motor habits controlling one arm are distinct from those of the other. People constantly learn skills involving different movements for each arm, so that this specificity of habit recalibration is not surprising.

If a situation could be devised in which the eyes have to modify their movements in order to reach a target, then one might expect a visual recalibration and not a recalibration of a limb. Howard, Craske, and Templeton have devised such a task. The subject was asked to place the index finger of one hand in a straight-ahead position. The lights were then put out and twelve degree laterally displacing prisms in spectacle frames were placed on the subject. He was asked to glance to one side keeping his head straight in the head clamp, and to return his eyes to his finger tip. The lights were put on, revealing any error to the subject. The lights were put out and the procedure repeated twenty times, the subject being asked to do all he could to succeed in having the correct fixation when the lights were put on. The learning transferred from one hand to the other. We could not test whether it transferred from one eye to the other, for our subjects could not dissociate their eye movements; the experiment ought to be repeated with one of those rare people who can do this.

Thus, considering the parts of the total control system involved in a particular visual–motor response, it seems that *recalibration occurs only in that part of the system which the training procedure demands.*

In a more recent publication Harris (1964) has gone some way to meet these objections to his proprioceptive theory of visual–motor adaptation. He admitted that under certain circumstances it may be the felt position of the eyes in their sockets or of the head on the body which is affected by adaptation to a displaced visual array, and further admitted that the felt position of the eyes may depend on motor outflow rather than proprioceptive feedback. He has assembled an imposing array of evidence that his modified theory can explain visual–motor adaptation and even curvature after-effects. This latter effect he put down to a change in the felt direction of eye movements as the eyes scan a straight line after having inspected a curved line. His theory cannot, however account for curvature after-effects produced with constant fixation, nor the occurrence of two opposed curvature after-effects at the same time (see section 8.1). Furthermore, there are other visual adaptation effects which cannot be explained in kinaesthetic–motor terms, for instance, the movement after-effect (especially two simultaneous, opposed movement after-effects), tilt adaptation, many geometrical illusions. Anomalous correspondence and monocular diplopia, and pseudo-fovea are further examples of displaced visual space values which it would be difficult to explain in every case in proprioceptive–motor terms (see sections 2.12 and 2.13). We do not suggest that these cases demonstrate that there has been a change in the anatomical projections from retina to visual cortex but only that the visual information becomes coded in terms of a new visual-spatial frame of reference. The crucial test is whether or not the new apparent field of view is recognized to be different from the old when both are simultaneously present. The case of binocular diplopia satisfies this condition—if the new space values were due to an altered sense of the position of the eyes, the new and the old impressions could not co-exist. Localized tilt adaptation and curvature adaptation are other cases of simultaneously present old and new space values.

We suggest that such simultaneous comparisons between new and old spatial judgments within a modality provide the only really adequate criterion for deciding in which part of the system the change has taken place. This criterion is not always available.

The criterion adopted by Harris and others is that of transfer of the new habits. The argument is that if the recalibration is limited to one component (e.g. an eye or an arm) in the control loop, when a component is replaced by the contralateral structure, the new calibration may or may not transfer, depending on whether or not that component is the one which has been recalibrated. But apart from the possibility of intramodal comparison which we have already mentioned, one cannot talk about localization in a single modality without reference to a motor act or some other modality; one probably cannot even find independent criteria (e.g. the median plane) to indicate the site of recalibration. *Transfer experiments do not provide an adequate criterion for deciding what is meant by the locus of recalibration along the sensory– motor control loop; one may be able to say only that the relationship between a particular input or set of inputs and a particular output or set of outputs has been changed.* The results of transfer experiments enable us to make this kind of identification: the identification of affected *linkages*, not of affected *loci*.

If the rearrangement involved no more than the learning of 'a new pattern of muscle contractions', Harris (1963b) argued, then, when the subject uses an arm movement different from the one he practised with, the adaptation should be less than when he uses the well-practised movement. He found that when the arm movement was modified by asking the subject to point at other targets, the adaptation was at least as great as when he pointed at the practised target. Adaptation is apparently not limited to particular sensory–muscular linkages, although it presumably could be so limited if appropriate training were given. Freedman, Hall, and Rekosh (1965) also found transfer, though not always full transfer, when the movement used in testing differed from that used in training.

We shall not discuss the neurological theories of which centres are involved in visual–motor spatial coordination. These matters have been discussed by Bonin (1950), Penfield (1954), Paillard (1960), and Myers, Sperry, and McCurdy (1962).

Smith and Smith (1962) describe what they call a neurogeometric theory. They stress the innate, specific nature of the muscular–neurological organization underlying spatially coordinated behaviour. The main points of this 'theory', as far as spatial behaviour is concerned, may be summarized by quoting from their book (pp. 126–127).

'The spatial organization of motion depends on the ability of the living system to react to differences in stimulation between specific points. These might be two points on the same receptor surface, two points located on two different receptors, or one point associated with an effector and another associated with a receptor. To carry out this function, the internuncial neurons of the central nervous system are associated at their dendrite endings with two specific points, and react only when a difference in neural activity exists between these two points. Thus the basic mode of action of internuncial neurons is that of differential detection instead of simple conduction.

'Motion is multidimensional; it is made up of three primary movement components—posture, transport, and manipulation—which are integrated into complex motion patterns. These components are differentially controlled at different levels of the nervous system, and in relation to different types of stimuli. Posture is regulated by gravitational stimulation; transport movements, by differences in stimulation between the two sides of the body; and manipulative movements, by the properties of hard space (objects, surfaces). In addition, motion integration demands that each component be regulated relative to the other components.

'The neurogeometric detectors of the brain are the heritable anatomical units which account for genetically determined behavior.'

It is not clear to what differences between stimulated points neurogeometric internuncial neurons respond. Do they code the distance between the points or do they record differences in the frequency, intensity, etc. of the neural activities at these points?

Neurogeometric theory seems to lack any identifiable features of its own. It is a collection of statements stressing certain aspects of behaviour and stressing the need to look at specific patterns of neuromuscular activity in behaviour. This approach is claimed by Smith and Smith to be superior to 'the general inadequacy of animal-based learning theory when we attempt to apply it to human behaviour organization' (p. 126). We would agree that the specific aspects of human neuromuscular organization need to be studied particularly when there is an applied problem, such as is met with in time and motion study (Barnes, 1949). But detailed, particularized studies of this kind cannot lead to important theoretical generalizations. The only generalization to emerge from Smith and Smith's book is that human skills are highly specific with respect to the variables they studied. But the mechanisms of general theoretical interest about animal movements are common to many animal species. Sherrington's experiments on the reflex organization of the spinal cord, Holst's on reafference, Granit's on the γ-fibre system, Magnus's on the labyrinthine reflexes, all these experiments could have been done on any mammal and they all made important contributions to our basic knowledge of motor coordination in man.

15.24   The conditions for visual–motor adaptation

We shall now discuss the conditions necessary for visual–motor adaptation to take place.

The first person to study this question seems to have been Wooster in 1923. She studied the effects of wearing prisms which displaced the optical array 21 degrees to the right. In the various experiments, 72 subjects were tested. Each subject was tested while wearing the prisms for a short period on each of ten days or for as long as was required to overcome the effects of the distortion, if less than ten days.

The subjects had to make rapid movements of the right arm towards the position of one of several small round discs. Normally, the arm and hand were hidden from view. In one condition it was not possible to touch the target and no knowledge of results was provided, at least not deliberately. In other conditions information regarding the true position of the disc was potentially available to the subject, in one of several forms. The disc emitted a sound in one condition. In another, the subject was allowed to move his finger about until it touched the disc. In a third condition the tip of the finger could be seen when the localizing response had been made. Finally, the tip of the other index finger was used as the target, and the subject was allowed to touch it if he made the correct localizing response.

After ten days of practice Wooster found that, even with no knowledge of results, accuracy had increased until the subject's mean deviation from true localization was 40·5 per cent less than the deviation on the first day. In spite of Wooster's efforts to eliminate knowledge of results, some information must have been reaching the subjects. Wooster herself suggested that there was 'unconscious adaptation of the reaching movements to the new kinaesthetic stimuli from the eye muscles'. Presumably what was meant was that the subject's body faced the true position of the visual target, while the eye was directed to its displaced position, and that gradually the subject came to behave as if he were looking straight ahead—an after-effect of asymmetrical eye position on the apparent median plane (see section 11.31). It is a pity that this factor was not controlled by making the displaced visual targets symmetrical relative to the body median plane for some of the subjects.

The sound of the disc buzzer was found not to contribute towards increased accuracy of pointing. When the subject was allowed to slide his finger along until it touched the disc or when he was allowed to see his finger, there was a rapid improvement in accuracy. However, the most rapid improvement occurred when the visual target was the tip of the other index finger and the subject was allowed to touch it. In this last condition, we suggest that the subject could have performed correctly by disregarding visual information, because he could 'feel' the position of the target. The task would have been a purely kinaesthetic–motor one and as such would have involved no distortion of sensory input. It is no wonder that this condition appeared to give the largest adaptation. This interpretation could have been tested by investigating the after-effect of this training on pointing at visual targets other than the finger.

Although Wooster enquired into the nature of the conditions necessary for adaptation of visual–motor coordination with prismatic distortion, very few definite conclusions emerged from her work.

Stratton, Kohler, Wooster, and others have stressed the importance of active movements in the adaptation of movements to optical distortions. However, Holst and Mittelstaedt (1950) were the first to formulate a definite hypothesis (see also Holst, 1954). On the basis of his observations on insects and fish, in which he rearranged the visual input, Holst concluded that the important thing in visual–motor coordination is the relation of actively produced movements of the body or parts of the body to changes in the pattern of stimulation of the sense organs which these movements produce. Such changes in sensory stimulation consequent upon self-produced movement he called '*reafference*'. Stimulation of the sense organs produced solely by changes in the external world were called '*exafference*'. An animal capable of orientating itself must be capable of distinguishing between reafferent and exafferent stimulation. It does this by making use of information from the neural centres which control the movements of the parts of its body. The changes in the stimulation of the exteroceptors which a given pattern of muscular innervation would normally produce is 'allowed for' in processing the information from the exteroceptors. This idea has something in common with Helmholtz's theory of unconscious inference.

Held has recently applied this hypothesis to the case of visual–motor adaptation and reported experimental evidence which is claimed to support it. The schematized process which he proposes is shown in figure 15.3. It is

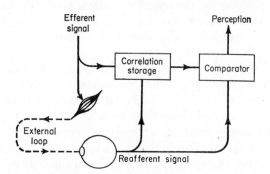

Figure 15.3 Schematized process assumed by Held to underlie the consequences of rearrangement, neonatal development, disarrangement, and deprivation on visual–motor coordination. [From Hein and Held, 1962]

similar to the one proposed by Holst except for the addition of the 'Correlation Storage'. The skeletal muscle represents any motor system that can be seen by the subject. In Held's words, '... the reafferent visual signal is compared (in the Comparator) with a signal selected from the Correlation

Storage by the monitored efferent signal. The Correlation Storage acts as a kind of memory which retains traces of previous combinations of concurrent efferent and reafferent signals. The currently monitored efferent signal is presumed to select the trace combination containing the identical efferent part and to activate the reafferent trace combined with it. The resulting revived reafferent signal is sent to the Comparator for comparison with the current reafferent signal. The outcome of this comparison determines further performance' (Held, 1961, p. 30).

Held has been responsible for designing several very ingenious experiments. His experiments with neonatal kittens (Hein and Held, 1962) we consider to be some of the neatest experiments in the psychological literature. His basic procedure was to compare the effectiveness of self-produced movement with that of passive movement in the readaptation of visual–motor coordination to a displaced visual input in adult human subjects. The experiments reported in Held and Hein (1958) and Held and Freedman (1963) are typical. They used an apparatus described by Held and Gottlieb (1958), which is shown in figure 15.4. This is similar to an apparatus described by Mowrer (1935b). The mirror (M) or the prism (P) could be moved into the subject's line of sight. The subject was first asked to mark the sheet under the

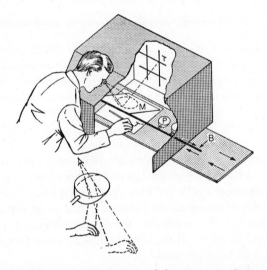

Figure 15.4 Schematic representation of the apparatus designed by Held and Gottlieb (1958) to study visual–motor adaptation. S views his hand through the prism (P) in the training period. In the test period, the bar (B) is moved across so that S views only the target (T) in the mirror, apparently at T'

mirror at the mirror-image positions of the four corners of a square. The subject was then allowed to see his hand through the prism for 3 min while the hand was motionless, moved passively from side to side by the experimenter, or moved actively. Only the active movement condition led to any significant shift in the mean position of aim when the subject was again asked to point with the unseen hand at the corners of the reflected target figure. The active exposure had led to a change in the relationship between the visual location of the targets and the localizing movements made to touch them, and Held and Hein concluded that reafference was necessary for such a change to take place. The failure of Weinstein, Sersen, and Weinstein (1964) to produce any adaptation even with an active condition was probably due to an experimental artifact as Held and Schlank (1964) pointed out. Weinstein et al. certainly produced adaptation with active training in their later studies, as we shall see.

We think that Held's conclusion that reafference is necessary for visual–motor adaptation to displaced vision is unwarranted. Some of the reasons for our view have been put forward in section 11.32. Other reasons will emerge in what follows. Held himself seems to have modified this extreme view recently.

15.25 The role of response inhibition and substitution in visual–motor adaptation

Anyone who tries to adjust his pointing to a displaced visual target will report that during the first few tries he has to actively inhibit his normal movement to the target, and deliberately make allowance for his error. When at last he 'gets the feel' of the correct movement, he has to practise it for a while before he is able to relax his active inhibition of the old habit. After a while the new habit becomes established firmly enough for him to report that he is responding 'naturally' to the position of the target. The after-effect produced when the prisms are removed surprises the subject. This demonstrates that, although the original recalibration was achieved only by deliberate inhibition and redirection, the new response, once established, acquires the status of an automatic habit. If it had to be maintained by a deliberate redirection of movement, the whole subject of visual–motor adaptation would be trivial. It is only this final automatic stage which we refer to as visual–motor adaptation.

We suggest that *where there is rapid adaptation of movements to distorted vision, over distances far greater than the normal range of error of those movements, an initial stage of gross inhibition of old habits and substitution of new responses must occur.* We shall refer to this stage as *response substitution,* and we suggest that it involves activity at a higher level in the neuraxis than the level at which practised habits operate. A person can be told of the extent of an optical distortion before he makes any movements at all, and as a result he may hit the displaced visual target on the first occasion. Clearly, then, the initial response substitution can occur no matter how the subject is informed of the distortion, and it is therefore meaningless to enquire into the necessary stimulus–response conditions for response substitution. Of course the information must be correct and the subject must be able to use it and be appropriately instructed.

Enquiries about the necessary stimulus–response conditions for visual–motor adaptation must be concerned, not with the essential initial response substitution stage, but rather with the subsequent stage in which the new response becomes automatic. *In any such studies, an opportunity and a demand for response substitution should be given.* If it is not, rapid, full adaptation cannot occur whatever the other conditions. If the opportunity for response substitution occurs in one condition of the experiment and not in another, the experiment will be futile.

When we talk of response substitution we do not imply that the response must be the same as that which is later tested. Training with one hand, for instance, may transfer to the other hand. It is reasonable to suppose that the type of response used in training must be linked by spatial habits to the type of response used in testing; that they must both be sensitive to visual–stimulus position.

Held and Hein should have optimized the conditions for response substitution in their passive condition. They did not do this; they did not even optimize these conditions in their active condition, as their results show. On average, the active adaptation was only one-third of the optical distortion. It is our experience that under different conditions of training, full adaptation occurs after about ten active hits at the target with visual knowledge of results. Held and Hein's training consisted of merely inspecting the actively moved arm. With no visual target in view, the subject was not called on to correct any error; he was therefore not called on to make a deliberate effort to recalibrate his movements. Wertheimer and Arena (1959) were at a loss to understand why they were able to get fuller adaptation in a much shorter time than Held and Hein. But Wertheimer and Arena's training procedure involved placing crosses in visible squares. Their subjects were required to deliberately correct their movements. No wonder they got more rapid adaptation than Held and Hein. But even Wertheimer and Arena's procedure did not produce full adaptation, and that was because they allowed their subjects to guide their hands visually to the target; they were not forced to recalibrate their visual–motor habits.

We suggest that the effectiveness of self-produced, error-guided movements in bringing about adaptation is due to the demand and opportunity for response substitution which they provide. If passive movements were accompanied by a demand and opportunity for response substitution, then they too, we suggest, would lead to adaptation. But this is what has not been done by Held and his coworkers. The subject in such an experiment must be repeatedly asked to judge the position of his passively moved, hidden arm in relation to a displaced visual target, and he must be given knowledge of results. If this is done, we make the following predictions. *A subject trained to make estimates of his passively moved arm in relation to a displaced visual target will acquire a set of new judgments of the position of his passively moved arm in relation to the target.* Secondly, we predict that his active pointing will be displaced significantly towards the real position of the visual target. In other words, *new habits of passive pointing transfer, to some extent at least, to active pointing, just as new active pointing habits transfer to passive pointing.* This is the crux of the question which Held and others have raised regarding active and passive training.

In order to test these predictions, we designed the following experiment (Templeton, Howard, and Lowman, in press). The subject wore 12° displacing prisms. His arm was passively swivelled horizontally about the shoulder, with the forearm and index finger extended at right angles from the body. A horizontal screen hid the arm from view, and carried a series of small rods on its outer rim which could be elevated one at a time into the subject's field of view. The subject's arm was swivelled by the experimenter towards the target until the subject reported that his finger was under the target. He was then shown his finger. A new target was substituted at random and the arm was again moved until the subject was satisfied he was on target, and he was again shown his finger. This procedure was repeated until the subject made consistent judgments, or for 16 trials, whichever was the shorter. We thus ensured that the subject was given information about the extent of the optical distortion and that he was called upon to use this information to make a response substitution.

The subject's ability to hit the target was tested without knowledge of results before and after the training procedure. This passive training led to a post-training shift in active pointing towards the position of the target of about ⅓ of the prismatic displacement. Thus, passive movement combined with knowledge of results produces visual–motor adaptation; not 100% adaptation under the conditions of this experiment, but longer training would probably have produced a greater effect.

Held and Mikaelian (1964) attempted to answer the criticism that in their wheel-chair experiment (see section 8.23) the passive subject was not motivated to make the effort necessary for adaptation. In the new experiment, all subjects wore 11° laterally displacing prisms. The active subjects were allowed to walk in a corridor, the 'passive' subjects propelled themselves in a wheel-chair. Only the 'active' subjects showed any evidence of a shift in their settings on a line to the median plane. There are several puzzling features about this experiment. Both groups of subjects were really active; what the experiment seems to show then is that reafference associated with 'normal' movements is necessary for adaptation. But even this conclusion is not valid, for we are not told about the precise nature of the passive subjects' experience. Were they allowed to see their bodies and the chair? If they were, they could visually guide the chair in relation to the seen sides of the corridor, and visual–motor adaptation would not be called for in order for them to succeed in avoiding collisions. Were they, on the other hand, prevented from seeing the chair or their bodies? If they were, they would not get visual feedback at the time and place of impact between chair and wall, and one of the essential conditions for adaptation would be absent. What is needed in these experiments, is that the part of the body which the subject is moving be hidden from view until after he has made his aiming movement, and that he then be allowed to see his error. The wheel-chair situation is much too cumbersome for controlling the information sequence which the subject is allowed to receive. Weinstein, Sersen, Fisher, and Weisinger (1964) repeated Held's earlier wheel-chair experiment, in a corridor, rather than outside. They got the same amount of adaptation in the passive condition as in the active condition. One would like to know what information the passive subjects had to enable them to even know they had prisms on, let alone adapt to them. Were they able to see their own apparently asymmetrically placed bodies? In any case they must have had a field of view which was asymmetrical with respect to the body median plane, and this alone could explain the adaptation which would then have little bearing on the problems which Held was studying.

It is easy to demonstrate the essential role of response substitution. If a subject wearing displacing prisms is asked to point to the visual position of a target he will repeatedly do so; little or no adaptation takes place. As soon as he is asked to try to actually hit the target, he very soon learns. In the first condition he behaves in a relaxed, automatic fashion, thinking only of the visual position of the target, in the second condition he concentrates on actually hitting the target.

Stereotyped behaviour is typical of submammalian species, which presumably lack a response substitution mechanism, although, as we shall see, the evidence for this view is questionable. Repeated claims have been made that submammalian species cannot adapt their movements to a disturbed optical array (Stone, 1944; Sperry, 1942, 1944, 1945, 1948; Hess, 1956;

Pfister, 1955; Holst, 1954). We do not intend to review these experiments in detail as our central interest is human orientation. However, we cannot allow these claims to go unchallenged.

Pfister, working at Innsbruck, placed right–left reversing prisms on a hen. It never relearned to peck at grain. The hen, of course, never had a chance, for when it reached what its habits indicated was the position of the grain, the actual piece of grain would be out of view, far off in the periphery of vision. The hen could therefore not detect its error, and could not be expected to learn.

Hess's design was slightly better: he used newly hatched chicks and introduced 7° of lateral visual displacement. Not one of the chicks modified its pecking towards the real position of the grain. The distortion was not so great here, but one still wonders whether the error could be visually detected by the chick, for when its beak touched the ground, the grain and beak were probably too near to be focused. Similar criticisms can be made of the experiments on amphibians by Stone and Sperry. Even if such animals could have visually detected the direction and extent of their error, it is asking a lot of such primitive nervous systems to store information about the direction of a reaching movement and substitute a new movement in accordance with a visually-detected error. These animals presumably behave like the human subject who lets himself be guided only by the apparent position of the target.

One should not conclude, however, even if submammalian species are shown to be incapable of a gross substitution of responses, that they are incapable of learning to adapt their behaviour to displaced vision. The training must be geared to their capacity. We propose the following principle: *in order to train submammalian species to adapt their motor behaviour, the change of habit required at any stage must be no greater than the range of normal variation in the animal's performance.* In practice, this means that the prismatic distortion must introduce a visual displacement just less than the range of pecking errors, or errors of other movements being trained. When the animal's mean position of pecking has shifted over, a further amount of prismatic distortion may be introduced, and so on. We predict that in the end the animal's pecking, or whatever, will be several degrees off the normal. With such a procedure it will not be necessary to demonstrate that the grain is in view at the time the peck is made.

Such a procedure of training could be used with humans also. If it were, we predict that motor adaptation would occur slowly and probably without the subject being able to report what was happening to him. This procedure is of course that of 'habit shaping' described by Skinner; the essential point is that one can utilize only those responses which the animal will make by chance.

15.26 Other forms of exafferent information

There is evidence that other forms of exafferent stimulation can lead to visual–motor adaptation to displaced vision. We have already described how Wooster obtained some adaptation of pointing to a displaced visual target under passive conditions, and it was probably the visual asymmetry of the displaced targets in relation to the body median plane which induced this passive adaptation. In addition, in section 10.21 we discussed Bruell and Albee's finding that visual symmetry of the field of view about the fixation point affects the judged position of the median plane. Held himself found that passive inspection of curved lines leads to a visual curvature after-effect. It is not known whether any of these factors affect active pointing behaviour, and Held has never denied that they may. It would be interesting to find out whether or not they do.

More recently Wallach, Kravitz, and Lindauer (1963) demonstrated that 10 minutes of inspecting the feet of one's own body seen through displacing prisms, led to some adaptation of pointing towards the real position of displaced visual targets. However, they did not run a control to reveal whether the effect of looking at the feet was due to the conflict of information from pro-prioceptive and visual inputs, or whether it was due to the visual asymmetry of the position of the feet relative to the body median plane. In the latter case, the effect would be the same as that reported by Wooster (see section 15.24.) Craske and Howard repeated this experiment by having the subject inspect his feet through prisms when his feet were physically off-centre by just the amount required for the prisms to restore them visually to the body median plane. No evidence of visual–motor adaptation was found, but the judgments of straight ahead which were used to reveal any adaptation effect were very erratic and a real shift may have been swamped. One would not expect much adaptation under these conditions, because one's idea of where the feet are when one is relaxing is very poor, and therefore the discrepancy between the felt position and the seen position would not be evident.

Howard, Craske, and Templeton (1965) have produced evidence that passive, exafferent, discordant stimulation induces visual–motor adaptation, even in the absence of the possible contaminating factors discussed above. This experiment was designed to test whether prodding a subject with a rod seen in a displaced position leads to visual–motor adaptation. The apparatus is shown in figure 15.5. The optical device consisted of two parallel mirrors which displaced the optical array 2 in to the left. Mirrors were used rather than prisms, because they do not introduce curvature, tilt, or colour fringes. The displacement is parallel rather than angular, which is essential for this purpose: with prismatic angular displacement the apparent displacement

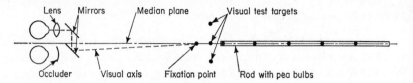

Figure 15.5 Apparatus used by Howard, Craske, and Templeton (1965) to study the effects of discordant exafferent stimulation on visual–motor coordination

reduces to zero as the viewed object comes towards the subject. A lens compensated for the increased optical path which the mirrors introduced. The subject's head was clamped and the right eye was occluded. In the pre-training condition the subject was asked to look through the optical device with his left eye and point to a target light in one of three positions in the frontal plane, symmetrical about the body median plane. The hand could not be seen. This initial test established the pre-training deviation of the subject's pointing. The subject was then told to fixate a light just above a rod which had five lights arranged along its length, and which appeared to be aligned with a point two inches to the left of his mouth. The rod was moved in towards the subject until one end of it hit him centrally on the lips. This was repeated 20 times. The subject was immediately retested on the pointing task. In a control condition, the same procedure was employed except that the rod did not quite touch the subject.

The results are set out in table 15.1. The 'being-hit' training procedure produced a significant mean change in pointing of 0·64 in towards the actual position of the target lights i.e. about ⅓ of the displacement.

The effect could not have been due solely to the visual asymmetry in the position of the rod and the target lights, for this was present in the control condition, where no adaptation occurred. The tactile stimulation was sym-

Table 15.1 Mean error in inches of pointing at targets optically displaced 2 in laterally, before and after 'being touched' and 'not being touched'. (From Howard, Craske, and Templeton, 1965)

	Not being touched	Being touched
Before	1·94	2·15
After	1·88	1·51
Adaptation	0·06	0·64

metrical, so that there was no need for a control condition where the subjects were touched without being able to see the rod. Apparently all active movement was prevented, even convergence of the eyes. We were even more careful in this respect than Held had been in his 'passive' conditions. We are forced to the conclusion therefore that *discordant exafferent stimulation, which gives a passive subject 'information' regarding optical distortion, may lead to at least some visual–motor adaptation.*

In a recent paper Held and Mikaelian (1964) have modified the categorical assertion that reafference is essential for visual–motor adaptation in conditions not involving intrafield distortions.

They wrote, 'The conditions which have so far been shown to produce adaptation to rearrangements without self-produced movement do not appear to have the generality shown by involvement of the motor–sensory feedback loop. As far as is known, these conditions do not yield full and exact compensation for rearrangement . . .' We have no quarrel with this statement; it does seem that passive training is not as effective as active training, and if this is Held's thesis, there is as yet no good evidence to refute it. Weinstein, Sersen, Weisinger, Fisher, and Richlin (1964) obtained 100% adaptation of active pointing after 10 minutes of passive inspection of the feet seen through 7° prisms. But we have already argued that his procedure produces an asymmetrical eye position which could be partly responsible for the reported effect.

The main issue is still to be settled by experiment: namely, are there conditions of passive training which are as effective as active training? Held, by his phrase 'As far as is known', clearly admits that there may be. Held's group did not explore ways of presenting exafferent information. In fact, in some of their experiments, it seems that no exafferent information was available at all. We have already discussed one case (Bossom and Held, 1957) in section 11.32. The experiment of Held and Hein (1963) on neonatal kittens is another case.

In these experiments, an active moving kitten was linked mechanically to a restrained passive kitten (see figure 15.6). They both had the same visual experience of moving stripes, but the active kitten could relate the visual inputs to its own self-produced movements. This was the only visual experience either kitten had. Only the active kitten developed the ability to avoid a visual cliff, blink to an approaching object, and extend its paws to a surface.

They showed in another experiment (unpublished) that this difference between the two animals could not be due to the effects of physical restraint on the passive animal. In this experiment, each animal was in turn active and passive, but when active, only one eye was open, and when passive, only the other eye was open. It was now found that the animals could perform on the three tests only when the 'active eye' was open (or both). This result is surprising in view of all the evidence that interocular transfer of visual–motor habits occurs unless both corpus callosum and optic chiasma are sectioned (Downer, 1958). Presumably the ability to transfer skills itself depends on learning or maturation.

Held and Hein concluded that reafferent stimulation is essential for the development of visual–motor coordination. We suggest that the passive kitten or 'passive eye' was never given usable exafferent stimulation. All it saw was a moving display of stripes. There were no other features of its environment to which it could relate this visual input. Held and Hein never tried to

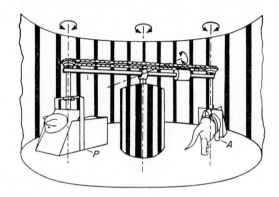

Figure 15.6 Apparatus used by Held and Hein (1963) for equating motion and consequent visual feedback for an actively moving animal (*A*) and a passively moving animal (*P*)

teach it anything. But there are a vast range of possibilities for correlated intersensory inputs which could be tried. For instance a visible object could be placed in the path of the animal; on some occasions the object could collide with the animal, and on other occasions the object could miss. To provide reinforcement (another thing Held and Hein failed to supply to the passive animal), the object could be food and sometimes hit the kitten in the mouth, or it could give an electric shock, or make a noise, pleasant or unpleasant. Another possibility would be to cause the passive animal to bump down a cliff and thus receive strong vestibular and tactile stimulation. In all this, one would merely have to ensure that the kitten could not move actively in such a way as to alter the visual signals. Eating movements, startle responses and the like would be permitted, for these would not affect the critical spatial feedback.

In view of all this, the surprising thing is the adequate performance of the active kitten on the tests. A possible explanation may be found in the work of Hubel and Wiesel (1963) and Wiesel and Hubel (1963a, 1963b) who showed that the visual receptor units which respond selectively to the direction and movement of stimuli are functional at birth but degenerate in a kitten which has been kept in the dark. Perhaps the experience that Held's active kittens were allowed to have was sufficient to prevent degeneration of these units, whereas the experience of the passive kittens was insufficient even though their visual experience was identical. If this were the case, experiments would need to be done to find out whether richer, purely exafferent stimulation would allow cortical units to develop normally. In any case, Held's evidence does not prove that the blink response, paw-placing reaction, and the visual-cliff responses depend on learning, for there may have been retrogressive development in the passive kittens.

Apparently a newly learned adaptation to an optical displacement is not stable when it has developed. Hamilton and Bossom (1964) found that subjects lose the prism after-effect, not only when they can view their own movements, as one would expect, but also when they sit quietly in the dark. Neither reafference nor exafference are necessary for the reestablishment of the old habits. This is presumably due to the vastly greater strength of the old habits relative to the new.

15.27 Kinaesthetic and motor components in visual–motor adaptation

In chapter 4, four types of afferent and efferent activity associated with muscular contraction were identified: motor outflow, activity of the muscle-spindle stretch receptors with their γ efferents, activity of Golgi tendon-tension receptors, and activity of skin and joint receptors.

The question is which, if any, of these four fundamental components is necessary or sufficient for visual–motor adaptation. It has already been shown that visual–motor adaptation can occur when none of these systems has been active during training, so that none of them is essential for adaptation. We have already enquired whether a recalibration of the judged position of a passively moved arm is sufficient; in this case it is presumably the joint receptors which are predominantly involved.

One may also ask whether any of the other possible combinations of the four efferent–afferent systems is sufficient to produce visual–motor adaptation, assuming of course, that the subject has optimum instructions and knowledge of results.

The various combinations are set out in table 15.2 with brief descriptions of the techniques involved, of the known capabilities of each combination,

Table 15.2 Procedures for obtaining various combinations of efferent–afferent conditions of muscular activity, and their behavioural properties

Receptors active	Procedures	Known and predicted capabilities	Visual–motor adaptation
(1) None	No movement	—	Occurs if discordant exafferent information is present
(2) Motor outflow alone	Self-produced movement with anaesthesia of all afferents	Accurate sense of amplitude of self-produced movement possible if loading is normal (Lashley, 1917)	*To do* predicted with no load transfer
(3a) Spindle–Golgi receptors alone in passive movement	Passive movement of tongue or eye or anaesthetized joint	No position nor amplitude of passive movement sense (Ludvigh, 1952b; Merton, 1964)	*To do* not predicted
(3b) Ditto, in active (not self-produced) movement	Stimulation of motor neurons with anaesthetized joint	No position nor amplitude of movement sense	*To do*

To do

		To do	*To do*
(4) Joint receptors alone	Passive movement with severed tendons	Position and passive movement sense predicted	predicted
(5) Motor outflow and spindle–Golgi receptors	Self-produced movement of tongue or eye, or ischaemic paralysis of a joint	No position sense, but sense of amplitude of self-produced movement is possible if loading is normal (Merton, 1964)	predicted with no load transfer
(6) Motor outflow and joint receptors	Self-produced movement with paralysis of spindle–Golgi afferents	*To do*	predicted with load transfer if load change is not too great
(7) Spindle–Golgi receptors and joint receptors	No known procedure. Passive movement may be an approximation	Position sense and sense of amplitude of passive movement predicted	predicted
(8) All three	Normal self-produced movement	Full capabilities	Present

and of the known presence or absence of visual–motor adaptation in each case. The muscle-spindle system and the Golgi tendon receptors are grouped together; it is not easy to separate them in practice. No account is taken of skin receptors on the assumption that the skin is anaesthetized throughout. The procedures for eliminating the various components have been described fully in section 4.4.

Of these combinations, only (1), (7), and (8) have been studied in relation to visual–motor adaptation. One of Held and Hein's training procedures was to have the subject inspect his passively moved arm. They compared this training procedure with one in which the subject inspected his actively moved arm. It is not clear which systems are inactive in such a passive condition, compared with the active one. If the subject really relaxed, motor outflow would be inactive, and Held and Hein seem to have assumed that this is the only difference between the two conditions. However, although the joint receptors are probably active in a similar way in the two conditions, the activity of the muscle-spindle system and Golgi receptors is certainly different in the two conditions. These two systems will be active to some extent in passive movement but not to the same extent as in active movement. But it is unlikely that muscle spindles and Golgi organs have anything to do with position or movement sensitivity; so the crucial difference between the two conditions, as far as the four factors are concerned, is probably the presence or absence of motor outflow, as Held and Hein presumably believed. Even so, the fact that Held and Hein got adaptation only with active training could have been due to the way active movement tended to make the subject attend to the discrepancy between the seen and felt positions of his arm.

Held (1963a) went some way towards meeting this objection. He compared the amount of visual–motor adaptation to a 20 dioptre prism, with self-produced movement and with the subject ineffectively straining against a swivel which forced his arm in an arc. Only the normal, self-produced movement produced any significant change in pointing. In the other condition, the visual feedback was said to have been 'de-correlated' from the motor outflow. Held concluded that the effectiveness of normal self-produced movement is not due to any exertion of effort which 'somehow potientiates the system'. This does not really answer our objection, for de-correlated motor outflow may act as a distraction, inducing the subject to ignore his kinaesthetic inputs.

Although such passive training as Held and Hein applied did not affect pointing in an active test condition, this may have been because any 'recalibration' of the kinaesthetic system which such passive training may have produced was 'swamped' in the active test conditions by the old calibration of the motor outflow. The proper test for any recalibration of the kinaesthetic system is to ask the subject to judge the position of his passively moved arm in relation to a visual target.

It can be seen from the table that we predict at least some adaptation when motor outflow and/or joint receptors are active, assuming the other conditions are optimized. This is because both these systems have been found to signal amplitude of movement. The muscle-spindle system probably does not add anything to the ability to judge either position or amplitude of movement; its function may not be sensory at all in the usual sense (see section 4.4). It is unlikely, therefore, that muscle-spindle activity can either improve or reduce visual–motor adaptation under ordinary circumstances. A probable consequence of the absence of the spindle system would be that judgments based on motor outflow alone would be easily disturbed by changes in the mechanical properties of the muscle tissue; for the spindle system is probably concerned with compensating for such changes.

The predictions in the table also involve statements about load transfer. We refer here to whether or not adaptation, trained when the limb is loaded to one extent, transfers to a test situation in which the loading is different. There is a continuum of loading values: where the limb has to pull against a resistance that it cannot move, where only its own internal friction is present, where its own friction is just overcome by a pull in the direction of movement, and finally where the arm has to pull back against a force in the direction of movement.

A change of loading will obviously affect the motor outflow, and in the absence of joint receptors (case 2) we predict that position sense will be distorted accordingly (see evidence in section 4.43). Therefore transfer will probably not occur from one load to another when only motor outflow is present, or when only motor outflow and spindle-Golgi receptors are present.

When motor outflow and joint receptors are active together, there should be some defence against distortions of position sense by load changes, and hence some transfer of adaptation from one load condition to another. The presence or absence of load transfer in these circumstances will indicate which of the two systems is most involved in visual–motor adaptation. If full transfer occurs it would indicate that the joint receptors are primarily involved. If no transfer occurs, it would indicate that the motor outflow is primarily involved. This complex of problems has hardly begun to be investigated.

15.3 Eye and head movements with rotated optical arrays

We must first consider the basic geometry of the relationship between movements of the eyes and head, and the resulting movements of the retinal image when inverting and/or reversing devices are worn. There are three cases to be considered. The lenses may be attached (1) to the subject's eyes, (2) to the subject's head, and (3) to a stationary object outside the subject. We shall assume for simplicity that the field of view is only inverted, that only one eye is open, and that the eye and head rotate about the centre of the eye's lens, from which all angular measures are taken.

The geometrical consequences of case (1) are shown in figure 15.7(a) and (b). As the front of the eye is elevated through an angle ϕ, the optical system moves through the same angle, carrying with it the visual axis. If A and B are two distal stimuli, and B is $\phi°$ above A, then under normal conditions the image a is above image b on the retina and a change in fixation from A to B by means of an upward eye movement (downward retinal movement) causes a corresponding upward movement through $\phi°$ of images a and b on the retina. If, however, inverting prisms are attached to the eye, image b is above image a on the retina. In this case a change of fixation from A to B is achieved by means of a similar upward eye movement (downward retinal movement). But bringing image b, which is above image a, to the centre of the retina in this way must involve a *downward* movement of the two images on the retina, i.e. *relative to an outside standard the images move in the same direction as the retina and twice as far.*

Movement of images on the retina through the same angle and in the opposite direction to movement of the retina itself (the normal case) signifies a stationary distal stimulus; stationary images on the retina signify a stimulus moving at the same speed and in the same direction as the eye movements; and movement of images in the same direction as the retina and twice as fast (the case when wearing inverting prisms), normally signifies a stimulus moving in the same direction and twice as fast as the eye movements.

If the subject's head is tilted backwards or forwards, the consequences are the same as for eye movements. When a subject, wearing inverting lenses on his eye, attempts to move his gaze from point A to point B, his normal habits, which determine the direction of eye movements relative to the position of the image of the visual target on the retina, will cause his eye to move in the wrong direction. He will move his eye down and his gaze will retreat away from the point which he was instructed to fixate. However, there will be one sense in which his old habits will be appropriate. If he is commanded to look at, for example, his feet, and if he ignores the inverted optical array, then past habit will indicate that a downward movement of the gaze is required, as indeed it is, even with the inverting devices on. In practice, however, the habits governed by the geometry of the retinal image dominate the meaning-mediated habits, for subjects on first wearing inverting devices built on contact lenses (Taylor, 1962, p. 224) have to learn to direct their eyes to specified points in space.

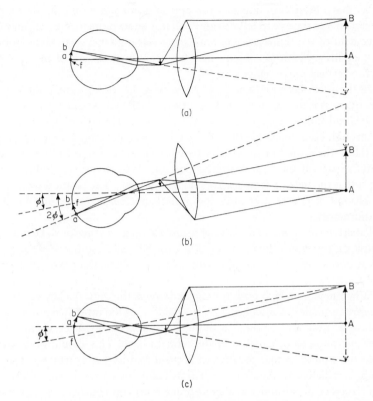

(a)

(b)

(c)

Figure 15.7 Diagrammatic representation of the effects on retinal-image motion of wearing an inverting optical device

(a) Initial position of eye and inverting lens. The object A–B is imaged at a–b on the retina, f is the fovea

(b) The eye and inverting lens move together through angle ϕ until the optic axis of the system is directed at B; the retinal image of the target moves through 2ϕ in the same direction as the eye, and the direction of gaze corresponds to the actual direction of the object imaged on the fovea

(c) The eye moves through angle ϕ while the lens remains stationary; the retinal image remains stationary relative to the target, and the direction of gaze does not correspond to the actual direction of the object imaged on the fovea

We have been assuming that the optical distortion is an inversion only. Movements of the eye to left or right will not be accompanied by an unusual movement of the retinal image. Similarly a left–right reversal of the optical array entails anomalous consequences for lateral movements of the eyes but not for vertical movements.

Both purely inverting and purely reversing devices introduce anomalous consequences if the eye is rotated about the visual axis. In practice, one must tilt the head and eye together. In this case, the retinal image rotates on the retina through the same angle that the eye describes, but in the same direction. Therefore the retinal image rotates twice as far as the eye relative to a fixed point in space. If the head rotates to one side through 45°, the subject will report that the field of view has rotated through 90°. The fixation point does not change of course, just as it does not change in normal vision in these circumstances.

Papert gave mathematical expression to these geometrical facts using complex number notation (Taylor, 1962, p. 189). The geometry of the situation is not so difficult to comprehend as Papert's treatment would seem to imply.

When devices which both reverse and invert the optical array are worn, there are anomalous consequences to both sideways and up–down movements of the eye. Rotations of the eye about the optic axis, however, do not now cause any anomalous rotation of the retinal image. This should be obvious when one considers that the distortion produced by an inverting–reversing device is radially symmetrical; a rotational shift of such a device relative to either subject or stimuli can therefore have no consequences. This is clear when one thinks of an ordinary astronomical telescope.

To summarize the case where the optical device is worn on the eye: the relation between the direction of eye or head movements and the direction of the change of fixation in actual space is the same as in normal vision. But the relation between eye or head movements and the direction of movement of the retinal image is the reverse of what it is in normal vision.

The geometrical consequences of case (2), where the device is attached to the subject's head, depend on whether the eye alone moves or the head and eye together. If they move together, the consequences are the same as case (1). If the eye alone is moved, the consequences are as shown in figure 15.7(c). As the line of sight is elevated the retina moves over an objectively stationary optical image in the opposite direction. This is just what happens in an eye under normal circumstances as far as the rays entering the eye are concerned. The subject receives the same proximal visual stimulation as he does when he scans a really inverted world without spectacles, that is, his retinal image moves in the usual way relative to the direction of his eye movements. However, the relation of the direction of his eye movements to the direction of the real objects in space is different to what it is with normal vision. When the eye is elevated, objects which are objectively lower than the initial point of gaze are brought into view. The situation is the reverse of case (1). The relation between the direction of eye movements and the direction of the change of fixation in actual space is the reverse of what it is in normal vision. But the relation between eye movements and the movement of the retinal image is the same as in normal vision.

In case (3) the optical device is attached to a stationary object outside the subject. The geometrical consequences of moving the eye or the head are the same as the consequences of moving the eye alone when the device is attached to the head. Table 15.3 summarizes this discussion.

We have avoided stressing the subject's judgments in this account: but have confined ourselves to the purely geometrical consequences of the various cases. What those judgments will be may be predicted for a naïve observer, using Helmholtz's maxim, that 'objects are always imagined as being present in the field of vision as would have to be there in order to produce the same impression on the nervous mechanism, the eyes being used under ordinary normal conditions'. (Helmholtz, 1962, vol. 3, p. 2.)

The usual experimental procedure is to wear inverting devices fixed to the head (case II in table 15.3) and, in accordance with Helmholtz's maxim, the disturbed relationship between direction of eye movement and direction of retinal-image movement results in reports that head movements cause the field of view to move through twice the angle in the opposite direction.

Whether these judgments will change as the subject continues to wear the device will depend on the behavioural interactions between him and his environment. There is ample evidence that after several days of continuous wearing of inverting spectacles subjects report a stable scene when the head is moved. Stratton (1897b) wrote on the third day of wearing inverting lenses, 'Head-movements were still accompanied by a slight swinging of the scene, although in a markedly less degree than on the first day. The movement was referred more to the observer, so that it seemed to be more a moving survey of stationary objects' (p. 349). By the fourth day, 'the swinging of the scene during movements of my body seemed greater or less, according to the way in which I represented to myself this movement of my body' (p. 354). By the sixth day, 'Movements of the head or of the body, which shifted the field of view, seemed now to be in entire keeping with the visual changes thus produced; the motion seemed to be towards that side on which objects entered the visual field, and not towards the opposite side, as the pre-experimental representation of the movement would have required. And when, with closed eyes, I rocked in my chair, the merely represented changes in the visual

Table 15.3 The geometrical consequences of wearing inverting or reversing devices in various ways

	Relation between direction of movement and movement of retinal image	Relation between direction of movement and direction of change of gaze in space
(I) Device worn on eye		
Eye or head movement	Retinal image moves through twice the angle in the same direction	Normal relationship
(II) Device worn on head		
(a) Head movement	As (I)	As (I)
(b) Eye movement	Normal relationship	Line of gaze in space moves through equal and opposite angle
(III) Device fixed externally		
Eye or head moves	Normal relationship	As (IIb)

field persisted with the same rhythmic variation of direction which they would have shown had I opened my eyes' (p. 358).

Ewert (1930) also noticed the gradual increase in apparent stability of the field of view as he moved his head after several days of wearing inverting spectacles.

Wundt (1894, p. 164) maintained that, 'If the position of objects in space is inferred from movement, the retinal image must be inverted, since only where this is the case is it possible for the movement to correspond with the actual position of the objects. So, far from being a paradox, the inverted retinal image is necessary for vision.'

Coyle (1907), an undergraduate, pointed out the fallacy in this and similar arguments in the literature. We have already shown that, whether or not an optical system attached to the eye produces an erect or inverted image, it does not upset the normal relationship between the direction of eye movements and the direction of movement of the line of sight in space.

Stratton (1907) was convinced that his experiments disproved the eye-movement theory of visual spatial localization. In those experiments, the lenses were attached to the head, so that the eyes had to move down to bring into central vision an object which was objectively above the initial fixation. In spite of this inversion of the normal relationship. Stratton was able to achieve a new and adequate visual–motor coordination, which he claimed would have been impossible on an eye-movement theory of localization. But Stratton has not disproved the eye-movement theory, he has only shown that the signals from the eye-movement centres do not have an immutable space value. Whether or not eye movements play an essential role in visual spatial localization is another question which is discussed in sections 2.5 and 3.5.

Recently Kottenhoff (1957b) has obtained quantitative data on adaptation to the anomalous motion of the visual image produced by right–left reversing spectacles. While wearing the spectacles a subject was rotated at a steady speed on a revolving chair placed inside patterned screening. He was asked to remember the apparent speed of the pattern and compare it with the speed of an actually moving pattern seen when rotation had stopped. Testing was apparently repeated at intervals over the three-hour period for which the spectacles were worn.

We are not told what the subjects did during these three hours; Kottenhoff's measure of the field motion would be contaminated by the visual after-effects of movement, and by nystagmus induced by the rotation, as well as by a time order error. He claimed to have demonstrated that only extroverted subjects show a decrease in the 'field motion.' His results could equally well have been due to his two groups of subjects having differential habituation to the after-effects of rotation (see section 5.5).

Taylor and Papert (1955) made much of the reduction of apparent motion in their discussion of the learning processes involved in adapting to inverted vision. They described how, with normal vision, there is a 'constancy' mechanism by which eye or head movements and the accompanying retinal-image movements are cancelled out to produce a stable judged field of view. When inverting spectacles are worn, a new set of equivalences must be built up between head movements and the movements of the retinal image. Apparently all subjects learn to stabilize their judgments, but some, according to Taylor and Papert, 'also eventually report that the perceived world no longer appears to be inverted'. It was predicted that those who continue to report an inverted world will, when they remove the spectacles, report an apparent rotation of the field of view at twice the angle in the opposite direction to tilts of the head. On the other hand, it was predicted that those who come to report an upright world will, after removing the spectacles, report a rotation of the field of view in the same direction as tilts of the head in the frontal plane. There is evidence to support Taylor and Papert's first hypothesis: Kohler (1951) reported that one of his subjects described the apparent movements of the field as opposite to the direction of head tilts. But Taylor and Papert could find no evidence in support of their second prediction. We are not surprised for we think the prediction is based on a false analysis.

We have already argued that once a subject wearing inverting spectacles has learnt to move correctly and to stabilize the field of view, then his answer to the question 'does the world appear erect?' is dependent on higher-order skills associated with mono-oriented objects in the visual field. A change in his answer to this question will not affect his visual–motor coordination, nor the apparent stability of the field of view, during the time the spectacles are worn. This being so, there is no reason to expect that it will affect them after the spectacles are removed. Taylor and Papert appear to think that adaptation produces an actual change in the geometry of the situation, and that there is a causal connection between the reported orientation of objects and the re-ported movements of the field of view during head movements. We have discussed this issue with Taylor, and while we understand each other's posi-tion, we have agreed to differ until there is more evidence.

To show that Taylor and Papert's second prediction is false, it is only necessary to consider what would happen in a world composed solely of polyoriented visible objects, such as cubes and spheres. Subjects would at no time report an experience of inversion; they would, however, have to learn to move correctly and to stabilize their judgments of movement, and no doubt, after removing the spectacles, they would experience the movement of the field in the opposite direction to their head movements. If mono-oriented objects were placed in the field of view after motor coordination and movement stability were completely adapted, these would be reported as being upside-down, and further learning would be necessary before they were reported as erect. But there is no reason to suppose that this learning would affect the already established skills.

Inverting optical devices may upset not only the normal relationship between eye movements and movements of the retinal image, but also that between optokinetic and vestibular nystagmus. We have discussed in section 5.31 how these two reflexes normally complement each other; but if left–right reversing devices are worn, the slow phase of optokinetic nystagmus will be in the opposite direction to the slow phase of vestibular nystagmus. Visually induced nystagmus will probably dominate the situation, so that there will still be compensation for retinal-image motion.

15.4 The behavioural effects of disturbed visual polarity

Ever since the seventeenth century when Kepler described the dioptrics of the eye and revealed that the retinal image is inverted relative to the distal stimulus, scientists and philosophers have disputed how it is that the visible world is not reported to be upside-down. This history has been recounted many times and need not be repeated here. The reader is referred to Hyslop (1897), Walls (1951a), and Polyak (1957).

It was against the background of these philosophical disputes that Stratton (1897a, 1897b) conducted his famous experiments in which he wore lenses which inverted and reversed the retinal image so that it became objectively erect. According to Giannitrapani (1958) the first experiment of this kind was conducted by Ardigo (1886) who reported that objects were eventually seen as upright, and that when the optical devices were removed, objects at first appeared upside-down.

The traditional question which these early studies attempted to answer was: does a person wearing inverting spectacles ever come to see the world right way up? This is a very ambiguous question and attempts to answer it have led to controversy and confusion. Before an attempt is made to analyse this issue, Stratton's reports while wearing inverting–reversing prisms will be briefly described.

On the fourth day of wearing his prisms Stratton wrote, 'Objects in sight called up the ideas of neighbouring objects in harmonious spatial relation with the things I saw . . . the movements of my legs and arms were, without my willing it, imaged in terms of the newer sight . . . the spatial reference of the touch perceptions was following with greater vividness the direction given by the new visualization.' Further on he reported,' . . . During active movements of the body . . . the feeling of the uprightness of the scene was much more vivid than when the body was quiet.' On the eighth day he wrote, 'As long as the new localization of my body was vivid, the general experience was harmonious, and everything was right side up. But when, for any of the reasons already given—an involuntary lapse into the older memory-materials, or a wilful recall of these older forms—the pre-experimental localization of my body was predominantly in mind, then as I looked out on the scene before me the scene was involuntarily taken as the standard of right direction, and my body was felt to be in an inharmonious position with reference to the rest. I seemed to be viewing the scene from an inverted body.'

Stratton's reports were ambiguous, not because he gave an ambiguous answer to an unambiguous question, but because the question which his protocols are supposed to answer is an ambiguous one. Stratton was not to blame, the confusion is not in his reports, but in the people who have expected to find in those reports a clear answer to a misleading question.

In the years following Stratton's experiments some writers (e.g. Carr, 1935) concluded that Stratton came to experience an upright world while others (Woodworth, 1934; Higginson, 1937; Ewert, 1930, 1937) concluded that he did not. Peterson and Peterson (1938) and Snyder and Pronko (1952) repeated Stratton's experiment but could not give a conclusive answer to the question. Snyder and Pronko's subject, when asked whether things looked upside-down, replied, 'I wish you hadn't asked me. Things were all right until you popped the question at me. Now when I recall how they *did* look *before* I put on these lenses, I must answer that they do look upside-down *now*. But until the moment that you asked me I was absolutely unaware of it and hadn't given a thought to the question of whether things were right-side-up or upside-down' (p. 113).

The question, 'does the world appear upright?' can mean at least three things. (1) It can refer to whether or not movements are effectively related to visual targets. We shall call this the *motor-coordination* upright. (2) It can refer to whether visual judgments of the direction of objects correspond to judgements based on other modalities. We shall call this the *intersensory upright*. Of particular significance here is the relation between vision and the gravity senses. This aspect of the question has already been discussed in chapter 7 and section 14.3. (3) It can refer to behaviour associated with mono-oriented objects such as chairs, people, houses, etc. The visible world is polarized, that is, under ordinary circumstances the sky, the ground, and most objects maintain a fairly constant orientation to gravity, to one another, and to the observer. There are situations, for instance when one is climbing a cliff face, where the polarity of the field of view is ambiguous, but, even in such circumstances, visual polarity is unambiguously defined by the direction in which objects heavier than air can be seen to fall and substances lighter than air, such as smoke, can be seen to rise. Many things are polarized left–right as well as up–down, for example, writing, traffic-flow, shoes. Left–right polarity is not geometrically analogous to up–down polarity, for one is defined with reference to the asymmetry of the human body and the other with reference to the centre of the earth. East–west and north–south polarities are analogous to up–down polarity; compasses and sunsets are examples of such polarities.

We shall refer to the objective, geometrical orientation of the visible world in relation to the earth's centre, body asymmetries, etc., as the *polarity of the visible world*. If the polarity is the usual one the distal stimuli are said to be upright, left–right correct, etc. Mono-oriented objects retain the same polarity with respect to each other, and this *intrafield polarity* can be appreciated by an observer even if his ability to detect the objective polarity of the whole field is absent.

People live in a consistent visible world most of the time, and consequently develop habits which enable them to behave adequately in such an environment, but inadequately when the polarity of the distal stimulus is altered. Left–right polarity can only be altered with reference to an observer, the up–down polarity of the visible world may be altered with reference to gravity and/or the observer. Behaviour is therefore polarized, and we shall refer to the observable consequences as *behavioural polarity*, i.e. *the tendency to behave towards mono-oriented objects in terms of earth- or body-based coordinates irrespective of the present orientation of the objects.*

One consequence of behavioural polarity is the use of words, such as 'upright', 'inside-out', 'back-to-front', 'wrong way round', etc. But these words are often ambiguous, and are best avoided. Simple discrimination tasks make the best behavioural indices of the polarity of behaviour, for they can be most precisely specified. We suggest the following tests.

(a) The speed of recognition of mono-oriented objects. A particularly good test of this kind is recognition of a person's face or identification of a facial expression as a smile or growl. A complex shape, such as a face, is particularly affected by changed orientation. The mouth of an erect smiling face is concave at the top like the mouth of an inverted growling face (see figure 15.8). The technique used by Rock (1956) of asking a subject to select a

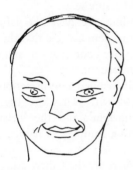 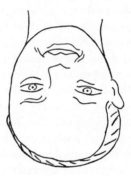

Figure 15.8 Showing the effect of the orientation of a face on the appearance of a smile

training shape from among several test shapes in various orientations is a useful one (see section 12.5).

(b) The correctness and speed of identification of the top and bottom of mono-oriented objects displayed in various orientations.

(c) The speed of recognition that a falling object is falling, or that smoke is rising—in other words, the ability to recognize 'polarized movements'.

(d) The first figure to be recognized in a composite ambiguous figure in which the alternative figures are separated by a specified angle (e.g. figures 12.7 and 12.12). Kohler (1953) used a Schröder staircase and asked the subjects which way they would approach it to climb the stairs.

It is not legitimate to use pointing or other directional movements to indicate behavioural polarity; for instance, if a subject were asked to indicate by pointing the direction in which he anticipates an object will fall, he may do one of two things. In the first place he may point objectively downwards because this is his usual response, and, of course, he would be correct. This aspect of his old behavioural polarity will not be disturbed by the visual inversion and therefore it can give no clue to those polarized habits which are affected by the inversion. On the other hand, if the object which is going to fall is seen against the background of a room, he may anticipate that it will fall in the direction of the displaced floor of the room. In purely visual terms, he will be correct, but if he points in that direction, he will be pointing in the objectively wrong direction. All this response will indicate, is that the subject expects the object to fall to what he can see is the floor. In a purely visual sense, he will be right, but it is not what we want to know. What we want to know is whether the fall, when it occurs, is discriminated speedily and fault-lessly as a 'fall' and not as a 'rise'. We can only get to know the answer to this question by eliciting discrimination responses such as correct verbal label-ling, or some other, equivalent, conditioned response.

We do not claim that these behavioural indices exhaust the definition of behavioural polarity, but they are sufficient to demonstrate that the concept is real and distinct from motor and intersensory coordination, and that dis-crimination responses are necessary for its measurement.

We thus have three broad operationally defined interpretations of the question, 'does the world appear upside-down?' They are the 'motor-coordination upright', the 'intersensory upright', and the 'behavioural-polarity upright'. Each one of these involves a complex of habits, and each habit may be retrained independently.

Most writers have ignored the fact that there are these three aspects to the question of the visual upright and endless dispute has resulted (Pickford, 1956).

We have already shown that people wearing inverting spectacles can adapt so that their 'motor-coordination upright' becomes correct. It also seems that their 'intersensory upright' adapts to the distortion. It remains to enquire whether their polarity behaviour can adapt.

Polarity is a purely visual matter, it has no necessary connection with other modalities nor with gravity. A world in which there was no gravity could still be polarized. A person with no gravity receptors other than vision could still appreciate that our world is polarized, and if he maintained a constant orientation of his body to his visual surroundings his behaviour would be-come polarized. Even if he did not maintain a constant orientation, he could still appreciate that mono-oriented objects remain in a constant relationship to one another, and he could still judge the direction of gravity in most visual surroundings, whatever he called it. If such a hypothetical person suddenly gained gravity receptors he would have to learn to relate the inputs from them with visual polarity. To see the direction in which things fall and hang is just as much gravity reception as interpreting signals from the otoliths. Both indicate the direction of the earth's centre. Visual signals mediate righting reflexes in man, and in animals (see section 9.13). Righting reflexes based on vision, known as dorsal light reactions, occur in many animal phyla: coelenterates, insects, crustacea, and fish (Fraenkel and Gunn, 1961, ch. X). They occur in such animals whether or not their other gravity receptors are functioning.

Vestibular signals also mediate unlearned righting reflexes in both men and animals. But, in spite of having these reflexes, men must learn to judge 'up' and 'down' on the basis of vestibular signals just as they must for visual ones. But Erisman (Pickford, 1956), and Gibson and Mowrer (1938) claim that we can only judge the direction of gravity visually if vision has been associated with signals from other gravity receptors. We do not agree, for a 'purely visual' person can be taught to judge 'up' and 'down' in most natural environments. The fact that it would be easy to fool him is not significant, for it is also easy to fool a purely vestibular man, by putting cold water in his ear for instance, or by putting him in a centrifuge. In fact, in ordinary circumstances visual judgments of the vertical, by a plumb-line for instance, are much more accurate and reliable than judgments based on the so-called gravity receptors. It is true that in order to utilize visual polarity for motor responses, the position of the head and body, of the eye in the head, and of the head on the body must be sensed; but vestibular stimuli are equally useless if the position of the head in relation to the body is not sensed. When Gibson and Mowrer wrote that 'visual lines are not in their own right stimuli for orientation', they should have added that vestibular signals are not adequate in their own right either. Normal response mechanisms are needed in both cases, but verbal and motor discriminations based on each modality can be taught independently of the other.

Only mono-oriented objects can be said to be upside-down in a purely visual sense, where questions of motor and intersensory coordination are not considered. Therefore, inverting spectacles cause only mono-oriented objects (and movements) to be reported as being 'upside-down'.

The world is 'polarized', and if the righting reflexes are unlearned this implies that the visual system itself is polarized with respect to certain features of the environment. Even so, we presumably learn to behave differentially to most of the polarized features of the world, and verbal responses such as 'up' and 'down' must be learned. This being so, it is reasonable to suppose that human beings can fully adapt most, if not all of their behaviour to inverting spectacles, so far as behaviour associated with visual polarity is concerned. Logically, of course, one cannot conclude that skills which were initially learned must be capable of drastic reorganization.

Walls (1951c) has argued, falsely, we think, that complete adaptation to inversion is not possible because the structural features of the visual system are innate and immutable. He conceded (p. 191 footnote) that behaviour associated with mono-oriented objects is entirely learned, so that he must have been thinking of something other than visual polarity when he concluded that full behavioural adaptation is impossible.

One of the reasons why Walls concluded that full adaptation is not possible may have been that he was looking for the wrong thing. He expected that full adaptation would imply in some way a geometrical shifting of the retinal image, what he called a 're-structuring of the visual field'. It is not clear what Walls meant, but perhaps he was referring to what Taylor insists happens to persons wearing inverting spectacles. Taylor (1962) maintains that when inverting spectacles have been worn for some time, objects which have been handled are reported to be erect, but objects which have not been handled are reported to be inverted. For instance, a person may be in a room and report that the contents of the room look erect, but that the scene outside the window looks inverted. Taylor maintains that this report implies that the subject will draw what he sees by drawing such a figure as figure 15.9. If this

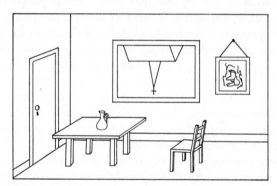

Figure 15.9 The kind of drawing which a person wearing inverting spectacles may make according to Taylor and Papert

is what Walls refused to believe, we sympathize with his views, for Taylor is surely wrong. It is an error which many people make when thinking about these problems. Taylor is wrong because he confuses geometry with what we have called behavioural polarity. The subject whom Taylor described could not reveal the nature of his polarity responses in a drawing. The distinction between the inside and outside of the room is that only for objects inside the room has the subject's polarity behaviour become adapted. In terms of our operational tests, he will recognize objects in the room quickly, identify their tops and bottoms, predict their direction of fall, etc. The geometry of their position on his retina is unchanged, he has simply learned new polarity habits. Objects outside the window, having been seen less and handled less, elicit the old polarity habits. The subject cannot depict his change of polarity behaviour in a drawing, for no geometrical change is involved. His drawing of the room and the view outside will retain the same relative orientation of all its parts (see figure 15.10).

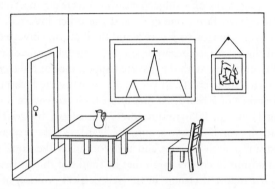

Figure 15.10 The kind of drawing which a person wearing inverting spectacles is most likely to make

This fallacy of regarding a change of polarity behaviour as a geometrical change equivalent to a geometrical righting of the image on the retina is the same fallacy which led Taylor and Papert to make false predictions about the consequences of head movements in inverted vision (see section 15.3).

Taylor and Papert had no justification for their error, for all the published protocols of subjects wearing inverting spectacles stress that the 'polarity righting' of the field of view is not to be thought of as a geometrical shift of the visual field. One of Kohler's subjects (Kottenhoff, 1961) reported that things sometimes looked upright but that this did not mean that things appeared to turn round.

He said, 'I see always the same but the interpretation is different.' For this subject, distant objects had an unusual or upside-down appearance, while nearby, familiar objects had a right-way-up look about them. Kohler himself (1953), when describing the left–right appearance of things when wearing reversing spectacles, wrote, '. . . but this isn't a sudden reversal; it remains the same picture experienced differently'. For this subject, inscriptions on buildings, or advertisements were still seen in mirror-writing, but the objects containing them were seen the right way round. Vehicles seen as driving on the right (in Austria this is correct) nevertheless carried licence numbers in mirror-writing, Kohler commented that this is optically impossible and his attempt to give a pictorial reconstruction of the subject's report is very misleading, as he realized when he wrote, 'the purely pictorial impression remains reversed' (Kohler, 1955). These effects are not at all geometrically paradoxical; it is simply a question of different left–right polarity habits holding simultaneously for different parts of the field of view. In the film which Erisman and Kohler (1953) produced, an experience is described (in a very misleading way) of a subject wearing inverting spectacles who was confronted with two faces, one erect and the other inverted. At first the inverted face was reported to be erect and the erect one inverted; but when the owner of the erect face began to smoke a cigarette, the direction of the smoke was incompatible with the inverted appearance of the face, and it was suddenly reported to be erect and yet retain some inverted features. The hair had the appearance of a beard. At one point both faces were reported to be erect. Taylor (1962, p. 206) misinterprets this report by concluding that, 'The erect face appeared to have acquired a beard, as if the crown of the head had failed to jump with the rest and now occupied the same space as the chin.' Taylor admits in conversation that he thinks of this situation as one in which there is a reported change in the geometrical position of one part of the face in relation to other parts. We are convinced that his interpretation is wrong.

It would be wrong to suppose that these paradoxical effects cannot be experienced unless one is prepared to wear inverting spectacles for long periods. It is possible, by simply looking through one's legs backwards, to gain some insight into what these reports mean. From this position, another person who is standing erect is reported as being upright in the intermodal sense and also in the motor-coordination sense, but many people say that his face has the same upside-down polarity which an inverted face has. In the first two senses the face 'looks' upright and yet it has an upside-down look about it. Some people are able to adopt either of two attitudes towards the polarity of a face seen between their legs, and this change of attitude may be brought about by a change in the orientation of the background. In the situation where two people look at each other through their legs, some people describe the other person as having upside-down polarity and others see him as having erect polarity. There is no question that any of these changes in behavioural polarity are accompanied by any geometrical change in what is reported.

If one stands erect and looks at an upside-down face, one may report that the hair has a 'beardy' look about it, and that the eyelids have a 'mouthy' look. The face, though familiar, may not be recognizable and certainly facial expressions will be very difficult to judge. If the upside-down face is seen in its proper relative orientation in an upside-down picture in which there is plenty of background, an observer may describe it as having upright polarity, and at the same time describe an erect face outside the picture, seen against the erect room, as also having upright polarity. Here are two faces, one 180° disoriented with respect to the other, and yet both eliciting the description of erect polarity. These are just the responses which one of Kohler's subjects made. According to Taylor (private conversation) this type of behaviour implies that the subject will, when asked to draw what he sees, draw two faces in the same geometrical orientation. We hope our account has made it clear that Taylor is wrong.

In spite of our disagreement with Taylor we have to admit that genuine geometrical shifts are sometimes reported. One of Kohler's subjects reported that after wearing left–right reversing spectacles, a sort of mirror-writing appeared between lines of print. Another subject reported two points of light when only one was present, one in the position of the light and a dimmer one in the symmetrical position on the other side, and these were seen even monocularly. Taylor (1962) reported that Papert, while wearing reversing spectacles, saw two chairs, one on one side and one on the other. It seems more likely, when one looks at the details of what Papert reported, that the 'two chairs' were not both seen, but rather that one was felt and the other seen. It is difficult to see how the cases of diplopia reported by Kohler can be explained this way. Rapid eye movements may have been taking place, or the dim second light may have been an after-image or eidetic image. The problems raised by these reports must be considered in relation to the problem of monocular diplopia which we have discussed in section 2.3.

Walls had to admit that monocular diplopia is a very difficult fact to accommodate. We also admit the difficulty, but insist that even if monocular diplopia does exist as a consequence of distorted vision, this would have no connection with the problem of visual polarity. Such diplopia would be the result of the changed 'space values' of retinal points in relation to motor movements and other sense modalities. A change of polarity does not involve a change in the geometrical space values of the retina. We predict that monocular diplopia, if it occurs at all, will result when inverting spectacles are worn in a purely polyoriented, unpolarized visual environment.

Thus the question, do things appear upside-down?, is a very ambiguous one; the answer a subject gives will depend on his criteria of inversion. However, no one would describe a polyoriented, or unpolarized field of view as either upright or upside-down. It is unlikely that anyone would use these terms in such surroundings even if they knew that motor behaviour and intersensory judgments were disturbed. Polarity seems to be a necessary basis for the application of any ordinary verbal judgments of inversion.

Kohler contends that, 'Only through manipulation of objects does the simultaneously seen world obtain its directions; ... he who wants to *see* correctly must first be able to *manipulate* correctly' (Kohler 1953, trans. by Gleitman, p. 19). Taylor's theory is also based on the necessity for movements and so also in a different way is Held's theory.

The experiments necessary to prove this point of view have not been done. The following are outlines of some possible crucial experiments.

The polarity of the optical array may be inverted by simply placing a person in objectively inverted surroundings. Kohler had an inverted room made, but he does not seem to have used it for testing whether a change in behavioural polarity is dependent on manipulation. To be fully convincing, objects in an inverted room would have to fall upwards and smoke would have to descend.

The question is whether visual inspection alone would lead to new polarity habits, such as rapid and accurate recognition of objects, reading, the anticipation of the direction of falling objects, and a change in the choice of ambiguous figures, etc. If such changes occurred they would demonstrate that a change in polarity behaviour does not necessarily involve any manipulative activity or reafferent stimulation (see section 15.24). The training, in other words, would be purely exafferent and not reafferent. We predict that learning would take place under these circumstances, and that new polarity habits would be built up. Of course eye movements would occur and, although these are not normally thought of as 'manipulations', they do give rise to reafferent stimulation. To control for this factor and at the same time use a less complex visual input, one could test whether the speed of reading inverted writing improves when the print is moved intermittently across the subject's field of view while he wears a device which stabilizes the position of the retinal image on the retina. We would be very surprised if reading did not improve under these circumstances and, if it did, one would have to abandon any narrowly based theories of so-called perceptual learning, in which muscular manipulations or reafference are thought to be essential.

This is not to say that in a mono-oriented, apparently inverted field of view, motor adaptation and changing intersensory judgments would not contribute to a change of behavioural polarity. It seems from most of the protocols that a change of behavioural polarity occurs after many motor and intermodal adjustments have been made, although one of Kohler's subjects (Marte) reported new polarity habits on the first day. On the other hand, Kottenhoff did not report a change of polarity after 40 days of inverted vision, even though his motor behaviour was well adjusted. However, Kottenhoff described to Taylor (1962, p. 180) the technique he employed, when he was asked to report on the left–right polarity of his visual surroundings while wearing left–right reversing spectacles. According to Taylor, 'Kottenhoff defined the positions of the edges of his field of vision as being next to his forehead, his nose, his right temple, and his left temple. Since these parts were not in his field of view, they constituted a frame of reference that remained invariant through the experiment.' Assuming that this invariance refers to the relationship between the felt position of the frame and the felt direction of gravity, it is not clear why this frame should necessarily have remained invariant throughout the experiment for this subject. It did not remain invariant for all subjects: Stratton and other subjects reported feeling as though they were standing on their heads.

We may have given the impression that we regard behavioural polarity as a unitary thing, but this is not so: a change in one aspect of polarized behaviour, for instance recognition speed, may occur without any change in another, for instance rapid prediction of the direction of fall. It is because of these multiple possibilities, that it is of little use to ask the subjects whether things look upright. If one does this, one will inevitably get ambiguous answers. The conflicting reports made by Kohler's subjects, and much of the dispute in the literature, are probably due to the use of a concept of polarity which is not operationally defined.

Our analysis so far has consisted in classifying the various habits which are affected by distortions of the optical array, and considering to what extent they become adapted to the distortion. It may seem that we have assumed that if all these habits became adapted to distorted vision, so that they functioned rapidly and accurately, the adult subject would in all senses be said to 'see the world the right way'. But this does not follow, because an adult subject will retain all the old habits which he has built up over the greater part of his lifetime. He can recall these habits, and when he does so, he will be able to report on the discrepancy between these old habits and the new ones. The old habits will remain the preferred standard of what is 'correct' because they have occupied the largest part of the subject's life. The new habits will, even when functioning as well as the old, be reported as upside-down, etc., when compared with the old. If the distorting devices were worn from birth or for many years, the adapted habits would be the only or the strongest standard of 'normality'. Such experiments have not been done, but it is difficult to see how they could do other than prove the correctness of our analysis.

A person who has had no other visual experience but through distorting devices, would, we suggest, be behaviourally indistinguishable from an ordinary person in almost all respects. His post-rotational nystagmus would probably be anomalous, and it is more than likely that he would be slower than the normal child in developing visual–motor skills, etc., and this would probably have a general retarding effect. Furthermore, it is probable that such a person would adapt to normal vision more quickly than a normal person adapts to distorted vision. These differences, if they were shown to exist, would demonstrate that the neonatal nervous system is structurally biased in favour of the normal visual–motor and intersensory relationships. In some respects, for instance in the case of vestibular-visual reflexes, this is known to be so. There are good reasons for supposing that head and eye fixation reflexes are also built into the system. It is unlikely that the nervous system is a *tabula rasa* as far as spatial skills are concerned, and however successfully a human being could adapt to visual distortion, it would not prove that the nervous system is initially unbiased.

Disturbances of visual polarity may apparently occur as a result of cerebral injury. Klopp (1951) reviewed 13 papers from the clinical literature in which there were reports of patients who described their visible surroundings as upside-down. Whether this affected their visual–motor coordination is not clear. The etiology and theoretical significance of this condition defy analysis at the present time.

16

Orientation in the weightless state

The age of human space travel has arrived and knowledge is accumulating about how man's behaviour will be affected by the conditions prevailing

in outer space. The most significant difference between a terrestrial environment and the environment of outer space is the absence of a gravitational
field in the latter. Serious attempts to study the effects of zero gravity on
human performance started about 1950. Reports are now available on the
experiences of the first Russian and American cosmonauts in orbital flights
(Henry *et al.*, 1962).

We shall briefly describe the methods which have been used to produce
weightlessness; they are reviewed in more detail by Haber and Haber (1950),
Loftus and Hammer (1961), and Gerathewohl (1960). We shall adopt the
convention suggested by Ritter and Gerathewohl (1959), and use the term
'zero-g' to refer to the physical state in which there is no gravitational field,
and the term 'weightlessness' to refer to the physiological and psychological
state which zero-g produces.

16.1 Methods of producing weightlessness

Free fall produces a state of weightlessness. In the atmosphere, air resistance prevents the fall from being completely 'free'. The feeling of falling
which the rush of air produces may be eliminated by placing the subject in
an enclosed cabin. Some attempts have been made to use a falling lift, but
only two seconds of zero-g have been produced in this way (Gerathewohl,
1963), although designs for falling capsules to produce up to 30 sec weightlessness have been proposed (Walton, 1957; Ordway, Gardner, and Sharpe,
1962, p. 559).

Diringshofen (1952) produced a ten-second period of zero-g by flying
an aircraft in a power dive. Haber and Haber (1950) suggested flying an
aircraft in a Keplerian parabolic trajectory. The principle of such a flight
is that at the push-over point to zero-g the free contents of the aircraft are
launched into a parabolic path. The aircraft is then flown (aerodynamically
controlled) so as to follow the falling contents until the recovery point. The
maximum period of zero-g possible with this method is about 50 sec, although, for reasons of fuel economy it is not usual to exceed 20 sec of zero-g.
The main features of such a flight are depicted in figure 16.1. It can be seen
that the zero-g state is preceded and succeeded by about two seconds of $2\frac{1}{2}$-g.
This is a severe limitation of the method, in that many of the observed effects
on behaviour may be due to the preceding period of excess g rather than to
the state of zero-g. Cargo aircraft are now used, in which there is ample room
for unrestrained subjects to float and soar. Orbital flight beyond the earth's
atmosphere is obviously the most satisfactory method for producing zero-g
conditions and is the only way to produce long periods of zero-g. Theoretically, an object in an orbital flight is in perpetual free fall; therefore all the

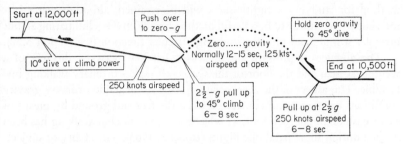

Figure 16.1 Flight profile of a typical zero-*g* manœuvre. [From Hammer, 1962]

methods so far mentioned are theoretically equivalent, the significant difference between them being the duration of weightlessness they produce.

Attempts have been made to approximate the zero-*g* condition by fully immersing a subject in water, at that depth where the upward thrust of the water exactly counters his body weight. This point is reached when the water pressure compresses his thorax by the amount necessary to bring his mean body density to that of the surrounding water. Kinaesthetic cues are never entirely absent, for the limbs do not have the same density as the body, and will therefore be differentially buoyant. Care must be taken to ensure that the subject cannot see his expired air, for otherwise the direction of movement of the bubbles would indicate the upward direction. Immersion does not eliminate the action of gravity on the otoliths. Several methods have been proposed for overcoming this limitation. Subjects with non-functioning otoliths can be used, but such an experiment does not seem to have been done. In any case, it is difficult to be certain that otoliths are completely non-functional.

Studying subjects on a gimballed frame, Quix (1928) described a position of the body in space in which there is apparently no sensory input from the otoliths. Graybiel (1954) noted the same 'blind spot' when his subjects were upside-down. Knight (1958) considered that this phenomenon provided a method for producing weightlessness, but it has not been used for this purpose. Muller (1958) proposed placing a subject horizontally in a rotating tank of water so that he is caused to rotate about his longitudinal body axis. He argued that some rate of revolution may be found where there would be 'fusion' of the stimulating effects of rotation on the utricles. But even if such a revolution rate could be found, the method would not allow the subject to move his head as this would produce a strong Coriolis effect (see section 16.51). Furthermore, centrifugal forces would operate on his limbs.

Now that manned space flight is possible it is doubtful whether any other method for studying weightlessness will be retained, although water immersion will continue to be a useful method for selectively eliminating all but utricular stimuli, and thus for studying utricular function (see section 5.22).

The absence of pressure and hence of friction, between the feet of a weightless man and the floor of the spacecraft makes ordinary walking impossible. This aspect of the zero-*g* state may be simulated in ordinary gravity conditions by preventing contact between the feet and ground by means of an air cushion under each foot. This has not been done, but walking has been studied during short parabolic flights (Roberts, 1963). The ability of subjects to position themselves whilst supported on a frictionless air-cushion platform has also been studied (Jacobs, 1960; Pigg, 1961).

16.2 The perceptual effects of weightlessness

Basic visual functions will probably be somewhat disturbed under weightlessness. Visual acuity has been found to be reduced by about 6% during short periods of weightlessness (Pigg and Kama, 1961). Whether acuity would return to normal or deteriorate further during longer periods of weightlessness is not known. Outside the spaceship important depth cues, such as the texture gradient over large receding surfaces, and aerial perspective, will be absent. The effects of lack of texture in the field of view have been described as 'empty field myopia'; because of the lack of small detail, there is a disturbance of accommodation which makes it difficult to detect small objects. The stars provide a visible textured backcloth, but whether this will prevent the development of empty field myopia is not known. There is a very wide range of light intensity; the background is black, but any near object is glaringly bright and will doubtless require the use of special anti-glare optical devices.

16.21 Sensations of falling

The otoliths of a weightless man will behave as they would in a fall. This fact led Gauer and Haber (1950) to speculate that zero-*g* would induce a sensation of falling. In parabolic zero-*g* flights carried out since 1950 by the U.S. Air Force, only a few subjects reported sensations of falling and these sensations were usually transitory. In fact many subjects reported a floating sensation (Ballinger, 1952; Gerathewohl, 1956, 1957; Schock, 1958b). The first human subject to be in full orbit was the Russian cosmonaut, Gagarin. He was in orbit for one and a half hours. According to the newspaper reports, he reported no sensory difficulties. Major Titov, the second Russian cosmonaut, was in orbit for a day. He reported no falling sensations. Neither did the other Russian and American cosmonauts.

The Russian cosmonauts reported no difficulty with hand movements or the use of controls; Titov ate three meals successfully and wrote notes. The American cosmonauts in the Mercury flights reported no disturbances in spatial orientation and performed manual tasks accurately (Results, 1961a, 1961b, 1962).

Thus Gauer and Haber's prediction has not been confirmed. The presence of a visual frame, and the absence of the air-flow sensations which normally accompany falling probably serve to prevent a sensation of falling. Furthermore, there is no reason to believe that the subjects consciously thought of the situation as one in which they were falling, and this cognitive factor probably helped to prevent a sensation of falling. Most people never fall more than a few feet; therefore they never have the opportunity of sampling the sensations produced by falling. Floating on water is the nearest approximation to the conditions of weightlessness which most people have, and so it is not surprising that most people at zero-g have reported floating sensations. Even parachutists report that the sensations before the parachute opens are more akin to floating than to falling.

16.22 Orientation judgments

Hammer (1962) is the only person to have studied the judgment of the visual vertical under reduced g conditions, although several studies have been done with submerged subjects (see section 5.22). Hammer asked his subjects to judge the apparent vertical position of a luminous line seen in the dark. The judgments were made inside an aircraft which was flown so as to produce 1·0, 0·5, 0·25, and zero-g. The mean variable error increased from 0·8° at 1·0-g to 3·5° at zero-g. In the zero-g condition in the dark, any reference to the gravitational vertical is meaningless, the subject can only have been aligning the light with some retinal or body axis. The task is similar to that required of Rock's subjects when they were asked to set a rod parallel to their body when lying on their backs (see section 7.52).

Conclusive experiments need to be done on human orientation in orbiting vehicles. We have as yet only the reports of the experiences of the first astronauts. Carpenter (1962) wrote, 'I was never disoriented. I always knew where the controls and other objects within the cabin were relative to myself. I could reach anything I needed. I did have one unusual experience. After looking out of the window for some time, I noticed that when I turned my head to the right to look at the special equipment storage kit, I would get the impression that it was oriented vertically, or from where I felt it should be, this impression was because of my training in the procedure trainer and lasted only temporarily' (p. 70).

A weightless, free-floating person is aware of the static position of his limbs. If he moves his limbs, however, the consequent reactive movement and rotation of his whole body may confuse him (Gerathewohl, 1954; Simons and Gardner, 1963). There is also a tendency for a free-floating subject to overshoot a target when pointing, as we shall see later. Beckh (1959) described how a subject, who was awakened when weightless, felt that his legs were floating away and felt otherwise disoriented. Subjects tend to underestimate their own rates of rotation and during such movements become disoriented, especially in the dark (Simons and Kama, 1962).

Gauer and Haber (1950) suggested that the Weber–Fechner law implies that vestibular sensitivity will be altered in passing from a one-g environment to a zero-g environment. Haber and Gerathewohl (1951) extrapolated the Weber–Fechner relationship to values below one-g, using one-g as corresponding to zero in the sensory scale. Gougerot (1953) challenged these contentions, and argued that the system would rapidly adapt to the zero-g condition. This last prediction seems to have been borne out by the reported experiences of weightless subjects (Gerathewohl, 1954), although precise measures have not yet been obtained. King (1961) showed that utricular head reflexes are absent in weightless pigeons, so it seems that the utricles do not operate under zero-g conditions.

Under zero-g a sense of up and down can originate only from either the visual frame provided by the spacecraft, or from the felt position of the feet and head, assuming that objects outside the spacecraft are not in view. Simons (1959) has shown that subjects are able to walk on an iron surface when wearing magnetic shoes, and that they accept the surface upon which they are walking as down. This suggests that space vehicles need not be visually arranged with a floor and ceiling but that the whole inside surface could be used for the 'floor'.

16.23 Reports of well-being

Haber (1951) predicted that, 'A man liberated from the shackles of gravity would most probably be in a constant state of physiological and psychological tension.' This prediction has not been borne out by the evidence. Those few subjects who experienced fear probably did so because they anticipated such fear (Simons and Gardner, 1963).

Many subjects show various symptoms of motion sickness during parabolic flight manoeuvres. However, the most probable cause for this sickness is the rapid changes in g at the start and finish of the manoeuvres, rather than the weightlessness itself (Gerathewohl, 1956; Simons and Kama, 1962; Wendt, 1963; Beckh, 1963). Labyrinth-defective subjects were found to be unaffected (Kellogg, Kennedy, and Graybiel, 1964). The Russian, Titov, reported unpleasant sensations of nausea after his sixth orbit, especially when he turned his head. After some sleep, these symptoms decreased but did not disappear altogether before re-entry. However, his symptoms could not have been too severe, for he ate a meal and carried out various tasks successfully.

Many subjects in parabolic flight, far from experiencing sickness, feel exhilerated by the state of weightlessness. They laugh and appear to enjoy the soaring and floating, and report feelings of euphoria. The absence of body weight, skin pressure, and clothes pressure induces a sense of comfort (Haber, 1951).

The cosmonauts of Vostocks III and IV suffered no symptoms of nausea during their orbiting flights of four and three days respectively (but see note on p. 444). The American cosmonauts reported no nausea; indeed, the period of weightlessness was described as 'pleasant' (Results, 1962).

16.24 Visual illusions of movement

Small fixed visible objects seen in dark surrounds have been reported to move downwards during weightlessness. Whiteside (1961) and Schock (1958a), on the other hand, reported that such objects appear to oscillate during weightlessness, but Roman, Warren, Niven, and Graybiel (1962) attributed this to an uneven state of zero-g in Schock's experiment. The apparent downward displacement of a visible object is complementary to the apparent upward displacement which has usually been reported in states of increased-g (Clark, Graybiel, and MacCorquodale, 1948; Whiteside, 1961; Roman et al., 1962). After-images seen in total darkness during weightlessness appear to move in the opposite direction to that in which real visible objects appear to move (Gerathewohl and Stallings, 1958; Whiteside, 1961; Roman et al., 1962); however, when an after-image is superimposed on a visible object, both appear to move together. These relationships are set out in table 16.1. Gerathewohl and Stallings called the apparent elevation of an after-image in weightlessness, the 'oculoagravic illusion'. This term suggests that the effect is related to the oculogravic illusion, but this is not so. The oculogravic illusion is the apparent tilt of a vertical line of light when the direction of the gravitational force is changed (see section 7.46), while the 'oculoagravic illusion' results from a change in the magnitude of the force of gravity. The term 'oculoagravic illusion' is therefore misleading. Whiteside has suggested the term 'elevator illusion' because he noticed the apparent elevation and depression of visual objects when accelerating up and down in an elevator.

Table 16.1 Vertical displacement of a visible object and an after-image during a change in the magnitude of g. Results of several investigators

Investigator	> 1·0-g		Zero-g	
	Visible object	After-image	Visible object	After-image
Clark *et al.* (1948)	↑			
Gerathewohl and Stallings (1958)		↓		↑
Schock (1958a)	↓		oscillation	
Whiteside (1961)	↑	↓	↓	
Roman *et al.* (1962)	↑	↓	↓	↑

Gerathewohl and Stalling's paper is confusing, for in their summary they referred to the apparent movement of 'an object in space', yet their experiment referred only to after-images. After-images, as we have already noted, behave differently from real visible objects. They present arguments against an explanation of their results in terms of nystagmus, but gave no good reason why the apparent movement of the after-image could not be due to an elevation of the eyes. We suggest the following explanation. If the centre of gravity of the eyeball is not at its centre of rotation, then under normal circumstances the muscles of the eye will have to counter a natural tendency of the eyeball to rotate. In the weightless condition, the eyeball will be released from the torque due to gravity, and any pattern of voluntary innervation necessary to maintain the eyes in a given direction of gaze will be different to the pattern in normal gravitational conditions. Further, it is known that the retinal space values change with the pattern of voluntary innervation, even if the eyes do not move (see section 3.5).

Weightless observers are often confused as to whether a given motion is due to their motion or to the movement of the aircraft. A free-floating soft mass (e.g. a pillow) serves to indicate to the observer whether he or the plane is moving relative to the orbit into which he was initially launched (Simons and Gardner, 1963).

16.25 Weight discrimination

Although objects have no weight in the zero-g state, their mass may still be perceived by the inertial forces they produce when moved. Simons and Kama (1962) asked subjects to match objects by weight by lifting them under ordinary-g conditions. He then asked them to match the objects by mass when the objects were supported on a frictionless air-cushioned table. In the mass judgment situation, the subjects were not allowed to lift the objects, but were allowed to push them over the frictionless surface. The inertial information they got in this way was equivalent to the information they would be able to get from objects in the zero-g state. The difference ratio for mass was found to be 0·1, which is twice what it was for weight. The relative difficulty of judging mass may have been due to the unfamiliarity of making such judgments. Perhaps with practice men could learn to make inertial mass judgments as accurately as they normally make weight judgments.

Thus, as far as the limited evidence allows, we may conclude that short periods of weightlessness produce no formidable sensory or perceptual complications. Whether weeks or months of weightlessness will produce profound perceptual derangements is not yet known, but we predict that they will not. The most disturbing consequence of long periods of weightlessness will probably be the difficulty of adapting back to 1-g on return to earth. The anti-gravity postural muscles will weaken through disuse and will have to be retrained to full strength on return to earth. The musculature of the vascular system will also have to readapt back to supporting the weight of the blood, and maintaining a normal blood pressure in the head. The pathophysiology of weightlessness is reviewed by McCally and Lawton (1963).

16.3 Rotary orientation of the free-floating man

16.31 Introduction

A free-floating, weightless man is free to rotate about any one of the three principal body axes. It has become accepted practice to describe rotations by reference to the Air Force aircraft-axis system which is shown in figure 1.3. The three axes are formed by the intersections of the three principal planes of the body, each passing through the centre of mass of the body. The centre of mass is that point in the body about which the body will always balance. The X axis is at the intersection of the sagittal and horizontal planes; the Y axis is at the intersection of the frontal and horizontal planes; and the Z axis is at the intersection of the sagittal and frontal planes. Rolling, pitching, and yawing are the names of the rotations about the X, Y, and Z axes respectively.

Classical mechanics may be used to analyse these rotations and their dynamic effects. For such an analysis it is necessary to know the centres of gravity and moments of inertia of the articulated segments of the human body, and the centre of gravity and moment of inertia of the body as a whole in various postures. The centre of gravity of the whole human body may be determined by one of three techniques: (1) By a balance technique, involving balancing the body in various planes (Swearingen, 1953). (2) By the determination of volume contour maps of the body, assuming that the body has a homogeneous density (Weinbach, 1938). (3) By suspending the body in a pendulum in various postures. Both the centre of gravity and the moment of inertia of the body may be determined in this last way, which has been used on both cadavers (Braune and Fischer, 1889, 1892, 1963), and on living subjects with and without space suits (Santschi, DuBois, and Omoto, 1963; DuBois, Santschi, Walton, Scott, and Mazy, 1964). The centres of gravity and moments of inertia of the body segments have been calculated for the U.S. Air Force 'mean man' (Hertzberg, Daniels, and Churchill, 1954) by Whitsett (1963) and by Hanavan (1964).

A human body floating in space is a dynamically closed system. This means that as long as mass is not expelled from the body a person is unable to alter his linear or angular momentum. In other words, no matter how he moves the parts of his body, he cannot shift his centre of gravity from its orbital path nor set his body spinning. In spite of this limitation, a free-floating man has some control over, (1) his angular velocity, (2) the relative angular position of the parts of his body, (3) the axis of rotation about which his body is spinning, and (4) his angular position in space. We shall consider each of these types of control in turn.

16.32 The control of angular velocity

The angular momentum of an object equals its angular velocity multiplied by its moment of inertia. The moment of inertia of an object about any given axis of rotation depends on the total mass of the object and the way in which the mass is distributed about the axis of rotation. If the mass of a body is considered to be composed of a large number of small masses (dm), then the moment of inertia (I) is equal the sum of each mass times the square of its distance (r) from the axis of rotation,

or $I = \int r^2 dm.$

This means that if the mass of a rotating body becomes more widely distributed the moment of inertia rapidly increases, and, in order that the total angular momentum (H) be conserved, the angular velocity (ω), must be decreased in proportion. It follows that a free-floating man, although unable to alter his angular momentum, can alter his angular velocity. To do this, he must alter the spatial distribution of his body mass (moment of inertia). This type of manœuvre is well illustrated by the somersaulting high diver. He starts his dive with his body extended; this gives him a high moment of inertia and low angular velocity. As he somersaults, he draws up his legs, tucks in his head and arms, and thus reduces his moment of inertia, and at the same time increases his rate of spin (see figure 16.2). The pirouetting

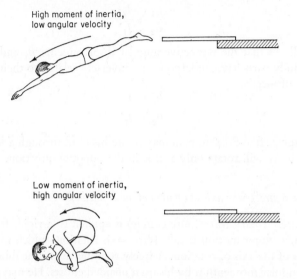

High moment of inertia, low angular velocity

Low moment of inertia, high angular velocity

Figure 16.2 Showing how the body's angular velocity is increased as its moment of inertia is decreased

ballet dancer and skater use a similar technique to produce rapid rotations of the body; they start to rotate with their arms extended, and spin faster and faster as they draw them in to the body.

The human body can tolerate rotations of at least 90 rev/min without undue physiological stress (H. S. Weiss, 1955), although for comfort and absence of dizziness, rotations of less than about 5 rev/min seem desirable (Simons and Gardner, 1960).

16.33 The control of the relative angular position of body parts

Rotations are brought about by the application of a torque (T). Torque is the rotational equivalent of force, and is the product of angular acceleration, a, and inertia.

or $$T = Ia.$$

This equation is analogous to the well known equation $F = ma$ for linear motion.

When a free-floating man rotates a part of his body, the applied torque reacts by an equal amount in the opposite direction on the rest of his body. The vector sum of the torques must be zero. It follows that the accelerations of the two parts are in inverse proportion to their moments of inertia,

or
$$\frac{a_1}{a_2} = \frac{I_2}{I_1},$$

It also follows that the respective angular displacements, θ_1 and θ_2, which the two body parts have undergone, are inversely related to their respective moments of inertia,

or
$$\frac{\theta_1}{\theta_2} = \frac{I_2}{I_1}.$$

For example, a free-floating man may rotate his head through a large angle, while his body will rotate only a little in the opposite direction.

16.34 The control of the axis of rotation of the whole body

If a purely rotary force (pure couple) is applied to a rigid, free-floating body, the resulting motion is called 'free-axis rotation' which may involve oscillation of the axis of rotation. A freely rotating man is unable to change his total angular momentum by his own unaided efforts. He may, however, alter the axis of rotation about which he is spinning in order to stabilize his rotation about one axis and so overcome the complex sensory effects of unstable, multiaxial rotations. A stable rotation is one which occurs about an axis which remains fixed in space. Rotation of a freely rotating body is stable only about an axis for which the moment of inertia is a minimum or a maximum (principal axes). Rotation about any axis of intermediate moment of inertia is always unstable.

Consider the human body as a rigid rectangular block; the maximum moment of inertia occurs about the X, or mid-sagittal axis, and the minimum occurs about the Z, or mid-body axis. Rotation about either of these axes is stable, that is, it will continue indefinitely with uniform velocity about the same axis. If, however, a torque is applied about another axis, the body will start to oscillate, that is, its axis of rotation will alter its position in space from instant to instant, describing a closed path in space. The more unstable a rotation is, the more affected the rotation is by a disturbing torque.

Furthermore, an object is more stable in its rotation about one of its stable axes the greater the difference between the moment of inertia of this axis and that of any other. A rectangular block with the principal dimensions of a human body can be in stable rotation only about the Z axis or the X

axis, but rotation about the Z axis is most stable of all because the moment of inertia about this axis is least like that about any other. A cube may be in stable rotation about each of the three principal axes at right angles to its sides, though the stability is not high because the maximum and minimum moments of inertia are equal. The cube has several other axes of stable rotation (across diagonals, for example). A sphere has an infinite number of axes of stable rotation, but a minimal disturbing torque will alter its axis of rotation.

It is possible to predict from these dynamic principles that if a weightless man wishes to achieve the maximum rotary stability, he should extend himself to the full and attempt to express whatever rotary momentum his body possesses, about his Z or mid-body axis. However, Whitsett (1963) has argued that if the body is dissipating kinetic energy, rotation about the Z axis becomes unstable and the only stable rotation would be about the X axis.

Such transfers of angular momentum between different axes of rotation may be achieved by manœuvring the limbs and trunk. But such manœuvres are difficult to learn and would be exhausting to apply for a man in a space suit, unless he were provided with some mechanical aids. Far from bringing stability, it is much more likely that movements of the body and limbs would lead to multiaxis rotations and consequent confusion of the cosmonaut.

16.35 The control of the angular position of the whole body

By manœuvres of body parts, skilfully applied, a man who is not spinning may change the direction in which he faces. By continually carrying out a sequence of body manœuvres he may cause his whole body to repeatedly change its attitude. At no instant during these manœuvres will his body as a whole acquire angular momentum nor will his centre of mass move.

Nine such manœuvres for rotating the body relative to each of the three principal axes have been described by Kulwicki, Schlei, and Vergamini (1962). Each of these manœuvres has been given a name by Simons. To illustrate the principles involved, we shall describe the so-called 'cat reflex' which changes the attitude of the body about the Z axis. It consists of a four-part cycle, the parts of which are illustrated in figure 16.3.

(1) Initially the body is straight, arms down, and legs spread to the sides, giving the lower part of the body a high moment of inertia and the upper part a low moment of inertia.

(2) The torso is twisted about the Z axis as far as possible; the upper part

of the body rotates further than the lower because of its lower moment of inertia.

(3) The moment of intertia of the upper part of the body is increased by spreading the arms out to the sides, and the moment of intertia of the lower part of the body is decreased by bringing the legs in.

(4) The torso is now straightened. During this process, the lower part of the body rotates further than the upper part, because it now has the lower moment of inertia.

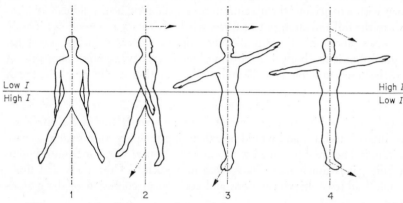

Figure 16.3 The four parts of one of the manœuvres by which a free-floating person may change his angular position

A little thought will show that there has been a net change in the angular position of the body relative to a fixed external reference point (a distant star for instance). Paradoxical though it seems, the body during these manœuvres has at no time any net angular momentum (i.e. the vector sum of the torques of the upper and lower parts of the body is always zero). If the cycle is repeated, the subject may rotate to any position he pleases.

In practice, cosmonauts working outside a spacecraft will have mechanical aids for controlling the orientation of their bodies. A single gyroscope is stable about two axes, so that two gyroscopes worn with their axes at right angles will give stability about three axes. Purposeful rotation can be achieved by applying a torque to the axis of a gyroscope and thereby precessing (rotating) the whole system at the expense of the angular momentum of the gyroscope (Simons and Kama, 1962). Tethers and jet units may also be used to control orientation.

The reported experiences of the first United States cosmonauts (Grissom 1961; Carpenter, 1962) suggest that for the accurate judgment of body rotations or rotations of a spacecraft, an instrumental display will have to be provided. In the words of Carpenter, 'I began the turnaround and wondered why I felt nothing. At this time, the angular accelerations of the spacecraft were not perceptible, and only the blackness of space could be seen through the window. The instruments provided the only reference. The turnabout proceeded just as in the trainer except that I was somewhat distracted initially by the new sensation of weightlessness. I followed the needles around and soon there was the horizon' (p. 70).

We thus complete this account of the rotary orientation of the free-floating man. With carefully designed mechanical aids, the problems should not prove to be too formidable. Effective body orientation without mechanical aids will require much skill but one can envisage this activity becoming a new form of sport when space travel becomes more general.

16.4 Locomotion in the weightless state

A weightless man cannot translate his centre of mass unless he applies a force to some external object, or expels mass. These two procedures involve, on the one hand, pushing and soaring, and on the other hand, jet propulsion. We shall consider these possibilities in turn.

16.41 Walking

A weightless man cannot walk; any attempt to push himself along a surface will only result in his propulsion away from the surface. If a series of handholds are provided by a ladder or a rope, he will be able to pull himself along. He may also proceed with his hands against one surface and his feet on a parallel surface.

Simons (1959) has designed magnetic sandals which enable a weightless man to walk on iron surfaces. These only work if they produce sufficient friction between the sandal and the 'floor'. This frictional force must be at least equal to the force necessary to accelerate (or decelerate) a man's body to a reasonable velocity in a reasonable time. If the man's mass is 200 lb, and he wishes to accelerate at $\frac{1}{3}$-g, then the force (F) required is given by,

$$F = ma$$

$$\text{or} \quad F = \frac{200}{g} \times \frac{g}{3} = 66 \cdot 7 \text{ poundals.}$$

This is also the minimum required frictional force which must oppose the force his foot applies to the surface. If the frictional force is less than this, either the man's foot will slip or he will have to be content with a slower acceleration. The frictional force is equal to the product of the coefficient of dynamic friction and the force normal to the surface (N),

$$\text{or } f = \mu N.$$

If the coefficient of friction is 0·8, then the minimum required magnetic force for an acceleration of $\frac{1}{3}$-g is,

$$N = \frac{66 \cdot 7}{0 \cdot 8} = 83 \cdot 4 \text{ poundals.}$$

If a gravitational field were generated by spinning the spacecraft, magnetic sandals would not be necessary, but this would introduce complications due to the fact that the strength of the gravititional field would depend on the direction in which the occupants walked in relation to the axis of rotation of the spacecraft. These matters are discussed under the heading of the Coriolis force. The minimum gravitational field necessary for ordinary walking on materials with various coefficients of friction may be calculated by using the above equations. There is certainly no point in having the gravitational field stronger than is needed for walking. One might as well take advantage of the comfort which a reduced gravitational field will afford.

The lower limit of gravity necessary for unaided walking is not known, but it has been established that a man can walk at a level of 0·2-g (Loret, 1961). In specifying the angular velocity necessary to generate such a gravitational field, allowance must be made for the effective reduction in angular velocity which would occur as the man walked in a direction opposite to the direction of spin of the vehicle.

16.42 Soaring

One of the potential advantages of the weightless state is that a person is able to traverse a given space by simply launching himself from any surface. The maximum speed which the average man is able to attain in this way is approximately 10 miles per hour (Simons and Gardner, 1963).

However, free soaring is not without its complications. Unless the launching thrust is applied directly in line with the centre of mass of the body, part of the force will generate a torque and a resultant spin of the body. Some practice is required before a person becomes capable of launching himself in a given direction without spin.

There is a danger from collisions with hard objects: a free-soaring person will not be able to slow down before impact with any object. Any attempt to shield the face with the hands may only disturb the attitude of the body in an unpredictable way. Soaring by inexperienced subjects has already produced some hard 'falls' (Simons and Gardner, 1963). These difficulties may be overcome using lifelines strung from one point to another with slip rings to hold.

Free soaring outside a spacecraft will introduce other difficulties. The most obvious danger is that the astronaut will not be able to get back to the spacecraft. This danger could be overcome by tethering, but this too has its complications. If the cosmonaut who is being pulled into a spacecraft has any angular momentum round the craft, his angular velocity will increase rapidly

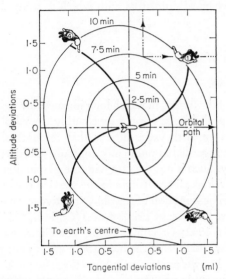

Figure 16.4 Predicted deviations from the initial direction of the trajectory of a man who has launched himself from a spacecraft at 10 m/h. [From Müller and Simons, 1962]

as he is pulled nearer the craft, with possibly disastrous consequences (Müller, 1962a). If the spacecraft were in orbit round the earth the trajectory of the soaring astronaut would, in any case, be curved. This is because he would depart from the orbital path of the spacecraft (Müller and Simons, 1962). The predicted deviations from the initial direction of the trajectory at successive moments of time are shown in figure 16.4.

16.43 Jet-aided progression

The most obvious way to facilitate transfer from one space vehicle to another is for the cosmonaut to wear small jet propulsion units. Various models have been designed and tested. A single nozzle device with pistol-grip control was among the early designs (Simons and Gardner, 1960). A more advanced design by Flexman, Seale, and Henderson (1963) for the Bell Aerosystems Co. has several nozzles fixed on a belt. Levers enable the astronaut to control his linear and angular movements. This so-called 'zero-g belt' is capable of lifting a man off the ground for a period of 26 sec. The propellant is compressed nitrogen; it is important that non-toxic propellants are used.

The problems associated with the relative motions of two spacecraft in orbital rendezvous have been analysed by Müller (1962b). Kasten (1962) has studied the human control problems in bringing about a successful rendezvous, and has built mechanical simulators with which to study the human factors empirically.

16.5 The design of spacecraft

16.51 Coriolis effects

In spacecraft of the future, in which long journeys are to be made, gravitational fields will probably be created by rotating the whole spacecraft. The gravitational field on earth varies little within the normal environment of man, and may be regarded as uniformly constant, and unaffected by movements of the body. Such is not the case with the gravitational field generated inside a rotating vehicle. The changes in the gravitational field acting on an object, due to the linear motion of the object relative to the axis of spin of the rotating vehicle are known as Coriolis forces (Coriolis, 1846; Schubert, 1932, 1933, 1954; Meda, 1952; Greening, 1962). The effects on the semicircular canals produced by rotations of the head about an axis not parallel to that of the spacecraft are known as cross-coupling effects (see section 16.52).

In a rotating spaceship, the total force acting on a small body at a point is given by

$$F = m \left[a + \omega^2 r + 2v \sin \theta \right]$$

where m = mass of the particle.

   a = linear acceleration of the particle with respect to the vehicle.

   ω = angular velocity of the vehicle.

   r = distance of the particle from the axis of rotation.

   v = linear velocity of the particle with respect to the vehicle.

   θ = angle between axis of rotation and direction of v.

It can be seen that the total force is the sum of three forces, indicated by the three terms in square brackets. The term 'a' is the acceleration of the body and is a measure of the force required to stop it relative to the vehicle, just as it would be in a stationary environment. The '$\omega^2 r$' term is a measure of the gravitational (centrifugal) force acting on the object and produced by the spin of the spacecraft. This depends only on the angular velocity, and distance of

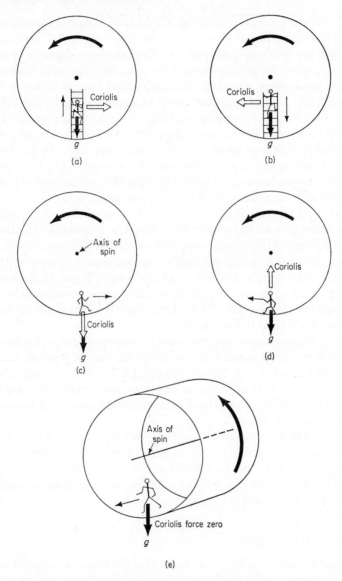

Figure 16.5 Diagrammatic representation of the direction of the Coriolis force acting on a man walking in various directions with respect to the axis of rotation of a spacecraft. (a) Man moving towards axis of spacecraft; (b) Man moving away from axis of spacecraft; (c) Man moving with spin of spacecraft; (d) Man walking against spin of spacecraft; (e) Man moving in axial direction. [Adapted from Loret, 1961]

the object from the axis of rotation. The '$2v\sin\theta$' term is a measure of the Coriolis force.

Unlike the gravitational force, the Coriolis force depends upon the direction in which the person moves in the space ship. For radial motion, the Coriolis force is perpendicular to the gravitational force as shown in figure 16.5(a) and (b). As the cosmonaut moves in towards the axis of rotation of the spacecraft, his angular velocity will tend to increase to compensate for his decreased moment of intertia about the centre of spin. If he is to stay on the same radial path he must counter this tendency to accelerate, by decelerating in the opposite direction. In other words, he will experience a force pulling him in the same direction as the spaceship's spin. When he moves out from the centre, he will experience a force in the opposite direction.

For tangential motion, the Coriolis force is parallel to the centrifugal force, making the man feel heavier if the direction of motion is with the spin and making him feel lighter if the direction of motion is against the spin. This is because, when walking one way, he increases his angular velocity, and when walking the other way, he decreases his angular velocity (figure 16.5(c) and (d)).

When a man walks parallel to the spin axis, there are no changes in either his distance or in his angular velocity, hence there is no change of any kind in the gravitational force (figure 16.5e).

The best design of spaceships, to minimize Coriolis effects, is that shown in figure 16.6. Most movements are parallel to the axis of rotation, and will produce no Coriolis forces. The torus (figure 16.7) is not such a good design, because Coriolis effects are high for tangential movements. At what value these variations of the gravitational field with body movement become intolerable is not known.

The larger the diameter of the revolving spacecraft, the smaller the angular velocity needs to be to achieve a given strength of gravitational field. It is an advantage to keep the angular velocity as low as possible so as to minimize the Coriolis forces, but practical and economic considerations demand that the craft be kept as small as possible.

16.52 Cross-coupling effects

Several investigators have concluded that the degree to which Coriolis effects can be tolerated is the central design problem (Dole, 1960; Lansberg, 1955a, 1955b; Guedry and Montague, 1961). This conclusion is unwarranted; the error arises from the confusion of Coriolis effects with cross-coupling effects (see section 5.12). It is toleration of cross-coupling effects which is the limiting design factor. The experiments conducted by Graybiel, Clark, and Zarriello (1960) give some guidance as to human cross-coupling tolerance

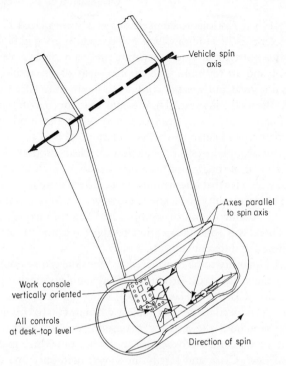

Figure 16.6 Compartment design to minimize adverse effects of Coriolis forces on crew inside rotating vehicle. [From Loret, 1961]

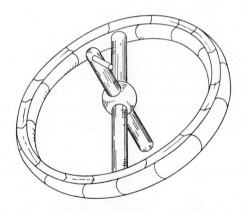

Figure 16.7 Illustration of torus as proposed by von Braun. [From Loret, 1961]

(erroneously called Coriolis tolerance). Subjects were placed in a room 15 feet in diameter and 7 feet high which was constantly rotated in a horizontal plane about its centre for 48 hours. Separate runs were made at various speeds between 1·71 and 10 rev/min. The displacement of the resultant force of gravity was not great and was not considered significant. The cross-coupling effects were the main interest. They found that the maximum vestibular symptoms (nausea, giddiness, etc.) occurred when the head was rotated about an axis perpendicular to the axis of spin. This is the movement in which the cross-coupling effect is maximum. Head motion along an axis parallel to the axis of rotation or head rotation about such an axis, produced no ill effects, which is what one would expect. There were marked individual differences in susceptibility to sickness. However, at 10 rev/min, all but one of the subjects became ill and that subject had a non-functioning vestibular apparatus. There was some adaptation to the environment after different periods of time for different subjects.

The crucial quantity to be considered, as far as the cross-coupling effect is concerned, is the vector cross-product of head angular velocity with vehicle angular velocity. Clark and Hardy (1960), using a centrifuge spinning at 1 radian per sec, produced nausea in a subject when he rotated his head at more than 0·6 rad/sec about the axis for maximum cross-coupling effect. This suggests that the maximum cross-product of velocities which man can tolerate is 0·6 rad²/sec². Clark and Hardy, however, used only one subject, and there was the incidental effect of a 2-g gravitational field in their centrifuge. Their figure is probably conservative. Normally, head rotations occur up to about 6 rad/sec. For such head rotations to occur without nausea, the angular velocity of the spacecraft would not have to exceed 0·1 rad/sec. The relationships between the design factors which have been considered are shown in figure 16.8. If a gravitational field of 1-g were desired in a spacecraft rotating at this speed the ship would have to have a radius of 100 feet. This size could be reduced by either accepting a less than normal gravitational field or by restricting the number and speed of head rotations about axes at right angles to the axis of the spacecraft. We have attempted to outline the basic principles by which the competing requirements of spacecraft design imposed by human factors may be resolved. The optimal values for the crucial variables have yet to be decided.

16.6 The performance of motor skills in the weightless state

16.61 Visual-motor coordination

In the earliest parabolic flights it was noticed that the hand tends to overshoot in the direction of the head on reaching for an object (Gerathewohl,

1954). This overshooting tendency was later investigated by means of an eye–hand coordination test (Gerathewohl, Strughold, and Stallings, 1957). Subjects thrust a stylus at a vertical paper target. At normal gravity the hits clustered round the bullseye, but at zero-*g* they hit the target 'above' the bullseye. After a few tries there was some improvement in the zero-*g* performance. The possibility of continuous visual guidance of the stylus to the bullseye was reduced in this experiment by having the subject bring the stylus rapidly to the target from out of sight.

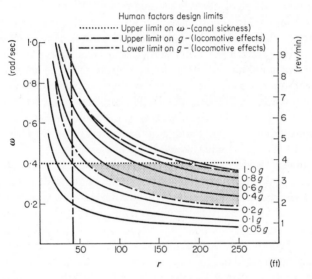

Figure 16.8 Human factor limits superimposed on plot of angular velocity (ω) versus radius of rotation (*r*) to achieve various levels of artificial gravity in spacecraft. The shaded area is the human factors design envelope. [Adapted from Loret, 1961]

A similar tendency for movements to overshoot visual targets was reported by Beckh (1954) who asked weightless subjects to place crosses in a series of squares arranged diagonally on a vertical piece of paper. At normal gravity and with eyes open, the crosses were accurately placed in the squares. With eyes closed after the target had been seen, the crosses were not so accurately placed. At zero-*g* with eyes open, the crosses tended to be displaced upwards, but the errors were small. With eyes closed the crosses drifted upwards and to the right. The significance of the drift to the right is impossible to assess, for Beckh did not state which hand was being used, though presumably it was the right hand, and perhaps the drift would have been the other way had he used the left hand. The upward drift was presumably independent of the hand used.

Beckh's experiments were done during a few seconds of weightlessness. They need to be repeated under conditions of prolonged weightlessness. Beckh did find that practice greatly improved performance at zero-g, although he did not report whether the subjects were given knowledge of results.

Whiteside (1961) found that a weightless subject pointed too low when asked to point to visible targets when his hands could not be seen. This finding contradicts those of other investigators, but Whiteside apparently used only one subject. No reports have yet appeared of quantitative studies of visual–motor coordination during prolonged periods of weightlessness.

Kama (1961) used a horizontal surface upon which objects could be supported by air cushions. In this way, the objects could be moved over the surface without friction at normal-g. The ability of subjects to position such objects on visible marks was tested. The subjects tended to undershoot, although in this case, only the objects were weightless (frictionless) and the movements were in the horizontal, not the vertical plane. Such a technique is not a valid indicator of what would happen at zero-g.

Simons and Gardner (1963) found that weightless subjects could accurately touch the nose with the two index fingers when blindfolded. Their subjects were experienced in weightless flight before the test, and may therefore have learned to compensate any tendency to overshoot by the time the test was given.

In zero-g conditions the muscular effort associated with reaching 'up' to a given seen locality will be less than under normal gravity and the output from the motor centres will be inappropriate until they have become adapted to the new conditions. This being so, overreaching is just what one would expect, when the arm has to reach 'up' (i.e. in the direction of the head). This effect may be reinforced by a short-term after-effect in the anti-gravity (abductor) muscle system when the arms are released from the need to support their own weight against gravity. This latter effect would produce the involuntary elevation of the arms which has been reported by Gurfinkell (Loftus and Hammer, 1961). The effect is the well-known post-contraction phenomenon which may be observed in ordinary conditions by pressing the arm upwards against a rigid object and then relaxing. The arm rises involuntarily; the effect decays after a few seconds. Any post-contraction effects in weightlessness would also decay in the first few seconds of weightlessness. Overshooting must also be influenced by the fact that objects appear displaced towards the feet in weightlessness (see section 16.24), although the directions of the two effects are not the same. If the hand is under the continuous guidance of vision, then any tendency to overshoot may be controlled, and performance should not suffer, except that movement would probably be slower. Ordinary tasks, such as eating, writing, and controlling instruments have been carried on at zero-g without special training.

It is most probable that, even without continuous visual guidance, all forms of visual–motor coordination will be adequately performed after a short training period at zero-g.

16.62 The use of tools and instruments

In space flights, cosmonauts may not always have a consistent orientation in relation to control panels. It may be advantageous to design such panels so that they can be controlled and read equally well from all directions. Simons and Gardner (1963) have suggested that a universally jointed switch may be useful, that is, a switch which is 'off' when centred, and 'on' when in any peripheral position. However, the ordinary push-button switch is radially symmetrical and has been shown to be the fastest switch to operate under both normal and zero-g conditions (Wade, 1961). A radially symmetrical dial may be advantageous. An expanding disc of light would be one possible design.

Perhaps the chief difficulty which a weightless person has in using tools is in applying a torque. In the absence of the normal frictional contact between his body and the 'ground', his whole body will be rotated by a torque equal and opposite to the torque he applies to the tool. Unless a hand-hold or other form of constraint is provided, the free-floating man will be able to apply only impulsive torques. Such impulsive torques will be performed with least counter-rotation of the body if the operator is positioned at right angles to the axis of rotation of the tool; in this position his body presents the maximum moment of inertia round that axis. Dzendolet and Rievley (1959) have investigated the torque that man can exert using impulsive forces when his whole body is supported on an air-bearing frictionless platform. Whitsett (1963) has calculated that the torque which a free-floating, average man should be able to apply is 2·7 ft-lbs over a period of 1·1 sec, which will result in a rotation of his body at 32·9 rev/min. Similar arguments apply to the task of pressing against objects in the weightless state. For instance, any attempt a free-floating man makes to drive a nail in will result in one impulsive blow at the nail and a subsequent backward movement of the man. A handhold or other form of constraint is clearly required for a weightless man to use tools efficiently (Dzendolet, 1960).

The weightless state will entail many incidental annoyances such as free-floating dust, objects floating from pockets, and tears adhering to the cornea.

The discussion of such aspects of space travel is beyond the scope of this book.

For further general information on human factors in space flight see Gantz (1959), Haber (1953), Hanrahan and Bushnell (1960), Helvey (1960), Ordway, Gardner, and Sharpe (1962), Pirie (1961), Proell and Bowman (1958), Seifert (1959), and Sells and Berry (1961).

In December 1965 the Soviet news agency Tass reported complaints of nausea and postural delusions (see p. 425) by non-pilots Feoktistov and Yegorov who accompanied cosmonaut Komarov on the three-man Voskhod flight in October 1964

Bibliography and author index

The pages on which the reference is mentioned are given in square brackets at the end of the entry.

Aarons, L., and Goldenberg, L., 1964. Galvanic stimulation of the vestibular system and perception of the vertical. *Percept. mot. Skills*, **19**, 59–66. [196]

Abderhalden, E., 1919. Beobachtungen zur Frage der morphologischen und functionellen Asymmetrie des menschlichen Körpers. *Pflüg. Arch. ges. Physiol.*, **177**, 213–216. [257, 258]

Abel, T. M., 1936. A comparison of tactual-kinaesthetic and visual perceptions of extent among adults, children and subnormals. *Amer. J. Psychol.*, **48**, 269–296. [357]

Abels, H., 1906. Über Nachempfindung im Gebiete des kinästhetischen und statischen Sinnes; ein Beitrag zur Lehre von Bewegungsschwindel (Drehschwindel). *Z. Psychol. Physiol. Sinnesorg.*, **43**, 268–289, 374–422. [127]

Adams, H. F., 1912. The autokinetic sensations. *Psychol. Rev. Monogr., Suppl.*, **14**, No. 2, 1–45. [25, 27, 30]

Adrian, E. D., Cattell, McK., and Hoagland, H., 1931. Sensory discharges in single cutaneous nerve fibres. *J. Physiol.*, **72**, 377–392. [81]

Aggazzotti, A., 1911. Sul più piccolo intervallo di tempo percettibile nei processi psichici. *Arch. Fisiol.*, **9**, 523–574. [158]

Akishige, Y., 1951. Experimental researches on the structure of the perceptual space. *Bull. Fac. Lit., Kyushu Univ.* [281, 288]

Alexander, S. J., Cotzin, M., Hill, C. J., Ricciuti, E. A., and Wendt, G. R., 1945. Wesleyan University studies of motion sickness: I. The effects of variation of time intervals between accelerations upon sickness rates. *J. Psychol.*, **19**, 49–62. [135]

Allen, M. J., 1954. Dependence of cyclophoria on convergence elevation and the system of axes. *Amer. J. Optom.*, **31**, 297–307. [45]

Allers, R., and Schmiedek, O., 1925. Über die Wahrnehmung der Schallrichtung. *Psychol. Forsch.*, **6**, 92–112. [360]

Alpern, M., 1957. The position of the eyes during prism vergence. *Arch. Ophthal., N.Y.*, **57**, 345–353. [64]

Anderson, D. C., and Moss, C. A., 1964. The auditory autokinetic effect. *Amer. J. Psychol.*, **77**, 502. [30]

Anderson, H. C., Jepson, O., and Kristiansen, F., 1956. The occurrence of directional preponderance in some intracranial disorders: A study of the Fitzgerald–Hallpike caloric test. *Acta oto-laryng., Stockh., Suppl.*, **118**, 19–31. [120]

Anderson, I., 1946. The effect of letter-position on range of apprehension scores, with special reference to reading disability. *Univ. Mich. Sch. Educ. Bull.*, **18**, 37–40. [302, 310]

Anderson, I., and Crosland, H. R., 1933. A method of measuring the effect of primacy of report in the range of attention experiment. *Amer. J. Psychol.*, **45**, 701–713. [303]

Andrew, B. L., 1954. The sensory innervation of the medial ligament of the knee joint. *J. Physiol.*, **123**, 241–250. [81]

Andrew, B. L., and Dodt, E., 1953. The development of sensory nerve endings at the knee joint of the cat. *Acta physiol. scand.*, **28**, 287–297. [81]

Angell, J. R., and Fite, W., 1901. The monaural localization of sound. *Psychol. Rev.*, **8**, 225–246. [158]

Angier, R. P., 1905. Die Schätzung von Bewegungsgrössen bei Vorderarmbewegungen. *Z. Psychol. Physiol. Sinnesorg.*, **39**, 429–448. [88, 93]

Angyal, A., 1930. Über die Raumlage vorgestellter Örter. *Arch. ges. Psychol.*, **78**, 47–94. [262]

Antonovsky, H. F., and Ghent, L., 1964. Cross-cultural consistency of children's preferences for the orientation of figures. *Amer. J. Psychol.*, **77**, 295–297. [297]

Ardigo, 1886. Cited in Giannitrapani, 1958. [407]

Arndts, F., 1924. Zur Frage nach der Lagewahrnehmung dienenden Sinnesfunctionen. *Pflüg. Arch. ges. Physiol.*, **204**, 539–540. [247]

Arnheim, R., 1954. *Art and Visual Perception*. Faber and Faber, London. [297]

Arnoult, M. D., 1950. Post-rotatory localization of sound. *Amer. J. Psychol.*, **63**, 229–236. [160]

Arnoult, M. D., 1952. Localization of sound during rotation of the visual environment. *Amer. J. Psychol.*, **65**, 48–58. [161]

Arnoult, M. D., 1954. Shape discrimination as a function of the angular orientation of the stimuli. *J. exp. Psychol.*, **47**, 323–328. [318]

Arslan, M., 1955. On the renewing of the methodology for the stimulation of the vestibular apparatus. *Acta oto-laryng.*, Stockh., Suppl. **122**. [115]

Asch, S. E., and Witkin, H. A., 1948a. Studies in space orientation: I. Perception of the upright with displaced visual fields. *J. exp. Psychol.*, **38**, 325–337. [203]

Asch, S. E., and Witkin, H. A., 1948b. Studies in space orientation: II. Perception of the upright with displaced visual fields and with body tilted. *J. exp. Psychol.*, **38**, 455–477. [203, 204]

Aschan, G., 1956. Nystagmography. Recording of nystagmus in clinical neuro-otological examinations. *Acta oto-laryng.*, Stockh., Suppl., **129**. [115]

Ashby, W. R., 1957. *An Introduction to Cybernetics*. Chapman and Hall, London. [372]

Aub, J., and Knapp, F., 1870. Finden Raddrehungen der Augen bei Seitwärtsneigungen des Kopfes statt. *Knapps Arch. Augen-Ohrenheilk.*, **1**, 232. [50]

Aubert, H., 1861. Eine scheinbare bedeutende Drehung von Objekten bei Neigung des Kopfes nach rechts oder links. *Virchows Arch.*, **20**, 381–393. [189, 194]

Aubert, H., 1887. Die Bewegungsempfindungen. *Pflüg. Arch. ges. Physiol.*, **40**, 459–480. [25]

Ayres, J. J., and Harcum, E. R., 1962. Directional response-bias in reproducing brief visual patterns. *Percept. mot. Skills*, **14**, 155–165. [309, 310]

Babcock, H. L., 1917. Some observations on the Bárány tests as applied to aviators. *Boston med. surg. J.*, **177**, 840–843. [127]

Bach, L., 1894. Über künstlich erzeugten Nystagmus bei normalen Individuen und bei Taubstummen. *Arch. Augenheilk.*, **30**, 10–14. [131]

Bahrick, H. P., Bennett, W. F., and Fitts, P. M., 1955. Accuracy of positioning responses as a function of spring loading in a control. *J. exp. Psychol.*, **49**, 437–444. [90]

Bahrick, H. P., Fitts, P. M., and Schneider, R., 1955. Reproduction of simple movements as a function of factors influencing proprioceptive feedback. *J. exp. Psychol.*, **49**, 445–454. [90]

Bailey, N. J., 1958. Locating the centre of visual direction by a binocular diplopia method. *Amer. J. Optom.*, **35**, 484–495. [277]

Bailey, N. J., 1959. Determination of the location of the centre, or centres of projection in anomalous correspondence. *Diss. Abstr.*, **20**. [277]

Bakay, E., and Schiller, P. H., 1948. Manipulative correction of visually presented figures. *Amer. J. Psychol.*, **61**, 487–501. [301]

Ballinger, E. R., 1952. Human experiments in subgravity and prolonged acceleration. *J. Aviat. Med.*, **23**, 319–321. [422]

Banister, H., 1925. The effect of binaural phase differences on the localization of tones at various frequencies. *Brit. J. Psychol.*, **15**, 280–307. [155]

Bárány, R., 1906a. Über die vom Ohrlabyrinth ausgelöste Gegenröllung der Augen bei Normalhörenden, Ohrenkranken und Taubstummen. *Arch. Ohrenheilk.*, **68**, 1–30. [127]

Bárány, R., 1906b. Untersuchungen über den vom Vestibularapparat des Ohres reflektorisch ausgelösten rhythmischen Nystagmus und seine Begleiterscheinungen. *Mschr. Ohrenheilk.*, **40**, 193–297. [127]

Bárány, R., 1906c. Beitrag zur Lehre von den Funktionen der Bogengänge. *Mschr. Ohrenheilk.*, **40**, 358–360. [115]

Bárány, R., 1907a. New methods of examination of the semi-circular canals and their practical significance. *Ann. Otol., etc.*, St Louis, **16**, 755–861. [112, 127, 131]

Bárány, R., 1907b. Weitere Untersuchungen über den vom Vestibularapparat des Ohres reflektorisch ausgelösten rhythmischen Nystagmus und seine Begleiterscheinungen. *Mschr. Ohrenheilk.*, **41**, 477–526. [61, 112, 124, 127]

Bárány, R., 1908. Die Untersuchungen der optischen und vestibulären reflektorischen Augenbewegungen in einem Falle von einseitiger Blicklähmung. *Mschr. Ohrenheilk.*, **42**, 109–113. [56]

Bárány, R., 1921. Zur Klinik und Theorie des Eisenbahn—Nystagmus. *Arch. Augenheilk.*, **87**, 139–142. [56, 59, 60, 196]

Bárány, R., 1922. Zur Klinik und Theorie des Eisenbahn—Nystagmus. *Acta otolaryng.*, Stockh., **2**, 260–265. [56]

Barker, D., 1948. The innervation of the muscle spindle. *Quart. J. micr. Sci.*, **89**, 143–186. [72, 74, 77]

Barker, D. (Ed.), 1962a. *Symp. Muscle Receptors.* Hong Kong Univ. Press, Hong Kong. [72, 73]

Barker, D., 1962b. Receptors in mammalian skeletal muscle. *Proc. Symp. Effect of Use and Disuse on Neuromuscular Functions, Liblice, Prague.* [77]

Barker, D., and Gidumal, J. L., 1960. Some observations on the morphology of the intrafusal muscle fibre. *J. Physiol.*, **153**, 28–29. [77]

Barker, D., and Ip, M. C., 1961. A study of single and tandem types of muscle-spindle in the cat. *Proc. roy. Soc., Ser. B*, **154**, 377–397. [73]

Barlow, H. B., 1963. Slippage of contact lenses and other artefacts in relation to fading and regeneration of supposedly stable retinal images. *Quart. J. exp. Psychol.*, **15**, 36–51. [47]

Barlow, H. B., and Levick, W. R., 1963. Are bipolar cells directionally selective? *J. Physiol.*, **170**, 53–54P. [15]

Barnes, R. M., 1949. *Motion and Time Study* 3rd ed. Wiley, New York. [382]

Bartels, M., 1920. Aufgaben der vergleichenden Physiologie der Augenbewegungen. *v. Graefes Arch. Ophthal.*, **101**, 299–331. [59]

Bartels, M., 1941. Reflexe, supranucleare Bahnen und Zentren des Augenmuskeltonus, insbesondere des Bergarbeiter—Nystagmus. *v. Graefes Arch. Ophthal.*, **144**, 1–24. [61]

Bartlett, F. C., and Mark, H., 1922. A note on local fatigue in the auditory system. *Brit. J. Psychol.*, **13**, 215–218. [162]

Bartlett, M. R., 1936. Suggestibility in psychopathic individuals: A study with psychoneurotic and dementia praecox subjects. *J. gen. Psychol.*, **14**, 241–251. [254]

Bartlett, M. R., 1944. Suggestibility in dementia praecox paranoid patients. *J. gen. Psychol.*, **30**, 97–102. [254]

Bartley, S. H., 1958. *Principles of Perception.* Harper, New York. [200]

Baruk, H., Leroy, B., Launay, J., and Vallancien, B., 1953. Les étapes du développement psychomoteur et de la préhension volontaire chez le nourrisson. *Arch. franç. Pédiat.*, **10**, 425–432. [359]

Battersby, W. S., Kahn, R. L., Pollack, M., and Bender, M. B., 1956. Effects of visual, vestibular, and somatosensori-motor deficit on autokinetic perception. *J. exp. Psychol.*, **52**, 398–410. [27]

Battig, W. F., 1954. The effect of kinaesthetic, verbal, and visual cues on the acquisition of a lever-positioning skill. *J. exp. Psychol.*, **47**, 371–380. [365]

Bauermeister, M., 1964. Effect of body tilt on apparent verticality, apparent body position, and their relation. *J. exp. Psychol.*, **67**, 142–147. [191, 194]

Bauermeister, M., Werner, H., and Wapner, S., 1964. The effect of body tilt on tactual-kinesthetic perception of verticality. *Amer. J. Psychol.*, **77**, 451–456. [192, 193]

Baumgarten, F., 1927. Die Orientierungstäuschungen. *Z. Psychol. Physiol. Sinnesorg.*, **103**, 111–122. [263]

Beckh, H. J. A. von, 1954. Experiments with animals and human subjects under sub- and zero-gravity conditions during the dive and parabolic flight. *J. Aviat. Med.*, **25**, 235–241. [441]

Beckh, H. J. A. von, 1959. Human reactions during flight to acceleration preceded by or followed by weightlessness. *Aerosp. Med.*, **30**, 391–409. [424]

Beckh, H. J. A. von, 1963. A summary of motion sickness experiences in weightless flights conducted by the aeromedical field laboratory. In Loftus, J. P., *Symp. Motion Sickness*, p. 67–72. [424]

Beeley, A. L., 1918. An experimental study in left-handedness. *Suppl. Educ. Monogr.*, **2**, 1–69. [347]

Beevor, C., 1903 (reprinted 1950). *The Croonian Lectures on Muscular Movement.* (Delivered to Roy. Coll. Physicians, London.) Macmillan, London. [255]

Begbie, G. H., 1959. Accuracy of aiming in linear hand-movements. *Quart. J. exp. Psychol.*, **11**, 65–75. [87]

Békésy, G. von, 1930. Zur Theorie des Hörens: Über das Richtungshören bei einer Zeitdifferenz oder Lautstarken-Ungleichheit der beidseitigen Schalleinwirkung. *Z. Phys.*, **31**, 824–835, 857–868. [172]

Békésy, G. von, 1953. Shearing microphonics produced by vibrations near the inner and outer hair cells. *J. acoust. Soc. Amer.*, **25**, 786–790. [109]

Békésy, G. von, 1960. *Experiments on Hearing.* McGraw-Hill, New York. [174]

Bell, C., 1826. On the nervous circle which connects the voluntary muscles with the brain. *Phil. Trans.*, **116**, 163–173. [72]

Beller, H. K., and Morant, R. B., 1963. Adaptation to prismatically rotated visual fields. Typescript from authors. [217]

Belzile, M., and Markle, D. M., 1959. A clinical comparison of monaural and binaural hearing aids worn by patients with conductive or perceptive deafness. *Laryngoscope, St Louis*, **69**, 1317–1323. [170]

Bender, M. B., 1945. Polyopia and monocular diplopia of cerebral origin. *Arch. Neurol. Psychiat., Chicago*, **54**, 323–338. [23]

Bender, M. B., 1952. *Disorders in Perception; With Particular Reference to the Phenomena of Extinction and Displacement.* Thomas, Springfield, Ill. [291]

Bender, M. B., 1955. The eye-centering system. *Arch. Neurol. Psychiat., Chicago.* **73**, 685–699. [61]

Bender, M. B. (Ed.), 1964. *The Oculomotor System.* Harper and Row, New York. [43, 62, 65]

Bender, M. B., and Jung, R., 1948. Abweichungen der subjektiven optischen Vertikalen und Horizontalen bei Gesunden und Hirnverletzten. *Arch. Psychiat. Nervenkr.*, **181**, 193–212. [211]

Bender, M. B., and O'Brien, 1946. Cited in Bender, 1955. [62]

Bender, M. B., Shapiro, M. F., and Teuber, H. L., 1949. Allesthesia and disturbances of the body scheme. *Arch. Neurol. Psychiat., Chicago*, **62**, 222–235. [293]

Bender, M. B., Teng, P., and Weinstein, E. A., 1954. Centering of eyes: a patterned eye movement. *Arch. Neurol. Psychiat., Chicago*, **72**, 282–295. [62]

Bender, M. B., and Teuber, H. L., 1946. Nystagmoid movements and visual perception: their interrelation in monocular diplopia. *Arch. Neurol. Psychiat., Chicago*, **55**, 511–529. [23]

Bender, M. B., and Teuber, H. L., 1947. Spatial organisation of visual perception following injury to the brain. *Arch. Neurol. Psychiat., Chicago*, **58**, 721–739. [40]

Bender, M. B., and Teuber, H. L., 1948. Spatial organisation of visual perception following injury to the brain. *Arch. Neurol. Psychiat., Chicago*, **59**, 39–62. [40, 332]

Bender, M. B., and Teuber, H. L., 1949. Disturbances in visual perception following cerebral lesions. *J. Psychol.*, **28**, 223–233. [40]

Benson, A. J., 1964. Comparison of post-rotatory sensation and nystagmus. Paper read to Exp. Psychol. Soc., London. [114, 129]

Bentley, M., and Dunlap, K., 1918. *Manual Med. Res. Lab.* p. 96–132, 163–199. [128]

Benton, A. L., 1955. Right–left discrimination and finger localization in defective children. *Arch. Neurol. Psychiat., Chicago*, **74**, 583–589. [292]

Benton, A. L., and Abramson, L. S., 1952. Gerstmann symptoms following electro-shock treatment. *Arch. Neurol. Psychiat., Chicago*, **68**, 248–257. [292]

Benton, A. L., Hutcheon, J. F., and Seymour, E., 1951. Arithmetic ability, finger-localization capacity and right–left discrimination in normal and defective children. *Amer. J. Orthopsychiat.*, **21**, 756–766. [292]

Bergstedt, M., 1961a. The effect of gravitational force on the vestibular caloric test. *Acta oto-laryng., Stockh.*, **53**, 551–562. [115]

Bergstedt, M., 1961b. Studies of positional nystagmus in the human centrifuge. *Acta oto-laryng., Stockh., Suppl.*, **165**. [121]

Bernadin, A. C., and Gruber, H. E., 1957. An auditory autokinetic effect. *Amer. J. Psychol.*, **70**, 133–134. [30, 162]

Berry, C. M., Karl, R. C., and Hinsey, J. C., 1950. Course of spinothalamic and medial lemniscus pathways in cat and rhesus monkey. *J. Neurophysiol.*, **13**, 149–156. [82]

Bessou, P., and Laporte, Y., 1962. Responses from primary and secondary endings of the same neuromuscular spindle of the tenuissimus muscle of the cat. In Barker, D. (Ed.), *Symp. Muscle Receptors*. Hong Kong Univ. Press, Hong Kong. [74]

Bianconi, R., and van der Meulen, J. P., 1963. The response to vibration of the end organs of mammalian muscle spindles. *J. Neurophysiol.*, **26**, 177–190. [74]

Biehler, W., 1896. Bieträge zur Lehre vom Augenmass für Winkel. *Diss.*, Freiburg (cited in Helmholtz, 1962, Vol. III, p. 234). [39]

Bielschowsky, A., 1898. Über monokulare Diplopia ohne physikalische Grundlage nebst Bemerkungen über das Sehen Schielender. *v. Graefes. Arch. Ophthal.*, **46**, 143–148. [21]

Bielschowsky, A., 1931. Der Sehakt bei Strungen im Bewegungsapparat der Augen. In Bethe, A., *Handbuch der Normalen und Pathologischen Physiologie* Vol. 12. Springer, Berlin. p. 1095–1112. [21]

Bilodeau, E. A., 1951. Modification of direction of movement preference with independent variation of two stimulus dimensions. Human Resources Res. Center. *Res. Bull.*, No. 51–12. [364]

Binet, M. A., 1894. Reverse illusions of orientation. *Psychol. Rev.*, **1**, 337–350. [263]

Birch, H. G., Belmont, I., Reilly, T., and Belmont, L., 1961. Visual verticality in hemiplegia. *Arch. Neurol., Chicago*, **5**, 444–453. [212]

Birch, H. G., Belmont, I., Reilly, T., and Belmont, L., 1962. Somesthetic influences on perception of visual verticality in hemiplegia. *Arch. phys. Med. Rehab.*, **43**, 556–560. [212]

Birch, H. G., Proctor, F., Bortner, M., and Lowenthal, M., 1960. Perception in hemiplegia: II. judgment of the median plane. *Arch. phys. Med. Rehab.*, **41**, 71–75. [289]

Birren, J. E., 1945. Static equilibrium and vestibular function. *J. exp. Psychol.*, **35**, 127–133. [254, 255]

Bishop, H. E., 1959. Innateness and learning in the visual perception of direction. *Ph.D. Diss.*, Univ. Chicago. [369]

Bitterman, M. E., and Worchel, P., 1953. The phenomenal vertical and horizontal in blind and sighted subjects. *Amer. J. Psychol.*, **66**, 598–602. [192, 208]

Blodgett, H. C., Wilbanks, W. A., and Jeffress, L. A., 1956. Effect of large interaural time differences upon the judgment of sidedness. *J. acoust. Soc. Amer.*, **28**, 639–643. [158, 168]

Blodi, F. C., and Van Allen, M. W., 1957. Electromyography of extraocular muscles in fusional movement: I. Electric phenomena at the breakpoint of fusion. *Amer. J. Ophthal.*, **44**, 136–144. [65]

Blomberg, L. H., 1960. The optokinetic fusion limit. *Acta oto-laryng., Stockh.*, **51**, 455–466. [57, 58]

Blumenthal, A., 1928. Über den Einfluss der Kopfhaltung auf die Gehrichtung. *Beitr. Anat. etc., Ohr.*, **26**, 390–422. [257]

Boeder, P., 1944. Image formation in the eye. *Amer. opt. Co.*, **28**, No. 1. [34]

Boenninghaus, G., 1926. Über das Versagen der labyrinthogenen statischen Kompensation im Affekt. *Mschr. Ohrenheilk.*, **60**, 1139–1144. [134]

Bonin, G. von, 1950. *Essay on the Cerebral Cortex.* Thomas, Springfield, Ill. [381]

Boring, E. G., 1926. Auditory theory with special reference to intensity, volume and localization. *Amer. J. Psychol.*, **37**, 157–188. [154, 169]

Boring, E. G., 1942. *Sensation and Perception in the History of Experimental Psychology.* Appleton-Century-Crofts, New York. [174]

Boring, R. O., 1952. The effect of visual stimulus variables upon the perception of the visual vertical. Proj. No. NM.001.063.01.28. U.S. Nav. Sch. aviat. Med., Pensacola, Fla. [204]

Bossom, J., and Hamilton, C. R., 1963. Interocular transfer of prism-altered co-ordinations in split-brain monkeys. *J. comp. physiol. Psychol.*, **56**, 769–774. [368, 378]

Bossom, J., and Held, R., 1957. Shifts in egocentric localization following prolonged displacement of the retinal image. Paper read to Amer. Psychol. Ass., New York. [285, 393]

Bourdon, B., 1902. *La Perception Visuelle de l'Espace.* Schleicher, Paris. [26]

Bourdon, B., 1904. La perception de la verticalité de la tête et du corps. *Rev. philo-math.*, **57**, 462–492. [247]

Bourdon, B., 1906a. Sur le rôle de la tête dans la perception de l'espace. *Rev. Philos.*, **61**, 526–529. [191]

Bourdon, B., 1906b. Influence de la force centrifuge sur la perception de la verticale. *Année psychol.*, **12**, 84–94. [198]

Bourdon, B., 1914. Recherches sur las perception des movements rectilignes de tout le corps. *Année psychol.*, **20**, 1–16. [117]

Bourdon, B., 1925. Quelques expériences sur des perceptions spatiales auditives. *Année psychol.*, **26**, 72–78. [162]

Bowditch, H. P., and Southard, W. F., 1880. A comparison of sight and touch. *J. Physiol.*, **3**, 232–245. [349]

Boyd, I. A., 1962. The structure and innervation of the nuclear bag muscle fibre system and the nuclear chain muscle fibre system in mammalian muscle spindles. *Phil. Trans., Ser. B.*, **245**, 81–136. [72]

Boyd, I. A., and Davey, M. R., 1962. The groups of origin in the nerves to skeletal muscle of the γ_1 and γ_2 fusimotor fibres present close to, and within mammalian muscle spindles. In Barker, D. (Ed.), *Symp. Muscle Receptors*. Hong Kong Univ. Press, Hong Kong. [77]

Boyd, I. A., and Roberts, T. D. M., 1953. Proprioceptive discharges from the stretch receptors in the knee-joint of the cat. *J. Physiol.*, **122**, 38–58. [81]

Bradley, J. V., 1957. Direction-of-knob-turn stereotypes. WADC Tech. Rep. 57–388. Wright-Patterson AFB, Ohio. [364]

Brain, W. R., 1941a. Visual object-agnosia with special reference to the Gestalt theory. *Brain*, **64**, 43–62. [40]

Brain, W. R., 1941b. Visual disorientation with special reference to lesions of the right cerebral hemisphere. *Brain*, **64**, 244–272. [268, 291]

Brain, W. R., 1952. The neurology of John Hunter's last illness. *Brit. med. J.*, **2**, 1371–1373. [212]

Brandt, H. F., 1940. Ocular patterns and their psychological implications. *Amer. J. Psychol.*, **53**, 260–268. [26]

Brandt, U., 1962. The cause and practical importance of oculogravic illusions. *Acta oto-laryng., Stockh.*, **54**, 127–135. [198]

Braune, W., and Fischer, O., 1885–1904. Various papers in *Abh. sächs. Ges. (Akad.) Wiss.* Reviewed in Fearing, 1924. [253]

Braune, W., and Fischer, O., 1889. Über den Schwerpunkt des menschlichen Körpers mit Rücksicht auf die Ausrüstung des deutschen Infanteristen. *Abh. sächs. Ges. (Akad.) Wiss.*, **15**, 561. [428]

Braune, W., and Fischer, O., 1892. Bestimmung der Trägheitsmomente des menschlichen Körpers und seiner Gleider. *Abh. sächs. Ges. (Akad.) Wiss.*, **18**, 409. [428]

Braune, W., and Fischer, O., 1963. Center of gravity of the human body. In *Human Mechanics.* AMRL-TDR-63-123. Wright-Patterson AFB, Ohio. [428]

Brecher, G. A., 1934. Die optokinetische Auslösung von Augenrollung und rotatorischem Nystagmus. *Pflüg. Arch. ges. Physiol.*, **234**, 13–28. [51, 56, 229]

Breinin, G. M., 1955. The nature of vergence revealed by electromyography. *Arch. Ophthal., N.Y.*, **54**, 407–409. [65]

Breinin, G. M., 1957. Electromyographic evidence for ocular proprioception in man. *Arch. Ophthal., N.Y.*, **57**, 176–180. [78]

Bremer, F., 1952. Les aires auditives de l'écorce cérébrate. In *La Surdité: sa misure et sa correction.* Maloine, Paris. [171]

Bremer, F., and Dow, R. S., 1939. The acoustic area of the cerebral cortex in the cat. *J. Neurophysiol.*, **2**, 308–318. [171]

Breuer, J., 1874. Über die Funktion der Bogengänge des Ohrlabyrinthes. *Wein. med. Jahrb.*, **4**, 72–124. [50, 101]

Breuer, J., 1875. Beiträge zur Lehre vom statischen Sinne. *Wien. med. Jahrb.*, **5**, 87–156. [130]

Breuer, J., and Kreidl, A., 1898. Über die scheinbare Drehung des Besichtfeldes während der Einwirkung einer Centrifugalkraft. *Pflüg. Arch. ges. Physiol.*, **70**, 494–507. [198]

Bridges, C. C., Bitterman, M. E., 1954. The measurement of autokinetic movement. *Amer. J. Psychol.*, **67**, 525–529. [25]

Brigden, R. L., 1935. The dynamics of spiral movement in man. *J. comp. Psychol.*, **20**, 59–74. [257]

Brindley, G. S., and Merton, P. A., 1960. The absence of position sense in the human eye. *J. Physiol.*, **153**, 127–130. [68]

Broadbent, D. E., 1958. *Perception and Communication*. Pergamon, London. [362]

Brogden, W. J., 1953. The trigonometric relationship of precision and angle of linear pursuit-movement as a function of amount of practice. *Amer. J. Psychol.*, **66**, 45–56. [87]

Bromleigh, R., 1961. Effect of letter-symmetry on distribution of errors in tachisto-scopic letter-targets. Paper read to Virginia Acad. Sci., Lexington. [308]

Brookhart, J. M., 1960. The cerebellum. In *Handbook of Physiology* Sec. 1, Vol. II. Amer. Physiol. Soc., Washington. [241]

Brown, D. R., Hitchcock, L., and Michels, K. M., 1962. Quantitative studies in form perception: an evaluation of the role of selected stimulus parameters in the visual discrimination performance of human subjects. *Percept. mot. Skills*, **14**, 519–529. [317]

Brown, J. L., 1961. Orientation to the vertical during water immersion. *Aerosp. Med.*, **32**, 209–217. [117]

Brown, J. S., Knauft, E. B., and Rosenbaum, G., 1948. The accuracy of positioning reactions as a function of their direction and extent. *Amer. J. Psychol.*, **61**, 167–182. [88]

Brown, J. S., and Slater-Hammel, A. T., 1949. Discrete movements in the horizontal plane as a function of their length and direction. *J. exp. Psychol.*, **39**, 84–95. [87]

Brown, K. T., 1953. Factors affecting differences in apparent size between opposite halves of a visual meridian. *J. opt. Soc. Amer.*, **43**, 464–472. [38]

Brown, K. T., 1955. An experiment demonstrating instability of retinal directional values. *J. opt. Soc. Amer.*, **45**, 301–307. [38]

Brown, R. H., and Guedry, F. E., 1951. Influence of visual stimulation on habituation to rotation. *J. gen. Psychol.*, **45**, 151–161. [129]

Brown, T. G., 1922. Reflex orientation of the optic axes and the influence upon it of the cerebral cortex. *Arch. néerl. Physiol.*, **7**, 571–578. [61]

Brown, W. R. J., 1949. Eye movements and the variation of visual acuity with test object orientation. *J. opt. Soc. Amer.*, **39**, A1057. [32]

Browne, K., Lee, J., and Ring, P. A., 1954. The sensation of passive movement at the metatarso-phalangeal joint of the great toe in man. *J. Physiol.*, **126**, 448–458. [93]

Bruell, J. H., 1958. Retinal local signs in homonymous hemianopsia, strabismus, and normal vision. *Amer. J. Ophthal.*, **45**, 662–666. [24]

Bruell, J. H., and Albee, G. W., 1955a. Effect of asymmetrical retinal stimulation on the perception of the median plane. *Percept. mot. Skills*, **5**, 133–139. [188, 281, 282]

Bruell, J. H., and Albee, G. W., 1955b. Notes towards a motor theory of visual egocentric localization. *Psychol. Rev.*, **62**, 391–399. [282, 284]

Bruell, J. H., and Peszczynski, M., 1958. Perception of verticality in hemiplegic patients in relation to rehabilitation. *Clin. Orthopaedics*, **12**, 124–130. [212]

Brunner, H., 1922. Zur klinischen Bedeutung des optischen Drehnystagmus. *Klin. Mbl. Augenheilk.*, **68**, 783–785. [60]

Bryden, M. P., 1960. Tachistoscopic recognition of non-alphabetical material. *Canad. J. Psychol.*, **14**, 78–86. [308]

Bryden, M. P., 1961. The role of post-exposural eye movements in tachistoscopic perception. *Canad. J. Psychol.*, **15**, 220–225. [312]

Bryden, M. P., 1964. Tachistoscopic recognition and cerebral dominance. *Percept. mot. Skills*, **19**, 686. [305]

Budkiewicz, J., 1926. Étude experimentale sur les processus de mesure spatiale linéaire. *Année psychol.*, **27**, 94–173. [357]

Bühler, K., 1913. *Die Gestaltwahrnehmungen*. Spemann, Stuttgart. [314]

Burckhardt, H., 1925. Veränderungen der Raumlage in Kinderzeichnungen. *Z. pädag. Psychol.*, **26**, 352–371. [341]

Burckhardt, H., 1933. Über Verlagerung räumlicher Gestalten. *N. psychol. Stud.*, **7**, 158. [332]

Burke, R. S., and Dallenbach, K. M., 1924. Position vs. intensity as a determinant of attention of left-handed observers. *Amer. J. Psychol.*, **35**, 267–269. [305]

Burow, A., 1841. Beiträge zur Physiologie und Physik des menschlichen Auges. Cited in Nagel, 1896. [50]

Burt, C., 1921. *Mental and Scholastic Tests*. King, London, p. 312. [347]

Burtt, H. E., 1917. Auditory illusions of movement: a preliminary study. *J. exp. Psychol.*, **2**, 63–75. [162]

Burtt, H. E., 1918. The perception of slight changes of equilibrium with especial reference to problems of aviation. *J. appl. Psychol.*, **2**, 101–115. [244]

Buys, E., 1924. Contribution à l'étude du nystagmus oculaire de la rotation chez l'homme. *Rev. Oto-Neuro-Ocul.*, **2**, 641–659, 721–749. [121]

Buys, E., 1937. Interrogatoire de l'appareil semicirculaire par déclanchment d'un nystagmus post-rotatoire 'primaire' au moyen du fauteuil Buys-Rijlant. *Valsalva*, **13**, 139–144. [112, 116]

Buys, E., and Rijlant, P., 1939. Le seuil d'excitation (accélération angulaire) des canaux semi-circulaires. *Arch. int. Physiol.*, **49**, 101–112. [116]

Buzzard, E. F., 1908. A note on the occurrence of muscle-spindles in ocular muscles. *Proc. R. Soc. Med. neurol. Sect.*, **1**, 83–88. [67]

Camis, M., 1930. *The Physiology of the Vestibular Apparatus*. Clarendon Press, Oxford. [138]

Camp, D., 1960. Attensity gradients in the perception of binary patterns. *Virginia J. Sci.*, **11**, 217–218. [310]

Camp, D. S., 1961. The effect of simultaneous vs. successive presentation on hemifield differences within the perceptual span. Paper read to Virginia Acad. Sci., Lexington. [310]

Cantrell, R. P., 1963. Body balance activity and perception. *Percept. mot. Skills*, **17**, 431–437. [254]

Carmichael, E. A., Dix, M. R., and Hallpike, C. S., 1954. Lesions of the cerebral hemispheres and their effect upon optokinetic and caloric nystagmus. *Brain*, **77**, 345–372. [62]

Carmichael, L., and Cashman, H., 1932. A study of mirror-writing in relation to handedness and perceptual and motor habits. *J. gen. Psychol.*, **6**, 296–329. [347]

Carpenter, M. B., Bard, D. S., and Alling, F. A., 1959. Anatomical connections between the fastigial nuclei, the labyrinth and the vestibular nuclei in the cat. *J. comp. Neurol.*, **111**, 1–25. [130]

Carpenter, M. S., 1962. Pilot's flight report. In *Results of the Second U.S. Manned Orbital Space Flight*. Manned Spacecraft Center, Nat. Aeronaut. and Space Admin. U.S. Govt. Printing Office, Washington, D.C. [423, 432]

Carr, H. A., 1910. The autokinetic sensation. *Psychol. Rev.*, **17**, 42–75. [25, 26, 27, 187]

Carr, H. A., 1935. *An Introduction to Space Perception*. Longmans, Green, New York. [15, 407]

Carterette, E. C., Friedman, M. P., Lindner, W., and Pierce, J., 1964. Lateralization of sounds at the unstimulated ear opposite to a noise-adapted ear. Tech. Rep. No. 24, Human Communication Lab., Dept. of Psychol. Univ., California, Los Angeles. [162]

Cass, E. E., 1941. Monocular diplopia occurring in cases of squint. *Brit. J. Ophthal.*, **25**, 565–577. [21]

Cattell, J. McK., 1895. The sense of equilibrium. *Science*, **2**, 99–100. [247]

Cawthorne, T., 1946. Vestibular injuries, *Proc. R. Soc. Med.*, **39**, 270–273. [134]

Cawthorne, T., Dix, M. R., Hallpike, C. S., and Hood, J. D., 1956. Vestibular function. *Brit. med. Bull.*, **12**, 131–142. [114]

Cawthorne, T., Fitzgerald, G., and Hallpike, C. S., 1942. Studies in human vestibular function: II. Observations on the directional preponderance of caloric nystagmus ('Nystagmus Bereitschaft') resulting from unilateral labyrinthectomy. *Brain*, **65**, 138–180. [118]

Chandler, K. A., 1953. The effect of moving and non-moving visual stimuli upon head torsion. *Ph.D. Diss.*, Clark Univ. [288]

Chandler, K. A., 1961. The effect of monaural and binaural tones of different intensities on the visual perception of verticality. *Amer. J. Psychol.*, **74**, 260–265. [195]

Charnwood, Lord, 1949. Some factors affecting physiological diplopia. *Optician*, January 6. [278]

Charnwood, Lord, 1950. Effect of posture on involuntary eye movements. *Nature, Lond.*, **166**, 348–349. [36]

Charpentier, A., 1886. Sur une illusion visuelle. *C.R. Acad. Sci., Paris*, **102**, 1155–1157. [25]

Chernikoff, R., and Taylor, F. V., 1952. Kinesthetic reaction time. *J. exp. Psychol.*, **45**, 1–8. [96]

Cherry, E. C., 1953. Some experiments on the recognition of speech, with one and with two ears. *J. acoust. Soc. Amer.*, **25**, 975–979. [170]

Cherry, E. C., 1961. Electro-acoustics for human listeners. *J. Brit. Instn. Radio Engrs.*, **21**, 5–15. [170]

Cherry, E. C., and Bowles, J. A., 1960. Contribution to a study of the 'cocktail party problem'. *J. acoust. Soc. Amer.*, **32**, 884. [169]

Cherry, E. C., and Sayers, B. Mc.A., 1956. 'Human cross correlator'—A technique for measuring certain parameters of speech perception. *J. acoust. Soc. Amer.*, **28**, 889–895. [170]

Cherry, E. C., and Sayers, B. Mc.A., 1959. On the mechanism of binaural fusion. *J. acoust. Soc. Amer.*, **31**, 535. [170]

Cherry, E. C., and Taylor, W. K., 1954. Some further experiments upon the recognition of speech with one and with two ears. *J. acoust Soc. Amer.*, **26**, 554–559. [158, 170]

Chinn, H. I., and Smith, P. K., 1955. Motion sickness. *Pharmacol. Rev.*, **7**, 33–82. [135]

Chou, S. K., 1935. Reading and legibility of Chinese characters: IV. An analysis of judgments of positions of Chinese characters by American subjects. *J. exp., Psychol.*, **18**, 318–347. [297]

Christian, P., 1939. Über unbewusste Vestibulariswirkung. *Z. ges. Neurol. Psychiat.*, **165**, 214–219. [116, 288]

Christian, P., 1940. Experimentelle Beiträge zur intermodalen vestibulo-optischen Wechselbeziehung der Sinnesorgane. *Pflüg. Arch. ges. Physiol.*, **243**, 370–387. [116]

Christiansen, J. A., 1964. On hyaluronate molecules in the labyrinth as mechano-electrical transducers, and as molecular motors acting as resonators. *Acta oto-laryng., Stockh.*, **57**, 33–49. [106]

Christman, E. H., and Kupfer, C., 1963. Proprioception in extraocular muscles. *Arch. Ophthal., N.Y.*, **69**, 824–829. [67]

Christman, R. J., and Victor, G., 1955. Reported in Whitworth and Jeffress, 1961. [165]

Claparède, E., 1903. La faculté d'orientation lointaine (sens de direction, sens de retour). *Arch. Psychol., Genève*, **2**, 133–180. [262]

Claparède, E., 1924. Note sur la localisation du moi. *Arch. Psychol., Genève*, **19**, 172–182. [262]

Claparède, E., 1943. L'Orientation Lointaine, *Nouveau Traité de Psychologie*, VIII. 3. Presse Universitaire, Paris. [257, 262, 265].

Clark, B., and Graybiel, A., 1949. The effect of angular acceleration on sound localization: the audiogyral illusion. *J. Psychol.*, **28**, 235–244. [159]

Clark, B., and Graybiel, A., 1951. Visual perception of the horizontal following exposure to radial acceleration on a centrifuge. *J. comp. physiol. Psychol.*, **44**, 525–534. [198]

Clark, B., and Graybiel, A., 1961. Human performance during adaptation to stress in the Pensacola slow rotation room. *Aerosp. Med.*, **32**, 93–106. [136]

Clark, B., and Graybiel, A., 1962. Visual perception of the horizontal during prolonged exposure to radial acceleration on a centrifuge. *J. exp. Psychol.*, **63**, 294–301. [199]

Clark, B., and Graybiel, A., 1963a. Contributing factors in the perception of the oculogravic illusion. *Amer. J. Psychol.*, **76**, 18–27. [199]

Clark, B., and Graybiel, A., 1963b. Perception of the postural vertical in normals and subjects with labyrinthine defects. *J. exp. Psychol.*, **65**, 490–494. [248, 249]

Clark, B., Graybiel, A., and MacCorquodale, K., 1948. The illusory perception of movement caused by angular acceleration and by centrifugal forces during flight: II. Visually perceived motion and displacement of a fixed target during turns. *J. exp. Psychol.*, **38**, 298. [425, 426]

Clark, B., and MacCorquodale, K., 1949. The effects of repeated rotary acceleration on the oculo-gyral illusion. *J. exp. Psychol.*, **39**, 219–227.

Clark, B., and Stewart, J. P., 1962. Perception of angular acceleration about the yaw axis of a flight simulator. *Aerosp. Med.*, **33**, 1426–1432. [116]

Clark, C. C., and Hardy, J. D., 1960. Gravity problems in manned space stations. In *Proc. Manned Space Stations Symp.*, Inst. Aeronaut. Sci., New York. [440]

Clark, W. E. Le Gros, 1932. A morphological study of the lateral geniculate body. *Brit. J. Ophthal.*, **16**, 264–284. [15]

Clegg, W. C., 1954. Non-visual perception of the postural vertical: III. diagonal planes. *Canad. J. Psychol.*, **8**, 209–213. [242, 244, 246, 247]

Clegg, W. C., and Dunfield, N. M., 1954a. Non-visual perception of the postural vertical: I. sagittal plane. *Canad. J. Psychol.*, **8**, 1–8. [242, 243, 246, 247]

Clegg, W. C., and Dunfield, N. M., 1954b. Non-visual perception of the postural vertical: II. lateral plane. *Canad. J. Psychol.*, **8**, 80–86. [242, 243, 246, 247]

Cleghorn, T. E., and Darcus, H. D., 1952. The sensibility to passive movement of the human elbow joint. *Quart. J. exp. Psychol.*, **4**, 66–77. [83]

Cogan, D. G., 1956. *Neurology of the Ocular Muscles*. Thomas, Springfield, Ill. [42, 43, 49, 62]

Cogan, D. G., and Loeb, D. R., 1949. Optokinetic responses and intracranial lesions. *Arch. Neurol. Psychiat., Chicago*, **61**, 183–187. [57]

Cohen, B., Suzuki, J. I., Shanzer, S., and Bender, M. B., 1964. Semicircular canal control of eye movements. In Bender, M. B. (Ed.), *The Oculomotor System*. Harper and Row, New York. [123]

Cohen, L. A., 1955. Activity of knee joint proprioceptors recorded from the posterior articular nerve. *Yale J. Biol. Med.*, **28**, 225–232. [81]

Cohen, L. A., 1958a. Analysis of position sense in human shoulder. *J. Neurophysiol.*, **21**, 550–562. [84]

Cohen, L. A., 1958b. Contribution of tactile-musculo-tendino and joint mechanisms to position sense in human shoulder. *J. Neurophysiol.*, **21**, 563–568. [94]

Cohen, W., and Tepas, D., 1958. Temporal factors in the perception of verticality. *Amer. J. Psychol.*, **71**, 760–763. [179, 210]

Collins, W. E., 1962. Effects of mental set upon vestibular nystagmus. *J. exp. Psychol.*, **63**, 191–197. [131]

Collins, W. E., 1963. Manipulation of arousal and its effects on human vestibular nystagmus induced by caloric irrigation and angular accelerations. *Aerosp. Med.*, **54**, 124–129. [131]

Collins, W. E., 1965. Interaction of visual and vestibular factors in the performance of figure skaters. Paper read to Psychonomics Soc., Chicago. [129, 134]

Collins, W. E., Crampton, G. H., and Posner, J. B., 1961. Effects of mental activity on vestibular nystagmus and the electroencephalogram. *Nature, Lond.*, **190**, 194–195. [131]

Collins, W. E., and Guedry, F. E., 1962. Arousal effects and nystagmus during prolonged constant angular acceleration. *Acta oto-laryng., Stockh.,* **54,** 349–362. [131]

Collins, W. E., Guedry, F. E., and Posner, J. B., 1962. Control of caloric nystagmus by manipulating arousal and visual fixation distance. *Ann. Otol., etc., St Louis,* **71,** 187–203. [131]

Collins, W. E., and Posner, J. B., 1963. Electroencephalogram alpha-activity during mild vestibular stimulation. *Nature, Lond.,* **199,** 933–934. [131]

Comalli, P. E., 1963. Body position and localization of a visual object. *Percept. mot. Skills,* **16,** 86. [187]

Comalli, P. E., Wapner, S., and Werner, H., 1959. Perception of verticality in middle and old age. *J. Psychol.,* **47,** 259–266. [191]

Conklin, J. E., 1957. The influence of figural inspection on the autokinetic illusion. *Amer. J. Psychol.,* **74,** 395–402. [29]

Connell, S., and Grether, W. F., 1948. Psychological factors in check-reading single instruments. Memorandum Rep. No. MCREXD-694-17A. U.S.A.F. Air Material Command, Dayton, Ohio. [363]

Contejean, Cn., and Delmas, A., 1894. Sur le 'mouvement de roue' du globe oculaire se produisant pendant l'inclination laterale de la tête. *Arch. Physiol.,* **6,** 687–692. [50]

Cook, T. W., 1933a. Studies in cross education: II. Further experiments in mirror tracing the star-shaped maze. *J. exp. Psychol.,* **16,** 679–700. [378]

Cook, T. W., 1933b. Studies in cross education: I. Mirror tracing the star-shaped maze. *J. exp. Psychol.,* **16,** 144–160. [378]

Cooksey, F. S., 1946. Rehabilitation in vestibular injuries. *Proc. R. Soc. Med.,* **39,** 273–278. [134]

Cooper, S., 1959. The secondary endings of muscle spindles. *J. Physiol.,* **149,** 27–28P. [74]

Cooper, S., 1961. The responses of the primary and secondary endings of muscle spindles with intact motor innervation during applied stretch. *Quart. J. exp. Physiol.,* **46,** 389–398. [74]

Cooper, S., and Daniel, P. M., 1949. Muscle spindles in human extrinsic eye muscles. *Brain,* **72,** 1–24. [67]

Cooper, S., and Daniel, P. M., 1956. Human muscle spindles. *J. Physiol.,* **133,** 1–3P. [77]

Cooper, S., Daniel, P. M., and Whitteridge, D., 1955. Muscle-spindles and other sensory endings in the extrinsic eye muscles; the physiology and anatomy of these receptors and of their connections with the brain-stem. *Brain,* **78,** 564–583. [67]

Corbin, H. H., Reese, E. P., Reese, T. W., and Volkmann, J., 1956. Experiments on visual discrimination 1952–1955. Rep. No. AF 18(600)-344. Mt. Holyoke College, Mass. [277, 278]

Cords, R., 1926a. Zur Theorie des optomotorischen Nystagmus. Eine Widerlegung Ohms. *Klin. Mbl. Augenheilk.,* **77,** 781–787. [56]

Cords, R., 1926b. Optisch-motorisches Feld und optisch-motorische Bahn. Ein Beitrag zur Physiologie und Pathologie der Rindeninnervation der Augenmuskeln. *v. Graefes Arch. Ophthal.,* **117,** 58–114. [60, 61]

Cords, R., and Nolzen, L., 1928. Weitere Untersuchungen über den optokinetischen (opto-motorischen) Nystagmus. *v. Graefes Arch. Ophthal.*, **120**, 506–525. [56]

Coriolis, G., 1846. Traité de mécanique des corps solides et du calcul de l'effect des machines. Paris. [436]

Corrigan, R. E., and Brogden, W. J., 1948. The effect of angle upon precision of linear pursuit-movements. *Amer. J. Psychol.*, **61**, 502–510. [87]

Corrigan, R. E., and Brogden, W. J., 1949. The trigonometric relationship of precision and angle of linear pursuit-movements. *Amer. J. Psychol.*, **62**, 90–98. [87]

Corso, J. F., and Soloyanis, G., 1962. Auditory stimulation and induced changes in autokinetic movement. *Proc. Penn. Acad. Sci.*, **36**, 140–144. [27]

Coyle, D., 1907. Upright vision and the inverted image. *Psychol. Bull.*, **4**, 97–99. [404]

Craig, E. A., and Lichtenstein, M., 1953. Visibility-invisibility cycles as a function of stimulus orientation. *Amer. J. Psychol.*, **66**, 554–563. [31]

Crampton, G. H., 1964. Habituation of ocular nystagmus of vestibular origin. In Bender, M. B. (Ed.), *The Oculomotor System*. Harper and Row, New York. [131]

Crampton, G. H., and Schwam, W. J., 1961. Effects of arousal reaction on nystagmus habituation in the cat. *Amer. J. Physiol.*, **200**, 29–33. [131]

Critchley, M., 1953. *The Parietal Lobes*. Arnold, London. [267, 268, 269, 270, 291, 293, 333]

Crosland, H. R., 1931. Letter-position effects, in the range of attention experiment, as affected by the number of letters in each exposure. *J. exp. Psychol.*, **14**, 477–507. [302]

Crovitz, H. F., 1962. Directional differences in autokinesis based on stimulation of the left versus the right eye. *Percept. mot. Skills*, **15**, 631–634. [27]

Crovitz, H. F., and Daves, W., 1962. Tendencies to eye movement and perceptual accuracy. *J. exp. Psychol.*, **63**, 495–498. [312]

Crum Brown, A., 1875. On the sense of rotation and the anatomy and physiology of the semicircular canals of the internal ear. *J. Anat., London*, **8**, 327–331. [101]

Crutchfield, R. S., and Edwards, W., 1949. The effect of a fixated figure on auto-kinetic movement. *J. exp. Psychol.*, **39**, 561–568. [29]

Culbert, S. S., 1954. Directional after-effects following systematic distortion of the visual field. *J. Psychol.*, **37**, 81–93. [219]

Curran, C. R., and Lane, H. L., 1962. On the relations among some factors that contribute to estimates of verticality. *J. exp. Psychol.*, **64**, 295–299. [206]

Dallenbach, K. M., 1923. Position vs. intensity as a determinant of clearness. *Amer. J. Psychol.*, **34**, 282–286. [305]

Daniel, P., 1946. Spiral nerve endings in extrinsic eye muscles of man. *J. Anat., Lond.*, **80**, 189–193. [67]

Darwin, C., 1859. *On the Origin of Species*. Univ. Penn. Press, Philadelphia. (1959 ed.). [265]

Darwin, E., 1801. *Zoonomia: on the Laws of Organic Life*. Johnson, London. [197]

David, E. E., 1959. Comment on the precedence effect. *Proc. 3rd int. Congr. Acoust.* Stuttgart, 144–146. [154]

David, E. E., 1962. Closing the binaural gap. Paper to Acoust. Soc. Amer. [154]

David, E. E., Guttman, N., and Van Bergeijk, W. A., 1958. On the mechanism of binaural fusion. *J. acoust. Soc. Amer.*, **30**, 801–802. [147]

David, E. E., Guttman, N., and Van Bergeijk, W. A., 1959. Binaural interaction of high-frequency complex stimuli. *J. acoust. Soc. Amer.*, **31**, 774–782. [155, 167, 172]

Davidson, H. P., 1934. A study of reversals in young children. *J. genet. Psychol.*, **45**, 452–465. [347]

Davidson, H. P., 1935. A study of the confusing letters, B, D, P, and Q. *J. genet. Psychol.*, **47**, 458–468. [346, 347]

Davies, A. D. M., and Leytham, G. W. H., 1964. Perception of verticality in adult life. *Brit. J. Psychol.*, **55**, 315–320. [192]

Davies, T., and Merton, P. A., 1958. Recording compensatory rolling of the eyes. *J. Physiol.*, **140**, 27–28P. [51, 54]

Davis, F. C., 1933. Effect of maze rotation upon subjects reporting different methods of learning and retention. *Publ. Univ. Calif. Los Angeles Educ., Philos., Psychol.*, **1**, 47–64. [264]

Davson, H. (Ed.), 1962. *The Eye. Vol. 3: Muscular Mechanisms.* Academic Press, New York. [65]

Dearborn, G. V. N., 1899. Recognition under objective reversal. *Psychol. Rev.*, **6**, 395–406. [317, 318]

Deatherage, B. H., 1961. Binaural interaction of clicks of different frequency content. *J. acoust. Soc. Amer.*, **33**, 139–145. [147, 155]

Deatherage, B. H., Eldredge, D. H., and Davis, H., 1959. Latency of action potentials in the cochlea of the guinea pig. *J. acoust. Soc. Amer.*, **31**, 479–486. [165, 166]

Deatherage, B. H., and Hirsh, I. J., 1959. Auditory localization of clicks. *J. acoust. Soc. Amer.*, **31**, 486–492. [166, 167]

De Boer, E., Carels, J., and Philipszoon, A. J., 1963. The torsion swing. A simple rotation test. *Acta oto-laryng., Stockh.*, **56**, 457–460. [115]

Deese, V., and Grindley, G. C., 1947. The transposition of visual patterns. *Brit. J. Psychol.*, **37**, 152–163. [317]

De Haan, P., 1959. The significance of optic stimuli in maintaining the equilibrium. *Acta oto-laryng., Stockh.*, **50**, 109–115.

De Kleyn, A., and Magnus, P., 1921. Über die Function der Otolithen. Labyrinth-reflex und Progressivebewegungen. *Pflüg. Arch. ges. Physiol.*, **186**, 6–81. [98]

De Kleyn, A., and Schenk, V., 1931. Über den Reflexbogen des vestibulären Augen-nystagmus beim Menschen. *Acta oto-laryng., Stockh.*, **15**, 439–450. [122]

Delabarre, E. B., 1891. *Über Bewegungsempfindungen.* Freiburg I. B. [88]

Denny-Brown, R. S., Eccles, J. C., Liddell, E. G. T., and Sherrington, C. S., 1938. *Reflex Activity of the Spinal Cord.* Oxford Univ. Press, London. [241]

De Rivera, J., 1959. The postural sway test and its correlations. Proj. MR005.13-3001, Subtask 7, Rep. No. 3. U.S. Nav. Sch. aviat. Med., Pensacola, Fla. [253]

De Silva, H. R., 1931. A case of a boy possessing an automatic directional orientation. *Science*, **75**, 393–394. [266]

Deutsch, J. A., 1960. *The Structural Basis of Behavior.* Cambridge Univ. Press, Cambridge. [336]

Diamant, H., 1946. Sound localization and its determination in connection with some cases of severely impaired function of vestibular labyrinth but with normal hearing. *Acta oto-laryng., Stockh.*, **34**, 576–586. [159]

Dietzel, H., 1924. Untersuchungen über die optische Lokalisation der Mediane. *Z. Biol.*, **80**, 289–316. [281]

Di Giorgio, A. M., 1936. Fenomeno di Aubert e orientamento del bulbo oculare rispetto ai prani fondamentali dell' orbita. *Arch. Fisiol.*, **36**, 257–299. [194]

Diringshofen, H. von, 1952. Medizinische Probleme der Raumfahrt. In Gartmann, H. (Ed.), *Raumfahrt Forschung*. Oldenberg Press, Munich. [420]

Ditchburn, R. W., 1955. Eye movements in relation to retinal action. *Opt. Acta*, **4**, 171–176. [47]

Ditchburn, R. W., 1963. A new apparatus for producing a stabilized retinal image. *Opt. Acta*, **10**, 325–331. [47]

Ditchburn, R. W., and Fender, D. H., 1955. The stabilized retinal image. *Opt. Acta*, **2**, 128–133. [47]

Ditchburn, R. W., and Ginsberg, B. L., 1952. Vision with a stabilized retinal image. *Nature, Lond.*, **170**, 36–38. [47]

Dodge, R., 1921. The latent time of compensatory eye-movements. *J. exp. Psychol.*, **4**, 247–269. [56, 121]

Dodge, R., 1923a. Habituation to rotation. *J. exp. Psychol.*, **6**, 1–34. [129, 132]

Dodge, R., 1923b. Adequacy of reflex compensatory eye-movements including the effects of neural rivalry and competition. *J. exp. Psychol.*, **6**, 169–181. [121]

Dodge, R., 1923c. Thresholds of rotation. *J. exp. Psychol.*, **6**, 107–137. [116]

Dodge, R., and Fox, J. C., 1928. Optic nystagmus: I. Technical introduction, with observations in a case with central scotoma in the right eye and external rectus palsy in the left eye. *Arch. Neurol. Psychiat., Chicago*, **20**, 812–823. [57]

Dodge, R., Travis, R. C., and Fox, J. C., 1930. Optic nystagmus: III. Characteristics of the slow phase. *Arch. Neurol. Psychiat., Chicago*, **24**, 21–34. [58]

Dodwell, P. C., 1963. Children's understanding of spatial concepts. *Canad. J. Psychol.*, **17**, 141–161. [345]

Dohlman, G., 1935. Towards a method for quantitative measurement of the functional capacity of the vestibular apparatus. *Acta oto-laryng., Stockh.*, **23**, 50–62. [114, 116, 124]

Dohlman, G., 1959. Modern concept of vestibular physiology. *Trans. Amer. laryng. rhin. otol. Soc.*, 508–518. [106]

Dohlman, G., 1960. On the case for repeal of Ewald's second law. *Acta oto-laryng., Stockh., Suppl.*, **159**, 15–24. [120]

Dohlman, G., Henriksson, N. G., and Andrén, G., 1956. A method for direct registration of the speed of the eye-movements in nystagmic reactions. *Acta oto-laryng., Stockh.*, **46**, 323–333. [114]

Dole, S. H., 1960. Design criteria for rotating space vehicles. Res. Memo. RM-2668, Proj. Rand. The Rand Corp., Santa Monica, Calif. [438]

Dolowitz, D. A., Forssman, B., and Henriksson, N. G., 1962. Studies of cristospinal relexes (laterotorsion): III. Patterns of cristoocular and cristopinal relexes in clinical oto-neurology. *Acta oto-laryng., Stockh.*, **55**, 496–504. [124]

Donders, F. C., 1846. *Ned. Lancet*, **47**, 110. Referred to by Nagel, 1896. [50]

Donders, F. C., 1870. Die Bewegungen des Auges, veranschaulicht durch das Phänophthalmotrop. *v. Graefes Arch. Ophthal.*, **16**, 154. [50]

Donders, F. C., 1875. Über das Gesetz der Lage der Netzhaut in Beziehung zu der Blickebene. *v. Graefes Arch. Ophthal.*, **21**, 125–130. [50]

Downer, J. L. de C., 1958. Role of corpus callosum in transfer of training in *Macaca mulatta*. *Fed. Proc.*, **17**, 37. [394]

Drever, J., 1955. Early learning and the perception of space. *Amer. J. Psychol.*, **68**, 605–614. [261]

Duane, A., 1931. Binocular vision and projection. *Arch. Ophthal.*, *N.Y.*, **5**, 734–753. [17]

DuBois, J., Santschi, W. R., Walton, D. M., Scott, C. O., and Mazy, F. W., 1964. Moments of inertia and centers of gravity of the living human body encumbered by a full-pressure suit. AMRL-T R-64-110. Wright-Patterson AFB, Ohio. [428]

Duke-Elder, W. S., 1939. *Textbook of Ophthalmology* Vol. 1. Mosby, St Louis. pp. 623–628. [50]

Duke-Elder, W. S., 1949. *Textbook of Ophthalmology* Vol. IV. Mosby, St Louis. [61, 65]

Du Mas, F., and Worchel, P., 1956. The influence of the spatial context on the relearning of a rotated perceptual motor task. *J. gen. Psychol.*, **54**, 65–80. [264]

Duncan, B. K., 1934. A comparative study of finger maze learning by blind and sighted subjects. *J. genet. Psychol.*, **44**, 69–95. [261]

Dunlap, K., 1919. The nystagmus test and practice. *J. Amer. med. Ass.*, **73**, 54–55. [128]

Dusser de Barenne, J. G., 1913. Zur Kenntnis der Alloästhesie. *Mschr. Psychiat. Neurol.*, **34**, 523–540. [293]

Dusser de Barenne, J. G., 1934. The labyrinthine and postural mechanisms. In Murchison, C., *Handbook of General Experimental Psychology*. Clark Univ. Press, Worcester, Mass., p. 204–246. [101, 138]

Dusser de Barenne, J. G., 1935. Central levels of sensory integration. In Sensation: Its Mechanism and Disturbances. *Proc. Ass. Res. nerv. Dis.*, **15**, 274–278. Williams and Wilkins, Baltimore. [293]

Dyer, D. W., and Harcum, E. R., 1961. Visual perception of binary patterns by preschool children and by school children. *J. educ. Psychol.*, **52**, 161–165. [303]

Dzendolet, E., 1960. Manual application of impulses while frictionless. WADC Tech. Rep. 60-129. Wright-Patterson AFB, Ohio. [443]

Dzendolet, E., and Rievley, J. F., 1959. Man's ability to apply certain torques while weightless. WADC Tech. Rep. 59-94. Wright-Patterson AFB, Ohio. [443]

Eastman, A. E., 1958. A new astigmatic test chart. *Amer. J. Optom.*, **45**, 461–468. [35]

Eccles, J. C., Fatt, P., and Koketsu, K., 1954. Cholinergic and inhibitory synapses in a pathway from motor-axon collaterals to motoneurones. *J. Physiol.*, **126**, 524–562. [80]

Eccles, J. C., and Sherrington, C. S., 1930. Numbers and contraction-values of individual motor units examined in some muscles of the limb. *Proc. roy. Soc.*, *Ser. B*, **106**, 326–357. [74, 77]

Edgington, E. S., 1953. Kinaesthetically guided movements of head and arm. *J. Psychol.*, **36**, 51–57. [350, 351]

Edgren, R. D., 1953. A developmental study of motion perception, size constancy, recognition speed and judgment of verticality. *Ph.D. Diss.*, Stanford Univ. [210]

Edwards, A. S., 1942. The measurement of static ataxia. *Amer. J. Psychol.*, **55**, 171–188. [253]

Edwards, A. S., 1943. Factors tending to decrease the steadiness of the body at rest. *Amer. J. Psychol.*, **56**, 599–602. [254]

Edwards, A. S., 1946. Body sway and vision. *J. exp. Psychol.*, **36**, 526–535. [254]

Edwards, W., 1954a. Two- and three-dimensional autokinetic movement as a function of size and brightness of stimuli. *J. exp. Psychol.*, **48**, 391–398. [29]

Edwards, W., 1954b. Autokinetic movement of very large stimuli. *J. exp. Psychol.*, **48**, 493–495. [29]

Edwards, W., 1959. Information and autokinetic movement. *J. exp. Psychol.*, **57**, 89–90. [29]

Edwards, W., and Crutchfield, R. S., 1951. Differential reduction of autokinetic movement by a fixated figure. *J. exp. Psychol.*, **42**, 25–31. [29]

Ehlers, H., 1926. On optically elicited nystagmus. *Acta ophthal., Kbh.*, **3**, 254–271. [58]

Ek, J., Jongkees, L. B. W., and Klijn, J., 1959. The threshold of the vestibular organ. *Acta oto-laryng., Stockh.*, **50**, 292–300. [116, 117]

Ek, J., Jongkees, L. B. W., and Klijn, J., 1960. On the effect of continuous acceleration. *Acta oto-laryng., Stockh.*, **51**, 416–419. [112, 127]

Eldred, E., 1960. Posture and locomotion. In *Handbook of Physiology* Sec. 1, Vol. II. Amer. Physiol. Soc., Washington. p. 1067. [255]

Eldred, E., Granit, R., Holmgren, B., and Merton, P. A., 1953. Proprioceptive control of muscular contraction and the cerebellum. *J. Physiol.*, **123**, 46–47P. [79]

Eldred, E., Granit, R., and Merton, P. A., 1953. Supraspinal control of the muscle spindles and its significance. *J. Physiol.*, **122**, 498–523. [77]

Eldridge-Green, F. W., 1920. *The Physiology of Vision*. Bell, London. [30]

Elliott, R., and McMichael, R. E., 1963. Effects of specific training on frame dependence. *Percept. mot. Skills*, **17**, 363–367. [210]

Ellis, W. D. (Ed.), 1938. *A Source Book of Gestalt Psychology*. Harcourt, New York. [24]

Emsley, H. H., 1925. Irregular astigmatism of the eye: effect of correcting lenses. *Trans. opt. Soc., Lond.*, **27**, 28–42. [30]

Emsley, H. H., 1946. *Visual Optics* 4th ed. Hatton Press, London. [50]

Engström, H., 1961. The innervation of the vestibular sensory cells. *Acta oto-laryng., Stockh., Suppl.*, **163**, 30–41. [102, 105]

Enoksson, P., 1956. Optokinetic nystagmus in brain lesions. *Acta ophthal., Kbh.*, **34**, 163–184. [61]

Enoksson, P., 1961. A method for investigation of ocular dominance based on optokinetic nystagmus. *Acta ophthal., Kbh.*, **39**, 115–140. [62]

Enoksson, P., 1963. Binocular rivalry and monocular dominance studied with optokinetic nystagmus. *Acta ophthal., Kbh.*, **41**, 544–563. [62]

Erb, M. B., and Dallenbach, K. M., 1939. Subjective colours from line patterns. *Amer. J. Psychol.*, **52**, 227–241. [30]

Erickson, M. H., 1962. An investigation of optokinetic nystagmus. *Amer. J. clin. Hypnosis.*, **4**, 181–183. [57]

Erisman, T., and Kohler, I., 1953. Upright vision through inverting spectacles. Penn. State College: Psychol. Cinema. Reg. No. 2070. [414]

Erulkar, S. D., 1959. The responses of single units of the inferior colliculus of the cat to acoustic stimulation. *Proc. roy. Soc., Ser. B*, **150**, 336–355. [171]

Ewald, J. R., 1892. *Physiologische Untersuchungen über das Endorgan des Nervus Octavus.* Bergmann, Wiesbaden. [107, 115]

Ewert, P. H., 1926. Bilateral transfer in mirror drawing. *J. genet. Psychol.*, **33**, 235–249. [378]

Ewert, P. H., 1930. A study of the effects of inverted retinal stimulation upon spatially co-ordinated behavior. *Genet. Psychol. Monogr.*, **7**, 177–363. [370, 404, 407]

Ewert, P. H., 1936. Factors in space localization during inverted vision: I. Interference. *Psychol. Rev.*, **43**, 522–546. [370]

Ewert, P. H., 1937. Factors in space localization during inverted vision: II. An explanation of interference and adaptation. *Psychol. Rev.*, **44**, 105–116. [370, 407]

Exner, S., 1896. Über autokinetische Empfindungen. *Z. Psychol. Physiol. Sinnesorg.*, **12**, 313–330. [26]

Eysenck, H. J., 1947. *Dimensions of Personality.* Routledge and Kegan Paul, London. [253]

Eysenck, H. J., and Furneaux, W. D., 1945. Primary and secondary suggestibility: An experimental and statistical study. *J. exp. Psychol.*, **35**, 485–503. [253]

Faistauer, A., 1926. Links und Rechts im Bilde. *Amicis Jb. Oesterr Galerien.* [300]

Fantz, R. L., 1958. Pattern vision in young infants. *Psychol. Rec.*, **8**, 43–47. [342]

Farrow, B. J., and Santos, J. F., 1962. Changes in autokinetic perception as a function of the transfer of conditioning effects. *Brit. J. Psychol.*, **53**, 331–337. [30]

Favauge-Bruyel, A. J. de, and Roelofs, C. O., 1924. Über das Zentrum der Sehrichtungen. *Arch. Augenheilk.*, **95**, 111–139.

Fearing, F. S., 1924. The factors influencing static equilibrium. *J. comp. Psychol.*, **4**, 91–121, 162–188. [253]

Fearing, F. S., 1925. Factors influencing static equilibrium: an experimental study of the effect of controlled and uncontrolled attention upon sway. *J. comp. Psychol.*, **5**, 1–24. [253]

Feddersen, W. E., Sandel, T. T., Teas, D. C., and Jeffress, L. A., 1957. Localization of high-frequency tones. *J. acoust. Soc. Amer.*, **29**, 988–991. [143, 145, 152]

Feilchenfeld, H., 1903. Zur Lageschätzung bei seitlichen Kopfneigungen. *Z. Psychol. Physiol. Sinnesorg.*, **31**, 127–150. [196]

Fender, D. H., 1955. Torsional motions of the eyeball. *Brit. J. Ophthal.*, **39**, 65–72. [51]

Fenn, W. O., and Hursh, J. B., 1937. Movements of the eyes when the lids are closed. *Amer. J. Physiol.*, **118**, 8–14. [122]

Fernald, M. R., 1913. The mental imagery of two blind subjects. *Psychol. Bull.*, **10**, 62–63. [261]

Ferraro, A., 1921. Ricerche sul valore della prova 'P. Marie-Béhague', diretta a svelare i disturbi dell' orientamento fine. *Riv. Pat., nerv., ment.*, **26**, 74–78 (Abs.). [270]

Ferree, C. E., 1908. The streaming phenomenon. *Amer. J. Psychol.*, **19**, 114–129. [30]

Ferree, C. E., and Collins, R., 1911. An experimental demonstration of the binaural ratio as a factor in auditory localization. *Amer. J. Psychol.*, **22**, 250–297. [148, 174]

Finger, F. W., and Spelt, D. K., 1947. The illustration of the horizontal–vertical illusion. *J. exp. Psychol.*, **37**, 243–250. [37]

Finkel, M. E., and Harcum, E. R., 1962. Tachistoscopic recognition of words and their mirror images. Paper read to Virginia Acad. Sci., Norfolk. [308]

Firestone, F. A., 1930. The phase difference and amplitude ratio at the ears due to a source of pure tone. *J. acoust. Soc. Amer.*, **2**, 260–270. [142]

Fischer, B., 1915. Der Einfluss der Blickrichtung und Änderung der Kopfstellung (Halsreflex) auf der Báranyshen Zeigversuch. *Jb. Psychiat. Neurol.*, **35**, 155–158. [288]

Fischer, F. P., 1924. Über Asymmetrien des Gesichtssinnes, speziell des Raumsinnes beider Augen. *Pflüg. Arch. ges. Physiol.*, **204**, 203–233. [38]

Fischer, J. J., 1956. *The Labyrinth. Physiology and Functional Tests.* Grune and Stratton, New York and London. [138]

Fischer, M. H., 1927. Messender Untersuchungen über die Gegenrollung der Augen und die lokalisation der scheinbaren Vertikalen bei seitlicher Neigung (des Kopfes, des Stammes und des Gesamtkörpers). I. Neigungen bis zu 40°. *v. Graefes Arch. Ophthal.*, **118**, 633–680. [194]

Fischer, M. H., 1928. Die Regulationsfunktionen des menschlichen Labyrinthes und die Zusammenhänge mit verwandten Funktionen. *Ergebn. Physiol.*, **27**, 209–379. [138]

Fischer, M. H., 1930a. Messende Untersuchungen über die Gegenrollung der Augen und die Lokalisation der scheinbaren Vertikalen bei seitlicher Neigung des Gesamt-körpers bis zu 360°: II Mitteilung. Untersuchungen an Normalen. *v. Graefes Arch. Ophthal.*, **123**, 476–508. [50, 52, 53, 54, 194]

Fischer, M. H., 1930b. Messende Untersuchungen über die Gegenrollung der Augen und die Lokalisation der scheinbaren Vertikalen bei seitlicher Neigung des Körpers, Kopfes und Stammes: III Mitteilung. Untersuchungen an einem Ertaubten mit Functionsuntüchtigkeit beider Vestibularapparate und einem einseitig Labyrinth-losen. *v. Graefes Arch. Ophthal.*, **123**, 509–531. [50, 194, 196]

Fisher, G. H., 1960a. Intersensory localisation in three modalities. *Bull. Brit. Psychol. Soc.*, **41**, 24–25A. [353].

Fisher, G. H., 1960b. Intersensory elements of phenomenal space. *Proc. 16th. int. Cong. Psychol.*, 840. [353]

Fisher, G. H., 1961. Autokinesis in the spatial senses. *Bull. Brit. Psychol. Soc.*, **44**, 16–17A. [355]

Fisher, G. H., 1962a. Resolution of spatial conflict. *Bull. Brit. Psychol. Soc.*, **46**, 3A. [361]

Fisher, G. H., 1962b. Intersensory localization. *Ph.D. Thesis*, Univ. Hull. [353]

Fisher, G. H., 1964. Spatial localization by the blind. *Amer. J. Psychol.*, **77**, 2–14. [359, 362]

Fisher, L., and Babcock, H. L., 1919. The reliability of the nystagmus test. *J. Amer. med. Ass.*, **72**, 779–782. [128]

Fitts, P. M., 1947. A study of location discrimination ability. In Fitts, P. M. (Ed.),

Psychological Research on Equipment Design. A.A.F. Aviat. Psychol. Res. Rep. No. 19. Govt. Printing Office, Washington, D.C. [185, 350]

Fitts, P. M., 1951. Engineering psychology in equipment design. In Stevens, S. S. (Ed.), *Handbook of Experimental Psychology.* Wiley, New York. p. 1287–1340. [362]

Fitts, P. M., and Crannell, C., 1949. Location discrimination: II. Effect of twelve days of practice on the accuracy of reaching movements to twenty-four different areas. Tech. Rep. No. 5833. U.S.A.F. Air Material Command, Dayton, Ohio. [350]

Fitts, P. M., and Deininger, R. L., 1954. S–R compatibility: correspondence among paired elements within stimulus and response codes. *J. exp. Psychol.,* **48**, 483–492. [365]

Fitts, P. M., and Seeger, C. M., 1953. S–R compatibility: spatial characteristics of stimulus and response codes. *J. exp. Psychol.,* **46**, 199–210. [364]

Fitts, P. M., and Simon, C. W., 1949. Effect of pointer position and of horizontal vs. vertical instrument separation on performance on a dual pursuit task. Tech. Rep. No. 5832. U.S.A.F. Air Material Command, Dayton, Ohio. [363]

Fitts, P. M., Weinstein, M., Rapaport, M., Anderson, N., and Leonard, J. A., 1956. Stimulus correlates of visual pattern recognition: a probability approach. *J. exp. Psychol.,* **51**, 1–11. [314, 315]

Fitzgerald, G., and Hallpike, C. S., 1942. Studies in human vestibular function: I. Observations on the directional preponderance ('Nystagmusbereitschaft') of caloric nystagmus resulting from cerebral lesions. *Brain,* **65**, 115–137. [115]

Fleishman, E. A., 1953. Perception of body position in the absence of visual cues. *J. exp. Psychol.,* **46**, 261–270. [242, 244, 245, 248]

Fletcher, D. E., Collins, C. C., and Brown, J. L., 1958. Effect of positive acceleration upon the performance of an air-to-air tracking task. *J. Aviat. Med.,* **29**, 891–897. [366]

Flexman, R. E., Seale, L. M., and Henderson, C., 1963. Development and test of the Bell zero-*g* belt. AMRL-TDR-63-23, Wright-Patterson AFB, Ohio. [436]

Flugel, J. C., 1921. On local fatigue in the auditory system. *Brit. J. Psychol.,* **11**, 105–134. [162]

Fluur, E., 1960. Vestibular compensation after labyrinthine destruction. *Acta oto-laryng., Stockh.,* **52**, 367–375. [134]

Fluur, E., 1961. Efferent influence on vestibular function following unilateral laby-rinthectomy. *Acta oto-laryng., Stockh.,* **53**, 571–577. [120]

Fluur, E., 1962. The mechanism of nystagmus. *Acta oto-laryng., Stockh.,* **54**, 181–188. [123]

Fluur, E., and Eriksson, L., 1961. Nystagmographic recording of vertical eye move-ments. *Acta oto-laryng., Stockh.,* **53**, 486–492. [185]

Fluur, E., and Mendel, L., 1962a. Habituation, efference, and vestibular interplay: I. Monaural caloric habituation. *Acta oto-laryng., Stockh.,* **55**, 65–80. [131, 132, 133]

Fluur, E., and Mendel, L., 1962b. Habituation, efference, and vestibular interplay: II. Combined caloric habituation. *Acta oto-laryng., Stockh.,* **55**, 136–144. [132]

Fluur, E., and Mendel, L., 1963. Habituation, efference and vestibular interplay: Threshold after habituation, habituation of horizontal and vertical semicircular ducts. Preliminary report. *Acta oto-laryng., Stockh.,* **56**, 521–522. [129]

Fluur, E., and Mendel, L., 1964. Habituation, efference, and vestibular interplay: III. Unidirectional rotatary habituation. *Acta oto-laryng., Stockh.*, **57**, 82–88. [129]

Foley, J. P., 1940. An experimental investigation of the effect of prolonged inversion of the visual field in the rhesus monkey (*Macaca multatta*). *J. genet. Psychol.*, **56**, 21–51. [368]

Foley, P. J., 1962. Stimulus orientation and retinal summation. *J. opt., Soc., Amer.*, **52**, 474–475. [33]

Forgays, D. G., 1953. The development of differential word recognition. *J. exp. Psychol.*, **45**, 165–168. [303]

Forssman, B., 1964. Studies on habituation of vestibular reflexes: VII. Habituation in light of calorically induced nystagmus, laterotorsion, and vertigo in man. *Acta oto-laryng., Stockh.*, **57**, 163–173. [129]

Forssman, B., Henriksson, N. G., and Dolowitz, D. A., 1963. Studies on habituation of vestibular reflexes. *Acta oto-laryng., Stockh.*, **56**, 663–671. [129]

Fox, B. H., 1951. Figural after-effects: 'satiation' and adaptation. *J. exp. Psychol.*, **42**, 317–326. [227]

Fox, J. C., 1932. Disorders of optic nystagmus due to cerebral tumors. *Arch. Neurol. Psychiat., Chicago*, **28**, 1007–1029. [60, 61]

Fox, J. C., and Dodge, R., 1929. Optic nystagmus: II. Variations in nystagmographic records of eye movement. *Arch. Neurol. Psychiat., Chicago*, **22**, 55–74. [57]

Fox, J. C., and Holmes, G., 1926. Optic nystagmus and its value in the localization of cerebral lesions. *Brain*, **49**, 333–372. [57, 60, 61]

Fraenkel, G. S., and Gunn, D. L., 1940. *The Orientation of Animals.* Clarendon Press, Oxford; Dover paper-back, New York, 1961. [4, 411]

Francis, J. L., and Harwood, K. A., 1951. The variation of the projection centre with differential stimulus and its relation to ocular dominance. *Trans. int. Congr., Brit. opt. Ass., London.* p. 75–87. [278]

Free, W. T., and Jones, G. M., 1960. A method for simultaneous resolution of horizontal, vertical and rolling components of eye movements recorded on ciné film. *J. Physiol.*, **155**, 34–35. [51]

Freedman, S. J., Hall, S. B., and Rekosh, J. H., 1965. Effects on hand–eye co-ordination of two different arm motions during adaptation to displaced vision. *Percept. mot. Skills*, **20**, 1054–1056. [381]

Freedman, S. J., and Stampfer, K., 1964. Changes in auditory localization with displaced ears. Paper presented to Psychonomic Soc., Niagara Falls, Ont. [163]

Freeman, H., and Rodnick, E. H., 1942. Effect of rotation on postural steadiness in normal and in schizophrenic subjects. *Arch. Neurol. Psychiat., Chicago*, **48**, 47–53. [254]

Freilicher, J., 1963. Effect of symmetrical extraneous stimulation on the position of the apparent median plane. *M.A. Thesis*, Clark Univ. [288]

French, R. S., 1953. The accuracy of discrimination of dot patterns as a function of angular orientation of the stimulus. *Res. Bull.*, 53–3. U.S.A.F., Air Training Command, H.R.R.C. [318]

Friedman, S. M., 1961. Effects of spatial–temporal sequencies in visual presentation of binary patterns. Paper read to Virginia Acad. Sci., Lexington. [311]

Fry, G. A., 1945. Specification of the direction of regard (Special Report No. 1, Comm. on Nomenclature and Standards, Amer. Acad. Optom.). *Amer. J. Optom.*, **22**, 353–362. [47]

Fry, G. A., 1947a. Definition and measurement of torsion. (Special Report No. 2, Comm. on Nomenclature and Standards, Amer. Acad. Optom.). *Amer. J. Optom.*, **24**, No. 7. [47]

Fry, G. A., 1947b. Definition and measurement of cyclophoria with converged and elevated lines of sight. (Special Report No. 3, Comm. on Nomenclature and Standards, Amer. Acad. Optom.). *Amer. J. Optom.*, **24**, No. 10. [47]

Fuchs, W., 1920. Untersuchung über das Sehen der Hemianopiker und Hemiamblyopiker: I. Verlagerungserscheinungen. *Z. Psychol. Physiol. Sinnesorg.* **84**, 67–169. [24, 283]

Fuchs, W., 1922. Eine Pseudofovea bei Hemianopikern. *Psychol. Forsch.*, **1**, 157–186. [23]

Fukuda, T., 1959a. The stepping test. *Acta oto-laryng., Stockh.*, **50**, 95–108. [112, 124]

Fukuda, T., 1959b. Vertical writing with eyes covered. A new test of vestibulospinal reaction. *Acta oto-laryng., Stockh.*, **50**, 26–36. [112]

Fukuda, T., 1959c. The unidirectionality of the labyrinthine reflex in relation to the unidirectionality of the optokinetic reflex. *Acta oto-laryng., Stockh.*, **50**, 507–516. [60]

Fukuda, T., 1961. Studies on human dynamic postures from the viewpoint of postural reflexes. *Acta oto-laryng., Stockh., Suppl.*, **161**. [235]

Fukuda, T., Hinoki, M., and Tokita, T., 1957. Provocation of labyrinthine reflex by visual stimuli. *Acta oto-laryng., Stockh.*, **48**, 425–432. [112, 122]

Fukuda, T., and Tokita, T., 1957. Über die Beziehung der Richtung der optischen Reize zu den Reflextypen der Augen- und Skelettmuskeln. *Acta oto-laryng., Stockh.*, **48**, 415–424. [60]

Fuller, G. B., and Laird, J. T., 1963. Comments and findings about rotations. *Percept. mot. Skills*, **16**, 673–679. [333]

Fulton, J. F., 1946. *Howell's Textbook of Physiology* 15th ed. Saunders, Philadelphia and London. [72]

Fulton, J. F., and Pi-Suñer, J., 1928. A note concerning the probable function of various afferent end-organs in skeletal muscle. *Amer. J. Physiol.*, **83**, 554–562. [75]

Funaishi, S., 1926. Über das Zentrum der Sehrichtungen. *v. Graefes Arch. Ophthal.*, **117**, 296–303. [277]

Funaishi, S., 1927. Über die falsche Lichtlokalisation bei geschlossenen Lidern sowie über das subjektive Zyklopenauge. *v. Graefes Arch. Ophthal.*, **119**, 227–234. [277]

Furneaux, W. D., 1946. The prediction of susceptibility to hypnosis. *J. Personality*, **14**, 281–294. [252, 253]

Furneaux, W. D., 1952. Primary suggestibility and hypnotic susceptibility in a group situation. *J. gen. Psychol.*, **46**, 87–91. [253]

Furneaux, W. D., 1961. Neuroticism, extroversion, drive, and suggestibility. *Int. J. clin. exp. Hypnosis*, **9**, 195–214. [253]

Gaffron, M., 1950. Right and left in pictures. *Art. Quart.*, **13**, 312–331. [300]

Galambos, R., Rose, J. E., Bromiley, R. B., and Hughes, J. R., 1952. Microelectrode studies on medial geniculate body of cat: II. Response to clicks. *J. Neurophysiol.*, **15**, 359–380. [165]

Galambos, R., Schwartzkopf, J., and Rupert, A., 1959. Micro-electrode study of superior olivary nuclei. *Amer. J. Physiol.*, **197**, 527–536. [171, 172]

Galebski, A., 1928. Vestibular nystagmus in newborn infants. *Acta oto-laryng., Stockh.*, **11**, 409–423. [134]

Gantz, K. F. (Ed.), 1959. *Man in Space.* Sloan and Pearce, New York. [444]

Gardner, E., 1944. The distribution and termination of nerves in the knee joint of the cat. *J. comp. Neurol.*, **80**, 11–32. [81]

Gardner, E., 1948. Conduction rates and dorsal root inflow of sensory fibres from the knee joint of the cat. *Amer. J. Physiol.*, **152**, 436–445. [81]

Gardner, E., 1950. Physiology of movable joints. *Physiol. Rev.*, **30**, 127–176. [81]

Gardner, E., and Haddad, B., 1953. Pathways to the cerebral cortex for afferent fibres from the hindleg of the cat. *Amer. J. Physiol.*, **172**, 475–482. [82]

Gardner, E., and Morin, F., 1953. Spinal pathways for projection of cutaneous and muscular afferents to the sensory and motor cortex of the monkey (*Macaca mulatta*). *Amer. J. Physiol.*, **174**, 149–154. [76]

Garten, S., 1920. Über die Grundlagen unserer Orientierung im Raum. *Abh. sächs. Ges. (Akad.) Wiss.*, **36**, 431–510. [247, 249]

Gauer, O., and Haber, H., 1950. Man under gravity-free conditions. In *German Aviation Medicine World War II.* U.S. Govt. Printing Office, Washington, D.C. [422, 424]

Gellerman, L. W., 1933. Form discrimination in chimpanzees and two-year-old children: I. Form (triangularity) per se. *J. genet. Psychol.*, **42**, 1–27. [336]

Gellhorn, E., 1921. Psychologische und physiologische Untersuchungen über Übung und Ermüdung. *Pflüg. Arch. ges. Physiol.*, **189**, 144–180. [249]

Gellhorn, E., 1948. The influence of alterations in posture of the limbs on cortically induced movements. *Brain*, **71**, 26–33. [78]

Gellhorn, E., 1949. Proprioception and the motor cortex. *Brain*, **72**, 35–62. [78]

Gemelli, A., 1951. The effect of illusory perception of movement on sound localization. In *Essays in Psychology*, dedicated to David Katz. Almqvist and Wiksell, Uppsala. p. 104–117. [161]

Gemelli, A., Tessier, G., and Galli, A., 1920. La percezione della posizioni del nostro corpo e dei suoi spostamenti. *Arch. ital. psichol.*, **1**, 107–182. [241]

George, F. H., and McIntosh, S. B., 1960. Experimental disorientation and conceptual confusion. *Quart. J. exp. Psychol.*, **12**, 141–148. [259]

Gerathewohl, S. J., 1954. Comparative studies on animals and human subjects in the gravity-free state. *J. Aviat. Med.*, **25**, 412–417. [424, 440]

Gerathewohl, S. J., 1956. Personal experiences during short periods of weightlessness reported by 16 subjects. *Astronautica Acta*, **2**, 203–217. [422, 424]

Gerathewohl, S. J., 1957. Weightlessness. *Astronautica Acta*, **2**, 32–34, 74–75. [422]

Gerathewohl, S. J., 1960. Zero-G devices and weightlessness simulators. Nat. Res. Coun., Publ. 781. Nat. Acad. Sci., Washington, D.C. [420]

Gerathewohl, S. J., 1963. Personal experiences during short periods of weightlessness in jet aircraft and on the subgravity tower. In Loftus, J. P., *Symp. Motion Sickness.* p. 73–80. [420]

Gerathwohl, S. J., and Stallings, H. D., 1958. Experiments during weightlessness: a study of the oculo-agravic illusion. *J. Aviat. Med.*, **29**, 504–516. [425, 426]

Gerathewohl, S. J., Strughold, H., and Stallings, H. D., 1957. Sensori-motor performance during weightlessness: eye–hand co-ordination. *J. Aviat. Med.*, **27**, 7–12. [441]

Gernandt, B., 1949. Response of mammalian vestibular neurones to horizontal rotation and caloric stimulation. *J. Neurophysiol.*, **12**, 173–184. [108]

Gernandt, B., 1950. The effect of the centrifugal force upon the nerve discharge from the horizontal canal. *Acta physiol. scand.*, **21**, 61–71. [98]

Gernandt, B., 1959. Vestibular mechanisms. In *Handbook of Physiology* Sec. 1, Vol. 1. Amer. Physiol. Soc., Washington. p. 549–564. [105, 138]

Gernandt, B. E., 1964. Vestibular connections in the brainstem. In Bender, M. B. (Ed.), *The Oculomotor System.* Harper and Row, New York. [111]

Gerstmann, J., 1927. Fingeragnosie und isolierte Agraphie—ein neues Syndrom. *Z. ges. Neurol. Psychiat.*, **108**, 152–177. [291]

Gerstmann, J., 1930. Zur Symptomatologie der Hirnläsionen im Übergangsgebiet der unteren Parietal—und mittleren Occipitalwindung. (Das Syndrom: Fingeragnosie, Rechts—Links—Störung, Agraphie, Akalkulie). *Nervenarzt*, **3**, 691–695. [291]

Gerstmann, J., 1940. Syndrome of finger agnosia; disorientation for right and left, agraphia and acalculia. *Arch. Neurol. Psychiat., Chicago*, **44**, 398–408. [291]

Gerstmann, J., and Kestenbaum, A., 1930. Monokuläres Doppeltsehen bei cerebralen Erkrankungen. *Z. ges. Neurol. Psychiat.*, **128**, 42–56. [23]

Ghent, L., 1960. Recognition by children of realistic figures presented in various orientations. *Canad. J. Psychol.*, **14**, 249–256. [337]

Ghent, L., 1961. Form and its orientation: a child's-eye view. *Amer. J. Psychol.*, **74**, 177–190. [297, 298, 299]

Ghent, L., and Bernstein, L., 1961. Influence of the orientation of geometric forms on their recognition by children. *Percept. mot. Skills*, **12**, 95–101. [315, 324]

Ghent, L., Bernstein, L., and Goldweber, A. M., 1960. Preferences for orientation of form under varying conditions. *Percept. mot. Skills*, **11**, 46. [299, 331]

Giannitrapani, D., 1953. Effects of brightness gradients on the position of the apparent median plane. *M.A. Thesis*, Clark Univ. [283]

Giannitrapani, D., 1958. Changes in adaptation to prolonged perceptual distortion: a developmental study. *Ph.D. Diss.*, Clark Univ. [407]

Gibbs, C. B., 1954. The continuous regulation of skilled responses by kinesthetic feedback. *Brit. J. Psychol.*, **45**, 25–39. [90]

Gibson, E. J., Gibson, J. J., Pick, A. D., and Osser, H., 1962. A developmental study of the discrimination of letter-like forms. *J. comp. physiol. Psychol.*, **55**, 897–906. [339]

Gibson, J. J., 1933. Adaptation, after-effect and contrast in the perception of curved lines. *J. exp. Psychol.*, **16**, 1–31. [213, 231]

Gibson, J. J., 1937a. Adaptation, after-effect, and contrast in the perception of tilted lines: II. Simultaneous contrast and the areal restriction of the after-effect. *J. exp. Psychol.*, **20**, 553–569. [215]

Gibson, J. J., 1937b. Adaptation with negative after-effects. *Psychol. Rev.*, **44**, 222–244. [215]

Gibson, J. J., 1950a. The relation between visual and postural determinants of the phenomenal vertical. In Witkin, H. A. (Ed.), *Psychophysiological Factors in Spatial Orientation*. Office of Naval Res. p. 77–80. [14, 203]

Gibson, J. J., 1950b. *The Perception of the Visual World*. Houghton-Mifflin, Boston.

Gibson, J. J., 1952. The relation between visual and postural determinants of the phenomenal vertical. *Psychol. Rev.*, **59**, 370–375. [203, 208]

Gibson, J. J., and Mowrer, O. H., 1938. Determinants of the perceived vertical and horizontal. *Psychol. Rev.*, **45**, 300–323. [201, 411]

Gibson, J. J., and Radner, M., 1937. Adaptation, after-effect, and contrast in the perception of tilted lines. I. Quantitative studies. *J. exp. Psychol.*, **20**, 453–467. [179, 180, 202, 214, 215, 216, 219, 221, 226]

Gibson, J. J., and Robinson, D., 1935. Orientation in visual perception: the recognition of familiar plane forms in differing orientations. *Psychol. Monogr.*, **46**, No. 210, 39–47. [320]

Glanville, A. D., and Dallenbach, K. M., 1929. The range of attention. *Amer. J. Psychol.*, **41**, 207–236. [302]

Glick, J., 1959. The effects of static extraneous stimuli upon the localization of the apparent horizon. *M.A. Thesis*, Clark Univ. [187]

Gloster, J., 1953. Factors influencing the visual judgment of the vertical direction. *Trans. ophthal. Soc. U.K.*, **73**, 421–433. [193]

Goldhamer, H., 1934. The influence of area, position, and brightness in the visual perception of a reversible configuration. *Amer. J. Psychol.*, **46**, 189–206. [313]

Goldman, A. E., 1953. Studies in vicariousness: degree of motor activity and the autokinetic phenomenon. *Amer. J. Psychol.*, **66**, 613–617. [28]

Goldmeier, E., 1937. Über Ähnlichkeit bei gesehen Figuren. *Psychol. Forsch.*, **21**, 146–208. [296]

Goldscheider, A., 1889. Untersuchungen über den Muskelsinn. *Arch. Anat. Physiol.*, *Lpz.*, 369–502. Ministry Supply Trans. No. 20825T. [82, 93]

Goldscheider, A., 1898. *Physiologie des Muskelsinnes*. Barth, Leipzig. [255]

Goldstein, A. G., and Andrews, J., 1962. Perceptual uprightness and complexity of random shapes. *Amer. J. Psychol.*, **75**, 667–669. [298]

Goldstein, K., 1925. Über induzierte Tonusveränderungen beim Menschen (sog. Hals-reflexe, Labyrinthreflexe, usw.). VIII. Über den Einfluss unbewusster Bewegungen resp. Tendenzen zu Bewegungen auf die taktile und optische Raumwahrnehmung. *Klin. Wschr.*, **4**, 294–299. [160]

Goldstein, K., 1926. Über induzierte Veränderungen des 'Tonus', *Schweiz. Arch. Neurol. Psychiat.*, **17**, 203–228. [160]

Goldstein, K., 1939. *The Organism; a Holistic Approach to Biology Derived from Pathological Data in Man*. American Book Co., New York. [211]

Goldstein, K., and Riese, W., 1923. Über induzierte Veränderungen des Tonus (Halsreflexe, Labyrinthreflexe und ähnliche Erscheinungen): III. Blickrichtung und Zeigeversuch. *Klin. Wschr.*, **2**, 2338–2340. [288]

Goldstein, K., and Rosenthal-Veit, O., 1926. Über akustische Lokalisation und deren

Beeinflussbarkeit durch andere Sinnesreize. *Psychol. Forsch.*, **8**, 318–335. [161]

Gordon, H., 1920. Left-handedness and mirror-writing, especially among defective children. *Brain*, **43**, 313. [347]

Górska, T., and Jankowska, E., 1959. Instrumental conditioned reflexes of the deafferentated limb in cats and rats. *Bull. Acad. polon. Sci.*, *Ser. Sci. biol.*, **7**, 161–164. [78]

Górska, T., and Jankowska, E., 1960. The effect of deafferentation on instrumental conditioned reflexes established in dogs by reinforcing passive movements. *Bull. Acad. polon. Sci.*, *Ser. Sci. biol.*, **8**, 527–530. [78]

Górska, T., and Jankowska, E., 1963. The effects of deafferentation of a limb on instrumental reflexes. *Proc. Conf. Central and Peripheral Mechanisms of Motor Functions, Liblice, Prague*, 1961. Czech. Acad. Sci., Prague. [78]

Göthlin, G. F., 1927. Die Bewegungen und die physiologischen Konsequenzen der Bewegungen eines zentralen optischen Nachbildes in dunklem Blickfeld bei postrotatorischer und kalorischer Reizung des Vestibularapparates. *Nova Acta Soc. Sci. upsal.*, Almqvist and Wiksell, Stockholm. [125]

Göthlin, G. F., 1946. Entoptic analysis of vestibular nystagmus. *Acta oto-laryng., Stockh.*, **34**, 230–245. [125]

Gougerot, L., 1953. Lois de Weber—Fechner et variations de la pesanteur apparante. *Med. Aeronaut.*, **8**, 119. [424]

Graefe, A. von, 1854. Beiträge zur Physiologie und Pathologie der schiefen Augenmuskeln. *v. Graefes Arch. Ophthal.*, **1**, 28–50. [50]

Granit, R., 1950. Reflex self-regulation of muscle contraction and autogenetic regulation. *J. Neurophysiol.*, **13**, 351–372. [80]

Granit, R., 1955. *Receptors and Sensory Perception*. Yale Univ. Press, New Haven. [75, 76, 80]

Granit, R., Holmgren, B., and Merton, P. A., 1955. The two routes for excitation of muscle and their subservience to the cerebellum. *J. Physiol.*, **130**, 213–224. [79]

Granit, R., and Kaada, B. R., 1952. Influence of stimulation of central nervous structures on muscle spindles in cat. *Acta physiol. scand.*, **27**, 130–160. [79]

Granit, R., and Suursoet, V., 1949. Self regulation of the muscle contraction by facilitation and inhibition from its proprioceptors. *Nature, Lond.*, **164**, 270–271. [80]

Gray, R. F., 1960. Functional relationships between semicircular canals and otolith organs. *Aerosp. Med.*, **31**, 413–418. [98]

Gray, R. F., and Crosbie, R. J., 1958. Variations in direction of oculogyral illusions as a function of the radius of turn. Rep. No. MA-5806. U.S. Nav. Air Devel. Cen., Johnsville. [98]

Graybiel, A., 1952a. The oculogravic illusion. *Arch. Ophthal.*, *N.Y.*, **48**, 605–615. [199]

Graybiel, A., 1952b. The effect on vision produced by stimulation of the semicircular canals by angular acceleration and stimulation of the otolith organs by linear acceleration. In White, C. S., and Benson, O. O., *Physics and Medicine of the Upper Atmosphere*. Univ. of Mexico Press. [124]

Graybiel, A., 1954. Thresholds of stimulation of the otolith organs as indicated by the oculogravic illusion. Res. Rep. No. NM.001.059.01.38. U.S. Nav. Sch. aviat. Med., Pensacola, Fla. [421]

Graybiel, A., 1956. The importance of the otolithic organs in man based upon a specific test for utricular function. *Ann. otol., etc., St Louis*, **65**, 470–487. [199]

Graybiel, A., and Brown, R. H., 1951. The delay in visual reorientation following exposure to a change in direction of resultant force on a human centrifuge. *J. gen. Psychol.*, **45**, 143–150. [199]

Graybiel, A., Clark, B., MacCorquodale, K., and Hupp, D. I., 1946. Role of vestibular nystagmus in the visual perception of a moving target in the dark. *Amer. J. Psychol.*, **59**, 259–266. [125]

Graybiel, A., Clark, B., and Zarriello, J. J., 1960. Observations on human subjects, living on a slow rotation room for periods of two days. *Arch. Neurol., Lond.*, **3**, 55–73. [135, 136, 438]

Graybiel, A., Guedry, F. E., Johnson, W., and Kennedy, R., 1961. Adaptation to bizarie stimulation of the semicircular canals as indicated by the oculogyral illusion. *Aerosp. Med.*, **32**, 321–327. [129]

Graybiel, A., and Hupp, D. I., 1946. The oculo-gyral illusion; a form of apparent motion which may be observed following stimulation of the semicircular canals. *J. Aviat. Med.*, **17**, 3–27. [124, 287]

Graybiel, A., Hupp, D. I., and Patterson, J. L., Jr., 1946. The law of the otolith organ. *Fed. Proc.*, **35**, 35 (Abs.). [199]

Graybiel, A., and Johnson, W. H., 1962. A comparison of the symptomatology experienced by healthy persons and subjects with loss of labyrinthine function when exposed to unusual patterns of centripetal force in a counter-rotating room. Proj. MR005.13-6001, Subtask I, Rep. No. 70. U.S. Nav. Sch. aviat. Med., Pensacola, Fla. [135]

Graybiel, A., Kerr, W. A., and Bartley, S. H., 1948. Stimulus thresholds of the semicircular canals as a function of angular acceleration. *Amer. J. Psychol.*, **61**, 21–36. [116, 127]

Graybiel, A., and Niven, J. I., 1951. The effect of a change in direction of resultant force on sound localization: the audiogravic illusion. *J. exp. Psychol.*, **42**, 227–230. [160]

Graybiel, A., Niven, J., and MacCorquodale, K., 1956. The effect of linear acceleration on the oculogyral illusion. Proj. NM.001.110.100, U.S. Nav. Sch. aviat. Med., Pensacola, Fla. [99]

Graybiel, A., and Patterson, J. L., 1955. Thresholds of stimulation of the otolith organs as indicated by the oculogravic illusion. *J. appl. Physiol.*, **7**, 666–670. [117]

Graybiel, A., and Woellner, R. C., 1958. A new and objective method for measuring ocular torsion. *Amer. J. Ophthal.*, **47**, 349–352. [51]

Greenberg, G., 1960. Visual induction of eye torsion, as measured with an afterimage technique, in relation to visual perception of the vertical. *Ph.D. Diss.*, Duke Univ. [230]

Greene, T. C., 1929. The ability to localize sound (A study of binaural hearing in patients with tumor of the brain). *Arch. Surg., Chicago*, **18**, 1825–1841. [172]

Greening, C. P., 1962. Coriolis effects on operator movements in rotating vehicles. *Aerosp. Med.*, **33**, 579–582. [436]

Gregg, F. M., 1939. Are motor accompaniments necessary to orientational perception? *J. Psychol.*, **8**, 63–97. [262]

Gregg, F. M., 1940. Overcoming geographic disorientation. *J. cons. Psychol.*, **4**, 66–68. [267]

Gregory, R. L., 1959. Eye movements and the stability of the visual world. *Bull. Brit. Psychol. Soc.*, **38**, 23A. [27, 69]—*See also Nature, Lond.*, 1958, **182**, 1214–1216

Gregory, R. L., and Zangwill, O. L., 1963. The origin of the autokinetic effect. *Quart. J. exp. Psychol.*, **15**, 252–261. [27]

Grether, W. F., 1947. Efficiency of several types of control movements in the performance of a simple compensatory pursuit task. In Fitts, P. M. (Ed.), *Psychological Research on Equipment Design*. A.A.F. Aviat. Psychol. Res. Rep. No. 19. Govt. Printing Office, Washington, D.C. [366]

Griffith, C. R., 1920. Organic effects of repeated bodily rotation. *J. exp. Psychol.*, **3**, 15–46. [129]

Griffith, C. R., 1922. An historical survey of vestibular equilibrium. *Bull. Univ. Ill.*, **20**, 1–178. [138]

Griffith, C. R., 1924. A note on the persistence of the 'practice effect' in rotation experiments. *J. comp. Psychol.*, **4**, 137–149. [129]

Griffith, C. R., 1929. Vestibular sensations and the mechanisms of balance. *Psychol. Bull.*, **26**, 549–565. [129, 138]

Griffith, C. R., 1932. The perceptions and mechanisms of vestibular equilibrium. *Psychol. Bull.*, **29**, 279–303. [138]

Grissom, V. I., 1961. Pilot's flight report. In *Results of the Second U.S. Manned Suborbital Space Flight*. Manned Spacecraft Center, Nat. Aeronaut, and Space Admin., U.S. Govt. Printing Office, Washington, D.C. p. 47–58. [432]

Grodins, F. S., 1963. *Control Theory and Biological Systems*. Columbia Univ. Press. [3]

Groen, J. J., 1957. Cupulometry. *Laryngoscope, St Louis*, **67**, 894–910. [112]

Groen, J. J., 1960a. On the repeal of Ewald's second law. *Acta oto-laryng., Stockh., Suppl.*, **159**, 42–46. [108, 118]

Groen, J. J., 1960b. Problems of the semicircular canal from a mechanico-physiological point of view. *Acta oto-laryng., Stockh., Suppl.*, **163**, 59–67. [113, 114, 130]

Groen, J. J., 1961. The problems of the spinning top applied to the semi-circular canals *Confin. neurol., Basel*, **21**, 454–455. [100, 104]

Groen, J. J., 1963. Postnatal changes in vestibular reactions. *Acta oto-laryng., Stockh.*, **56**, 390–396. [134]

Groen, J. J., and Jongkees, L. B. W., 1948. The threshold of angular acceleration perception. *J. Physiol.*, **107**, 1–7. [116]

Gross, F., 1959. The role of set in perception of the upright. *J. Personality*, **27**, 95–103. [208]

Grosvenor, T., 1959. Eye movements and the autokinetic illusion. *Amer. J. Optom.*, **36**, 78–87. [25]

Grüttner, R., 1939. Experimentelle Untersuchungen über den optokinetischen Nystagmus. *Z. Sinnesphysiol.*, **68**, 1–48. [58]

Guedry, F. E., 1950a. Age as a factor in post-rotational phenomena. In *Psychophysiological Factors in Space Orientation*. U.S. Office of Nav. Res., Pensacola, Fla. p. 67–69. [134]

Guedry, F. E., 1950b. The effect of visual stimulation on the duration of post-rotational apparent motion effects. *J. gen. Psychol.*, **43**, 313–322. [124]

Guedry, F. E., and Beberman, N., 1957. Apparent adaptation effects in vestibular reactions. Rep. No. 293, U.S. Army Med. Res. Lab., Fort Knox. [127]

Guedry, F. E., Collins, W. E., and Sheffey, P. L., 1961. Perceptual and oculomotor reactions to interacting visual and vestibular stimulation. *Percept. mot. Skills*, **12**, 307–324. [122, 125]

Guedry, F. E., and Graybiel, A., 1962. Compensatory nystagmus conditioned during adaptation to living in a rotating room. *J. appl. Physiol.*, **17**, 398–404. [133]

Guedry, F. E., Graybiel, A., and Collins, W. E., 1962. Reduction of nystagmus and disorientation in human subjects. *Aerosp. Med.*, **33**, 1356–60. [133]

Guedry, F. E., and Lauver, L. S., 1961. Vestibular reactions during prolonged constant angular acceleration. *J. appl. Physiol.*, **16**, 215–220. [127]

Guedry, F. E., and Montague, E. K., 1961. Quantitative evaluation of the vestibular Coriolis reaction. *Aerosp. Med.*, **32**, 487–500. [105, 438]

Guilford, J. P., 1928. Autokinesis and the streaming phenomenon. *Amer. J. Psychol.*, **40**, 401–417. [25, 30]

Guilford, J. P., and Dallenbach, K. M., 1928. A study of the autokinetic sensation. *Amer. J. Psychol.*, **40**, 83–91. [25, 26, 30]

Guldberg, F. O., 1897. Die Circularbewegung als thierische Grundbewegung, ihre Ursache, Phänomenalität und Bedeutung. *Z. Biol.*, **17**, 419–458. [257, 258]

Gulliver, F. P., 1908. Orientation of maps. *J. Geogr.*, *N.Y.*, **7**, 55–59. [267]

Gullstrand, A., 1901. Die Konstitution des im Auge gebrochenen Strahlbundels. *v. Graefes Arch. Ophthal.*, **53**, 185. [34]

Gurnee, H., 1931. The effect of a visual stimulus upon the perception of bodily motion. *Amer. J. Psychol.*, **43**, 26–48. [126]

Gurnee, H., 1934. Thresholds of vertical movement of the body. *J. exp. Psychol.*, **17**, 270–285. [117]

Guttman, N., 1962. A mapping of binaural click lateralizations. *J. acoust. Soc. Amer.*, **34**, 87–92. [153, 158]

Guttman, N., Van Bergeijk, W. A., and David, E. E., 1960. Monaural temporal masking investigated by binaural interaction. *J. acoust. Soc. Amer.*, **32**, 1329–1336. [154]

Haber, F., and Haber, H., 1950. Possible methods of producing the gravity-free state for medical research. *J. Aviat. Med.*, **21**, 395–400. [420]

Haber, H., 1951. The human body in space. *Sci. Amer.*, **184**, 16–19. [424, 425]

Haber, H., 1953. *Man in Space*. Bobbs-Morrill, Indianapolis. [444]

Haber, H., and Gerathewohl, S. J., 1951. Physics and psychophysics of weightlessness. *J. Aviat. Med.*, **22**, 180–189. [424]

Hackman, R. B., 1940. An experimental study of variability in ocular latency. *J. exp Psychol.*, **27**, 546–558. [63]

Hagbarth, K. E., and Wohlfart, G., 1952. The number of muscle-spindles in certain muscles in cat in relation to the composition of the muscle nerves. *Acta anat.*, **15**, 85–104. [77]

Haggard, E. A., and Babin, R., 1948. On the problem of 'reinforcement' in conditioning the autokinetic phenomenon. *J. exp. Psychol.*, **38**, 511–525. [30]

Haggard, E. A., and Rose, G. J., 1944. Some effects of mental set and active participation in the conditioning of the autokinetic phenomenon. *J. exp. Psychol.*, **34**, 45–59. [30]

Hall, G. S., and Hartwell, E. M., 1884. Bilateral asymmetry of function. *Mind*, **9**, 93–109. [84, 281]

Hallpike, C. S., and Hood, J. D., 1953. The speed of the slow component of ocular nystagmus induced by angular acceleration of the head; its experimental determination and application to the physical theory of the cupular mechanism. *Proc. roy. Soc., Ser. B*, **141**, 216–230. [114, 125, 127]

Halpern, L., 1949. Sensorimotor induction in disturbed equilibrium. *Arch. Neurol. Psychiat., Chicago*, **62**, 330–354. [211]

Halpern, L., 1954a. Biological significance of head posture in unilateral disequilibrium. *Arch. Neurol. Psychiat., Chicago*, **72**, 160–168. [254]

Halpern, L., 1954b. Optic function and postural attitude. *Neurology*, **4**, 831–836. [256]

Halpern, L., 1956. Additional contributions to the sensorimotor induction syndrome in unilateral disequilibrium with special reference to the effect of colors. *J. nerv. ment. Dis.*, **123**, 334–350. [254]

Halpern, L., and Kidson, D. P., 1954. Sensorimotor induction syndrome in unilateral disequilibrium. *Neurology*, **4**, 233–240. [254]

Halpin, V. G., 1955. Rotation errors made by brain-injured and familial children in two visual-motor tests. *Amer. J. ment. Defic.*, **59**, 485–489. [332]

Halverson, H. M., 1922. Binaural localization of tones as dependent upon differences of phase and intensity. *Amer. J. Psychol.*, **33**, 178–212. [152, 155, 164]

Halverson, H. M., 1927. The upper limit of auditory localization. *Amer. J. Psychol.*, **38**, 97–106. [155]

Ham, G. C., 1943. Effects of centrifugal acceleration on living organisms. *War Med., Chicago*, **3**, 30–56. [198]

Hamberger, C. A., and Hydén, H., 1949. Production of nucleoproteins in the vestibular ganglion. *Acta oto-laryng., Stockh., Suppl.*, **75**, 53–81. [130]

Hamblin, J. R., and Winser, T. H., 1927. On the resolution of gratings by the astigmatic eye. *Trans. Opt. Soc., Lond.*, **29**, 28–42. [33]

Hamilton, C. R., 1964. Intermanual transfer of adaptation to prisms. *Amer. J. Psychol.*, **77**, 457–462. [378]

Hamilton, C. R., and Bossom, J., 1964. Decay of prism after-effects. *J. exp. Psychol.*, **67**, 148–150. [395]

Hammer, L. R., 1961. Aeronautical systems division studies in weightlessness. 1959–1960. WADC Tech. Rep. 60–715. Wright-Patterson AFB, Ohio.

Hammer, L. R., 1962. Perception of the visual vertical under reduced gravity. AMRL-TDR-62-55. Wright-Patterson AFB, Ohio. [421, 423]

Hammond, P. H., Merton, P. A., and Sutton, G. G., 1956. Nervous gradation of muscular contraction. *Brit. med. Bull.*, **12**, 214–218. [80]

Hanavan, E. P., 1964. A mathematical model of the human body. AMRL-TDR-64-102. Wright-Patterson AFB, Ohio. [428]

Hanfmann, E., 1933. Some experiments on spatial position as a factor in children's perception and reproduction of simple figures. *Psychol. Forsch.*, **17**, 319–329. [301, 314, 344]

Hanrahan, J. S., and Bushnell, D., 1960. *Space Biology, The Human Factor in Space Flight.* Basic Books, New York. [444]

Hanson, R. L., and Kock, W. E., 1957. Interesting effect produced by two loudspeakers under free space conditions. *J. acoust. Soc. Amer.*, **29**, 145L. [147]

Hanvick, L. J., and Anderson, A. L., 1950. The effect of focal brain lesions on recall and on the production of rotations in the Bender gestalt test. *J. cons. Psychol.*, **14**, 197–198. [332]

Harcum, E. R., 1957a. Visual recognition along four meridians of the visual field: preliminary experiments. Proj. Rep. 2144-50-T. Univ. Michigan. [303, 306]

Harcum, E. R., 1957b. Three inferred factors in the visual recognition of binary targets. In Wulfeck, J. W., and Taylor, J. H. (Eds.), *Form Discrimination as Related to Military Problems.* Nat. Res. Coun. Publ., 561. Nat. Acad. Sci., Washington, D.C. p. 32–37. [303, 306]

Harcum, E. R., 1958a. Visual recognition along various meridians of the visual field: XII. Acuity for open and blackened circles. Proj. Rep. 2144-315-T. Univ. Michigan. [304]

Harcum, E. R., 1958b. Visual recognition along various meridians of the visual field: XIII. Linear binary patterns at known eccentricities. Proj. Rep. 2144-316-T. Univ. Michigan. [310]

Harcum, E. R., 1958c. Visual recognition along various meridians of the visual field: V. Binary patterns along twelve meridians. Proj. Rep. 2144-302-T. Univ. Michigan. [306]

Harcum, E. R., 1958d. Visual recognition along various meridians of the visual field: VI. Eight-element and ten-element binary patterns. Proj. Rep. 2144-303-T. Univ. Michigan. [307]

Harcum, E. R., 1958e. Visual recognition along various meridians of the visual field: VII. Effect of target length measured in angular units. Proj. Rep. 2144-304-T. Univ. Michigan. [307, 310]

Harcum, E. R., 1958f. Visual recognition along various meridians of the visual field: IX. Monocular and binocular recognition of patterns of squares and circles. Proj. Rep. 2144-307-T. Univ. Michigan. [305]

Harcum, E. R., 1958g. Visual recognition along various meridians of the visual field: X. Binary patterns of the letters 'H' and 'O'. Proj. Rep. 2144-308-T. Univ. Michigan. [307]

Harcum, E. R., 1958h. Visual recognition along various meridians of the visual field: II. Nine-element typewritten targets. Proj. Rep. 2144-293-T. Univ. Michigan. [306]

Harcum, E. R., 1962. Recognition vs. recall of tachistoscopic patterns. *Percept. mot. Skills*, **15**, 238. [309]

Harcum, E. R., 1964. *Reproduction of Linear Visual Patterns Tachistoscopically Exposed in Various Orientations.* The College of William and Mary, Williamsburg, Virginia. [304]

Harcum, E. R., and Blackwell, H. R., 1958. Visual recognition along various meridians of the visual field: XI. Identification of the number of blackened circles presented. Proj. Rep. 2144-314-T. Univ. Michigan. [311]

Harcum, E. R., and Dyer, D. W., 1962. Monocular and binocular reproduction of binary stimuli appearing right and left of fixation. *Amer. J. Psychol.*, **75**, 56–65. [305]

Harcum, E. R., and Filion, R. D. L., 1963. Effects of stimulus reversals on lateral dominance in word recognition. *Percept. mot. Skills*, **17**, 779–794. [308]

Harcum, E. R., Filion, R. D. L., and Dyer, D. W., 1962. Distribution of errors in tachistoscopic reproduction of binary patterns after practice. *Percept. mot. Skills*, **15**, 83–89. [307]

Harcum, E. R., and Friedman, S. M., 1963. Reversal reading by Israeli observers of visual patterns without intrinsic directionality. *Canad. J. Psychol.*, **17**, 361–369. [310]

Harcum, E. R., and Hartman, R. R., 1961. A serial-learning effect within the perceptual span. Paper read to Virginia Acad. Sci., Lexington. [311]

Harcum, E. R., Hartman, R. R., and Smith, N. F., 1963. Pre- versus post-knowledge of required reproduction sequence for tachistoscopic patterns. *Canad. J. Psychol.*, **17**, 264–273. [309, 310]

Harcum, E. R., and Rabe, A., 1958a. Visual recognition along various meridians of the visual field: III. Patterns of blackened circles in an eight-circle template. Proj. Rep. 2144-294-T. Univ. Michigan. [307]

Harcum, E. R., and Rabe, A., 1958b. Visual recognition along various meridians of the visual field: IV. Linear binary patterns at 36 orientations. Proj. Rep. 2144-296-T. Univ. Michigan. [304, 310]

Harcum, E. R., and Rabe, A., 1958c. Visual recognition along various meridians of the visual field: VIII. Patterns of solid circles and squares. Proj. Rep. 2144-306-T. Univ. Michigan. [305, 307].

Harcum, E. R., and Smith, N. F., 1963. Effect of pre-known stimulus reversals on apparent cerebral dominance in word recognition. *Percept. mot. Skills*, **17**, 799–810. [308]

Harker, G. S., 1962. Apparent frontoparallel plane, stereoscopic correspondence, and induced cylotorsion of the eyes. *Percept. mot. Skills*, **14**, 75–87. [23]

Harris, C. S., 1963a. Adaptation to displaced vision. A proprioceptive change. *Ph.D. Diss.*, Harvard Univ. [376]

Harris, C. S., 1963b. Adaptation to displaced vision: Visual, motor, or proprioceptive change? *Science*, **140**, 812–813. [376, 378, 381]

Harris, C. S., 1964. Proprioceptive changes underlying adaptation to visual distortions. *Amer. Psychologist*, **19**, 562A. [380]

Harris, G. G., 1960. Binaural interactions of impulsive stimuli and pure tones. *J. acoust. Soc. Amer.*, **32**, 685–692. [149, 155, 164, 168]

Hartley, R. V. L., and Fry, T. C., 1921. The binaural location of pure tones. *Phys. Rev.*, **18**, 431–442. [142]

Hartmann, F., 1902. *Die Orientierung*. Vogel, Leipzig. [269]

Hartridge, H., 1950. *Recent Advances in the Physiology of Vision*. Churchill, London. p. 137, 142. [30, 31, 33]

Harvey, R. J., and Matthews, P. B. C., 1961. The response of de-efferented muscle spindle endings in the cat's soleus to slow extension of the muscle. *J. Physiol.*, **157**, 370–392. [74]

Hassler, R., 1960. The extrapyramidal system. In *Handbook of Physiology* Sec. 1, Vol. II. Amer. Physiol. Soc., Washington. p. 863. [241]

Hatwell, Y., 1960. Étude de quelques illusions geometriques tactiles chez les aveugles. *Année psychol.*, **60**, 11–27. [37]

Hauty, G. T., 1953. Psychological adaptability: investigation of mirror vision performance. Proj. 21-0202-0005. Rep. No. 4. U.S.A.F. Sch. aviat. Med., Randolf Field, Texas. [378]

Head, H., 1926. *Aphasia and Kindred Disorders of Speech.* (2 vols.) Cambridge Univ. Press, Cambridge. [270]

Hecht, S., 1928. The relation between visual acuity and illumination. *J. gen. Physiol.*, **11**, 255–281. [32]

Hein, A., and Held, R., 1962. A neural model for labile sensorimotor coordinations. In *Biological Prototypes and Synthetic Systems* Vol. 1. Plenum Press, New York. [384, 385]

Heinemann, E. G., and Marill, T., 1954. Tilt adaptation and figural after-effects. *J. exp. Psychol.*, **48**, 468–472. [222]

Held, R., 1955. Shifts in binaural localization after prolonged exposures to atypical combinations of stimuli. *Amer. J. Psychol.*, **68**, 526–548. [163]

Held, R., 1961. Exposure history as a factor in maintaining stability of perception and coordination. *J. nerv. ment. Dis.*, **132**, 26–32. [385]

Held, R., 1963a. Correlated and de-correlated visual feedback in modifying eye–hand coordination. Paper read to Exp. Psychol. Ass., Bryn Mawr, August, 1963. [398]

Held, R., 1963b. Movement-produced stimulation is important in prism-induced after-effects: a reply to Hochberg. *Percept. mot. Skills*, **16**, 764. [219]

Held, R., 1963c. Localized normalization of tilted lines. *Amer. J. Psychol.*, **76**, 146–148. [222, 223]

Held, R., and Bossom, J., 1961. Neonatal deprivation and adult rearrangement: complementary techniques for analysing plastic sensory-motor coordinations. *J. comp. physiol. Psychol.*, **54**, 33–37.

Held, R., and Freedman, S. J., 1963. Plasticity in human sensorimotor control. *Science*, **142**, 455–462. [385]

Held, R., and Gottlieb, N., 1958. Technique for studying adaptation to disarranged hand–eye coordination. *Percept. mot. Skills*, **8**, 83–86. [385]

Held, R., and Hein, A., 1958. Adaptation of disarranged hand–eye coordination contingent upon re-afferent stimulation. *Percept. mot. Skills*, **8**, 87–90. [385]

Held, R., and Hein, A., 1963. Movement-produced stimulation in the development of visually guided behaviour. *J. comp. physiol. Psychol.*, **56**, 872–876. [393, 394]

Held, R., and Mikaelian, H., 1964. Motor-sensory feedback versus need in adaptation to rearrangement. *Percept. mot. Skills*, **18**, 685–688. [388, 393]

Held, R., and Rekosh, J., 1963. Motor-sensory feedback and the geometry of visual space. *Science*, **141**, 722–723. [219]

Held, R., and Schlank, M., 1964. An attempt that failed to reproduce a study of disarranged eye–hand coordination. *Percept. mot. Skills*, **19**, 301. [386]

Hellebrandt, F. A., 1944. Postural adjustments in convalescence and rehabilitation. *Fed. Proc.*, **3**, 243–246. [252]

Hellebrandt, F. A., 1953. Kinesthetic awareness in motor learning. *Cerebral Palsy Rev.*, **14**, 3–5. [72]

Hellebrandt, F. A., and Franseen, E. B., 1943. Physiological study of the vertical stance of man. *Physiol. Rev.*, **23**, 220–255. [252]

Hellebrandt, F. A., Fries, E. C., Larsen, E. M., and Kelso, L. E. A., 1944. The influence of the army pack on postural stability and stance mechanics. *Amer. J. Physiol.*, **140**, 645–655. [252]

Hellebrandt, F. A., Nelson, B. G., and Larsen, E. M., 1943. The eccentricity of standing and its cause. *Amer. J. Physiol.*, **140**, 205–211. [253]

Helmholtz, H. von, 1962. *Treatise on Physiological Optics.* Dover, New York. [15, 38, 39, 47, 56, 59, 65, 66, 194, 201, 376, 379, 403]

Helson, H., and Howe, W. H., 1942. A study of factors determining accuracy of tracking by means of handwheel control. The Foxboro. Co., OSRD Report No. 3453. Foxboro, Mass. [366]

Helvey, T. C., 1960. *Moon Base: Technical and Physiological Aspects.* Rider, New York. [444]

Henderson, J. W., and Crosby, E. C., 1952. An experimental study of optokinetic responses. *Arch. Ophthal., N.Y.*, **47**, 43–54. [61]

Hendrickson, L. N., and Muehl, S., 1962. The effect of attention and motor response pretraining on learning to discriminate B and D in kindergarten children. *J. educ. Psychol.*, **53**, 236–241. [339, 347]

Henle, M., 1942. An experimental investigation of past experiences as a determinant of visual form perception. *J. exp. Psychol.*, **30**, 1–27. [321]

Hennebert, P. E., 1960. Nystagmus audiocinétique. *J. aud. Res.*, **1**, 84–87. [62]

Henriksson, N. G., 1955a. The correlation between the speed of the eye in the slow phase of nystagmus and vestibular stimulus. *Acta oto-laryng., Stockh.*, **45**, 120–136. [121]

Henriksson, N. G., 1955b. An electrical method for registration and analysis of the movements of the eyes in nystagmus. *Acta oto-laryng., Stockh.*, **45**, 25–41. [57, 115]

Henriksson, N. G., 1956. Speed of slow component and duration in caloric nystagmus. *Acta oto-laryng., Stockh., Suppl.*, **125**. [114, 129]

Henriksson, N. G., Dolowitz, D. A., and Forssman, B., 1962. Studies of cristospinal reflexes (laterotorsion): I. A method for objective recording of cristospinal reflexes. *Acta oto-laryng., Stockh.*, **55**, 33–40. [124]

Henriksson, N. G., Forssman, B., and Dolowitz, D. A., 1962. Studies of cristospinal reflexes (laterotorsion): II. Caloric nystagmus and laterotorsion in normal individuals. *Acta oto-laryng., Stockh.*, **55**, 116–128. [124]

Henriksson, N. G., Kohut, R., and Fernández, C., 1961. Studies on habituation of vestibular reflexes: I. Effect of repetitive caloric test. *Acta oto-laryng., Stockh.*, **53**, 332–349. [129]

Henry, J. P., Augerson, W. S., Belleville, R. E., Douglas, W. K., Grunzke, M. K., Johnson, R. S., Laughlin, P. C., Mosely, J. D., Rohles, F. H., Voas, R. B., and

White, S. C., 1962. Effects of weightlessness in ballistic and orbital flight. A progress report. *Aerosp. Med.*, **33**, 1056–1068. [420]

Hering, E. (Trans. by Radde, A.), 1942. *Spatial Sense and Movements of the Eye.* Amer. Acad. Optom., Baltimore. [16, 65, 66]

Hermelin, B., and O'Connor, N., 1961. Shape perception and reproduction in normal children and mongol and non-mongol imbeciles. *J. ment. Defic. Res.*, **5**, 67–71. [333]

Heron, W., 1957. Perception as a function of retinal locus and attention. *Amer. J. Psychol.*, **70**, 38–48. [302]

Hertzberg, H. T. E., Daniels, G. S., and Churchill, E., 1954. Anthropometry of flying personnel—1950. WADC-TDR-52-321. Wright-Patterson AFB, Ohio. [428]

Herzberger, M., 1963. Some recent ideas in the field of geometrical optics. *J. opt. Soc. Amer.*, **53**, 661–671. [36]

Hess, E. H., 1956. Space perception in the chick. *Sci. Amer.*, **195**, 71–80. [389]

Hess, W. R., 1957. *The Functional Organization of the Diencephalon.* Grune and Stratton, New York. [235, 240]

Hick, W. E., 1945. The precision of incremental muscular forces with special reference to manual control design. Rep. No. 642. Flying Personnel Res. Comm., Great Britain. [90]

Hick, W. E., 1953. Some features of the after-contraction phenomenon. *Quart. J. exp. Psychol.*, **5**, 166–170. [85]

Higgins, D. C., and Glaser, G. H., 1964. Stretch responses during chronic cerebellar ablation. A study of reflex instability. *J. Neurophysiol.*, **27**, 49–62. [80]

Higgins, D. C., Partridge, L. D., and Glaser, G. H., 1962. A transient cerebellar influence on stretch responses. *J. Neurophysiol.*, **25**, 684–692. [80]

Higgins, G. C., and Stultz, K., 1948. Visual acuity as measured with various orientations of a parallel-line test object. *J. opt. Soc. Amer.*, **38**, 756–758. [31, 304]

Higgins, G. C., and Stultz, K., 1950. Variation of visual-acuity with various test-object orientations and viewing conditions. *J. opt. Soc. Amer.*, **40**, 135–137. [32, 33]

Higginson, G. D., 1936. Human learning with a rotated maze. *J. Psychol.*, **1**, 277–294. [264]

Higginson, G. D., 1937. An examination of some phases of space perception. *Psychol. Rev.*, **44**, 77–96. [407]

Hilding, A. C., 1953. Studies on the otic labyrinth III: On the threshold of minimum perceptible angular acceleration. *Ann. Otol., etc., St Louis*, **62**, 5–14. [116]

Hinsey, J. C., 1934. The innervation of skeletal muscle. *Physiol. Rev.*, **14**, 514–585. [72]

Hirsh, I. J., 1950. The relation between localization and intelligibility. *J. acoust. Soc. Amer.*, **22**, 196–200. [170]

Hixson, W. C., and Niven, J. I., 1961. Application of the system transfer function concept to a mathematical description of the labyrinth: I. steady state nystagmus response to semicircular canal stimulation by angular acceleration. Bur. Med. Surg., NR005.13-6001, Subtask 1, Rep. No. 57, and NASA order No. R-1. U.S. Nav. Sch. aviat. Med., Pensacola, Fla. [103]

Hixson, W. C., and Niven, J. I., 1962. Frequency response of the human semicircular canals: II. Nystagmus phase shift as a measure of nonlinearities. Bur. Med. Surg.,

Project MR005.13-6001, Subtask 1, Rep. No. 73, and NASA order No. R-37. U.S. Nav. Sch. aviat. Med., Pensacola, Fla. [103]

Hochberg, J., 1963. On the importance of movement-produced stimulation in prism-induced after-effects. *Percept. mot. Skills*, **16**, 544. [219]

Hoff, H., and Schilder, P., 1925. Über Lagebeharrung. *Mschr. Psychiat. Neurol.*, **58**, 257. [84]

Hoffman, E. L., Swander, D. V., Baron, S. H., and Rohrer, J. H., 1953. Generalization and exposure time as related to autokinetic movement. *J. exp. Psychol.*, **46**, 171–177. [30]

Hofmann, F. B., 1926. Über die Sehrichtungen. *v. Graefes Arch. Ophthal.*, **116**, 135–142.

Hofmann, F. B., and Bielschowsky, A., 1909. Über die Einstellung der scheinbaren Horizontalen und Vertikalen bei Betrachtung eines von schrägen Konturen erfullten Gesichtsfeldes. *Pflüg. Arch. ges. Physiol.*, **126**, 453–475. [220]

Hoffman, P., 1922. *Untersuchungen über die Eigenreflexe (Sehnenreflexe) Menschlicher Muskeln*. Springer, Berlin. [75]

Hoffman, P., 1934. Die physiologishen Eigenschaften der Eigenreflexe. *Ergebn. Physiol.*, **36**, 15–108. [67]

Högyes, A., 1880. On the nervous mechanism of the involuntary associated movements of the eyes. *Orv. Hétil.*, **23**, 17–29. [123]

Holbrook, T. J., and de Gutiérrez-Mahoney, C. G., 1947. Diffusion of painful stimuli over segmental, infrasegmental and suprasegmental levels of the spinal cord. *Fed. Proc.*, **6**, 131. [293]

Holding, D. H., 1957a. Direction of motion relationship between controls and displays moving in different planes. *J. appl. Psychol.*, **41**, 93–97. [362, 363]

Holding, D. H., 1957b. The effect of initial pointer position on display-control relationships. *Occup. Psychol.*, **31**, 127–130. [364]

Holding, D. H., and Dennis, J. P., 1957. An unexpected effect in sound localization. *Nature, Lond.*, **180**, 1471–1472. [159]

Hollingworth, H. L., 1909. The inaccuracy of movement. *Arch. Psychol., N.Y.*, **2**, 1–87. [86]

Holmes, G., 1919. Disturbances of visual space perception. *Brit. med. J.*, **2**, 230–233. [40]

Holmgren B., and Merton, P. A., 1953. Local feedback control of motoneurones. *J. Physiol.*, **123**, 47P. [80]

Holmqvist, B., Lundberg, A., and Oscarsson, O., 1956. Functional organisation of the dorsal spino-cerebellar tract in the cat: V. Further experiments on convergence of excitatory and inhibitory actions. *Acta physiol. scand.*, **38**, 76–90. [76]

Holsopple, J. Q., 1923a. Some effects of duration and direction of rotation on post-rotation nystagmus. *J. comp. Psychol.*, **3**, 85–100. [129, 132]

Holsopple, J. Q., 1923b. Factors affecting the duration of post-rotation nystagmus. *J. comp. Psychol.*, **3**, 282–304. [129]

Holsopple, J. Q., 1924. An explanation for the unequal reductions in post-rotation nystagmus following rotation practice in only one direction. *J. comp. Psychol.*, **4**, 185–193. [132]

Holst, E. von, 1954. Relations between the central nervous system and the peripheral organs. *Brit. J. anim. Behav.*, **2**, 89–94. [384, 390]

Holst, E. von, and Grisebach, E., 1951. Einfluss des Bogengangsystems auf die 'subjektive Lotrechte' beim Menschen. *Naturwissenschaften*, **38**, 67–68. [198]

Holst, E. von, and Mittelstaedt, H., 1950. Das Reafferenzprinzip. *Naturwissenschaften*, **37**, 464–476. [384]

Honeyman, W. M., Cowper, M. C., and Rose, E. W., 1946. The autokinetic illusion. Flying Personnel Research Committee, Rep. No. 664. Air Ministry, London. [29, 30]

Hongo, T., Kubota, K., and Shimazu, H., 1963. EEG spindle and depression of gamma motor activity. *J. Neurophysiol.*, **26**, 568–580. [80]

Honisett, J., and Oldfield, R. C., 1961. Movement and distortion in visual patterns during prolonged fixation. *Scand. J. Psychol.*, **2**, 49–55. [29]

Hood, J. D., 1960. The neuro-physiological significance of cupular adaptation and its bearing upon Ewald's second law. *Acta oto-laryng., Stockh., Suppl.*, **159**, 50–55. [133]

Hood, J. D., and Pfaltz, C. R., 1954. Observations upon the effects of repeated stimulation upon rotational and caloric nystagmus. *J. Physiol.*, **124**, 130–144. [134]

Hoppeler, P., 1913. Über den Stellungsfaktor der Sehrichtungen; eine experimentelle Studie. *Z. Psychol. Physiol. Sinnesorg.*, **66**, 249–262. [185]

Hornbostel, E. M. von, 1926. Das räumliche Hören. In Bethe, A. (Ed.), *Handbuch der Normalen und Pathologischen Physiologie* Vol. II. Springer, Berlin. [158, 165]

Hornbostel, E. M. von, and Wertheimer, M., 1920. Über die Wahrnehmung der Schallrichtung. *S.B. preuss. Akad. Wiss.*, 388–396. [154, 158]

Horsley, V., 1905. The cerebellum, its relation to spatial orientation and to locomotion. (Boyle Lecture for 1906.) Bale, Sons and Danielsson, London. [84]

Howard, I. P., 1959. Some new subjective phenomena apparently due to interocular transfer. *Nature, Lond.*, **184**, 1516–1517. [22, 30]

Howard, I. P., 1966. The motor system. In Deutsch, J. A., and Deutsch, D., *Textbook of Physiological Psychology*. Dorsey, Homewood, Ill. [241]

Howard, I. P., Craske, B., and Templeton, W. B., 1965. Visuo-motor adaptation to discordant ex-afferent stimulation. *J. exp. Psychol.*, **70**, 189–191. [286, 391, 392]

Howard, I. P., and Evans, J. A., 1963. The measurement of eye torsion. *Vis. Res.*, **3**, 447–455. [50, 51, 53]

Howard, I. P., and Templeton, W. B., 1963. A critical note on the use of the human centrifuge. *Amer. J. Psychol.*, **76**, 150–152. [197, 200]

Howard, I. P., and Templeton, W. B., 1964a. The effect of steady fixation on the judgment of relative depth. *Quart. J. exp. Psychol.*, **16**, 193–203. [23, 207]

Howard, I. P., and Templeton, W. B., 1964b. Visually-induced eye torsion and tilt adaptation. *Vis. Res.*, **4**, 433–437. [53, 56, 229]

Howe, G. F., 1931. A study of children's knowledge of directions. *J. Geogr., N.Y.*, **30**, 298–304. [267]

Howe, G. F., 1932. The teaching of directions in space. *J. Geogr., N.Y.*, **31**, 207–210. [267]

484 Bibliography and author index

Hubel, D. H., and Wiesel, T. N., 1959. Receptive fields of single neurones in the cat's striate cortex. *J. Physiol.*, **148**, 574–591. [15, 306, 395]

Hubel, D. H., and Wiesel, T. N., 1963. Receptive fields of cells in striate cortex of very young, visually inexperienced kittens. *J. Neurophysiol.*, **26**, 994–1002. [395]

Hudson, W. H., 1922. On the sense of direction. *Cent. Mag.*, **104**, 693–701. [265]

Hueck, A., 1838. Die Arendrehung des Auges. Dorpat. Cited in Nagel, 1896. [50]

Hughes, J. W., 1939. Binaural localization with two notes differing in phase by 180°. *Brit. J. Psychol.*, **30**, 52–56. [155]

Hughes, J. W., 1940. The upper frequency limit for the binaural localization of a pure tone by phase difference. *Proc. R. Soc. Med.*, **128**, 293–305. [156]

Hull, C. L., 1933. *Hypnosis and Suggestibility*. Appleton-Century-Croft, New York. [253]

Humphries, M., 1958. Performance as a function of control-display relations, positions of the operator, and locations of the control. *J. appl. Psychol.*, **42**, 311–316. [366]

Hunt, C. C., 1952. The effect of stretch receptors from muscle on the discharge of motoneurones. *J. Physiol.*, **117**, 359–379. [80]

Hunt, C. C., and Kuffler, S. W., 1951a. Further study of efferent small-nerve fibers to mammalian muscle spindles. Muscle spindle innervation and activity during contraction. *J. Physiol.*, **113**, 283–297. [77]

Hunt, C. C., and Kuffler, S. W., 1951b. Stretch receptor discharges during muscle contraction. *J. Physiol.*, **113**, 298–315. [77]

Hunt, C. C., and Perl, E. R., 1960. Spinal reflex mechanisms concerned with skeletal muscle. *Physiol. Rev.*, **40**, 538–579. [76]

Hunter, J., 1786. Cited in Nagel, 1896. [50]

Hunton, V. D., 1955. The recognition of inverted pictures by children. *J. genet. Psychol.*, **86**, 281–288. [336]

Husband, R. W., 1934. The effects of musical rhythm and pure rhythms on bodily sway. *J. gen. Psychol.*, **11**, 328–336. [253]

Hyde, J. E., 1959. Some characteristics of voluntary human ocular movements in the horizontal plane. *Amer. J. Ophthal.*, **48**, 85–95. [63]

Hyde, J., and Eliasson, S., 1955. Centering of the eyes. *Amer. J. Physiol.*, **183**, 628–629A [62]

Hyde, J., and Gellhorn, E., 1949. Influence of deafferentation on stimulation of motor cortex. *Amer. J. Physiol.*, **156**, 311–316. [78]

Hyslop, J. H., 1897. Upright vision. *Psychol. Rev.*, **4**, 71–73, 142–163. [406]

Ingham, J. G., 1954. Body sway and suggestibility. *J. ment. Sci.*, **100**, 432–441. [253]

Ireland, W. W., 1881. On mirror writing and its relation to left-handedness and cerebral disease. *Brain*, **4**, 361–367. [348]

Irvine, S. R., and Ludvigh, E., 1936. Is ocular proprioceptive sense concerned in vision? *Arch. Ophthal., N.Y.*, **15**, 1037–1049. [68]

Jaccard, P., 1931. *Le Sens de Direction et L'Orientation Lointain chez L'Homme*. Payot, Paris. [265]

Jackson, C. V., 1953. Visual factors in auditory localization. *Quart. J. exp. Psychol.*, **5**, 52–65. [360]

Jackson, C. V., 1954. The influence of previous movement and posture on subsequent posture. *Quart. J. exp. Psychol.*, **6**, 72–78. [85]

Jackson, J. H., and Paton, L., 1909. On some abnormalities of ocular movements. *Lancet*, **176**, 900–905. [66]

Jacobs, H. L., 1960. The lack of bearing contact and the problem of weightlessness: The effect of past experiences on human performance on a free-rotating, low-friction turntable. *Ann. N.Y. Acad. Sci.*, **84**, 303–328. [422]

Jaensch, E. R., 1911. Cited in Kleint, 1911. [207]

Jaffe, K. M., 1952. Effect of asymmetrical position and directional dynamics of configurations on the visual perception of the horizon. *M.A. Thesis*, Clark Univ. [188]

James, W., 1882. The sense of dizziness in deaf-mutes. *Amer. J. Otol.*, **4**, 239–254. [135, 255]

James, W., 1890. *The Principles of Psychology* Vol. 2. Macmillan, London. [66]

Jansen, J. K. S., and Matthews, P. B. C., 1961. The dynamic responses to slow stretch of muscle spindles in the decerebrate cat. *J. Physiol.*, **159**, 20–22P. [77]

Jansen, J. K. S., and Matthews, P. B. C., 1962. The central control of the dynamic response of muscle spindle receptors. *J. Physiol.*, **161**, 357–378. [77]

Jastrow, J., 1889. Perception of space by disparate senses. *Mind*, **11**, 539–554. [357]

Jastrow, J., 1892. On the judgment of angles and positions of lines. *Amer. J. Psychol.*, **5**, 220–323. [179]

Javal, E., 1865. De la neutralisation dans l'acte de la vision. *Ann. Oculist.*, Paris, **54**, 5–16. [21, 50]

Jeffress, L. A., 1948. A place theory of sound localization. *J. comp. physiol. Psychol.*, **41**, 35–39. [172]

Jeffress, L. A., and Blodgett, H. C., 1962. Effect of switching earphone channels upon the precision of centering. *J. acoust. Soc. Amer.*, **34**, 1275–1276. [149]

Jeffress, L. A., Blodgett, H. C., and Deatherage, B. H., 1952. The masking of tones by white noise as a function of the interaural phases of both components. *J. acoust. Soc. Amer.*, **24**, 523–527. [170]

Jeffress, L. A., and Blodgett, H. C., and Deatherage, B. H., 1962. Effect of interaural correlation on the precision of centering a noise. *J. acoust. Soc. Amer.*, **34**, 1122–1126. [156]

Jeffress, L. A., and Taylor, R. W., 1961. Lateralization vs. localization. *J. acoust. Soc. Amer.*, **33**, 482–483. [149]

Jeffrey, W. E., 1958. Variables in early discrimination learning. I. Motor responses in the training of left–right discrimination. *Child Develpm.*, **29**, 269–275. [291, 339, 347]

Jenkins, W. O., 1947a. A psychophysical investigation of ability to reproduce pressures. In Fitts, P. M. (Ed.), *Psychological Research on Equipment Design*. A.A.F. Aviat. Psychol. Res. Rep. No. 19. Govt. Printing Office, Washington, D.C. [366]

Jenkins, W. O., 1947b. The discrimination and reproduction of motor adjustments, with various types of aircraft controls. *Amer. J. Psychol.*, **60**, 397–406 [366]

Jensen, C. E., Koefoed, J., and Vilstrup, T., 1954. Flow potentials in hyaluronate solutions. *Nature, Lond.*, **174**, 1101–1102. [106]

Johnson, W. H., 1954. Head movements and motion sickness. *Int. Rec. Med.*, **167**, 638–640. [136]

Johnson, W. H., 1956. Head movement measurements in relation to spatial disorientation and vestibular stimulation. *J. Aviat. Med.*, **27**, 148–152. [136]

Johnson, W. H., and Taylor, N. B. G., 1961. The importance of head movements in studies involving stimulation of the organ of balance. *Acta oto-laryng.*, *Stockh.*, **53**, 211–218. [136]

Jones, E., 1907. The precise diagnostic value of allochiria. *Brain*, **30**, 490–532. [293]

Jones, F. N., and Bunting, E. B., 1949. Displacement effect in auditory localization. *Amer. Psychologist*, **4**, 389A. [162]

Jones, I. H., 1918. *Equilibrium and Vertigo*. Lippincott, Philadelphia. [128]

Jongkees, L. B. W., 1960. On positional nystagmus. *Acta oto-laryng.*, *Stockh.*, *Suppl.*, **159**, 78–83. [121]

Jongkees, L. B. W., and Groen, J. J., 1946. The nature of the vestibular stimulus. *J. Laryng.*, **61**, 529–541. [98, 136]

Jongkees, L. B. W., Oosterveld, W. J., and Zelig, S., 1964. On nystagmus provoked by central stimulation. Preliminary note. *Acta oto-laryng.*, *Stockh.*, **57**, 313–319. [123]

Jongkees, L. B. W., and Philipszoon, A. J., 1963. The influence of position upon the eye-movements provoked by linear acceleration. *Acta oto-laryng.*, *Stockh.*, **56**, 414–420. [121]

Jongkees, L. B. W., and Van de Veer, R. A., 1957. Directional hearing capacity in hearing disorders. *Acta oto-laryng.*, *Stockh.*, **48**, 465–474. [158]

Jongkees, L. B. W., and Van de Veer, R. A., 1958. On directional sound localization in unilateral deafness and its explanation. *Acta oto-laryng.*, *Stockh.*, **49**, 119–131. [158]

Juba, A., 1948. Über nach Elektroschock auftretende kortikale Funktionsstörungen (Gerstmann'sches Syndrom, Gesichts- und Raumagnosien). *Schweiz. Arch. Neurol. Psychiat.*, **61**, 217–226. [292]

Jung, R., 1953. Nystagmographie. Zur Physiologie und Pathologie des optisch—vestibulären Systems beim Menschen. In von Bergmann, H. G., Frey, W., and Schwiegk, H., *Handbuch der Inneren Medizin* Vol. 5. Springer, Berlin. p. 1325. [57]

Jung, R., and Kornmuller, H. H., 1964. Results of electronystagmography in man: the value of optokinetic, vestibular, and spontaneous nystagmus for neurologic diagnosis and research. In Bender, M.B. (Ed.), *The Oculomotor System*. Harper and Row, New York. [62]

Kaden, S. E., 1953. Effect of directional dynamics of configurations and visually perceived words on the position of the apparent horizon. *M.A. Thesis*, Clark Univ. [188]

Kama, W. N., 1961. The effect of simulated weightlessness upon positioning responses. AMRL-TDR-61-555. Wright-Patterson AFB, Ohio. [442]

Kanzer, M., and Bender, M. B., 1939. Spatial disorientation with homonymous defects of the visual field. *Arch. Ophthal.*, *N.Y.*, **21**, 439–449. [24]

Karrer, E., and Stevens, H. C., 1930. The response of negative after-images to passive motion of the eyeball and the bearing of these observations on the visual perception of motion. *Amer. J. Physiol.*, **94**, 611–614. [66]

Karwoski, T. F., Redner, H., and Wood, W. O., 1948. Autokinetic movement of large stimuli. *J. gen. Psychol.*, **39**, 29–37. [29]

Kasten, D. F., 1962. Human performance in a simulated short orbital transfer. AMRL-TDR-62-138. Wright-Patterson AFB, Ohio. [436]

Katsui, A., 1962. A developmental study on the perception of direction in two-dimensional space. A mathematical expression of the developmental curve and a qualitative analysis of perceptual errors. *Jap. J. Psychol.*, **33**, 8. [183, 341]

Kaufman, E. L., Reese, E. P., Volkmann, J., and Rogers, S., 1949. In Reese, E. P. (Ed.), 1953. Summary Rep. No. SDC 131-1-5. Psychophysical Res. Unit, Mt. Holyoke College. [179]

Keene, G. C., 1963. The effect of response codes on the accuracy of making absolute judgments of linear inclinations. *J. gen. Psychol.*, **69**, 37–50. [182]

Keith, A., 1933. *The Engines of the Human Body*. Lippincott, Philadelphia. [252]

Keleman, G., 1926. Zur Bewertung des von der Körperlage abhängigen Nystagmus und Schwindels. *Mschr. Ohrenheilk.*, **60**, 1156–1161. [121]

Keller, R., 1942. The right–left problem in art. *Ciba Symp.* Summit, N.J. [300]

Kellogg, R. S., Kennedy, R. S., and Graybiel, A., 1964. Motion sickness symptomatology of labyrinthine defective and normal subjects during zero gravity maneuvers. AMRL-TDR-64-47. Wright-Patterson AFB, Ohio. [425]

Kelvin, R. P., and Mulik, A., 1958. Discrimination of length by sight and touch. *Quart. J. exp. Psychol.*, **10**, 187–192. [357]

Kestenbaum, A., 1930a. Zur Entwicklung der Augenbewegungen und des optokinetischen Nystagmus. *v. Graefes Arch. Ophthal.*, **124**, 113–127. [59]

Kestenbaum, A., 1930b. Zur Klinik des optokinetischen Nystagmus. *v. Graefes Arch. Ophthal.*, **124**, 339–369. [61]

Kestenbaum, A., 1947. *Clinical Methods of Neuro-Ophthalmology*. Williams and Witkins, Baltimore. [57, 61]

Kestenbaum, A., 1957. Nystagmus: Review of the literature in 1946–1954. *Bibl. ophth.*, **49**, 221–286. [62]

Khomskoya, E. D., 1962. K. probleme afferentatsü drizhenii glaz. *Vop. Psikhol.*, **3**, 73–84. [58]

Kikuchi, Y., 1957. Objective allocation of sound-image from binaural stimulation. *J. acoust. Soc. Amer.*, **29**, 124–128. [149, 164]

Kimura, D., 1959. The effect of letter position on recognition. *Canad. J. Psychol.*, **13**, 1–10. [304]

King, B. G., 1961. Physiological effects of postural disorientation by tilting during weightlessness. *Aerosp. Med.*, **32**, 137–140. [424]

King, B. G., and Wade, J. E., 1961. Vestibular functions. In Hammer, L. R., *Aeronautical Systems Division Studies in Weightlessness*. 1959–1960. WADC Tech. Rep. 60-715. Wright-Patterson AFB, Ohio. [55, 138]

Kirk, S. A., 1934. A study of the relation of ocular and manual preference to mirror reading. *J. genet. Psychol.*, **44**, 192–205. [347]

Kirk, W. D., and Kirk, S. A., 1935. The influence of the teacher's handedness on children's reversal tendencies in writing. *J. genet. Psychol.*, **47**, 473–477. [348]

Kirschensteiner, 1905. Die Entwicklung der zeichnerischen Begabung. Cited in Stern, 1909. [341]

Kiss, J., 1921. Über das Vorbeizeigen bei forciertem Seitwärtsschauen. *Z. ges. Neurol. Psychiat.*, **65**, 14–17. [288]

Klein, E., and Schilder, P., 1929. The Japanese illusion and the postural model of the body. *J. nerv. ment. Dis.*, **70**, 241–263. [249]

Klein, R., and Stein, R., 1934. Über einen Tumor des Kleinhirns mit anfallsweise auftretendem Tonusverlust und monokulärer Diplopie bzw. binokulärer Triplopie. *Arch. Psychiat. Nervenkr.*, **102**, 478–492. [23]

Kleinknecht, F., 1922. Ein weiterer Beitrag zur Frage des Ubungseinflusses und der Ubungsfestigkeit am Neigungsstuhl. *Z. Biol.*, **77**, 11–28. [244, 249]

Kleinknecht, F., and Lueg, W., 1924. Weitere Untersuchungen über Lagen-bedächtnis und Empfindung am Neigungsstuhl. *Z. Biol.*, **81**, 22–36. [249]

Kleint, H., 1936. Versuche über die Wahrnehmung. *Z. Psychol.*, **138**, 1–34. [207, 210, 220]

Kleint, H., 1937. Versuche über die Wahrnehmung. *Z. Psychol.*, **140**, 109–138. [195]

Klemm, O., 1909. Lokalisation von Sinneseindrücken bei disparaten Nebenreizen. *Psychol. Stud.* (*Wundt*), **5**, 73–161. [360]

Klemm, O., 1918. Untersuchungen über die Lokalisation von Schallreizen: III Mitteilung: Über den Anteil des beidohrigen Hörens. *Arch. ges. Psychol.*, **38**, 71–114. [158]

Klemm, O., 1920. Über den Einfluss des binauralen Zeitunterschiedes auf die Lokalisation. *Arch. ges. Psychol.*, **40**, 117–146. [154, 158, 164]

Klingelhage, H., 1933. Mit welcher Sicherheit wird ein den Tastwerkzeugen dargebotener Raumpunkt haptisch wieder aufgezeigt? *Z. Sinnesphysiol.*, **64**, 192–228. [84]

Klopp, H. W., 1951. Über Ungekehrt und Verkehrtsehen. *Dtsch. Z. Nervenheilk.*, **165**, 231–260. [212, 418]

Klumpp, R. G., 1953. Discriminability of interaural time difference. *J. acoust. Soc. Amer.*, **25**, 823A. [155, 157]

Klumpp, R. G., and Eady, H. R., 1956. Some measurements of interaural time difference thresholds. *J. acoust. Soc. Amer.*, **28**, 859–860. [157]

Knapp, H. D., Taub, E., and Berman, A. J., 1958. Effects of deafferentation on a conditioned avoidance response. *Science*, **128**, 842–843. [78]

Knapp, H. D., Taub, E., and Berman, A. J., 1959. Conditioned responses following deafferentation in the monkey. *Trans. Amer. neurol. Ass.*, **84**, 185–187. [78]

Knight, L. A., 1958. An approach to the physiologic simulation of the null-gravity state. *J. Aviat. Med.*, **29**, 283–286. [421]

Knotts, J. R., and Miles, W. R., 1929. The maze-learning ability of blind compared with sighted children. *J. genet. Psychol.*, **36**, 21–50. [261]

Kobayashi, Y., Oshima, K., and Tasaki, I., 1952. Analysis of afferent and efferent systems in the muscle nerve of the toad and cat. *J. Physiol.*, **117**, 152–171. [77]

Koch, H., Henriksson, N. G., Lundgren, A., and Andrén, G., 1959. Directional preponderance and spontaneous nystagmus in eye-speed recording. *Acta oto-laryng.*, *Stockh.*, **50**, 517–525. [133]

Koch, H. L., and Ufkess, J., 1926. A comparative study of stylus maze learning by blind and seeing subjects. *J. exp. Psychol.*, **9**, 118–131. [261]

Kock, W. E., 1950. Binaural localization and masking. *J. acoust. Soc. Amer.*, **22**, 801–804. [170]

Koenig, W., 1950. Subjective effects of binaural hearing. *J. acoust. Soc. Amer.*, **22**, 61. [170]

Koffka, K., 1935. *Principles of Gestalt Psychology.* Routledge and Kegan Paul, London. [200]

Kohler, I., 1951. *Über Aufbau und Wandlungen der Wahrnehmungswelt, insbesondere über 'bedingte' Empfindungen.* Rohrer, Vienna. [370, 405]

Kohler, I., 1953. Umgewöhnung in Wahrnehmungsbereich. *Pyramide*, **5**, 92–95; **6**, 109–113. [370, 372, 409, 413, 416]

Kohler, I., 1955. Experiments with prolonged optical distortions. *Acta psychol.*, *Hague*, **11**, 176–178. [370, 414]

Kohler, I., 1956a. Orientierung durch den Gehörsinn. *Pyramide*, **5**, 81–93. [370]

Kohler, I., 1956b. Die Methode des Brillenversuches in der Wahrnehmungspsychologie; mit Bemerkungen zur Lehre der Adaptation. *Z. exp. angew. Psychol.*, **3**, 381–417. [370, 372]

Kohler, I., 1962. Experiments with goggles. *Sci. Amer.*, **206**, 62–86. [370]

Köhler, W., 1940. *Dynamics in Psychology.* Liveright, New York. [323]

Köhler, W., and Dinnerstein, D., 1947. Figural after-effects in kinaesthesis. In *Miscellanea Psychologia Albert Michotte.* Librairie Philosophique, Paris. [85, 231]

Köhler, W., and Wallach, H., 1944. Figural after-effects: an investigation of visual processes. *Proc. Amer. phil. Soc.*, **88**, 269–357. [162, 219, 221, 224, 226]

Koike, Y., 1959. An observation on the eye-speed of nystagmus. *Acta oto-laryng.*, *Stockh.*, **50**, 377–390. [123]

Kölliker, A., 1862. Untersuchungen über die letzten Endigungen der Nerven. *Z. wiss. Zool.*, **12**, 149–164. [72]

Kompanejetz, S., 1924. Die Beteiligung des mechanischen Factors bei der Gegenrollung der Augen. *Arch. Ohr.-, Nas.-, u. KehlkHeilk.*, **112**, 1–11. [54]

Kompanejetz, S., 1925. On compensatory eye movements in deaf mutes. *Acta otolaryng.*, *Stockh.*, **7**, 323. [55]

Kompanejetz, S., 1928. Investigation on the counterrolling of the eyes in optimum head-positions. *Acta oto-laryng.*, *Stockh.*, **12**, 332–350. [50, 55]

Kopfermann, H., 1930. Psychologische Untersuchungen über die Wirkung zweidimensionaler Darstellungen körperlicher Gebilde. *Psychol. Forsch.*, **13**, 293–364. [325]

Kornmuller, A. E., 1930. Eine experimentalle Anästhesie der äusseren Augenmuskeln am Menschen und ihre Auswirkungen. *J. Psychol. Neurol.*, *Lpz.*, **41**, 354–366. [66]

Kottenhoff, H., 1957a. Situational and personal influences on space perception with experimental spectacles. I. Prolonged experiments with inverting glasses. *Acta psychol.*, *Hague*, **13**, 79–97. [370]

Kottenhoff, H., 1957b. Situational and personal influences on space perception with experimental spectacles. II. Semi-prolonged tests with inverting glasses. *Acta Psychol.*, *Hague*, **13**, 151–161. [370, 405]

Kottenhoff, H., 1961. *Was ist Richtiges Sehen mit Umkehrbrillen und in Welchem Sinne Stellt Sich das Sehen um?* Anton Hain, Meisenheim am Glan, Germany. [413]

Kramer, F., and Moskiewicz, G., 1901. Beiträge zur Lehre von den Lage- und Bewegungsempfindungen. *Z. Psychol. Physiol. Sinnesorg.*, **25**, 114–115. [89]

Krantz, F., 1930. Experimentell strukturpsychologische Untersuchungen über die Abhängigkeit der Wahrnehmungswelt vom Persönlichkeitstypus. *Z. Psychol.*, **16**, 105–214. [220]

Kraus, R. N., 1960. Evaluation of a simple coriolis test for vestibular sensitivity. *Aerosp. Med.*, **31**, 852–855. [129]

Krause, 1843. Cited in Nagel, 1896. [50]

Krauskopf, J., 1954. Figural after-effects in auditory space. *Amer. J. Psychol.*, **67**, 278–287. [162]

Kreidl, A., and Gatscher, S., 1923. Über die dichotische Zeitschwelle. *Pflüg. Arch. ges. Physiol.*, **200**, 366–373. [158]

Krus, D. M., Wapner, S., and Freeman, H., 1958. Effects of reserpine and iproniazid (Marsilid) on space localization. *Arch. Neurol. Psychiat.*, *Chicago*, **80**, 768–770. [188]

Kubie, L. S., and Beckmann, J. W., 1929. Diplopia without extra-ocular palsies, caused by heteronymous defects in the visual fields associated with defective macular vision. *Brain*, **52**, 317–333. [21]

Kuffler, S. W., and Hunt, C. C., 1952. The mammalian small-nerve fibres: A system for efferent nervous regulation of muscle spindle discharge. *Res. Publ., Ass. nerv. ment. Dis.*, **30**, 24–47. [77]

Kuffler, S. W., Hunt, C. C., and Quilliam, J. P., 1951. The function of small-nerve fibers in mammalian ventral roots. Efferent muscle spindle innervation. *J. Neurophysiol.*, **14**, 29–54. [77]

Kühne, W., 1863. Über die Endigung der Nerven in den Muskeln. *Virchows Arch.*, **27**, 508–533. [72]

Kulwicki, P. A., Schlei, E. J., and Vergamini, P. L., 1962. Weightless man: self-rotation techniques. AMRL-TDR-62-129. Wright-Patterson AFB, Ohio. [431]

Kundt, A., 1863. Untersuchungen über Augenmass und optische Täuschungen. *Pog. Ann. Phys. Chem.*, **120**, 118–129. [37]

Künnapas, T. M., 1955. An analysis of the vertical horizontal illusion. *J. exp. Psychol.*, **49**, 134–140. [37]

Künnapas, T. M., 1957. The vertical–horizontal illusion and the visual field. *J. exp. Psychol.*, **53**, 405–407. [37]

Künnapas, T. M., 1958. Influence of head inclination on the vertical–horizontal illusion. *J. Psychol.*, **46**, 179–185. [37]

Künnapas, T. M., 1959. The vertical–horizontal illusion in artificial visual fields. *J. Psychol.*, **47**, 41–48. [37]

L'Abate, L., 1960. Recognition of paired trigrams as a function of associative value and associative strength. *Science*, **131**, 984–985. [303]

Lachmann, J., and Bergmann, F., 1961. Mutual influence of nystagmogenic centres during labyrinthine or central nystagmus. *Acta oto-laryng., Stockh.*, **53**, 295–310. [123]

Lachmann, J., Bergmann, F., and Monnier, M., 1957. Localisation d'un centre nystagmogène dans le tronc cérébral. *J. Physiol. Path. gén.*, **49**, 248. [123]

Laidlaw, R. W., and Hamilton, M. A., 1937a. The quantitative measurement of apperception of passive movement. *Bull. neurol. Inst. N.Y.*, **6**, 145–153. [83]

Laidlaw, R. W., and Hamilton, M. A., 1937b. A study of thresholds in apperception of passive movement among normal control subjects. *Bull. neurol. Inst. N.Y.*, **6**, 268–273. [83]

Lancaster, W. B., 1943. Terminology in ocular motility and allied subjects. *Amer. J. Ophthal*, **26**, 122–133. [47, 50]

Langhorne, M. C., 1948. The effects of maze rotation on learning. *J. gen. Psychol.*, **38**, 191–205. [264]

Lansberg, M. P., 1955a. On the origin of the unpleasant sensations elicited by head movements during after sensations. *Aeromed. Acta*, **4**, 67–80. [438]

Lansberg, M. P., 1955b. The function of the vestibular sense and the construction of a satellite. *Aeromed. Acta*, **4**, 172–180. [438]

Laporte, Y., and Lundberg, A., 1956. Functional organisation of the dorsal spinocerebellar tract in the cat. III. Single fibre recording in Flechig's Fasciculus on adequate stimulation of primary afferent neurons. *Acta physiol. scand.*, **36**, 204–218. [76]

Laporte, Y., Lundberg, A., and Oscarsson, O., 1956a. Functional organisation of the dorsal spinocerebellar tract in the cat. I. Recording of mass discharge in dissected Flechig's Fasciculus. *Acta physiol. scand.*, **36**, 175–187. [76]

Laporte, Y., Lundberg, A., and Oscarsson, O., 1956b. Functional organisation of the dorsal spinocerebellar tract in the cat. II. Single fibre recording in Flechig's Fasciculus on electrical stimulation of various peripheral nerves. *Acta physiol. scand.*, **36**, 188–203. [76]

Lashley, K. S., 1917. The accuracy of movement in the absence of excitation from the moving organ. *Amer. J. Physiol.*, **43**, 169–194. [95, 396]

Law, T., and DeValois, R. L., 1958. Periorbital potentials recorded during small eye movements. *Pap. Mich. Acad. Sci.*, **43**, 171–180. [57]

Leakey, D. M., 1959. Some measurements on the effects of interchannel intensity and time differences in two channel sound systems. *J. acoust. Soc. Amer.*, **31**, 977–986. [148]

Leakey, D. M., and Cherry, E. C., 1957. Influence of noise upon the equivalence of intensity differences and small time delays in two loudspeaker systems. *J. acoust. Soc. Amer.*, **29**, 284–286. [164, 166]

Leakey, D. M., Sayers, B. McA., and Cherry, E. C., 1958. Binaural fusion of low- and high-frequency sounds. *J. acoust. Soc. Amer.*, **30**, 222–223. [155]

Lebensohn, J. E., 1931. Nystagmus of ocular origin. *Arch. Ophthal., N.Y.*, **5**, 638–644. [58, 59]

Leibowitz, H., 1952. The effect of pupil size on visual actuity for photometrically equated test fields at various levels of luminance. *J. opt. Soc. Amer.*, **42**, 416–422. [33, 34]

Leibowitz, H., 1953. Some observations and theory on the variation of visual acuity with the orientation of the test object. *J. opt. Soc. Amer.*, **43**, 902–905. [33, 34, 35]

Leibowitz, H., 1955. Some factors influencing the variability of vernier adjustments. *Amer. J. Psychol.*, **68**, 266–273. [34]

Leibowitz, H., Myers, N. A., and Grant, D. A., 1955a. Frequency of seeing and radial localization of single and multiple visual stimuli. *J. exp. Psychol.*, **50**, 369–373. [35]

Leibowitz, H., Myers, N. A., and Grant, D. A., 1955b. Radial localization of a single stimulus as a function of luminance and duration of exposure. *J. opt. Soc. Amer.*, **45**, 76–78. [181]

Leiri, F., 1927. Über optokinetisch hervorgerufene visuelle Täuschungen. *v. Graefes Arch. Ophthal.*, **119**, 719–732. [59]

Leksell, L., 1945. The action potential and excitatory effects of the small ventral root fibers to skeletal muscle. *Acta physiol. scand.*, **10**, Suppl. **31**, 84 pp. [77]

Lenkner, H., 1934. *Die Psychologischen Grundlagen der Fortbewegung des Menschen in der Zweidimensionalen unter Besonderer Berücksichtigung der Verkehrstechnik (das Drall-Problem)*. Trilsch, Würzburg. [258]

Lenz, H., 1949. Über zentral bedingte Störungen des Grössensehens, *Poetzl Festschrift*, 316–323. Wagner, Innsbruck. [211]

Leriche, R., 1930. Recherches sur le rôle de l'innervation sensitive des articulations et de leur appareil ligamentaire dans la physiologie pathologique articulaire. *Pre. méd.*, **38**, 417–418. [81]

Levinstein, S., 1905. *Kinderzeichnungen bis zum 14 Lebensjahre*. Tafel, Leipzig. [343, 344]

Levy, L., 1919. Vestibular reactions in five hundred and forty-one aviators. *J. Amer. med. Ass.*, **72**, 716. [128]

Lewis, P., 1944. Bilateral monocular diplopia with amblyopia. *Amer. J. Ophthal*, **27**, 1026–1027. [21]

Licklider, J. C. R., and Webster, J. C., 1949. The discriminability of interaural phase relations in two-component tones. *J. acoust. Soc. Amer.*, **21**, 62A. [155]

Licklider, J. C. R., Webster, J. C., and Hedlum, J. M., 1950. On the frequency limits of binaural beats. *J. acoust. Soc. Amer.*, **22**, 468–473. [155]

Liddle, D., and Foss, B. M., 1963. A vertical–horizontal illusion for movement perceived tactually. *Nature, Lond.*, **197**, 108. [37]

Lidén, G., and Nordlund, B., 1960. Stereophonic or monaural hearing aids. *Acta oto-laryng., Stockh., Suppl.*, **158**. [170]

Lidvall, H. F., 1961a. Vertigo and nystagmus responses to caloric stimuli repeated at short intervals. *Acta oto-laryng., Stockh.*, **53**, 33–44. [129]

Lidvall, H. F., 1961b. Vertigo and nystagmus responses to caloric stimuli repeated at short and long intervals. *Acta oto-laryng., Stockh.*, **53**, 507–518. [131]

Lidvall, H. F., 1962. Specific and non-specific traits of habituation in nystagmus responses to caloric stimuli. *Acta oto-laryng., Stockh.*, **55**, 315–325. [131, 132]

Liebert, H., 1940. Über die Schwankungen beim Stehen. *Arbeitsphysiologie*, **11**, 151–157. [253]

Liebert, R. S., and Rudel, R. G., 1959. Auditory localization and adaptation to body tilt: A developmental study. *Child Develpm.*, **30**, 81–90. [160]

Liebert, R. S., Wapner, S., and Werner, H., 1957. Studies in the effects of lysergic acid diethylamide (L.S.D. 25): Visual perception of verticality in schizophrenic and normal adults. *Arch. Neurol. Psychiat.*, *Chicago*, **77**, 193–201. [192]

Liebig, F. G., 1933. Über unsere Orientierung im Raume bei Ausschluss der Augen. *Z. Sinnesphysiol.*, **64**, 251–282. [259]

Lincoln, R. S., and Averbach, E., 1956. Spatial factors in check reading of dial groups. *J. appl. Psychol.*, **40**, 105–108. [303]

Ling, B.-C., 1941. Form discrimination as a learning cue in infants. *Comp. Psychol. Monogr.*, **17**, No. 86. [335]

Lissman, H. W., 1950. Proprioception. In *Physiological Mechanisms in Animal Behaviour*, *Soc. exp. Biol. Symp. IV*. Cambridge Univ. Press, Cambridge. [72]

Lloyd, D. P. C., 1943. Neuron patterns controlling transmission of ipsilateral hindlimb reflexes in cat. *J. Neurophysiol.*, **6**, 298–315. [74]

Lloyd, D. P. C., 1960. Spinal mechanisms involved in somatic activities. In *Handbook of Physiology* Sec. 1, Vol. II. Amer. Physiol. Soc., Washington. p. 929. [241]

Lloyd, D. P. C., and McIntyre, A. K., 1950. Dorsal column conduction of group I muscle afferent impulses and their relay through Clarke's column. *J. Neurophysiol.*, **13**, 39–54. [76]

Loeb, J., 1890. Untersuchungen über die Orientirung im Fühlraum der Hand und im Blickraum. *Pflüg. Arch. ges. Physiol.*, **46**, 1–46. [88]

Loemker, K. K., 1930. Certain factors determining the accuracy of a response to the direction of a visual object. *J. exp. Psychol.*, **13**, 500–518. [350]

Loftus, J. P. (Ed.), 1963. Symp. on motion sickness with special reference to weightlessness. AMRL-TDR-63-25. Wright-Patterson AFB, Ohio. [135]

Loftus, J. P., and Hammer, L. R., 1961. Weightlessness and performance: a review of the literature. ASD Tech. Rep. 61-166. Wright-Patterson AFB, Ohio. [420, 442]

Long, G. E., and Grether, W. F., 1949. Directional interpretation of dial, scale and pointer movements. Tech. Rep. No. 5910. U.S.A.F. Air Material Command, Dayton, Ohio. [363]

Lord, F. E., 1941. A study of spatial orientation of children. *J. educ. Res.*, **34**, 481–505. [267]

Lord, M. P., and Wright, W. D., 1950. The investigation of eye movements. *Rep. Progr. Phys.*, **13**, 1–23. [65]

Lorente de Nó, R., 1931. Ausgewählte Kapitel aus der vergleichenden Physiologie des Labyrinthes. *Ergebn. Physiol.*, **32**, 73–242. [61, 114]

Loret, B. J., 1961. Optimization of manned orbital satellite vehicle design with respect to artificial gravity. ASD Tech. Rep. 61-688. Wright-Patterson AFB, Ohio. [434, 437, 440, 441]

Loucks, R. B., 1949. The relative effectiveness with which various types of azimuth indicators can be interpreted by novices: I. Tech. Rep. No. 5825. U.S.A.F. Air Material Command, Dayton, Ohio. [363]

Loveless, N. E., 1962. Direction-of-motion stereotypes: A review. *Ergonomics*, **5**, 357–383. [362]

Lowenstein, O., 1950. Labyrinth and equilibrium. In *Physiological Mechanisms in Animal Behaviour, Soc. exp. Biol. Symp. IV.* Cambridge Univ. Press, Cambridge. [108]

Lowenstein, O., 1956a. Comparative physiology of the otolith organs. *Brit. med. Bull.,* **12,** 110–113. [108]

Lowenstein, O., 1956b. Peripheral mechanisms of equilibrium. *Brit. med. Bull.,* **12,** 114–118. [108]

Lowenstein, O., 1961. Problems concerning the mechanism of the hair cells of the vestibular receptors. *Acta oto-laryng., Stockh., Suppl.,* **163,** 56–58. [106]

Lowenstein, O., and Wersäll, J., 1959. A functional interpretation of the electron-microscopic structure of the sensory hairs in the cristae of the elasmobranch, *Raja clavata,* in terms of directional sensitivity. *Nature, Lond.,* **184,** 1807–1808. [109]

Lucannas, F. von, 1924. On the sense of locality in men and animals. *Rev. Revs.,* **70,** 218 (cited by Smith, 1933). [265]

Luchins, A. S., 1954a. Relation of size of light to autokinetic effect. *J. Psychol.,* **38,** 439–452. [29]

Luchins, A. S., 1954b. The autokinetic effect in central and peripheral vision. *J. gen. Psychol.,* **50,** 39–44. [27]

Luchins, A. S., 1954c. The autokinetic effect and gradients of illumination of the visual field. *J. gen. Psychol.,* **50,** 29–37. [28, 29]

Luchins, A. S., and Luchins, E. H., 1963. Half views and autokinetic effect. *Psychol. Rec.,* **13,** 415–444. [28]

Luciani, L., 1884. On the sensorial localisations in the cortex cerebri. *Brain,* **7,** 145–160. [171]

Ludvigh, E., 1952a. Possible role of proprioception in the extra ocular muscles. *Arch. Ophthal., N.Y.,* **48,** 436–441. [67, 68]

Ludvigh, E., 1952b. Control of ocular movements and visual interpretation of environment. *Arch. Ophthal., N.Y.,* **48,** 442–448. [64, 66, 68, 396]

Lund, F. H., 1930. Physical asymmetries and disorientation. *Amer. J. Psychol.,* **42,** 51–62. [257, 258]

Lundberg, A., and Oscarsson, O., 1956. Functional organisation of the dorsal spino-cerebellar tract in the cat. IV. Synaptic connections of afferents from Golgi tendon organs and muscle spindles. *Acta physiol. scand.,* **38,** 53–75. [76]

Luria, S. M., 1963. The effect of body-position on meridional variations in scotopic acuity. *Amer. J. Psychol.,* **75,** 598–606. [32]

McCabe, B. F., 1960. Vestibular suppression in figure skaters. *Trans. Amer. Acad. Ophthal. Oto-laryng.,* **64,** 264–268. [129]

McCabe, B. F., and Lawrence, M., 1959. Suppression of vestibular sequelae following rapid rotation. *J. Aviat. Med.,* **30,** 194A. [128]

McCally, M., and Lawton, R. W., 1963. The pathophysiology of disuse and the problem of prolonged weightlessness: a review. AMRL-TDR-63-3. Wright-Patterson AFB, Ohio. [427]

McCord, F., 1953. The measurement of adjustive eye movements. Joint Proj. NM. 001.063.01, Rep. No. 31. U.S. Nav. Sch. aviat. Med., Pensacola, Fla. [51]

MacDougall, R., 1903. The subjective horizon. *Psychol. Rev. Monogr., Suppl.*, **4**. [185, 187]

McEwen, P., 1958. Figural after-effects. *Brit. J. Psychol. Monogr., Suppl.*, **31**. [85, 231]

McFarland, J. H., 1962. Visual and proprioceptive changes during visual exposure to a tilted line. *Percept. mot. Skills*, **15**, 322. [216]

McFarland, J. H., Wapner, S., and Werner, H., 1962. Relation between perceived location of objects and perceived location of one's own body. *Percept. mot. Skills*, **15**, 331–341. [194]

McFarland, J. H., Werner, H., and Wapner, S., 1962. The effect of postural factors on the distribution of tactual sensitivity and the organization of tactual-kinaesthetic space. *J. exp. Psychol.*, **63**, 148–154. [288]

McFarland, R. A., Holway, A. J., and Hurvich, L. M., 1942. *Studies of Visual Fatigue.* Harvard Univ., Boston. [36]

McFie, J., Piercy, M. F., and Zangwill, O. L., 1950. Visual-spatial agnosia associated with lesions of the right cerebral hemisphere. *Brain*, **73**, 167–190. [270]

McGinnis, J. M., 1930. Eye movements and optic nystagmus in early infancy. *Genet. Psychol. Monogr.*, **8**, 321–430. [56, 59]

McGough, G. P., Deering, I. D., and Stewart, W. B., 1950. Inhibition of knee jerk from tendon spindles of crureus. *J. Neurophysiol.*, **13**, 343–350. [76]

McGraw, M. B., 1941. Development of rotary–vestibular reactions of human infants. *Child Develpm.*, **12**, 17–19. [134]

Mach, E., 1873. Physikalische Versuche über den Gleichgewichtssinn des Menschen *S.B. Akad. Wiss. Wien*, **68**, 124–140. [198]

Mach, E., 1874. Versuche über den Gleichgewichtessinn *S.B. Akad. Wiss. Wien*, **69**, 121. [198]

Mach, E., 1875. *Grundlinien der Lehre von den Bewegungsempfindungen.* Engelmann, Leipzig. [101, 116, 124, 198]

Mach, E., 1886. *Beiträge zur Analyse der Empfindungen* 1st ed. Fischer, Jena. English trans. 1958. *The Analysis of sensations.* Dover, New York. [66, 296]

Mach, E., 1897. *Contributions to the Analysis of the Sensations.* Trans. C. M. Williams. Open Court Publishing, Chicago. [31]

MacKay, D. M., 1958. Perceptual stability of a strobscopically lit visual field containing self-luminous objects. *Nature, Lond.*, **181**, 507–508. [69, 70]

Mackensen, G., 1953. Untersuchungen zur Physiologie des optokinetischen Nystagmus. *Klin. Mbl. Augenheilk.*, **123**, 133–143. [57]

Mackensen, G., 1954. Untersuchungen zur Physiologie des optokinetischen Nystagmus. *v. Graefes Arch. Ophthal.*, **155**, 284–313. [56, 58]

Mackensen, G., and Wiegman, O., 1959. Studies on the physiology of optokinetic after-nystagmus: I. Relation to the direction and velocity of the stimulus. *v. Graefes Arch. Ophthal.*, **160**, 497–509. [59]

McLay, K., Madigan, M. F., and Ormerod, F. C., 1957. Anomalies in the recorded movements of the eye during opto-kinetic, rotatory and caloric stimulation in normal subjects. *Ann. Otol., etc., St Louis*, **66**, 473–486. [59, 131]

McNally, W. J., 1944. The otoliths and the part they play in man. *Laryngoscope, St Louis*, **54**, 304–323. [135]

McNally, W. J., and Stewart, E. A., 1942. Physiology of the labyrinth reviewed in relation to sea sickness and other forms of motion sickness. *War Med., Chicago*, **2**, 683–771. [135, 138]

McReynolds, J., and Worchel, P., 1954. Geographic orientation in the blind. *J. gen. Psychol.*, **51**, 221–236. [261, 263]

Magnus, R., 1924. *Körperstellung*. Springer, Berlin. [109, 235]

Magnus, R., 1926. Some results of studies in the physiology of posture. The Cameron Prize Lectures. *Lancet*, **2**, 531–536, 583–588. [235]

Mahoney, J. L., Harlan, W. L., and Bickford, R. G., 1957. Visual and other factors influencing caloric nystagmus in normal subjects. *Arch. Otolaryng., Chicago*, **66**, 46–53. [122]

Malán, M., 1940. Zur Erblichkeit der Orientierungsfähigkeit im Raum. *Z. Morph. Anthr.*, **39**, 1–23. [266]

Mallock, A., 1908. Note on the sensibility of the ear to the direction of explosive sounds. *Proc. roy. Soc., Ser. A.*, **80**, 110–112. [158]

Mann, C. W., 1951. The effects of auditory-vestibular nerve pathology on space perception. *J. exp. Psychol.*, **42**, 450–456. [196, 247]

Mann, C. W., 1952a. Visual factors in the perception of verticality. *J. exp. Psychol.*, **44**, 460–464. [204, 205]

Mann, C. W., 1952b. An analysis of the oculogyral effect. *J. Aviat. Med.*, **23**, 246–253. [103]

Mann, C. W., Berthelot-Berry, N. H., and Dauterive, H. J., 1949. The perception of the vertical: I. Visual and non-labyrinthine cues. *J. exp. Psychol.*, **39**, 538–547. [179, 192, 199, 247]

Mann, C. W., and Boring, R. O., 1953. The role of instruction in experimental space perception. *J. exp. Psychol.*, **45**, 44–48. [207]

Mann, C. W., Guedry, F. E., and Ray, J. T., 1951. Post-rotational perception of apparent bodily rotation. *J. exp. Psychol.*, **41**, 114–120. [125]

Mann, C. W., and Passey, G. E., 1951. The perception of the vertical: V. Adjustment to the postural vertical as a function of the magnitude of postural tilt and duration of exposure. *J. exp. Psychol.*, **41**, 108–113. [241, 242, 243, 244, 245, 246]

Mann, C. W., Passey, G. E., and Ambler, R. K., 1950. The perception of the vertical: VII. Effect of varying intervals of delay in a tilted position upon the perception of the postural vertical. Jnt. Rep. No. 12. U.S. Nav. Sch. aviat. Med. and Tulane Univ. [242, 244, 245]

Mann, C. W., and Ray, J. T., 1956a. The perception of the vertical: XIII. An investigation of quadrant differences. Jnt. Proj. No. 39. Rep. No. 39. U.S. Nav. Sch. aviat. Med. Pensacola, Fla. [242, 244, 245, 246]

Mann, C. W., and Ray, J. T., 1956b. The perception of the vertical: XIV. The effect of rate of movement on the judgment of the vertical. Proj. NM.001.110.500 Rep. No. 40. U.S. Nav. Sch. aviat. Med., Pensacola, Fla. [244, 245, 246]

Marie, P., and Béhague, B., 1919. Syndrome de désorientation dans l'espace consécutif aux plaies profondes du lobe frontal. *Rev. neurol.*, **26**, 1–14. [270]

Marks, M. R., 1949. Some phenomena attendant on long fixation. *Amer. J. Psychol.*, **62**, 392–398. [29]

Mathes, R. C., 1955. Monaural direction finding. *J. acoust. Soc. Amer.*, **27**, 792. [159]

Matin, L., and MacKinnon, G. E., 1964. Autokinetic movement: selective manipulation of directional components by image stabilization. *Science*, **143**, 147–148. [26]

Matsumoto, M., 1897. Researches on auditory space. *Stud. Yale psychol. Lab.*, **5**. [146]

Matthews, B. H. C., 1931a. The response of a single end organ. *J. Physiol.*, **71**, 64–110. [72]

Matthews, B. H. C., 1931b. The response of a muscle spindle during active contraction of a muscle. *J. Physiol.*, **72**, 153–174. [72]

Matthews, B. H. C., 1933. Nerve endings in mammalian muscle. *J. Physiol.*, **78**, 1–53. [75]

Matthews, P. B. C., 1962. The differentiation of two types of fusimotor fibre by their effects on the dynamic response of muscle spindle primary endings. *Quart. J. exp. Physiol.*, **47**, 324–333. [77]

Matthews, P. B. C., 1964. Muscle spindles and their motor control. *Physiol. Rev.*, **44**, 219–288. [72, 74, 77]

Matzker, J., and Welker, H., 1959. Die Prüfung des Richtungshörens zum Nachweis und zur topischen Diagnostik von Hirnerkrankungen. *Z. Laryng.- Rhin.- Oto.* **38**, 277–294. [172]

Maxwell, S. S., 1923. *Labyrinth and Equilibrium.* Lippincott, Philadelphia. [138]

Mayne, R., 1950. The dynamic characteristics of the semicircular canals. *J. comp. Physiol. Psychol.*, **43**, 309–319. [103]

Meda, E., 1952. A research on the threshold for the Coriolis and Purkinje phenomena of excitation of the semi-circular canals. *Arch. Fisiol.*, **52**, 116. Trans. by E. R. Hope. Canada, Def. Sci. Inf. Service, DRB. T171. [436]

Merton, P. A., 1956. Compensatory rolling movements of the eye. *J. Physiol.*, **132**, 25–27P. [54]

Merton, P. A., 1958. Compensatory rolling movements of the eyes. *Proc. R. Soc. Med.*, **52**, 184–185. [54]

Merton, P. A., 1961. The accuracy of directing the eyes and the hand in the dark. *J. Physiol.*, **156**, 555–577. [67, 84, 354]

Merton, P. A., 1964. Absence of conscious position sense in the human eyes. In Bender, M. B. (Ed.), *The Oculomotor System*, Harper and Row, New York. [396, 397]

Metzger, E., 1927, Untersuchungen über die Wirkungsweise der Hemianopsie-Brillen. *v. Graefes Arch. Ophthal.*, **118**, 487–499. [25]

Meyer, O., 1900. Ein- und doppelseitige homonyme Hemianopsie mit Orientierungs-störungen. *Mschr. Psychiat. Neurol.*, **8**, 440–456. [269]

Meyer, P., 1913. Über die Produktion eingepraegter Figuren usw. *Z. Psychol.*, **64**, 34–91. [341]

Mikaelian, H., and Held, R., 1964. Two types of adaptation to an optically-rotated visual field. *Amer. J. Psychol.*, **77**, 257–263. [218]

Miller, B. L., and Harcum, E. R., 1963. Left–right redundancy and the perception of visual patterns. Paper read to Virginia Acad. Sci., Roanoke. [307]

Miller, E. F., 1962. Counter-rolling of the human eyes produced by head tilt with respect to gravity. *Acta oto-laryng., Stockh.*, **54**, 479–501. [53]

Miller, E. F., and Graybiel, A., 1962. Comparison of autokinetic movement perceived by normal persons and deaf subjects with bilateral labyrinthine defects.
Proj. MR005. 13-6001, Subtask 1, Rep. No. 66. U.S. Nav. Sch. aviat. Med., Pensacola, Fla. [28]

Miller, E. F., and Graybiel, A., 1963. Rotary autokinesis and displacement of the
visual horizontal associated with head (body) position. Proj. MR005.13-6001,
Subtask 1, Rep. No. 77. U.S. Nav. Sch. aviat. Med., Pensacola, Fla. [192]

Mills, A. W., 1958. On the minimum audible angle. *J. acoust. Soc. Amer.*, **30**, 237-246.
[149, 150, 151]

Mills, A. W., 1960. Lateralization of high-frequency tones. *J. acoust. Soc. Amer.*, **32**,
132-134. [151, 152, 153, 156]

Mishkin, M., and Forgays, D. G., 1952. Word recognition as a function of retinal
locus. *J. exp. Psychol.*, **43**, 43-48. [307]

Mitchell, M. J. H., and Vince, M. A., 1951. The direction of movement of machine
controls. *Quart. J. exp. Psychol.*, **3**, 24-35.

Miyakawa, T., 1944. Experimental research on the structure of visual space when we
bend forward and look backward between the spread legs. *Jap. J. Psychol.*, **18**,
289-309. [325]

Miyakawa, T., 1950. Experimental research on the structure of visual space when we
bend forward and look backward between the spread legs, II. *Jap. J. Psychol.*, **20**,
14-23. [325]

Montandon, A., 1954. A new technique for vestibular investigation. *Acta oto-laryng.*,
Stockh., **44**, 594-596. [115]

Montandon, A., and Russbach, A., 1955. L'épreuve giratoire liminaire. *Pract. oto-
rhino-laryng.*, **17**, 224-236. [116]

Moore, E. W., and Cramer, R. L., 1962. Perception of postural verticality: effects of
flying experience upon reduction of error. AFSC Proj. 7756, Task No. 59722.
[249]

Morant, R. B., 1958. The effect of labyrinthian and figural stimulation on the perception of the apparent median plane. Paper read to East. Psychol. Ass., Philadelphia. [286, 287]

Morant, R. B., 1959a. Displacement and configurational effects induced by labyrinthian stimulation. Paper read to East. Psychol. Ass., Atlantic City. [126]

Morant, R. B., 1959b. The visual perception of the median plane as influenced by
labyrinthian stimulation. *J. Psychol.*, **47**, 25-35. [287]

Morant, R. B., and Aronoff, J. C. Tilt after-effects with and without a visual frame
of reference. (In press.) [210]

Morant, R. B., and Beller, H. K. Adaptation to prismatically rotated visual fields.
Science (in press). [219]

Morant, R. B., and Harris, J. R., 1965. Two different after-effects of exposure to visual
tilts. *Amer. J. Psychol.*, **78**, 218-226. [226, 227, 228]

Morant, R. B., and Mikaelian, H. H., 1960. Inter-field tilt after-effects. *Percept. mot.
Skills*, **10**, 95-98. [217, 228]

Morant, R. B., and Mistovich, M., 1960. Tilt after-effects between the vertical and
horizontal axes. *Percept. mot. Skills*, **10**, 75-81. [221, 226, 227]

Morant, R. B., and Mistovich, M. Interaction between kinaesthetic and visual space. I. Kinaesthetic and inter-modal tilt after-effects. *Acta psychol., Hague* (in press). [229, 232, 233]

Morgan, M. W., 1955. A unique case of double monocular diplopia. *Amer. J. Optom.*, **32**, 70–87. [21]

Morinaga, S., Noguchi, K., and Ohishi, A., 1962. The horizontal–vertical illusion and the relation of spatial and retinal orientations. *Jap. psychol. Res.*, **4**, 25–29. [37]

Mountcastle, V. B., 1957. Modality and topographic properties of single neurons of cat's somatic sensory cortex. *J. Neurophysiol.*, **20**, 408–434. [76, 82]

Mountcastle, V. B., Covian, M. R., and Harrison, C. R., 1950. The central representation of some forms of deep sensibility. *Proc. Ass. Res. nerv. Dis.*, **30**, 339–370. [76, 82]

Moushegian, G., and Jeffress, L. A., 1959. Role of interaural time and intensity differences in the lateralization of low-frequency tones. *J. acoust. Soc. Amer.*, **31**, 1441–1445. [164, 166, 167, 168]

Mouzon, J. C., 1955. Stereophonic hearing with one earphone. *J. acoust. Soc. Amer.*, **27**, 381L [159]

Mowrer, O. H., 1934a. Influence of 'excitement' on duration of post-rotational nystagmus. *Acta oto-laryng., Stockh.*, **19**, 46–54. [131]

Mowrer, O. H., 1934b. The modification of vestibular nystagmus by means of repeated elicitation. *Comp. Psychol. Monogr.*, **9**, 1–48. [128, 129, 130]

Mowrer, O. H., 1935a. Some neglected factors which influence the duration of post-rotational nystagmus. *Acta oto-laryng., Stockh.*, **22**, 1–23. [122]

Mowrer, O. H., 1935b. A device for studying eye–hand co-ordination without visual guidance. *Amer. J. Psychol.*, **47**, 493–495. [385]

Mowrer, O. H., 1936. 'Maturation' vs. 'learning' in the development of vestibular and optokinetic nystagmus. *J. genet. Psychol.*, **48**, 383–404. [59]

Mowrer, O. H., 1937. The influence of vision during bodily rotation upon the duration of post-rotational vestibular nystagmus. *Acta oto-laryng., Stockh.*, **25**, 351–364. [122]

Mowrer, O. H., Ruch, T. C., and Miller, N. E., 1935. The corneo-retinal potential difference as the basis of the galvanometric method of recording eye movements. *Amer. J. Physiol.*, **114**, 433–428. [57]

Mudd, S. A., and McCormick, E. J., 1960. The use of auditory cues in a visual search task. *J. appl. Psychol.*, **44**, 184–188. [303]

Mulder, M. E., 1874. Over parallele Rolbewegingen der Oogen. *Onderz. psychiol. Lab. Utrecht. Hoogesch.*, **3**, 168. [50, 52, 53, 54, 194]

Mulder, M. E., 1875. Über parallele Rollbewegung der Augen. *v. Graefes Arch. Ophthal.*, **20**, 68–90.

Mulder, M. E., 1897. De la rotation compensatrice de l'oeil en cas d'inclination à droit ou à gauche de la tête. *Arch. Ophtal.*, Paris, **17**, 465–475. [54]

Müller, D. D., 1962a. A digital computer analysis of the behavior of long tetherlines in space. AMRL-TDR-62-123. Wright-Patterson AFB, Ohio. [435]

Müller, D. D., 1962b. Relative motion in the docking phase of orbital rendezvous. AMRL-TDR-62-124. Wright-Patterson AFB, Ohio. [436]

Müller, D. D., and Simons, J. C., 1962. Weightless man: single-impulse trajectories for orbital workers. AMRL-TDR-62-103. Wright-Patterson AFB, Ohio. [435]

Müller, G. E., 1961. Über das Aubertsche Phänomenon. Z. Psychol. Physiol. Sinnesorg., 49, 109–246. [190]

Muller, H. J., 1958. Approximation to a gravity-free situation for the human organism achievable at moderate expense. Science, 128, 772. [421]

Muller, P. F., Sidorsky, R. C., Slivinske, A. J., Alluisi, E. A., and Fitts, P. M., 1955. The symbolic coding of information on cathode ray tubes and similar displays. U.S.A.F. WADC Tech. Rep. No. 55–375. [181]

Münsterberg, H., 1889. Augenmass. Beit. exp. Psychol., 2, 125–181. [38]

Münsterberg, H., and Pierce, A. H., 1894. The localization of sound. Psychol. Rev., 1, 461–476. [159]

Mussen, A. T., 1927. Experimental investigations on the cerebellum. Brain, 50, 313–349. [238]

Myers, R. E., Sperry, R. W., and McCurdy, N. M., 1962. Neural mechanisms in visual guidance of limb movement. Arch. Neurol., Lond., 7, 195–202. [381]

Nachmias, J., 1953. Figural after-effects in kinaesthetic space. Amer. J. Psychol., 66, 609–612. [84]

Nachmias, J., 1959. Two-dimensional motion of the retinal image during monocular fixation. J. opt. Soc. Amer., 49, 901–908. [32, 47]

Nachmias, J., 1960. Meridional variations in visual acuity and eye movements during fixation. J. opt. Soc. Amer., 50, 569–571. [32]

Nachmias, J., 1961. Determiners of the drift of the eye during monocular fixation. J. opt. Soc. Amer., 51, 761–766. [47]

Nagel, W. A., 1896. Über kompensatorische Raddrehungen der Augen. Z. Psychol. Physiol. Sinnesorg., 12, 331–354. [50, 52, 53, 55, 193]

Nagel, W. A., 1898. Über das Aubertsche Phänomen und verwandte Täuschungen über die vertikale Richtung. Z. Psychol. Physiol. Sinnesorg., 16, 373–398. [192, 193]

Nair, P. J., 1958. Relationships between postural and conative aspects of organismic state and perceptual localization of the apparent horizon. M.A. Thesis, Clark Univ. [186]

Naylor, G. F. K., 1963. Effects of stress on the perception of direction. Aust. J. Psychol., 15, 17–28. [196]

Neal, E., 1926. Visual localization of the vertical. Amer. J. Psychol., 37, 287–291. [179, 201]

Neff, W. D., and Diamond, I. T., 1958. The neural basis of auditory discrimination. In Harlow, H. F., and Woolsey, C. N. (Eds.), Biological and Biochemical Bases of Behavior. Univ. Wisconsin Press, Madison. p. 101–126. [171]

Neilson, J. M., 1938. Gerstmann Syndrome; finger agnosia, agraphia, confusion of right and left and acalculia; comparison of this syndrome with disturbances of body scheme resulting from lesions of right side of brain. Arch. Neurol. Psychiat., Chicago, 39, 536–560. [291]

Newhall, S. M., 1937. Identification by young children of differentially oriented visual forms. Child Develpm., 8, 105–111. [334]

Nielsen, T. I., 1963. Volition: a new experimental approach. *Scand. J. Psychol.*, **4**, 225–230. [360]

Niven, J. I., and Hixson, W. C., 1961. Frequency response of the human semicircular canals: I. Steady-state ocular nystagmus response to high-level, sinusoidal angular rotations. Proj. MR005.13-6001, Subtask 1, Rep. No. 58. U.S. Nav. Sch. aviat. Med., Pensacola, Fla. [103]

Noble, C. E., 1949. The perception of the vertical: III. The visual vertical as a function of centrifugal and gravitational forces. *J. exp. Psychol.*, **39**, 839–850. [198]

Noble, R. L., 1945. Observations on various types of motion causing vomiting in animals. *Canad. J. Res.*, Sec. E, **23**, 212. [136]

Noji, R., 1929. Über optisch erzwungene parellele Rollungen der Augen. *v. Graefes Arch. Ophthal.*, **122**, 562–571. [56, 229]

Nordlund, B., 1962. Physical factors in angular localization. *Acta oto-laryng., Stockh.*, **54**, 75–93. [143]

Nordlund, B., 1963. Studies of stereophonic hearing. Dept. Otolaryngol. Univ. Göteborg, Sweden. [158]

Nystrom, C. O., and Grant, D. A., 1955. Performance on a key pressing task as a function of the angular correspondence between stimulus and response elements. *Percept. mot. Skills*, **5**, 113–125. [365]

Obersteiner, H., 1881. On allochiria, a peculiar sensory disorder. *Brain*, **4**, 153–163. [292]

Oetjen, F., 1915. Die Bedeutung der Orientierung des Lesestoffes für das Lesen und der Orientierung von sinnlosen Formen für das Wiedererkennen derselben. *Z. Psychol. Physiol. Sinnesorg.*, **71**, 321–355. [324]

Ogilvie, J. C., and Taylor, M. M., 1958. Effect of orientation on the visibility of fine wires. *J. opt. Soc. Amer.*, **48**, 628–629. [32]

Ogle, K. N., 1950. *Researches in Binocular Vision*. Saunders, Philadelphia. [229]

Ohm, J., 1922. Die klinische Bedeutung des optischen Drehnystagmus. *Klin. Mbl. Augenheilk.*, **69**, 323–355. [60]

Ohm, J., 1925. *Das Augenzittern als Gehirnstrahlung*. Urban and Schwarzenberg, Berlin and Vienna. [56]

Ohm, J., 1927a. Zur Theorie des optischen Drehnystagmus. Eine Antwort an Cords. *Klin. Mbl. Augenheilk.*, **78**, 218–227. [56]

Ohm, J., 1927b. Zur Augenzitternkunde, 7 Mitteilung. Der optische Drehnach-nystagmus. *v. Graefes Arch. Ophthal.*, **118**, 103–117. [56, 57, 59]

Ohm, J., 1928. Die Hebelnystagmographie. *v. Graefes Arch. Ophthal.*, **120**, 235–252. [56]

Ohm, J., 1931a. Zur Augenzitternkunde, 26 Mitteilung. Über den Einfluss zentraler und parazentraler Blenden auf den optokinetischen Nystagmus. *v. Graefes Arch. Ophthal.*, **127**, 373–394. [57]

Ohm, J., 1931b. Zur Augenzitternkunde. *v. Graefes Arch. Ophthal.*, **126**, 372–408. [59]

Ohm, J., 1932. Optokinetischer Nystagmus und Nystagmographie im Dienste der Hirndiagnostik. *Arch. Augenheilk.*, **106**, 185–220, 531–554. [60]

Ohm, J., 1936. Cited in Carmichael, Dix, and Hallpike, 1954. [62]

Ohm, J., 1939. Frequenz und Bahn des Augenzitterns der Bergleute in langer Beobachtung. *v. Graefes Arch. Ophthal.*, **141**, 604–620. [61]

O'Leary, J., Heinbecker, P., and Bishop, G. H., 1934. Analysis of function of a nerve to muscle. *Amer. J. Physiol.*, **110**, 636–658. [77]

Onley, J. W., and Volkman, J., 1958. The visual perception of perpendicularity. *Amer. J. Psychol.*, **71**, 504–516. [39]

Orbach, J., 1952. Retinal focus as a factor in recognition of visually perceived words. *Amer. J. Psychol.*, **65**, 555–562. [302]

Ordway, F. I., Gardner, J. P., and Sharpe, M. R., 1962. *Basic Astronautics*. Prentice Hall, Englewood Cliffs, N.J. [420, 444]

Oscarsson, O., 1956. Functional organisation of the ventral spino-cerebellar tract in the cat: I. Electrophysiological identification of the tract. *Acta physiol. scand.*, **38**, 144. [76]

Paillard, J., 1960. The patterning of skilled movements. In *Handbook of Physiology* Vol. 3. Amer. Physiol. Soc., Washington. p. 1679–1708. [381]

Park, R. S., and Park, G. E., 1933. The center of ocular rotation in the horizontal plane. *Amer. J. Physiol.*, **104**, 545–552. [44]

Partridge, L. D., and Glaser, G. H., 1960. Adaptation in regulation of movement and posture. A study of stretch responses in spastic animals. *J. Neurophysiol.*, **23**, 257–268. [79]

Pasik, T., Pasik, P., and Bender, M. B., 1959. Electro-oculogram and corneoretinal potentials. *Fed. Proc.*, **18**, 118. [57]

Passey, G. E., 1950a. The perception of the vertical: IV. Adjustment to the vertical with normal and tilted visual frames of reference. *J. exp. Psychol.*, **40**, 738–745. [241, 248]

Passey, G. E., 1950b. The perception of the vertical: IX. Adjustment of the visual vertical from various magnitudes of body tilt. Jnt. Rep. No. 15. U.S. Nav. Sch. aviat. Med. Res. and Tulane Univ. [192]

Passey, G. E., and Guedry, F. E., 1949. The perception of the vertical: II. Adaptation effects in four planes. *J. exp. Psychol.*, **39**, 700–707. [242, 244]

Passey, G. E., and Ray, J. T., 1950. The perception of the vertical: X. Adaptation effects in the adjustment of the visual vertical. Jnt. Rep. No. 17. U.S. Nav. Sch. aviat. Med. Res. and Tulane Univ. [191]

Paterson, A., and Zangwill, O. L., 1944. Recovery of spatial orientation in the post-traumatic confusional state. *Brain*, **67**, 54–68. [269]

Paterson, A., and Zangwill, O. L., 1945. A case of topographical disorientation associated with a unilateral cerebral lesion. *Brain*, **68**, 188–212. [269]

Pearson, R. G., and Hauty, G. T., 1959. Adaptive processes determining proprioceptive perception of verticality. *J. exp. Psychol.*, **57**, 367–371. [250]

Pearson, R. G., and Hauty, G. T., 1960. Role of postural experience in proprioceptive perception of verticality. *J. exp. Psychol.*, **59**, 425–428. [246, 250]

Pechuel-Loescher von, 1907. *Volkskunde von Loango*. Stuttgart. p. 76 (cited in Stern, 1909b). [265, 332]

Peiper, A., 1963. *Cerebral Function in Infancy and Childhood*. Pitman, London. [50, 122, 235, 236, 237, 238]

Pendleton, M. E., and Paine, R. S., 1961. Vestibular nystagmus in newborn infants. *Neurology*, **11**, 450–458. [131, 134]

Penfield, W., 1954. Mechanisms of voluntary movement. *Brain*, **77**, 1–17. [381]

Penfield, W., and Rasmussen, T., 1950. *The Cerebral Cortex of Man*. Macmillan, New York. [171]

Perkins, F. T., 1932. Symmetry in visual recall. *Amer. J. Psychol.*, **44**, 473–490. [301]

Perrin, F. A. C., 1914. An experimental and introspective study of the human learning process in the maze. *Psychol. Monogr.*, **16**, No. 70. [264]

Pestalozza, G., and Davis, H., 1956. Electric responses of the guinea pig ear to high audio frequencies. *Amer. J. Physiol.*, **185**, 595–609. [165]

Peterson, J., 1916. Illusions of direction orientation. *J. Phil. Psychol. sci. Meth.*, **13**, 225–238. [263]

Peterson, J., and Peterson, J. K., 1938. Does practice with inverting lenses make vision normal? *Psychol. Monogr.*, **50**, No. 225, 12–37. [370, 407]

Pfaltz, C. R., and Richter, H. R., 1956. Photoelektrische Nystagmusregistrierung. *Pract. oto-rhino-laryng.*, **18**, 263–271. [56]

Pfister, H., 1955. Über das Verhalten der Hühner beim Tragen von Prismen. *Ph.D. Thesis*, Innsbruck. [390]

Piaget, J., 1926. *Judgment and Reasoning in the Child*. Harcourt Brace, New York. [290]

Piaget, J., and Inhelder, B., 1956. *The Child's Conception of Space*. Routledge and Kegan Paul, London. [340, 344, 345]

Pickford, R. W., 1956. Inverting spectacles and inverting vision. *Bull. Brit. psychol. Soc.*, No. **28**, 68–71. [410, 411]

Pierce, A. H., 1901. *Studies in Auditory and Visual Space Perception*. Longmans, Green, New York. [149, 161, 174]

Piercy, M., 1957. Experimental disorientation in the horizontal plane. *Quart. J. exp. Psychol.*, **9**, 65–77. [259]

Piéron, H., 1922. L'orientation auditive latérale. *Année psychol.*, **23**, 186–213. [158]

Pigg, L. D., 1961. Frictionless devices. In Hammer, L. R., Aeronautical systems division studies in weightlessness 1959–1960. WADC Tech. Rep. 60-715. Wright-Patterson AFB, Ohio. [422]

Pigg, L. D., and Kama, W. N., 1961. The effect of transient weightlessness on visual acuity. WADC Tech. Rep. 61-184. Wright-Patterson AFB, Ohio. [422]

Pigg, L. D., and Kama, W. N., 1962. Visual acuity in relation to body orientation and *g*-vector. AMRL-TDR-62-74. Wright-Patterson AFB, Ohio. [36]

Pillsbury, W. B., 1901. Does the sensation of movement originate in the joints. *Amer. J. Psychol.*, **12**, 346–353. [83, 93]

Pirie, N. W. (Ed.), 1961. *The Biology of Space Travel*. Inst. of Biology, London. [444]

Pollack, I., and Trittipoe, W. J., 1959. Binaural listening and interaural noise cross correlation. *J. acoust. Soc. Amer.*, **31**, 1250–1252. [156]

Pollock, F., 1938. Zur Pathologie und Klinik der Orientierung (Isolierte Orientierungsstörung im Raum infolge übergrossen, linksseitigen Stirnhirntumors). *Schweiz. Arch. Neurol. Psychiat.*, **42**, 141–164. [270, 291]

Pollock, W. T., and Chapanis, A., 1952. The apparent length of a line as a function of its inclination. *Quart. J. exp. Psychol.*, **4**, 170–178. [36]

Polyak, S., 1957. *The Vertebrate Visual System*. Univ. Chicago Press, Chicago. [406]

Prentice, W. C. H., and Beardslee, D. C., 1950. Visual 'normalization' near the vertical and horizontal. *J. exp. Psychol.*, **40**, 355–364. [221, 224, 226]

Preyer, W., 1895. *Zur Psychologie des Schreibens*. Voss, Hamburg and Leipzig. p. 40. [347]

Proctor, L. R., and Fernández, C., 1963. Studies on habituation of vestibular reflexes: IV. Effect of caloric stimulation in blindfolded cats. *Acta oto-laryng., Stockh.*, **56**, 500–508. [129]

Proell, W., and Bowman, N. J., 1958. A *Handbook of Space Flight* 2nd ed. Perastadion Press, Chicago. [444]

Provins, K. A., 1958. The effect of peripheral nerve block on the appreciation and execution of finger movements. *J. Physiol.*, **143**, 55–67. [94]

Purdy, D. M., 1934. Double monocular diplopia. *J. gen. Psychol.*, **11**, 311–327. [21, 22, 23]

Purkinje, J. E., 1820. Beiträge zur näheren Kenntniss des Schwindels aus häutognostischen Daten. *Med. Jb. (Osterreich)*, **6**, 79–125. [124, 197]

Quereau, J., 1954. Some aspects of torsion. *Arch. Ophthal., N.Y.*, **51**, 783–788. [45]

Quereau, J., 1955. Rolling of the eye around its visual axis during normal ocular movements. *Arch. Ophthal., N.Y.*, **53**, 807. [51]

Quix, F. H., 1928. Un nouvel appareil pour l'examen du nystagmus de position *J. Neurol., Brux.*, **3**, 160–180. [421]

Rademaker, G. G. J., 1935. *Reactions Labyrinthiques et Equilibre: L'Ataxie Labyrinthique*. Masson, Paris. [254]

Rademaker, G. G. J., and Ter Braak, J. W. G., 1948. On the central mechanism of some optic reactions. *Brain*, **71**, 48–76. [58, 60]

Radner, M., and Gibson, J. J., 1935. Orientation in visual perception. The perception of tip-character in forms. *Psychol. Monogr.*, **46**, No. 210, 48–65. [301, 302]

Raffel, G., 1936. Visual and kinaesthetic judgments of length. *Amer. J. Psychol.*, **48**, 331–334. [357]

Rählmann, E., 1878. Über den Nystagmus and seine Ätiologie. *v. Graefes Arch. Ophthal.*, **24**, 237–242. [56]

Rashbass, C., 1960. New method for recording eye movements. *J. opt. Soc. Amer.*, **50**, 642–644. [56]

Ratliff, F., and Riggs, L. A., 1950. Involuntary motions of the eye during monocular fixation. *J. exp. Psychol.*, **40**, 687–701. [47]

Rauth, J. E., and Sinnott, J. J., 1937. A new eidetic phenomenon. *Child Develpm.*, **8**, 112–113. [325]

Ray, B. S., and Wolff, H. G., 1945. Studies on pain: 'spread of pain'; evidence on site of spread within the neuraxis of effects of painful stimulation. *Arch. Neurol. Psychiat., Chicago*, **53**, 257–261. [293]

Rayleigh, Lord, 1875. On our perception of the direction of a source of sound. *Proc. Mus. Ass.*, 75–84. [155]

Rayleigh, Lord, 1907. Acoustical notes, sensations of right and left from a revolving magnet and telephone. *Phil. Mag.*, **13**, 316–319. [155]

Rayleigh, Lord, 1945. *Theory of Sound* Vol. 2. Dover, New York. [174]

Rebelsky, F., 1964. Adult perception of the horizontal. *Percept. mot. Skills*, **19**, 371–374. [344]

Reed, J. D., 1949. Factors influencing rotary performance. *J. Psychol.*, **28**, 65–92. [366]

Reese, E. P. (Ed.), 1953. Summary Rep. No. SDC 131-1-5. Psychophysical Res. Unit, Mt. Holyoke College. [39, 180, 181, 183, 206]

Reid, R. L., 1954. An illusion of movement complementary to the horizontal–vertical illusion. *Quart. J. exp. Psychol.*, **6**, 107–111. [37]

Reinecke, R. D., 1961. Review of optokinetic nystagmus from 1954–1960. *Arch. Ophthal.*, *N.Y.*, **65**, 609–615. [62]

Rekosh, J. H., and Held, R., 1963. Visual–spatial distortion produced by the sensory feedback accompanying locomotion. Paper read to the East. Psychol. Ass. [219]

Renshaw, B., 1941. Influence of discharge of motoneurons upon excitation of neighbouring motoneurons. *J. Neurophysiol.*, **4**, 167–183. [80]

Results 1961a of the first U.S. manned suborbital space flight: A compilation of the papers presented. Nat. Aeronautics and Space Admin. in cooperation with the Nat. Inst. of Hlth, and Nat. Acad. Sci. [432]

Results 1961b of the second U.S. manned suborbital space flight. Manned Spacecraft Center, Nat. Aeronautics and Space Admin. U.S. Govt. Printing Office, Washington, D.C. [423]

Results 1962 of the first U.S. manned orbital space flight. Manned Spacecraft Center, Nat. Aeronautics and Space Admin. U.S. Govt. Printing Office, Washington, D.C. [423, 425]

Revusky, B. T. L., Moore, J. W., and Dzendolet, E., 1965. Conditioning of the human vestibular sway response. *Percept. mot. Skills*, **20**, 593–600.

Rhule, W., and Smith, K. U., 1959a. Effect of visual pretraining in inverted reading on perceptual-motor performance in inverted visual fields. *Percept. mot. Skills*, **9**, 327–331. [373, 374]

Rhule, W., and Smith, K. U., 1959b. Effects of inversion of the visual field on human motions. *J. exp. Psychol.*, **57**, 338–343. [373]

Rice, C., 1930. The orientation of plane figures as a factor in their perception. *Child Develpm.*, **1**, 111–143. [333, 337, 341]

Ridgley, D., 1922. The teaching of directions in space and on maps. *J. Geogr.*, *N.Y.*, **21**, 66–72. [267]

Riesen, A. H., and Kinder, E. F., 1952. *Postural Development of Infant Chimpanzees.* Yale Univ. Press, New Haven. [236]

Riggs, L. A., Ratliff, F., Cornsweet, J. C., and Cornsweet, T. N., 1953. The disappearance of steadily fixated visual test objects. *J. opt. Soc. Amer.*, **43**, 495–501. [32, 47]

Ritter, O. L., and Gerathewohl, S. J., 1959. The concept of weight and stress in human flight. Rep. No. 58-154. U.S.A.F. Sch. aviat. Med., Randolf Field, Texas. [420]

Ritter, S. M., 1917. The vertical–horizontal illusion. *Psychol. Monogr.*. **23**, No. 101. [36, 37]

Ritterich, 1843. Das Schielen und seine Heilung. Cited in Nagel, 1896. [50]

Rivers, W. H. R., 1900. Vision. In Schäfer, E. A., *Textbook of Physiology*. Pentland, Edinburgh and London. p. 1134. [68]

Roberts, J. F., 1963. Walking responses under lunar and low gravity conditions. AMRL-TDR-63-112. Wright-Patterson AFB, Ohio. [422]

Roberts, T. D. M., 1963. Rhythmic excitation of a stretch reflex, revealing (a) hysteresis and (b) a difference between the responses to pulling and to stretching. *Quart. J. exp. Physiol.*, **48**, 328–345. [79]

Rochlin, A. M., 1955. The effect of tilt on the visual perception of parallelism. *Amer. J. Psychol.*, **68**, 223–236. [31]

Rock, I., 1954. The perception of the egocentric orientation of a line. *J. exp. Psychol.*, **48**, 367–374. [206]

Rock, I., 1956. The orientation of forms on the retina and in the environment. *Amer. J. Psychol.*, **69**, 513–528. [325, 326, 327, 330, 409]

Rock, I., and Heimer, W., 1957. The effect of retinal and phenomenal orientation on the perception of form. *Amer. J. Psychol.*, **70**, 493–511. [325, 326, 327]

Rock, I., and Leaman, R., 1963. An experimental analysis of visual symmetry. *Acta psychol.*, *Hague*, **21**, 171–183. [296]

Rock, I., and Victor, J., 1963. Vision and touch: an experimentally created conflict between the two senses. *Science*, **143**, 594–596. [359]

Roelofs, C. O., 1935. Optische Lokalisation. *Arch. Augenheilk.*, **109**, 395–415. [281]

Roelofs, C. O., 1959. Considerations on the visual egocentre. *Acta psychol.*, *Hague*, **16**, 226–234. [274, 277, 278]

Roelofs, C. O., and van der Bend, I. H., 1930. Betrachtungen und Untersuchungen über den optokinetischen Nystagmus. *Arch. Augenheilk.*, **102**, 551–625. [56, 57, 59]

Rogers, S., 1941. The anchoring of absolute judgments. *Arch. Pediat.*, **37**, No. 261. [182]

Rogers, S., Volkmann, J., Reese, T. W., Kaufman, E. L., 1947. Accuracy and variability of direct estimates of bearing from large display screens. Memorandum Rep. 166-I-MHCI. Special Devices Center, O.N.R. [182]

Roggeveen, L. J., and Nijhoff, P., 1956. The normal and pathological thresholds of the perception of angular accelerations for the opto-gyral illusion and the turning sensation. *Acta oto-laryng.*, *Stockh.*, **46**, 533–541. [125]

Roman, J. A., Warren, B. H., Niven, J. I., and Graybiel, A., 1962. Some observations on the behavior of a visual target and a visual after-image during parabolic flight maneuvers. SAM-TDR-62-66. U.S. Nav. Sch. aviat. Med., Pensacola, Fla. [425, 426]

Ronchi, L., 1961. May a single stimulus evoke two sensations separate in space? *Pubbl. Ist. Ottica*, **16**, 77–80. [23]

Rose, J. E., and Mountcastle, V. B., 1959. Touch and kinaesthesis. In *Handbook of Physiology* Sec. 1, Vol. 1. Amer. Physiol. Soc., Washington. p. 387–429. [76]

Rosenberg, M., 1912. Zur Pathologie der Orientierung nach rechts und links. *Z. Psychol. Physiol. Sinnesorg.*, **61**, 25–60. [291]

Rosenblatt, B. P., 1956. The influence of affective states upon the body-image and upon the perceptual organization of external space. *Diss. Abstr.*, **16**, 1721. [189]

Rosenzweig, M. R., 1951. Representation of the two ears at the auditory cortex. *Amer. J. Physiol.*, **167**, 147–158. [171]

Rosenzweig, M. R., 1954. Cortical correlates of auditory localization and of related perceptual phenomena. *J. comp. physiol. Psychol.*, **47**, 269–276. [165, 171]

Rosenzweig, M. R., 1961. Development of research on the physiological mechanisms of auditory localization. *Psychol. Bull.*, **58**, 376–389. [172]

Rosenzweig, M. R., and Amon, A. H., 1955. Binaural interaction in the medulla of the cat. *Experientia*, **11**, 498–504. [171]

Rosenzweig, M. R., and Rosenblith, W. A., 1950. Some electrophysiological correlates of the perception of successive clicks. *J. acoust. Soc. Amer.*, **22**, 878–880. [171]

Rosenzweig, M. R., and Sutton, D., 1958. Binaural interaction in lateral lemniscus of cat. *J. Neurophysiol.*, **21**, 17–27. [171]

Rosenzweig, M. R., and Wyers, E. J., 1955. Binaural interaction at the inferior colliculi. *J. comp. physiol. Psychol.*, **48**, 426–431. [171]

Rosman, R. R., 1960. The tilting-chair tilting-rod task: a methodological note. *Percept. mot. Skills*, **10**, 9–10. [192]

Ross, E. L., and Olsen, A., 1936. Readjustment of equilibrium following unilateral labyrinthectomy. *Arch. Otolaryng., Chicago*, **24**, 190–198. [134]

Royce, J. R., Stayton, W. R., and Kinkade, R. G., 1962. Experimental reduction of autokinetic movement. *Amer. J. Psychol.*, **75**, 221–231. [28]

Rudel, R. G., and Teuber, H. L., 1963. Discrimination of direction of line in children. Rep. Psychophys. Lab., M.I.T. [183]

Ruetes, 1846. Cited in Nagel, 1896. [50]

Ruffini, A., 1898. On the minute anatomy of the neuromuscular spindles of the cat, and on their physiological significance. *J. Physiol.*, **23**, 190–208. [72]

Ryan, T. A., and Ryan, M. S., 1940. Geographical orientation. *Amer. J. Psychol.*, **53**, 204–215. [263]

Ryan, T. A., and Schehr, F., 1941. The influence of eye movement and position on auditory localization. *Amer. J. Psychol.*, **54**, 243–252. [161]

Sachs, M., and Meller, J., 1901. Über die optische Orientirung bei Neigung des Kopfes gegen die Schulter. *v. Graefes Arch. Ophthal.*, **52**, 387–401. [193]

Sachs, M., and Meller, J., 1903. Untersuchungen über die optische und haptische Lokalisation bei Neigungen um eine sagittale Achse. *Z. Psychol. Physiol. Sinnesorg.*, **31**, 89–109. [192]

Saechi, U., 1950. La percezione della verticale durante it nistagmo: II. Valore della sede e della dimensione dell'immagine retinica. *Sist. nerv.*, **2**, 213–216. [198]

Sanchez-Longo, L. P., and Forster, F. M., 1958. Clinical significance of impairment of sound localization. *Neurology*, **8**, 119–125. [172]

Sandel, T. T., Teas, D. C., Feddersen, W. E., and Jeffress, L. A., 1955. Localization of sound from single and paired sources. *J. acoust. Soc. Amer.*, **27**, 842–852. [151, 156, 158]

Sandström, C. I., 1951. *Orientation in the Present Space*. Almqvist and Wiksell, Uppsala. [186, 352, 353]

Sandström, C. I., 1952. Tactile kinaesthetic determination of the vertical position of a pivoting rod, with tilted head. *Nord. Psykol.*, 156–165. [192]

Sandström, C. I., 1954. A note on the Aubert Phenomenon. *J. exp. Psychol.*, **48**, 209–210 [191, 192]

Sandström, C. I., 1956. Sex differences in tactile-kinaesthetic and visual perception of verticality. *Quart. J. exp. Psychol.*, **8**, 1–7. [191]

Sandström, C. I., 1959. The lability of the tactile-kinaesthetic framework. *Quart. J. exp. Psychol.*, **11**, 33–38. [230, 231]

Santschi, W. R., DuBois, J., and Omoto, C., 1963. Moments of inertia and centres of gravity of the living human body. AMRL-TDR-63-36. Wright-Patterson AFB, Ohio. [428]

Sarnoff, S. J., and Arrowhead, J. G., 1947. Differential spinal block: III. The block of cutaneous and stretch reflexes in the presence of unimpaired position sense. *J. Neurophysiol.*, **20**, 205–210. [94]

Sato, C., 1960. Orientation in the perception of space. *Jap. J. Psychol.*, **31**, 153–160. [264, 317]

Sayers, B. Mc.A., and Cherry, E. C., 1957. Mechanism of binaural fusion in the hearing of speech. *J. acoust. Soc. Amer.*, **29**, 973–987. [170]

Schaeffer, A., 1928. Spiral movement in man. *J. Morph.*, **45**, 293–398. [258]

Schäfer, E. A. (Ed.), 1900. *Text-book of Physiology*. Young J. Pentland, Edinburgh. [252]

Schilder, P., 1912. Über autokinetische Empfindungen. *Arch. ges. Psychol.*, **25**, 36–77. [26]

Schilder, P., 1935. *The Image and Appearance of the Human Body*. Routledge and Kegan Paul, London. [211]

Schilder, P., 1942. *Mind: Perception and Thought in their Constructive Aspects*. Columbia Univ. Press, New York. [138, 211, 212, 359]

Schlosser, J. W., 1930. Inlorno alla lettura dei quadri. *Critica*, **28**, 72. [300]

Schmaltz, G., 1932. Physical phenomena occurring in semicircular canals during rotatory and thermic stimulation. *Proc. R. Soc. Med.*, **25**, 359–381. [102]

Schneider, C. W., and Bartley, S. H., 1962. A study of the effects of mechanically induced tension of the neck muscles on the perception of verticality. *J. Psychol.*, **54**, 245–248. [195]

Schock, G. J. D., 1958a. Apparent motion of a fixed luminous target during subgravity trajectories. AFMDC Tech. Rep. 58-3. Holloman AFB, New Mexico. [425, 426]

Schock, G. J. D., 1958b. Sensory reactions related to weightlessness and their implications to space flight. AFMDC Tech. Rep. 58-6. Holloman AFB, New Mexico. [422]

Schock, G. J. D., 1959. Perception of the horizontal and vertical in simulated subgravity conditions. AFMDC Tech. Rep. 59-13. Holloman AFB, New Mexico. [117]

Schöne, H., 1962. Über den Einfluss der Schwerkraft auf die Augenrollung und auf die Wahrnehmung der Lage im Raum. *Z. vergl. Physiol.*, **46**, 57–87. [52, 53, 55]

Schubert, E. D., 1963. Interpretation of the Butler–Naunton localization shifts. *J, acoust. Soc. Amer.*, **35**, 113. [166]

Schubert, E. D., and Schultz, M. C., 1962. Some aspects of binaural signal selection. *J. acoust. Soc. Amer.*, **34**, 844–849. [170]

Schubert, G., 1924. Studien über das Listingsche Bewegungsgesetz am Auge. I. *Pflüg. Arch. ges. Physiol.*, **205**, 637–668.

Schubert, G., 1932. Die physiologischen Auswirkungen der Coriolisbeschleunigungen bei Flugzeugsteuerung. *Z. Hals- Nas.- u. Ohrenheilk.*, **30**, 595–604. [436]

Schubert, G., 1933. Labyrinthreizung durch Zusatzbeschleunigung bei Einwerkung von Zentrifugalkraft. *Pflüg. Arch. ges. Physiol.*, **233**, 537–548. [436]

Schubert, G., 1954. Coriolis-nystagmus. *J. Aviat. Med.*, **25**, 257–259. [436]

Schubert, G., and Brecher, G. A., 1934. Über optische Lokalisation und Augenstellung bei Vor-Rückwärtsneigung oder exzentrischer Rotation des Körpers. *Z. Sinnesphysiol.*, **65**, 1–26. [187, 192]

Schwab, R. S., 1954. The nonlabyrinthine causes of motion sickness. *Int. Rec. Med.*, **167**, 631–637. [137]

Schweizer, G., 1858. Über das Sternschwanken. Referred to in Adams, 1912. [25, 29]

Scott, D. M., 1962. An annotated bibliography of research on eye movements published during the period 1932–1961. Defence Res. med. Labs. Proj. No. 246, Rep. No. 256-11. Dept. of National Defence, Toronto. [65]

Scott, D. M., 1963. Supplement I to an annotated bibliography of research on eye movements published during the period 1932–1961. Defence Res. med. Labs. Proj. No. 246, Rep. No. 246-11. Dept. of National Defence, Toronto. [65]

Searle, L. V., and Taylor, F. V., 1948. Studies in tracking behaviour: I. Rate and time characteristics of simple corrective movements. *J. exp. Psychol.*, **38**, 615–631. [87]

Sedee, G. A., 1957. *Over Stereo-akoesie.* Smits, Utrecht. [158]

Seifert, H. S. (Ed.), 1959. *Space Technology.* Wiley, New York. [444]

Selling, L. S., 1930. An experimental investigation of the phenomenon of postural persistence. *Arch. Psychol.*, *N.Y.*, **118**. [84]

Sells, S. B., and Berry, C. A., 1961. *Human Factors in Jet and Space Travel.* Ronald, New York. [444]

Semmes, J., Weinstein, S., Ghent, L., and Teuber, H. L., 1955. Spatial orientation in man after cerebral injury: I. Analysis by locus of lesion. *J. Psychol.*, **39**, 227–244. [270]

Semmes, J., Weinstein, S., Ghent, L., and Teuber, H. L., 1963. Correlates of impaired orientation in personal and extrapersonal space. *Brain*, **86**, 747–772. [271]

Shanzer, S., Teng, P., Krieger, H. P., and Bender, M. B., 1958. Defects in optokinetic after-nystagmus in lesions of the brain stem. *Amer. J. Physiol.*, **194**, 419–422. [59]

Shapiro, M. B., 1952. Experimental studies of a perceptual anomaly. II. Confirmatory and explanatory experiments. *J. ment. Sci.*, **98**, 605–617. [332]

Sharp, W. L., 1934. An experimental study concerning visual localization in the horizontal plane. *J. exp. Psychol.*, **17**, 787–797. [185]

Shaxby, J. H., and Gage, F. H., 1932. Studies in the localization of sound. M.R.C. Spec. Rep. Ser. No. 166, 1–32. [164]

Shephard, A. H., and Cook, T. W., 1959. Body orientation and perceptual-motor performance. *Percept. mot. Skills*, **9**, 271–280. [365]

Sherrington, C. S., 1894. On the anatomical constitution of nerves of skeletal muscles:

some remarks on recurrent fibres in the ventral spinal nerve roots. *J. Physiol.*, **17**, 211–258. [72, 74]

Sherrington, C. S., 1898. Further note on the sensory nerves of the eye muscles. *Proc. roy. Soc.*, **64**, 120–121. [67]

Sherrington, C. S., 1906. On the proprio-ceptive system, especially in its reflex aspect. *Brain*, **29**, 467–482. [71]

Sherrington, C. S., 1918. Observations on the sensual rôle of the proprioceptive nerve-supply of the extrinsic ocular muscles. *Brain*, **41**, 332–343. [67]

Sherrington, C., 1947. *The Integrative Action of the Nervous System*. Cambridge Univ. Press, Cambridge. [241]

Shipley, W. C., Nann, B. M., Penfield, M. J., 1949. The apparent length of tilted lines. *J. exp. Psychol.*, **39**, 548–551. [36]

Shlaer, S., 1937. The relation between visual acuity and illumination. *J. gen. Physiol.*, **21**, 165–188. [30, 32]

Siddall, G. J., Holding, D. H., and Draper, J., 1957. Errors of aim and extent in manual point to point movement. *Occup. Psychol.*, **31**, 185–195. [87]

Silver, R. J., and Morant, R. B., 1962. Tactile and kinaesthetic tilt after-effects. Paper read to East. Psychol. Ass., Atlantic City. [229, 231, 232]

Simon, C. W., 1948. Proactive inhibition as an effect of handedness in mirror drawing. *J. exp. Psychol.*, **38**, 697–707. [378]

Simon, R., 1904. Über Fixation im Dämmerungssehen. *Z. Psychol. Physiol. Sinnesorg.*, **36**, 186–193. [26]

Simons, J. C., 1959. Walking under zero-gravity conditions. WADC Tech. Rep. 59-327. Wright-Patterson AFB, Ohio. [424, 433]

Simons, J. C., and Gardner, M. S., 1960. Self maneuvering for the orbital worker. WADC Tech. Rep. 60-748. Wright-Patterson AFB, Ohio. [429, 435]

Simons, J. C., and Gardner, M. S., 1963. Weightless man: a survey of sensations and performance while free-floating. AMRL-TDR-62-114. Wright-Patterson AFB, Ohio. [424, 426, 434, 435, 442, 443]

Simons, J. C., and Kama, W., 1962. A review of the effects of weightlessness on selected human motions and sensations. Rep. No. R147687. Wright-Patterson AFB, Ohio. [424, 426, 432]

Sivian, L. J., and White, S. D., 1933. On minimum audible sound fields. *J. acoust. Soc. Amer.*, **4**, 288–321. [145]

Skoglund, S., 1956. Anatomical and physiological studies of knee joint innervation in the cat. *Acta physiol. scand.*, **36**, Suppl. 124. [81, 94]

Skolnick, A., 1940. The role of eye movements in the autokinetic phenomenon. *J. exp. Psychol.*, **26**, 373–393. [26]

Skramlik, E. von, 1933. Über die Beeinflussung unserer Tastwahrnehmungen durch Richtung und Schnelligkeit der Tastbewegung. *Z. Sinnesphysiol.*, **64**, 97–114. [83]

Skrebitzky, A., 1871. Ein Beitrag zur Lehre von den Augenbewegungen. *v. Graefes Arch. Ophthal.*, **17**, 107. [50, 52]

Slinger, R. T., and Horsley, V., 1906. Upon the orientation of points in space by the muscular, arthrodial, and tactile senses of the upper limbs in normal individuals and in blind persons. *Brain*, **29**, 1–27. [84]

Sloan, L. L., 1947. Rate of dark adaptation and regional threshold gradient of the dark-adapted eye; physiologic and clinical studies. *Amer. J. Ophthal.*, **30**, 705–720. [305]

Smedslund, J., 1963. The effect of observation on children's representation of the spatial orientation of a water surface. *J. genet. Psychol.*, **102**, 195–202. [344]

Smith, J. L., 1962. Vertical optokinetic nystagmus. *Neurology*, **12**, 48–52. [56, 373]

Smith, J. L., and Cogan, D. G., 1960. Optokinetic nystagmus in cerebral disease: A report of 14 autopsied cases. *Neurology*, **10**, 127–137. [61, 62]

Smith, K. U., 1937. The relation between visual acuity and the optic projection centers of the brain. *Science*, **86**, 564–565. [57]

Smith, K. U., and Bojar, S., 1938. The nature of optokinetic reactions in mammals and their significance in the experimental analysis of the neural mechanisms of visual functions. *Psychol. Bull.*, **35**, 193–219. [62]

Smith, K. U., and Bridgman, M., 1943. The neural mechanisms of movement vision and optic nystagmus. *J. exp. Psychol.*, **33**, 165–187. [60]

Smith, K. U., and Greene, P., 1963. A critical period in maturation of performance with space-displaced vision. *Percept. mot. Skills*, **17**, 627–639. [375]

Smith, K. U., Kappauf, W. E., and Bojar, S., 1940. The functions of the visual cortex in optic nystagmus at different velocities of movement in the visual field. *J. gen. Psychol.*, **22**, 341–357. [58]

Smith, K. U., and Smith, W. M., 1962. *Perception and Motion.* Saunders, Philadelphia and London. [252, 374, 375, 381]

Smith, W. F., 1933. Direction orientation in children. *Genet. Psychol. Monogr.*, **42–43**, 154–166. [266]

Smythies, J. R., 1959a. The stroboscopic patterns. I. The dark phase. *Brit. J. Psychol.*, **50**, 106–116. [30]

Smythies, J. R., 1959b. The stroboscopic patterns. II. The phenomenology of the bright phase and after-images. *Brit. J. Psychol.*, **50**, 305–324. [30]

Snell, A. C., 1939. The optokinetoscope. *Trans. Amer. Acad. Ophthal. Oto-laryng.*, **44**, 396. [62]

Snow, W. B., 1954. Effect of arrival time on stereophonic localization. *J. acoust. Soc. Amer.*, **26**, 1071–1074. [164]

Snyder, F. W., and Pronko, N. H., 1952. *Vision with Spatial Inversion.* McCormick-Armstrong, Wichita, Kansas. [370, 407]

Solley, C. M., 1956. Reduction of error with practice in perception of the postural vertical. *J. exp. Psychol.*, **52**, 329–337. [248, 249]

Solley, C. M., 1960. Influence of head tilt, body tilt, and practice on reduction of error in perception of the postural vertical. *J. gen. Psychol.*, **62**, 69–74. [248, 249]

Sperry, R. W., 1942. Reestablishment of visuo-motor coordinations by optic nerve regeneration. *Anat. Rec.*, **84**, 470A. [389]

Sperry, R. W., 1944. Optic nerve regeneration with return of vision in anurans. *J. Neurophysiol.*, **7**, 57–69. [389]

Sperry, R. W., 1945. Restoration of vision after crossing of optic nerves and after contralateral transplantation of eye. *J. Neurophysiol.*, **8**, 15–28. [389]

Sperry, R. W., 1948. Orderly patterning of synaptic associations in regeneration of intracentral fiber tracts mediating visuomotor coordination. *Anat. Rec.*, **102**, 63–76. [389]

Spiegel, E. A., 1932. The cortical centers of the labyrinth. *J. nerv. ment. Dis.*, **75**, 504–512. [124]

Spiegel, E. A., 1933. Role of vestibular nuclei in the cortical innervation of the eye muscles. *Arch. Neurol. Psychiat.*, *Chicago*, **29**, 1084–1098. [124]

Spiegel, E. A., and Aronson, L., 1934. The interaction of cortical and labyrinthine impulses to ocular muscle movements. *Amer. J. Physiol.*, **109**, 693–703. [122]

Spiegel, E. A., and Price, J. B., 1939. Origin of the quick component of labyrinthine nystagmus. *Arch. Otolaryng.*, *Chicago*, **30**, 576–588. [61, 122]

Spiegel, E. A., and Scala, N. P., 1943. Response of the labyrinthine apparatus to electrical stimulation. *Arch. Otolaryng.*, *Chicago*, **38**, 131–138. [115]

Spiegel, E. A., and Sommer, I., 1944a. *Medical Physics: Vestibular Mechanisms*. The Year Book Publishers, Chicago. p. 1638. [122, 138]

Spiegel, E. A., and Sommer, I., 1944b. *Neurology of the Eye, Ear, Nose and Throat*. Grune and Stratton, New York. [138]

Spigel, I. M., 1963. Autokinetic movement of an intermittent luminance. *Psychol. Rec.*, **13**, 149–153. [29]

Spitz, R. A., and Wolfe, K. M., 1946. The smiling response: A contribution to the ontogenesis of social relations. *Genet. Psychol. Monogr.*, **34**, 57–125. [342]

Starch, D., 1905. Perimetry of the localization of sound. *Psychol. Rev. Monogr. Suppl.*, **6**, No. 28, 1–45; 1908, **9**, No. 38, 1–55. [149]

Stein, J., 1910. *Schwindel*. Leiner, Leipzig. [254]

Steinhausen, W., 1931. Über den Nachweis der Bewegung der Cupola in der intakten Bogengansampulle des Labyrinths bei der natürlichen rotatorischen und calorischen Reizung. *Pflüg. Arch. ges. Physiol.*, **228**, 322–328. [102]

Stengel, E., 1944. Loss of spatial orientation, constructional apraxia and Gerstmann's syndrome. *J. ment. Sci.*, **90**, 753–760. [292]

Stenvers, H. W., 1924. Über die klinische Bedeutung des optischen Nystagmus für die zerebrale Diagnostik. *Schweiz. Arch. Neurol. Psychiat.*, **14**, 279–288. [60, 61]

Stern, W., 1909a. Die Entwicklung der Raumwahrnehmung in der ersten Kindheit. *Z. exp. angew. Psychol.*, **2**, 412–423. [347, 348]

Stern, W., 1909b. Über verlagte Raumformen. *Z. exp. angew. Psychol.*, **2**, 498–526. [332, 340, 341, 343, 344, 347]

Stevens, H. C., and Ducasse, C. J., 1912. The retina and righthandedness. *Psychol. Rev.*, **19**, 3–31. [38]

Stevens, S. S., and Davis, H., 1938. *Hearing: Its Psychology and Physiology*. Wiley, New York. [174]

Stevens, S. S., and Galanter, E. H., 1957. Ratio scales and category scales for a dozen perceptual continua. *J. exp. Psychol.*, **54**, 377–411. [182]

Stevens, S. S., and Newman, E. B., 1934. The localization of pure tones. *Proc. nat. Acad. Sci.*, *Wash.*, **20**, 593–596. [146]

Stevens, S. S., and Newman, E. B., 1936. The localization of actual sources of sound. *Amer. J. Psychol.*, **48**, 297–306. [146, 148, 149, 151]

Stewart, G. W., 1920a. The function of intensity and phase in the binaural localization of pure tones. I. Intensity. *Phys. Rev.*, **15**, 425–432. [142, 155]

Stewart, G. W., 1920b. The function of intensity and phase in the binaural localization of pure tones. II. Phase. *Phys. Rev.*, **15**, 432–445. [142, 155]

Stewart, G. W., 1922. The intensity logarithmic law and the difference of phase effect in binaural audition. *Psychol. Monogr.*, **31**, No. 140, 30–44. [152, 168]

Stewart, G. W., and Hovda, O., 1918. The intensity factor in binaural sound localization: an extension of Weber's law. *Psychol. Rev.*, **25**, 242–251. [152]

Stiefel, J. W., and Smith, J. L., 1962. Vertical optokinetic nystagmus: The normal response. *Neurology*, **12**, 245–249. [56]

Stigler, R., 1912. Versuche über die Beteiligung der Schwereemfindung an der Orientierung des Menschen im Raume. *Pflüg. Arch. ges. Physiol.*, **148**, 573–584. [117]

Stock, B., 1933. Über die symmetrische haptische Einstellung von Raumpunkte. *Z. Sinnesphysiol.*, **64**, 229–250. [84]

Stone, L. S., 1944. Functional polarization in retinal development and its reestablishment in regenerating retinae of rotated grafted eyes. *Proc. Soc. exp. Biol.*, *N.Y.*, **57**, 13–14. [389]

Stotler, W. A., 1953. An experimental study of the cells and connections of the superior olivary complex of the cat. *J. comp. Neurol.*, **98**, 401–432. [172]

Stratton, G. M., 1896. Some preliminary experiments in vision without inversion of the retinal image. *Psychol. Rev.*, **3**, 611–617. [359, 368]

Stratton, G. M., 1897a. Upright vision and the retinal image. *Psychol. Rev.*, **4**, 182–187. [407]

Stratton, G. M., 1897b. Vision without inversion of the retinal image. *Psychol. Rev.*, **4**, 341–360, 363–481. [361, 369, 403, 407]

Stratton, G. M., 1907. Eye-movements and visual direction. *Psychol. Bull.*, **4**, 155–158. [404]

Strauss, A., and Werner, H., 1938. Deficiency in the finger scheme in relation to arithmetic disability (Finger agnosia and acalculia). *Amer. J. Orthopsychiat.*, **8**, 719–725. [292]

Strauss, H., 1925. Die diagnostische Bedeutung des optomotorischen (Eisenbahn) Nystagmus für die Neurologie. *Z. ges. Neurol. Psychiat.*, **98**, 93–101. [61]

Strümpell, A., 1903. Über die Störungen der Bewegungen bei fast vollständiger Anästhesie eines Armes durch Stichverletzung des Rückenmarks. *Dtsch. Z. Nervenheilk.*, **23**, 1–38. [93]

Sutherland, N. S., 1957. Visual discrimination of orientation and shape by octopus. *Nature, Lond.*, **179**, 11–13. [183, 317]

Suto, Y., 1960. Study on the interdependence of the horizontal–vertical illusion and the divided illusion. *Jap. psychol. Res.*, **2**, 81–93. [37]

Suzuki, J., and Totsuka, G., 1960. Post-rotatory nystagmus: Modifications observed in experiments with repeated rotatory stimulation. *Acta oto-laryng.*, *Stockh.*, **51**, 570–578. [131]

Swanson, R., and Benton, A. L., 1955. Some aspects of the genetic development of right–left discrimination. *Child Develpm.*, **26**, 123–133. [290]

Swearingen, J. J., 1953. Determination of centers of gravity of man. CAA Proj. No. 53-203, Civil Aeronautical Med. Res. Lab., Oklahoma. [428]

Sylvester, R. H., 1913. The mental imagery of the blind. *Psychol. Bull.*, **10**, 210-211. [261]

Szafran, J., 1951. Changes with age and with exclusion of vision in performance at an aiming task. *Quart. J. exp. Psychol.*, **3**, 111-118. [349]

Szentágothai, J., 1950. The elementary vestibulo-ocular reflex arc. *J. Neurophysiol.*, **13**, 395-407. [123]

Sziklai, C., 1961. Effect of body position and muscular strain on space localization, as measured by the apparent eye-line. *M.A. Thesis*, Clark Univ. [187]

Szymanski, J. S., 1913. Versuche über den Richtungssinn beim Menschen. *Pflüg. Arch. ges. Physiol.*, **151**, 158-170. [257]

Takala, M., 1951a. On constant errors in the judgment of the degree of inclinations. *Acta Psychol. fenn.*, **1**, 129-142. [180]

Takala, M., 1951b. Asymmetries of the visual space. *Ann. Acad. Sci. fenn.*, **72**. [180, 301, 313, 314]

Tampieri, G., 1963. Il problema dell' indifferenza infantile per l'orientamento nello spazio visivo. *Estra. Riv. Psicol.*, **62**, 125-177. [337]

Tanaka, T., 1960. Developmental study on the comparison of similarity of figures which change in direction and arrangement of elements: V. recognition and direction. *Jap. J. Psychol.*, **31**, 222-227. [334]

Tanaka, T., 1962. Developmental study of the comparison of similarity of figures which change in direction and arrangement of elements: VIII. through recognition method. *Jap. J. Psychol.*, **32**, 388-394. [334]

Taub, E., Bacon, R. C., and Berman, A. J., 1965. The acquisition of a trace conditioned avoidance response after deafferentation of the responding limb. *J. comp. physiol. Psychol.*, **59**, 275-279. [78]

Taylor, J. G., 1962. *The Behavioural Basis of Perception.* Yale Univ. Press, New Haven and London. [372, 400, 402, 412, 414, 415, 416]

Taylor, J. G., and Papert, S., 1955. A theory of perceptual constancy. *Brit. J. Psychol.*, **47**, 216-224. [405]

Taylor, M. M., 1962. The distance paradox of the figural after-effect in auditory localization. *Canad. J. Psychol.*, **16**, 278-282. [162]

Taylor, M. M., 1963. Visual discrimination and orientation. *J. opt. Soc. Amer.*, **53**, 763-765. [36]

Teas, D. C., 1962. Lateralization of acoustic transients. *J. acoust. Soc. Amer.*, **34**, 1460-1465. [154]

Templeton, W. B., Howard, I. P., and Easting, G., 1965. Satiation and the tilt after-effect. *Amer. J. Psychol.*, **78**, 656-659. [224]

Templeton, W. B., Howard, I. P., and Lowman, A. E., 1966. Passively generated adaptation to prismatic distortion. *Percept. mot. Skills*, **22**, 140-142. [388]

Ten Cate, J., 1934. Akustische und optische Reaktionen der Katzen nach teilweisen und totalen Extirpationen des Neopallismus. *Arch. néerl. Physiol.*, **19**, 191-264. [171]

Terazawa, I., 1927. The relation of pathological changes in labyrinth to the loss of nystagmus and rotatory illusion. *Jap. J. Psychol.*, **2**, 591-611. [135]

Ter Braak, J. W. G., 1936. Untersuchungen über optokinetischen Nystagmus. *Arch. néerl. Physiol.*, **21**, 310–375. [57, 61]

Terrace, H. S., 1959. The effects of retinal locus and attention on the perception of words. *J. exp. Psychol.*, **58**, 382–385. [303]

Teuber, H. L., and Diamond, S., 1956. Effects of brain injury on binaural localization of sounds. Paper read at East. Psychol. Ass., Atlantic City. Reviewed in Rosenzweig, 1961. [171]

Teuber, H. L., and Mishkin, M., 1954. Judgment of visual and postural vertical after brain injury. *J. Psychol.*, **38**, 161–175. [211]

Thetford, P. E., and Guedry, F. E., 1952a. The postural vertical in unilaterally labyrinthectomized individuals. Proj. No. NM.001.063.01.26 (Joint Rep. No. 26). U.S. Nav. Sch. aviat. Med., Pensacola, Fla. [248]

Thetford, P. E., and Guedry, F. E., 1952b. Judgment of the postural vertical during exposure to a misleading visual framework in unilaterally labyrinthectomized subjects. Proj. No. NM.001.063.01.27 (Joint Rep. No. 27). U.S. Nav. Sch. aviat. Med., Pensacola, Fla. [248]

Thomas, G. J., 1941. Experimental study of the influence of vision on sound localization. *J. exp. Psychol.*, **28**, 163–177. [360]

Thompson, S. P., 1877. The phenomena of binaural audition I. *Phil. Mag.*, **4**, 274–276. [155]

Thompson, S. P., 1878. The phenomena of binaural audition II. *Phil. Mag.*, **6**, 386–387. [155]

Thouless, R. H., 1947. The experience 'upright' and 'upside-down' in looking at pictures. In *Miscellanea Psychologica Albert Michotte*. Univ. Louvain, Louvain. p. 130–137. [323, 324]

Thurlow, W. R., and Elfner, L. F., 1959. Pure-tone cross-ear localization effects. *J. acoust. Soc. Amer.*, **31**, 1606–1608. [168]

Thurlow, W. R., Gross, N. B., Kemp, E. H., and Lowy, K., 1951. Microelectrode studies of neural auditory activity of cat. I. Inferior colliculus. *J. Neurophysiol.*, **14**, 289–304. [165]

Tiegs, O. W., 1953. Innervation of voluntary muscle. *Physiol. Rev.*, **33**, 90–94. [72]

Tinker, M. A., 1946. The study of eye movements in reading. *Psychol. Bull.*, **43**, 93–120. [65]

Tobias, J. V., and Zerlin, S., 1959. Lateralization threshold as a function of stimulus duration. *J. acoust. Soc. Amer.*, **31**, 1591–1594. [157]

Tourtual, J., 1840. Bericht über die Leistungen im Gebiete der Physiologie der Sinne, insbesondere des Gesichtssinnes. *Arch. Anat., Physiol. Med. (Müller)*, **56**, 1. [50]

Travis, R. C., 1929. Reciprocal inhibition and reinforcement in the visual and vestibular systems. *J. exp. Psychol.*, **12**, 415–430. [122]

Travis, R. C., 1936. The latency and velocity of the eye in saccadic movements. *Psychol. Monogr.*, **47**, No. 212, 242–249. [62]

Travis, R. C., 1944. A new stabilometer for measuring dynamic equilibrium in the standing position. *J. exp. Psychol.*, **34**, 418–424. [252]

Travis, R. C., 1945. An experimental analysis of dynamic and static equilibrium. *J. exp. Psychol.*, **35**, 216–234. [253]

Trimble, O. C., 1928. Some temporal aspects of sound localization. *Psychol. Monogr.*, **28**, No. 4, 172–224. [158]

Trimble, O. C., 1929. The relative roles of the temporal and the intensity factor in sound localization. *Amer. J. Psychol.*, **41**, 564–576. [152, 164]

Trimble, O. C., 1935. Intensity-difference and phase-difference as conditions of stimulation in binaural sound-localization. *Amer. J. Psychol.*, **47**, 264–274. [152, 165, 168]

Trincker, D. E. W., 1961. Neuere Aspekte der Mechanismus der Haarzell-Erregung. *Acta oto-laryng.*, *Stockh.*, *Suppl.* **163**, 67–75. [105]

Trincker, D. E. W., 1962. The transformation of mechanical stimulus into nervous excitation by the labyrinthine receptors. In *Biological Receptor Mechanisms. Symp. Soc. exp. Biol.*, *No. 16*. Cambridge Univ. Press, Cambridge. [105, 109, 111]

Trowbridge, C. C., 1913. On fundamental methods of orientation and 'imaginary maps'. *Science*, **38**, 888–897. [262]

Tschermak-Seysenegg, A. von., 1899. Über anomale Sehrichtungsgemeinschaft der Netzhäute bei einem Schielenden. *v. Graefes Arch. Ophthal.*, **47**, 508–550. [21]

Tschermak-Seysenegg, A. von, 1952. *Introduction to Physiological Optics*. Thomas, Springfield, Ill. [186, 187, 200, 281]

Tschermak-Seysenegg, A. von, and Schubert, G., 1931. Über Vertikalorientierung im Rotatorium und in Flugzeuge. *Pflüg. Arch. ges. Physiol.*, **228**, 234–257. [198]

Tumarkin, I. A., 1937. Some observations on the function of the Labyrinth. *Proc. R. Soc. Med. otol. Sect.*, **30**, 599–610. [116]

Tunturi, A. R., 1944. Audiofrequency localization in the acoustic cortex of the dog. *Amer. J. Physiol.*, **141**, 397–403. [171]

Tunturi, A. R., 1946. A study of the pathway from the medial geniculate body to the acoustic cortex in the dog. *Amer. J. Physiol.*, **147**, 311–319. [171]

Tyler, D. B., and Bard, P., 1949. Motion sickness. *Physiol. Rev.*, **29**, 311–369. [135]

Valentine, C. W., 1912–1913. Psychological theories of the horizontal–vertical illusion. *Brit. J. Psychol.*, **5**, 8–35. [36]

Van Bergeijk, W. A., 1962. Variations on a theme of Békésy: a model of binaural interaction. *J. acoust. Soc. Amer.*, **34**, 1431–1437. [172, 173, 174]

Van Dishoeck, H. A. E., Spoor, A., and Nijhoff, P., 1954. The opto-gyral illusion and its relation to the nystagmus of the eyes. *Acta oto-laryng.*, *Stockh.*, **44**, 597–607. [125, 126]

Van Egmond, A. A. J., and Groen, J. J., 1955. Cupulometrie. *Pract. oto-rhino-laryng.*, **17**, 206–223. [112]

Van Egmond, A. A. J., Groen, J. J., and Jongkees, L. B. W., 1949a. The mechanics of the semi-circular canal. *J. Physiol.*, **110**, 1–17. [103, 114]

Van Egmond, A. A. J., Groen, J. J., and Jongkees, L. B. W., 1949b. The turning test with small regulable stimuli: V. Is Ewald's law valid in men? *J. Laryng.*, **63**, 299–305. [118]

Van Egmond, A. A. J., Groen, J. J., and de Wit, G., 1954. The selection of motion sickness-susceptible individuals. *Int. Rec. Med.*, **167**, 651–660. [136]

Van Egmond, A. A. J., and Tolk, J., 1954. On the slow phase of the caloric nystagmus. *Acta oto-laryng.*, *Stockh.*, **44**, 589–593. [114]

Velzeboer, C. M. J., 1952. Bilateral cortical hemianopsia and optokinetic nystagmus. *Ophthalmologica, Basel*, **123**, 187–189. [60]

Verhoeff, F. H., 1925. The theory of binocular perspective. *Amer. J. physiol. Opt.*, **6**, 416. [214]

Vernon, M. D., 1934. The perception of inclined lines. *Brit. J. Psychol.*, **25**, 186–196. [214]

Vernon, M. D., 1957. *Backwardness in Reading: A Study of its Nature and Origin.* Cambridge Univ. Press, London. [348]

Viguier, C., 1882. Le sens de l'orientation et ses organs chez les animaux et chez l'homme. *Rev. philomath.*, **14**, 1–36. [265]

Vilstrup, T., and Jensen, C. E., 1961. On the displacement potential in acid mucopolysaccharides. *Acta oto-laryng., Stockh., Suppl.*, **163**, 42–46. [106]

Vogelsang, C. J., 1961. The perception of a visual object during stimulation of the vestibular system. *Acta oto-laryng., Stockh.*, **53**, 461–469. [125]

Voth, A. C., 1941. Individual differences in the autokinetic phenomenon. *J. exp. Psychol.*, **29**, 306–322. [25]

Wade, J. E., 1961. Psychomotor performance: operation of switches. In Hammer, L. R., *Aeronautical systems division studies in weightlessness:* 1959–1960. WADC Tech. Rep. 60-715. Wright-Patterson AFB, Ohio. p. 53–54. [443]

Wallach, H., 1940. The role of head movements and vestibular and visual cues in sound localisation. *J. exp. Psychol.*, **27**, 339–368. [158]

Wallach, H., Kravitz, J. H., and Lindauer, J., 1963. A passive condition for rapid adaptation to displaced visual direction. *Amer. J. Psychol.*, **76**, 568–578. [391]

Wallach, H., Newman, E. B., and Rosenzweig, M. R., 1949. The precedence effect in sound localization. *Amer. J. Psychol.*, **62**, 315–336. [154]

Walls, G. L., 1951a. The problem of visual direction. I. The history to 1900. *Amer. J. Optom.*, **28**, 55–83. [16, 406]

Walls, G. L., 1951b. The problem of visual direction. II. The tangible basis for nativism. *Amer. J. Optom.*, **28**, 115–146. [15]

Walls, G. L., 1951c. The problem of visual direction. III. Experimental attacks and their results. *Amer. J. Optom.*, **28**, 173–212. [412]

Walls, G. L., 1962. The evolutionary history of eye movements. *Vis. Res.*, **2**, 69–80. [48, 49]

Walsh, E. G., 1957. An investigation of sound localization in patients with neurological abnormalities. *Brain*, **80**, 222–250. [56, 171]

Walsh, E. G., 1960. Perception of linear acceleration following unilateral labyrinthectomy: variation of threshold according to orientation of the head. *J. Physiol.*, **153**, 350–357. [135]

Walsh, E. G., 1961. Role of the vestibular apparatus in the perception of motion on a parallel swing. *J. Physiol.*, **155**, 506–513. [136]

Walsh, E. G., 1962. The perception of rhythmically repeated linear motion in the horizontal plane. *Brit. J. Psychol.*, **53**, 439–445. [118, 119, 136]

Walsh, F. B., 1957. *Clinical Neuro-Ophthalmology* 2nd ed. Williams and Wilkins, Baltimore. [62]

Walton, H. W., 1957. A device for artificial production of alternating gravitational forces. *J. Aviat. Med.*, **28**, 297. [420]

Walton, W. G., 1948. Compensatory cyclo-torsion accompanying head tilt. *Amer. J. Optom.*, **25**, 525–534. [50, 51, 52]

Wang, S. C., and Tyson, R. L., 1954. Central nervous pathways of experimental motion sickness. *Int. Rec. Med.*, **167**, 641–650. [137, 138]

Wapner, S., and Krus, D. M., 1959. Behavioral effects of lysergic acid diethylamine (L.S.D.-25). Space localization in normal adults as measured by the apparent horizon. *Arch. gen. Psychiat.*, *Chicago*, **1**, 417–419. [188]

Wapner, S., and Werner, H., 1952. Experiments on sensory-tonic field theory of perception: V. Effect of body status on the kinaesthetic perception of verticality. *J. exp. Psychol.*, **44**, 126–131. [192]

Wapner, S., and Werner, H., 1955. Gestalt laws of organisation and organismic theory of perception: effect of asymmetry induced by the factor of similarity on the position of the apparent median plane and apparent horizon. *Amer. J. Psychol.*, **58**, 258–265. [188, 283]

Wapner, S., and Werner, H., 1957. *Perceptual Development. An Investigation Within the Framework of Sensory-Tonic Field Theory.* Clark Univ. Press, Worcester, Mass. [186, 188, 191]

Wapner, S., Werner, H., Bruell, J. H., and Goldstein, A. G., 1953. Experiments on sensory-tonic field theory of perception: VII. Effect of asymmetrical extent and starting positions of figures on the visual apparent median plane. *J. exp. Psychol.*, **46**, 300–307. [282]

Wapner, S., Werner, H., and Chandler, K. A., 1951. Experiments on sensory-tonic field theory of perception: I. Effect of extraneous stimulation on the visual perception of verticality. *J. exp. Psychol.*, **42**, 341–343. [195]

Wapner, S., Werner, H., and Krus, D. M., 1957. The effect of success and failure on space location. *J. Personality*, **25**, 752–756. [188]

Wapner, S., Werner, H., and Morant, R. B., 1951. Experiments on sensory-tonic field theory of perception: III. Effect of body rotation on the visual perception of verticality. *J. exp. Psychol.*, **42**, 351–357. [198]

Wapner, S., and Witkin, H. A., 1950. The role of visual factors in the maintenance of body-balance. *Amer. J. Psychol.*, **63**, 385–408. [253, 254]

Warkentin, J., and Smith, K. U., 1937. The development of visual acuity in the cat. *J. genet. Psychol.*, **50**, 371–399. [59]

Warren, H. C., 1895. Sensations of rotation. *Psychol. R ev.*, **2**, 273–276. [126]

Warren, H. C., 1908. Magnetic sense of direction. *Psychol. Bull.*, **5**, 376–377. [265, 266]

Warrick, M. J., 1947. Direction of movement in the use of control knobs to position visual indicators. In Fitts, P. M. (Ed.), *Psychological Research on Equipment Design.* A.A.F. Aviat. Psychol. Res. Rep. No. 19. Govt. Printing Office, Washington, D.C. [364]

Warrick, M. J., and Grether, W. F., 1948. The effect of pointer alignment on check-reading of engine instrument panels. Memorandum Rep. No. MCREXD-694-17. U.S.A.F. Air Material Command, Dayton, Ohio. [363]

Wartenberg, R., 1953. *Diagnostic Tests in Neurology.* The Yearbook Publishers, Chicago. [189]

Weber, C. O., and Dallenbach, K. M., 1929. Properties of space in kinaesthetic fields of force. *Amer. J. Psychol.*, **41**, 95–105. [89]

Weene, P. L., 1962. Changes in perceived size of angles as a function of orientation. Paper read to East. Psychol. Ass. [40]

Weinbach, A. P., 1938. Contour maps, center of gravity, moment of inertia and surface area of the human body. *Hum. Biol.*, **10**, 356–371. [428]

Weiner, M., 1955a. The effects of differentially structured visual fields on the perception of verticality. *Amer. J. Psychol.*, **68**, 291–293. [205]

Weiner, M., 1955b. Effects of training in space orientation on perception of the upright. *J. exp. Psychol.*, **49**, 367–373. [209]

Weinstein, E. A., and Bender, M. B., 1948. The mid-position phenomenon in eye movements. *Trans. Amer. neurol. Ass.*, **73**, 163–165. [61, 62]

Weinstein, S., Semmes, J., Ghent, L., and Teuber, H. L., 1956. Spatial orientation in man after cerebral injury: II. Analysis according to concomitant defects. *J. Psychol.*, **42**, 249, 263. [270]

Weinstein, S., Sersen, E. A., Fisher, L., and Weisinger, M., 1964. Is reafference necessary for visual adaptation? *Percept. mot. Skills*, **18**, 641–648. [389]

Weinstein, S., Sersen, E. A., and Weinstein, D. S., 1964. An attempt to replicate a study of disarranged eye–hand coordination. *Percept. mot. Skills*, **18**, 629–632. [386]

Weinstein, S., Sersen, E. A., Weisinger, M., Fisher, L., and Richlin, M., 1964. Total adaptation to prismatic displacement in the absence of reafference. Typescript. [393]

Weiss, B., 1954. The role of proprioceptive feedback in positioning responses. *J. exp. Psychol.*, **47**, 215–224. [88]

Weiss, B., 1955. Movement error, pressure variation, and the range effect. *J. exp. Psychol.*, **50**, 191–196. [88]

Weiss, H. S., 1955. The human electrocardiogram during tumbling. *J. Aviat. Med.*, **26**, 206–213. [429]

Wendt, G. R., 1936a. The form of the vestibular eye-movement response in man. *Psychol. Monogr.*, **47**, No. 212, 311–328. [121]

Wendt, G. R., 1936b. An interpretation of inhibition of conditioned reflexes as competition between reaction systems. *Psychol. Rev.*, **43**, 258–281. [134]

Wendt, G. R., 1951. Vestibular functions. In Stevens, S. S., *Handbook of Experimental Psychology.* Wiley, New York. p. 1191–1293. [101, 131, 138]

Wendt., G. R., 1963. The etiology of vomiting during a weightless manoeuvre. In Loftus, J. P., *Symp. Motion Sickness.* p. 33–35. [424]

Werner, H., 1938. Binocular depth contrast and the conditions of the binocular field. *Amer. J. Psychol.*, **51**, 489–497. [207]

Werner, H., 1942. Binocular vision—normal and abnormal. *Arch. Ophthal.*, *N.Y.*, **28**, 834–844. [22, 23]

Werner, H., and Wapner, S., 1949. Sensory-tonic field theory of perception. *J. Personality*, **18**, 88–107. [178, 195]

Werner, H., and Wapner, S., 1952. Experiments on sensory-tonic field theory of perception: IV. Effects of initial position of a rod on apparent verticality. *J. exp. Psychol.*, **43**, 68–74. [178, 179, 211, 216]

Werner, H., and Wapner, S., 1954. Studies in physiognomic perception: I. Effect of configurational dynamics and meaning induced sets on the position of the apparent median plane. *J. Psychol.*, **38**, 51–65. [286, 287]

Werner, H., Wapner, S., and Bruell, J. H., 1953. Experiments on sensory-tonic field theory of perception: VI. Effect of position of head, eyes, and of object on position of the apparent median plane. *J. exp. Psychol.*, **46**, 293–299. [281, 288]

Werner, H., Wapner, S., and Chandler, K. A., 1951. Experiments on sensory-tonic field theory of perception: II. Effect of supported and unsupported tilt of the body on the visual perception of verticality. *J. exp. Psychol.*, **42**, 346–350. [195]

Wersäll, J., 1956. Studies on the structure and innervation of the sensory epithelium of the cristae ampullaris in the guinea pig. *Acta oto-laryng., Stockh., Suppl.*, **126**. [101,105]

Wertheimer, M., 1912. Experimentelle Studien über das Sehen von Bewegung. *Z. Psychol. Physiol. Sinnesorg.*, **61**, 161–265. [200, 217]

Wertheimer, M., 1961. Psychomotor coordination of auditory and visual space at birth. *Science*, **134**, 1692. [359]

Wertheimer, M., and Arena, A. J., 1959. Effect of exposure time on adaptation to disarranged hand–eye coordination. *Percept. mot. Skills*, **9**, 159–164. [387]

Westheimer, G., 1954a. Mechanism of saccadic eye movements. *Arch. Ophthal., N.Y.*, **52**, 710–724. [63]

Westheimer, G., 1954b. Eye movement responses to a horizontally moving visual stimulus. *Arch. Ophthal., N.Y.*, **52**, 932–941. [58, 59]

Westheimer, G., and Mitchell, A. M., 1956. Eye movement responses to convergence stimuli. *Arch. Ophthal., N.Y.*, **55**, 848–856. [64]

Weymouth, F. W., 1959. Stimulus orientation and threshold; an optical analysis. *Amer. J. Ophthal.*, **48**, 6–10. [34]

White, A. M., and Dallenbach, K. M., 1932. Position vs. intensity as a determinant of attention of left-handed observers. *Amer. J. Psychol.*, **44**, 175–179. [305]

White, C. T., Eason, R. G., and Bartlett, N. R., 1962. Latency and duration of eye movements in the horizontal plane. *J. opt. Soc. Amer.*, **52**, 210–213. [63]

White, W. J., and Jorve, W. R., 1956. The effects of gravitational stress upon visual acuity. Tech. Doc. Rep. 56-247. Wright-Patterson AFB, Ohio. [36]

White, W. J., and Monty, R. A., 1963. Vision and unusual gravitational forces. *Human Factors*, **131**, 239–263. [198]

Whiteside, T. C. D., 1960. The effect of weightlessness on some postural mechanisms. *Aerosp. Med.*, **31**, 324. [117]

Whiteside, T. C. D., 1961. Hand–eye co-ordination in weightlessness. *Aerosp. Med.*, **32**, 719–725. [425, 426, 442]

Whitsett, C. E., 1963. Some dynamic response characteristics of weightless man. AMRL-TDR-63-18. Wright-Patterson AFB, Ohio. [428, 431, 443]

Whitteridge, D., 1959. The effect of stimulation of intrafusal muscle fibres on sensitivity to stretch of extraocular muscle spindles. *Quart. J. exp. Physiol.*, **44**, 385–393. [78]

Whitworth, R. H., and Jeffress, L. A., 1961. Time vs. intensity in the localization of tones. *J. acoust. Soc. Amer.*, **33**, 925–929. [166, 168]

Wiener, F. M., and Ross, D. A., 1946. The pressure distribution in the auditory canal in a progressive sound field. *J. acoust. Soc. Amer.*, **18**, 248A. [153]

Wiesel, T. N., and Hubel, D. H., 1963a. Single-cell responses in striate cortex of kittens deprived of vision in one eye. *J. Neurophysiol.*, **26**, 1003–1017. [395]

Wiesel, T. N., and Hubel, D. H., 1963b. Effects of visual deprivation on morphology and physiology of cells in the cat's lateral geniculate body. *J. Neurophysiol.*, **26**, 978–993. [395]

Wilcott, R. C., 1955. Variables affecting the angular displacement threshold of simulated auditory movement. *J. exp. Psychol.*, **49**, 68–72. [149]

Williams, G. W., 1932. A study of the response of three psychotic groups to a test of suggestibility. *J. gen. Psychol.*, **7**, 302–309. [254]

Wilson, H. A., and Myers, C. S., 1908. The influence of binaural phase differences on the localization of sounds. *Brit. J. Psychol.*, **2**, 363–385. [169]

Wing, C. W., and Passey, G. E., 1950. The perception of the vertical: XI. The visual vertical under conflicting visual and acceleratory factors. Proj. NR.143-455, Rep. No. 20. U.S. Nav. Sch. aviat. Med., Pensacola, Fla. [199]

Wing, M. E., 1963. The response of the otolith organs to tilt. *Acta oto-laryng., Stockh.*, **56**, 537–545. [110]

Winter, J. E., 1912. The sensation of movement. *Psychol. Rev.*, **19**, 374–385. [83, 93]

Witkin, H. A., 1946. Studies in geographic orientation. *Yearb. Amer. phil. Soc.*, 152–155. [257, 260]

Witkin, H. A., 1948. The effect of training and of structural aids on performance in three tests of space orientation. Rep. No. 80. Civil Aeronautics Administration, Washington, D.C. [208]

Witkin, H. A., 1949. Perception of body position and of the position of the visual field. *Psychol. Monogr.*, **63**, No. 302. [204, 217]

Witkin, H. A., 1950. Perception of the upright when the direction of the force acting on the body is changed. *J. exp. Psychol.*, **40**, 93–106. [199, 200]

Witkin, H. A., 1952. Further studies of perception of the upright when the direction of the force acting on the body is changed. *J. exp. Psychol.*, **43**, 9–20. [199]

Witkin, H. A., 1953. Comment on 'The role of instruction in experimental space orientation'. *J. exp. Psychol.*, **46**, 135–136. [208]

Witkin, H. A., 1964. Uses of the centrifuge in studies of the orientation of space. *Amer. J. Psychol.*, **77**, 499–501. [200]

Witkin, H. A., and Asch, S. E., 1948a. Studies in space orientation: III. Perception of the upright in the absence of a visual field. *J. exp. Psychol.*, **38**, 603–614. [179, 191, 192]

Witkin, H. A., and Asch, S. E., 1948b. Studies in space orientation: IV. Further experiments on perception of the upright with displaced visual fields. *J. exp. Psychol.*, **38**, 762–782. [199, 203]

Witkin, H. A., Lewis, H. B., Hertzman, M., Machover, K., Meissner, P. B., and Wapner, S., 1954. *Personality Through Perception*. Harper, New York. [204, 210]

522   Bibliography and author index

Witkin, H. A., and Wapner, S., 1950. Visual factors in the maintenance of upright posture. *Amer. J. Psychol.*, **63**, 31–50. [254]

Witkin, H. A., Wapner, S., Leventhal, T., 1952. Sound localization with conflicting visual and auditory cues. *J. exp. Psychol.*, **43**, 58–67. [360]

Wittmann, J., 1925. Beiträge zur Analyse des Hörens bei dichotischer Reizaufnahme. *Arch. ges. Psychol.*, **51**, 21–222. [158, 164]

Woellner, R. C., 1957. The perception of vertical in the presence of increased accelerative forces. Proj. No. NM.17.01.11, Subtask 1, Rep. No. 45. U.S. Nav. Sch. aviat. Med., Pensacola, Fla. [199]

Woellner, R. C., and Graybiel, A., 1958. Reflex ocular torsion in healthy males. Proj. NM.17.01.11, Subtask 1, Rep. No. 47. U.S. Nav. Sch. aviat. Med., Pensacola, Fla. [51, 52, 55]

Woellner, R. C., and Graybiel, A., 1959. Counterrolling of the eyes and its dependance on the magnitude of gravitational or inertial force acting laterally on the body. *J. appl. Physiol.*, **14**, 632–634. [55]

Wohlgemuth, A., 1911. On the after-effect of seen movement.*Brit. J. Psychol. Monogr.*, *Suppl.*, No. 1. [15, 25]

Wohlwill, J. F., 1960. Developmental studies of perception. *Psychol. Bull.*, **57**, 249–288. [334]

Wohlwill, J. F., and Wiener, M., 1964. Discrimination of form orientation in young children. *Child Develpm.*, **35**, 1113–1125. [337, 338]

Woinow, M., 1871. Beiträge zur Lehre von den Augenbewegungen. *v. Graefes Arch. Ophthal.*, **17**, 233. [50]

Wolfe, H. K., 1923. On the estimation of the middle of lines. *Amer. J. Psychol.*, **34**, 313–358. [38]

Wölfflin, H., 1941. Über das Rechts und Links im Bilde. Gedanken zur Kunstgeschichte, Basel, p. 82. [300]

Wood, R. W., 1895. The 'haunted-swing' illusion. *Psychol. Rev.*, **2**, 277–278. [201]

Woodworth, R. S., 1899. Accuracy of voluntary movement. *Psychol. Rev. Monogr.*, *Suppl.*, **3**, 13. [85, 89]

Woodworth, R. S., 1934. *Psychology* 2nd ed. Holt, New York. [407]

Woodworth, R. S., 1938. *Experimental Psychology*. Holt, New York. [302]

Woodworth, R. S., and Schlosberg, H., 1955. *Experimental Psychology* 3rd ed. Methuen, London. [320]

Wooster, M., 1923. Certain factors in the development of a new spatial coordination. *Psychol. Monogr.*, **32**, No. 4, (whole No. 146). [382]

Worchel, P., 1951. Space perception and orientation in the blind. *Psychol. Monogr.*, **65**, No. 332. [261]

Worchel, P., 1952. The role of vestibular organs in space orientation. *J. exp. Psychol.*, **44**, 4–10. [260]

Worchel, P., and Dallenbach, K. M., 1948. The vestibular sensitivity of deaf–blind subjects. *Amer. J. Psychol.*, **61**, 94–99. [135, 255]

Worchel, P., and Dallenbach, K. M., 1950. Vestibular sensitivity in the deaf. *Amer. J. Psychol.*, **63**, 161–175. [135]

Worchel, P., and Rockett, F. C., 1955. The frame of reference in perceptual and motor skill: I. The effect of changing frames of reference. *Percept. mot. Skills,* **4,** 115–121. [264]

Worth, C., 1903. *Squint.* Blakiston, Philadelphia. [21]

Wundt,W., 1894. *Lectures on Human and Animal Psychology.* Sonnenschein. Eng. Trans., London, p. 114. [404]

Wycis, H. T., and Spiegel, E. A., 1953. Effect of cortical lesions and elimination of retinal impulses on labyrinthine nystagmus. *Arch. Otolaryng., Chicago,* **57,** 1–11. [61]

Wyke, M., and Ettlinger, G., 1961. Efficiency of recognition in left and right visual fields: its relation to the phenomenon of visual extinction. *Arch. Neurol., Chicago,* **5,** 659–665. [305]

Wyndham, R., 1936. *The Gentle Savage.* Morrow, New York. [332]

Yarbus, A. L., 1957. The perception of an image fixed in respect to the retina. *Biophysics,* **2,** 683–690. (Trans. from *Biofizikia,* **2,** 703–712.) [47]

Young, L. R., and Stark, L., 1963. Variable feedback experiments testing a sampled data model for eye tracking movements. *IEEE Trans. Human Factors Electronics,* **4,** 38–50. [59]

Young, P., 1928. Auditory localization with acoustical transposition of the ears. *J. exp. Psychol.,* **11,** 399–429. [360]

Young, P., 1931. The role of head movements in auditory localization. *J. exp. Psychol.,* **14,** 95–124. [150]

Zacks, J. L., and Freedman, S. J., 1963. Active and passive movement in the production of kinesthetic tilt after-effect. *Percept. mot. Skills,* **16,** 702. [232]

Zangwill, O. L., 1951. Discussion on parietal lobe syndromes. *Proc. R. Soc. Med.,* **44,** 343–346. [268, 269, 270]

Zusne, L., and Michels, K. M., 1962. Geometricity of visual form. *Percept. mot. Skills,* **14,** 147–154. [296, 301]

Zwislocki, J., and Feldman, R. S., 1956. Just noticeable differences in dichotic phase. *J. acoust. Soc. Amer.,* **28,** 860–864. [155, 156, 157]

Subject index

f following a page number indicates that the discussion continues on the next page.
ff following a page number indicates that the discussion continues on subsequent pages.